Psychiatric Mental Health Nursing

Sheila L. Videbeck, PhD, RN

Nursing Instructor
Des Moines Area Community College
Ankeny, Iowa

Illustrations by Cathy J. Miller

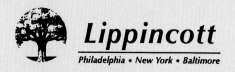
Lippincott
Philadelphia • New York • Baltimore

Acquisitions Editor: Margaret Zuccarini
Managing Editor: Barbara Ryalls
Developmental Editors: Sarah Kyle/Carole Wonsiewicz
Editorial Assistant: Helen Kogut
Senior Production Manager: Helen Ewan
Senior Production Coordinator: Nannette Winski
Art Director: Carolyn O'Brien
Manufacturing Manager: William Alberti
Indexer: Maria Coughlin
Compositor: Circle Graphics
Printer: RR Donnelley Willard
Prepress: Jay's Publishers Services, Inc.

9 8 7 6 5 4 3 2 1

Library of Congress Cataloging-in-Publication Data

Videbeck, Sheila L.
  Psychiatric mental health nursing / Sheila L. Videbeck ; illustrations by Cathy J. Miller.
    p. ; cm.
  Includes bibliographical references and index.
  ISBN 0-7817-1451-6 (alk. paper)
  1. Psychiatric nursing, I. Title.
  [DNLM: 1. Psychiatric Nursing. 2. Mental Disorders—nursing. WY 160 V652p 2001]
  RC440 .V536 2001
  610.73′68—dc21   00-045386

Care has been taken to confirm the accuracy of the information presented and to describe generally accepted practices. However, the authors, editors, and publisher are not responsible for errors or omissions or for any consequences from application of the information in this book and make no warranty, express or implied, with respect to the content of the publication.

The authors, editors, and publisher have exerted every effort to ensure that drug selection and dosage set forth in this text are in accordance with the current recommendations and practice at the time of publication. However, in view of ongoing research, changes in government regulations, and the constant flow of information relating to drug therapy and drug reactions, the reader is urged to check the package insert for each drug for any change in indications and dosage and for added warnings and precautions. This is particularly important when the recommended agent is a new or infrequently employed drug.

Some drugs and medical devices presented in this publication have Food and Drug Administration (FDA) clearance for limited use in restricted research settings. It is the responsibility of the health care provider to ascertain the FDA status of each drug or device planned for use in his or her clinical practice.

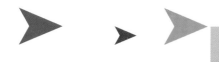

Reviewers

David J. Anna, MSN
Assistant Professor
Medical College of Georgia
Augusta, Georgia

Barbara Amendola, RN, MS, CS
Professor of Nursing
Ocean County College
Department of Nursing and Allied Health
Toms River, New Jersey

Kathleen C. Banks, MSN, CNS
Assistant Professor
Kent State University
ADN Program, East Liverpool Regional Campus
East Liverpool, Ohio

M. Claire Blanton, RN, BSN, BA, MHA, MS
Associate Professor of Nursing
Finger Lakes Community College
Canandaigua, New York

Daphne L. Boatright, BSN, MEd
Nursing Education Instructor and Assistant Director
 of Registered Nursing Program
Allan Hancock College
Santa Maria, California

Linda L. Breidigam, RN, BSN, MSN, CCE
Assistant Professor
Alvernia College
Reading, Pennsylvania

Paula H. Bryant, BSN, MSN
Associate Professor of Nursing
Georgia College and State University
Middle Georgia College
Cochran, Georgia

Wendy L. M. Carlson, MSN
Nursing Instructor
Jamestown Community College
Jamestown, New York

Elizabeth-Ellen Clark, BSN, MS
Associate Professor of Nursing
University of Maine at Augusta
Augusta, Maine

Nancy L. Cowan, RN, MSN, EdD
Director/Coordinator, Nursing Program
Chabot College
Hayward, California

Melanie Daniel, MSN, RN
Nursing Instructor, Walker Campus
Bevill State Community College
Sumiton, Alabama

Susan Dewey-Hammer, MN, RN, CS
Professor
Suffolk County Community College
Selden, New York

Brenda S. Edwards, BSN, RN
Instructor
Sanford-Brown College
St. Charles, Missouri

Rauda Gelazis, PhD, RN, CS, CTN
Associate Professor
Ursuline College
Pepper Pike, Ohio

Bonnie Gnadt, MSN
Faculty
Department of Nursing, Southwestern Adventist University
Keene, Texas

Patricia A. Goeden, RN, MSN
Assistant Professor, Department of Nursing
Mount Marty College
Yankton, South Dakota

Brigitte F. Haagen, MSN, RN, CS, DNSc candidate
Instructor, School of Nursing
Penn State University
Hershey, Pennsylvania

Alice R. Kemp, PhD, RN, CS
Associate Professor
Ursuline College
Pepper Pike, Ohio

Gwen Larsen, RN, PhD
Assistant Professor
University of Nebraska Medical Center
College of Nursing
Lincoln, Nebraska

Joanne Lavin, RN, CS, EdD
Professor
Nursing Department,
    Kingsborough Community College
Brooklyn, New York

Wanda Mohr, PhD, RN, FAAN
Associate Professor
Psychiatric Mental Health Nursing
Indiana University School of Nursing
Indiana, Pennsylvania

Elaine Mordoch, RN, BN, MN
Lecturer
University of Manitoba
Winnipeg, Manitoba, Canada

Pat Nashef, MHSc, BA, RN
Program Manager, Post-Diploma,
    Mental Health Nursing
Mohawk College
Hamilton, Ontario

Nancy Sonne, RN, MS
Associate Professor of Nursing
Huron University
Huron, South Dakota

Charlotte Spade, MS, RN, CS, CNS
Professor
Community College of Denver
Denver, Colorado

Martha B. Spear, RN, BS, MS
Associate Professor of Nursing
Harrisburg Area Community College
Harrisburg, Pennsylvania

Janet Mattson Starr, RN, BS, BSN, MEd
Nursing Education Consultant
Georgia Board of Examiners of Licensed Practical Nurses
Atlanta, Georgia

Deborah V. Thomas, EdD, ARNP, CS
Faculty
University of Louisville, School of Nursing
Louisville, Kentucky

Connie K. Ward, RN
Nurse Educator
Lamar University at Orange
Orange, Texas

Ulana Zinych, RN, MSN, MS
Professor of Nursing
Naugatuck Valley Community-Technical College
Waterbury, Connecticut

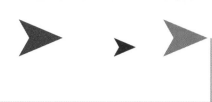

Contributors

Barbara Amendola, RN, MS, CS
Chapter 6:   Therapeutic Communication
Chapter 12: Anxiety and Stress-Related Illness
Chapter 14: Mood Disorders
Professor of Nursing
Ocean County College
Toms River, New Jersey

Charlotte Spade, MS, RN, CS
Chapter 9: Grief and Loss
Associate Professor, Nursing Program
Community College of Denver
Denver, Colorado

Special Consultants

Clinical Developmental Editor
Helene K. Nawrocki, RN, MSN
Executive Director
Potter County Education Council
Nurse Specialist
Private Practice Holistic Care
Genessee, Pennsylvania

Illustrator
Cathy J. Miller, RN
School Nurse
Washington Community School District
Washington, Iowa

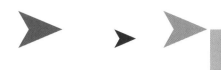

Preface

This first edition of **Psychiatric Mental Health Nursing** was written to make theory come alive for nursing students. It presents sound nursing theory, therapeutic modalities, and clinical applications across the treatment continuum. The chapters are short, to the point, and easy to read and understand. This text uses the nursing process framework and emphasizes assessment, therapeutic communication, neurobiologic theory, and pharmacology throughout. Interventions focus on all aspects of client care, including communication, client and family teaching, and community resources, and their practical application in a variety of clinical settings.

Organization of the Text

Unit I: Current Theories and Practice provides a strong foundation for students. Current issues in psychiatric nursing are addressed, as well as the variety of treatment settings where clients are encountered. Neurobiologic theories and psychopharmacology and psychosocial theories and therapy are thoroughly discussed as a basis for understanding mental illness and its treatment.

Unit II: Building the Nurse-Client Relationship presents the basic elements essential to the practice of mental health nursing. Chapters on therapeutic relationships and therapeutic communication prepare students to begin working with clients both in mental health settings and in all other areas of nursing practice as well. The chapter on the client's response to illness provides a framework for understanding the individual client. An entire chapter is devoted to assessment, emphasizing its importance in nursing.

Unit III: Current Social and Emotional Concerns covers topics that are not exclusive to mental health settings, including grief and loss, anger and aggression, and abuse and violence. Nurses in all practice settings find themselves confronted with clients whose lives are touched by loss and violence.

Unit IV: Nursing Practice for Psychiatric Disorders covers all the major categories identified in the DSM-IV-TR. Each chapter provides current information on etiology, onset and clinical course, treatment, and nursing care.

Pedagogical Features

Psychiatric Mental Health Nursing incorporates a number of pedagogical features designed to facilitate student learning, including:

- Learning objectives to focus the student's reading and study.
- Key terms that identify new terms used in the chapter. Each of these terms is identified in bold and defined in the text.
- Application of the nursing process using the assessment framework presented in Chapter 8, so students can compare and contrast the various disorders more easily.
- Critical thinking questions to stimulate students' thinking about current dilemmas and issues in mental health.
- Key points that summarize chapter content to reinforce important concepts.
- Chapter reviews that provide workbook-style questions for students to test their knowledge and understanding of each chapter.

Special Features

- Clinical vignettes are provided for each major disorder discussed in the text to "paint a picture" for better understanding.
- Drug alerts highlight essential points about psychotropic drugs.
- Cultural considerations are emphasized in a separate section of each chapter in response to increasing diversity.
- Therapeutic dialogues give specific examples of nurse-client interaction to promote therapeutic communication skills.
- Internet resources with URLs are located at the end of each chapter to further enhance their study.

- Client and family teaching checklists are highlighted to strengthen students' role as educators.
- Symptoms and interventions are highlighted for all chapters in Units III and IV.
- Sample nursing care plans are provided for all chapters in Units III and IV.
- Self-awareness feature at the end of each chapter encourages students to reflect upon themselves, their emotions, and their attitudes as a way to foster both personal and professional development.

To the Faculty

The following ancillary materials have been prepared to help you plan learning activities for class and clinical, and evaluate students' learning:

- Instructor's Resource Manual will include a variety of instructional support features for each chapter, including chapter summary, lecture outlines, and teaching–learning strategies that involve classroom, clinical, and self-awareness activities. In addition, guidelines are provided for leading class discussion relating to critical thinking questions included in the textbook. Transparency masters provide summary lists of symptoms, interventions, and Client and Patient Teaching checklists for each of the 12 disorder chapters.
- CD-ROM, included in the Instructor's Resource Manual, contains:
  - Testbank containing 350 NCLEX-style testing items
  - Lecture outlines for each chapter

To the Student

This textbook has been designed to be "student-friendly." Chapters are easy to read and understand, and pertinent information about caring for clients is presented in a practical, hands-on approach. Mental health nursing is an exciting and challenging field, and hopefully that attitude comes through in this text. The knowledge and skills you develop while studying mental health nursing will promote your growth as a nurse and improve the care you provide to clients in all settings.

Sheila L. Videbeck, PhD, RN

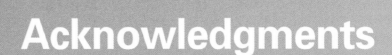

Acknowledgments

I owe a great deal of thanks to the people who helped and supported me throughout the creation of this text. Margaret Zuccarini, senior editor at Lippincott, provided guidance, answers to questions, and cheerful optimism when the going got rough. Helen Kogut, editorial assistant, coordinated and organized the exchange of materials and information. Carole Wonsiewicz and Sarah Anders Kyle, developmental editors, and Helene K. Nawrocki, RN, MSN, Nurse Educator and Clinical Developmental Editor, worked long and hard through many rewrites and revisions to help make this project a success. Diana Messersmith, librarian at Des Moines Area Community College, filled my numerous requests for articles. All the students I have worked with over the years helped make me a better teacher with their questions, feedback, and humor—they were the inspiration for this text. Finally, my husband, Mark, who provided the support and encouragement to make it all possible.

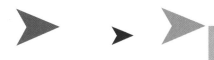

Contents

Client's Response to Illness   147

Assessment   167

Current Social and Emotional Concerns

Grief and Loss   186

Anger, Hostility, and Aggression   213

Abuse and Violence   232

➤ *Unit 4*
Nursing Practice for Psychiatric Disorders

Anxiety and Stress-Related Illness   260

Schizophrenia   296

Mood Disorders   330

Cognitive Disorders   383

Personality Disorders   414

Substance Abuse   451

Child and Adolescent Disorders   477

Somatoform Disorders   507

Eating Disorders   528

Current Theories and Practice

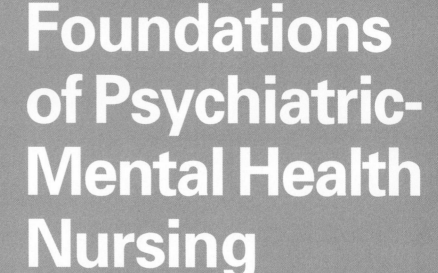

Foundations of Psychiatric-Mental Health Nursing

Mental health and mental illness are often difficult to define. When people are able to carry out their roles in society and their behavior is appropriate and adaptive, they are viewed as being healthy. Conversely, when a person fails to fulfill roles and carry out responsibilities, or his or her behavior is inappropriate, that person is viewed as ill. The culture of any society strongly influences its values and beliefs, and this in turn affects how health and illness are defined. What is viewed as acceptable and appropriate behavior in one society may be seen as maladaptive or inappropriate in another.

MENTAL HEALTH

The World Health Organization defines health as a "state of complete physical, mental, and social wellness, not merely the absence of disease or infirmity." This definition emphasizes health as a positive state of well-being, not just a lack of disease. People in a state of emotional, physical, and social well-being fulfill life responsibilities, function effectively in daily life, and are satisfied with their interpersonal relationships and themselves. No single, universal definition of mental health exists, but we can infer a person's mental health from his or her behavior. Because a person's behavior may be viewed or interpreted differently by others, depending on their values and beliefs, the determination of mental health may be difficult.

Mental health is a state of emotional, psychological, and social wellness evidenced by satisfying interpersonal relationships, effective behavior and coping, a positive self-concept, and emotional stability. Mental health has many components and is influenced by a wide variety of factors (Johnson, 1997):

- Autonomy and independence: The individual can look within for guiding values and rules to live by. The opinions and wishes of others are considered but do not dictate the person's decisions and behavior. The person who is autonomous and independent can work interdependently or cooperatively with others without losing his or her autonomy.
- Maximizing one's potential: The person has an orientation toward growth and self-actualization. He or she is not content with the status quo and continually strives to grow as a person.
- Tolerating life's uncertainties: The person can face the challenges of day-to-day living with hope and a positive outlook, despite not knowing what lies ahead.
- Self-esteem: The person has a realistic awareness of his or her abilities and limitations.
- Mastering the environment: The person can deal with and influence the environment in a capable, competent, and creative manner.
- Reality orientation: The person can distinguish the real world from a dream, fact from fantasy, and act accordingly.
- Stress management: The person can tolerate life stresses, experience feelings of anxiety or grief appropriately, and experience failure without devastation. He or she uses support from family and friends to cope with crises, knowing that the stress will not last forever.

There is constant interaction among these factors; thus, a person's mental health is a dynamic or ever-changing state.

Factors influencing a person's mental health can be categorized as individual, interpersonal, and social/cultural factors. Individual factors include a person's biologic makeup, having a sense of harmony in one's life, vitality, finding meaning in life, emotional resilience or hardiness, spirituality, and having a positive identity (Seaward, 1997). Interpersonal factors include effective communication, helping others, intimacy, and maintaining a balance of separateness and connection. Social/cultural factors include having a sense of community, access to adequate resources, intolerance of violence, and support of diversity among people. These factors are discussed in Chapter 7.

MENTAL ILLNESS

Historically, mental illness has been viewed as possession by demons, punishment for religious or social transgressions, weakness of will or spirit, and violations of societal norms. Persons who were mentally ill were persecuted, punished, shunned, ridiculed, and locked away from "normal" society. Until the 19th century, persons with mental illness were deemed incurable and were manacled in prisons without adequate food, shelter, or clothing.

Today, mental illness is identified and treated as a medical problem. The American Psychiatric Association (1994) defines a **mental disorder** as "a clinically significant behavioral or psychological syndrome or pattern that occurs in an individual and that is associated with present distress (e.g., a painful symptom) or disability (i.e., impairment in one or more important areas of functioning) or with a significantly increased risk of suffering death, pain, disability, or an important loss of freedom."

General criteria to diagnose mental disorders include dissatisfaction with one's characteristics, abilities, and accomplishments; ineffective or unsatisfying relationships; dissatisfaction with one's place in the world; or ineffective coping with life events and lack of personal growth. In addition, the person's behavior must not be culturally expected or sanctioned, nor is deviant behavior necessarily indicative of a mental disorder (DSM-IV, 1994).

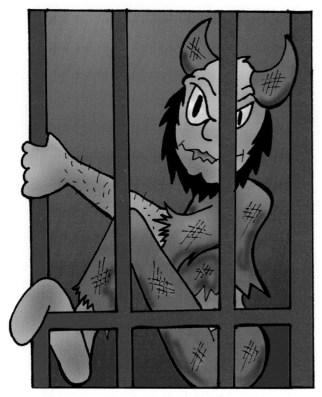

Demons

Factors contributing to mental illness can also be viewed in three categories. Individual factors include biologic makeup, anxiety, worries and fears, a sense of disharmony in life, and a loss of meaning in one's life (Seaward, 1997). Interpersonal factors include ineffective communication, excessive dependency or withdrawal from relationships, and loss of emotional control. Cultural and social factors include lack of resources, violence, homelessness, poverty, and discrimination such as racism, classism, ageism, and sexism.

DIAGNOSTIC AND STATISTICAL MANUAL OF MENTAL DISORDERS (DSM-IV-TR)

The *Diagnostic and Statistical Manual of Mental Disorders-Text Revision* (DSM-IV-TR), now in its fourth edition, is a taxonomy published by the American Psychiatric Association that describes all the mental disorders with specific diagnostic criteria. The DSM-IV-TR is used by all mental health disciplines for the diagnosis of psychiatric disorders and has three purposes:

- To provide a standardized nomenclature and language for all mental health professionals
- To present defining characteristics or symptoms that differentiate specific diagnoses
- To assist in identifying the underlying causes of disorders.

Specific diagnostic criteria are outlined for every disorder based on clinical experience and research. The diagnostic categories are listed in Appendix A. A multiaxial classification system that involves assessment on several axes, or domains of information, allows the practitioner to identify all the factors that relate to the person's condition:

- Axis I is for identifying all major psychiatric disorders, except mental retardation and personality disorders, such as depression, schizophrenia, anxiety, and substance-related disorders.
- Axis II is for reporting mental retardation and personality disorders, as well as prominent maladaptive personality features and defense mechanisms.
- Axis III is for reporting current medical conditions that are potentially relevant to the understanding or management of the person's mental disorder, as well as medical conditions that might contribute to the understanding of the person.
- Axis IV is for reporting psychosocial and environmental problems that may affect the diagnosis, treatment, and prognosis of mental disorders. Included are problems with primary support group, social environment, education, occupation, housing, economics, access to health care, and legal system.
- Axis V presents a Global Assessment of Functioning (GAF) that rates the overall psychological functioning of the person on a scale of 0 to 100. This represents the clinician's assessment of the person's current level of functioning, and a score may also be given for prior functioning (for instance, highest GAF in past year, or GAF 6 months ago).

Although student nurses do not use the DSM-IV to diagnose clients, it can be a helpful resource to describe the characteristics (diagnostic criteria) of the various disorders.

HISTORICAL PERSPECTIVES OF THE TREATMENT OF MENTAL ILLNESS

Ancient Times

In ancient times, it was believed that any sickness indicated displeasure of the gods and in fact was a punishment for sins and wrongdoing. Persons with mental disorders were viewed as being either demonic or divine, depending on their behavior. Individuals seen as divine were worshipped and adored; those seen as demonic were ostracized, punished, and sometimes burned at the stake. Later, Aristotle (382–322 BC) attempted to relate mental disorders to physical disorders and developed his theory that emotions were controlled by the amounts of blood, water, and yellow and black bile in the body. These four substances, or humors, corresponded to emotions of happiness, calmness, anger, and sadness. Imbalances of the four humors were believed to cause mental disorder, so treatment was aimed at restoring balance through bloodletting, starving, and purging. Such "treatments" persisted well into the 19th century (Baly, 1982).

In early Christian times (1–1000 AD), primitive beliefs and superstitions were strong. All diseases were again blamed on demons, and the mentally ill were viewed as possessed. Priests performed exorcisms to rid the person of the evil spirits. When that failed, more severe measures, such as incarceration in dungeons, flogging, starving, and other brutal treatments, were used.

During the Renaissance (1300–1600), persons with mental illness were distinguished from criminals in England. Those who were considered harmless were allowed to wander the countryside or live in rural communities, but the more "dangerous lunatics" were still thrown in prison, chained, and starved (Rosenblatt, 1984). In 1547, the Hospital of St. Mary of Bethlehem was officially declared a hospital for the insane, the first of its kind. By 1775, visitors at the institution were charged a fee for the privilege of viewing and ridiculing the inmates, who were seen as animals, less than human (McMillan, 1997). During this same period in the colonies, later the United States, the mentally ill were considered evil or possessed and were punished. Witch hunts were conducted, and offenders were burned at the stake.

Period of Enlightenment and Creation of Mental Institutions

In the 1790s, a period of enlightenment began concerning persons with mental illness. The establishment of the asylum is credited to Phillippe Pinel in France and William Tukes in England. The concept of **asylum** as a safe refuge or haven offering protection was instituted by these two men at institutions where people had been whipped, beaten, and starved just because they were mentally ill (Gollaher, 1995). This movement began the moral treatment of the mentally ill. In the United States, Dorothea Dix (1802–1887) began a crusade to reform the treatment of mental illness after a visit to Tukes' institution in England. She was instrumental in opening 32 state hospitals that offered asylum to the suffering. Dix believed that society had an obligation to persons who were mentally ill and promoted adequate shelter, nutritious food, and warm clothing (Gollaher, 1995).

The period of enlightenment was short-lived. Within 100 years after the first asylum was established, state hospitals were in trouble. Attendants were accused of abusing the patients, the rural location of hospitals was viewed as isolating patients from family and their homes, and the phrase "insane asylum" took on a negative connotation, rather than being a protective haven.

Sigmund Freud and Treatment of Mental Disorders

The period of scientific study and treatment of mental disorders began with Sigmund Freud (1856–1939). Along with others, such as Emil Kraepelin (1856–1926) and Eugene Bleuler (1857–1939), the study of psychiatry and the diagnosis and treatment of mental illnesses began in earnest. Kraepelin began classifying mental disorders according to their symptoms, and Bleuler coined the term "schizophrenia." Freud challenged society to look at human beings objectively and studied the mind and its disorders and their treatment as no one had before. Many other theorists built on Freud's pioneering work (see Chap. 3).

Development of Psychopharmacology

A great leap in the treatment of mental illnesses began in about 1950 with the development of **psychotropic drugs** (drugs used to treat mental illness). Chlorpromazine (Thorazine), an antipsychotic

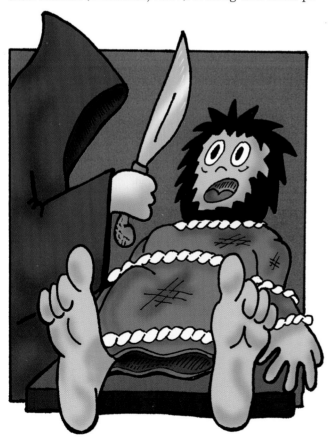

Bloodletting

drug, and lithium, an antimanic agent, were the first drugs to be developed. Monoamine oxidase inhibitor anti-depressants; haloperidol (Haldol), an antipsychotic; tricyclic antidepressants; and antianxiety agents called benzodiazepines were introduced over the next 10 years. For the first time, drugs that actually reduced agitation, psychotic thinking, and depression improved the condition of many patients. Hospital stays were shortened, and many people were well enough to go home. The level of noise, chaos, and violence was greatly diminished in the hospital setting (Trudeau, 1993).

Move Toward Community Mental Health

The movement toward treating persons with mental illness in less restrictive environments gained momentum in 1963 with the enactment of the Community Mental Health Centers Act. **Deinstitutionalization**, a deliberate shift from institutional care in state hospitals to community facilities, began. These community mental health centers served geographic catchment areas that provided less restrictive treatment, closer to the person's home, family, and friends. These centers provided emergency care, inpatient care, outpatient services, partial hospitalization, screening services, and education.

In addition to deinstitutionalization, federal legislation was passed to provide an income for disabled persons, Supplemental Security Income (SSI) and Social Security Disability Income (SSDI). This allowed persons with severe and persistent mental illnesses to be more independent financially, not having to rely on family for money. States were able to spend less money on care of the mentally ill than they had in state hospitals, because this was a federally funded program. Also, commitment laws changed in the early 1970s, making it more difficult to commit people for mental health treatment against their will. This further decreased the state hospital populations and therefore the money that states spent on them (Torrey, 1997).

Mental Illness in the 21st Century

The Department of Health and Human Services (1999) estimates that 51 million Americans have a diagnosable mental illness. Of that number, 6.5 million are disabled by severe mental illness, and 4 million of those disabled are children and adolescents. For example, 3% to 5% of school-age children are affected by attention deficit/hyperactivity disorder. More than 10 million children under age 7 grow up in homes where at least one parent suffers from significant mental illness or substance abuse that hinders their readiness to start school.

Deinstitutionalization is viewed by some as having negative as well as positive effects (Torrey, 1997). Although the number of public hospital beds was reduced by 80%, there was a corresponding 90% increase in the number of admissions to those beds (Appleby & Desai, 1993). This has led to the term "revolving door effect." Persons with severe and persistent mental illnesses have shorter hospital stays but are admitted more frequently. General hospital psychiatric units are overwhelmed with the continuous flow of patients being admitted and discharged quickly. Emergency room visits for acutely disturbed persons have increased by 400% to 500% in some cities.

Today's patients are seen by many to be more aggressive. Four to eight percent of patients seen in psychiatric emergency rooms are armed (Ries, 1997), and about 1,000 homicides a year are committed by persons with severe and persistent mental illness who are not receiving adequate care (Torrey, 1997). Ten to fifteen percent of persons in state prisons have severe and persistent mental illness (Lamb & Weinberger, 1998).

Homelessness is a major problem in the United States today. The Department of Health and Human Services (1999) estimates that 750,000 people live and sleep in the streets. Estimates of the prevalence of mental illness among the homeless population are that 25% to 50% of adult homeless persons have a psychosis and 33% to 50% have substance abuse problems (Haugland et al., 1997). Those who are homeless and mentally ill are found in parks, airport and bus terminals, alleys and stairwells, jails, and other public places. Some use shelters, halfway houses, or board-

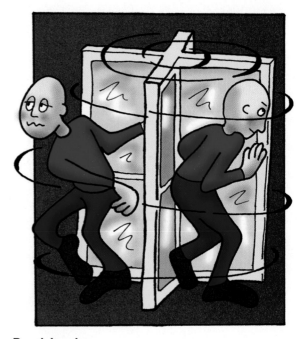

Revolving door

and-care rooms; others rent cheap hotel rooms when they can afford it (Haugland et al., 1997). Many people with mental illness who end up on the streets have their psychiatric problems worsened by homelessness, so it becomes a vicious cycle.

Many of the problems of the homeless mentally ill, as well as those who pass through the revolving door of psychiatric care, stem from the lack of adequate community resources. Money saved by states when state hospitals were closed has not been transferred to community programs and support. Inpatient psychiatric treatment still accounts for the majority of spending in mental health in the United States, so community mental health has never been given the financial base it needs to be effective (Keltner, Schwecke, & Bostrom, 1999).

In 1993, the Access to Community Care and Effective Services and Support (ACCESS) was created and funded by the federal government to begin to address the needs of people with mental illness who were homeless either all or part of the time. The goals of ACCESS were to improve access to comprehensive services across a continuum of care, reduce duplication and cost of services, and improve the efficiency of services (Randolph et al., 1997). Programs such as these provide services to people who otherwise would not receive them.

Objectives for the Future

Unfortunately, only one in four affected adults and one in three children receive treatment (DHHS, 1999). Statistics like these underlie the *Healthy People 2010* objectives for mental health proposed by the U.S. Department of Health and Human Services (Box 1-1). These objectives, originally developed as *Healthy People 2000*, were revised in January 2000 to increase the number of people who are identified, diagnosed, treated, and helped to live healthier lives. The objectives also strive to decrease rates of suicide and homelessness, to increase employment among those with serious mental illness, and to provide more services for both juveniles and adults who are incarcerated and have mental health problems.

COMMUNITY-BASED CARE

After deinstitutionalization, the 2,000 community mental health centers (CMHCs) that were supposed to be built by 1980 had not materialized. By 1990, only

---

Box 1-1

▶ HEALTHY PEOPLE 2010 MENTAL HEALTH OBJECTIVES

- Reduce suicides to no more than 6 per 100,000 people
- Reduce the incidence of injurious suicide attempts by 1% in 12 months for adolescents ages 14–17
- Reduce the proportion of homeless adults who have serious mental illness to 19%
- Increase the proportion of persons with serious mental illnesses who are employed to 51%
- Reduce the relapse rate for persons with eating disorders, including anorexia nervosa and bulimia nervosa
- Increase the number of persons seen in primary health care who receive mental health treatment screening and assessment
- Increase the proportion of children with mental health problems who receive treatment
- Increase the proportion of juvenile justice facilities that screen new admissions for mental health problems
- Increase the proportion of adults with mental disorders who receive treatment by 17%
  - Adults 18–54 with serious mental illness to 55%
  - Adults 18 and older with recognized depression to 50%
  - Adults 18 and older with schizophrenia to 75%
  - Adults 18 and older with anxiety disorders to 50%
- Increase the population of persons with concurrent substance abuse problems and mental disorders who receive treatment for both disorders
- Increase the proportion of local governments with community-based jail diversion programs for adults with serious mental illness
- Increase the number of states that track consumers' satisfaction with the mental health services they receive to 30 states
- Increase the number of states with an operational mental health plan that addresses cultural competence
- Increase the number of states with an operational mental health plan that addresses mental health crisis intervention, ongoing screening, and treatment services for elderly persons

U.S. Department of Health and Human Services. (2000). Healthy people 2010: National health promotion and disease prevention objectives. *Washington, DC: DHHS.*

1,300 programs provided various types of psychosocial rehabilitation services. Persons with severe and persistent mental illness were either ignored or underserved by the CMHCs (International Association of Psychosocial Rehabilitation Services, 1990). This meant that many people needing service were, and still are, in the general population with their needs unmet.

Community support services programs were developed to meet the needs of persons with mental illness outside the walls of an institution. These programs focus on rehabilitation, vocational needs, education, and socialization, as well as management of symptoms and medication. These services are funded by states (or counties) and some private agencies. Therefore, the availability and quality of services vary among different areas of the country. For example, rural areas may have limited funds to provide mental health services and smaller numbers of people needing them. Large metropolitan areas, while having larger budgets, also have thousands of people in need of service. Rarely is there enough money to provide all the services needed by the population. Chapter 4 provides a detailed discussion of community-based programs.

Still, community-based programs are preferred for treating persons with mental illness. Clients can remain in their communities, maintain contact with family and friends, and enjoy personal freedom that is not possible in an institution. People in institutions often lose motivation and hope, as well as functional daily living skills, such as shopping and cooking. Therefore, treatment in the community is a trend that will continue.

COST CONTAINMENT AND MANAGED CARE

Health care costs spiraled upward throughout the 1970s and 1980s in the United States. Managed care began in the early 1970s in the form of health maintenance organizations (HMOs), which were successful in some areas with healthier populations of people. In the 1990s, a new form of managed care called **utilization review firms** or **managed care organizations** were developed to control the expenditure of insurance funds by requiring providers to seek approval before the delivery of care. **Case management**, or management of care on a case-by-case basis, represented an effort to provide necessary services while containing costs. In reality, expenditures are often reduced by withholding services deemed unnecessary or substituting less expensive treatment alternatives for more expensive care, such as hospital admission (Mechanic, 1996).

Psychiatric care is costly because of the long-term nature of the disorders. A single hospital stay can cost $20,000 to $30,000. Also, there are fewer objective measures of health or illness. For example, when a person is suicidal, the clinician must rely on the person's report of suicidality; no laboratory tests or other diagnostics exist that can identify suicidal ideas. Mental health care is separated from physical health care in terms of insurance coverage: there are often specific dollar limits or permitted numbers of hospital days in a calendar year. When private insurance limits are met, public funds through the state are used to provide care. Legislation has been proposed in some states, such as New York, to provide parity between mental and physical health coverage, meaning that mental health care would get equal amounts of insurance coverage as physical illnesses, which often have no monetary caps. However, this has not yet happened.

Mental health care is managed through privately owned behavioral health care firms that often provide the services as well as manage their cost. Persons without private insurance must rely on their county of residence to provide funding through tax dollars. These services and the money to fund them often lag far behind the need that exists. In addition, many persons with mental illness do not seek care and in fact avoid treatment. These persons are often homeless or in jail. Two of the greatest challenges for the future are to provide effective treatment to all who need it and to find the resources to pay for this care.

CULTURAL CONSIDERATIONS

By the year 2020, most U.S. residents will trace their ancestry to Africa, Asia, or the Arab or Hispanic worlds rather than Europe. This represents a change from European Americans as the majority (Miller, 1996). Nurses must be prepared to care for this culturally diverse population, and that includes being aware of cultural differences that influence mental health and the treatment of mental illness. See Chapter 7 for a discussion of cultural differences.

Diversity is not limited to culture; the structure of families in America has changed as well. With a divorce rate of 50% in the United States, many families are headed by single parents, and many blended families are created when divorced persons remarry. Twenty-five percent of households consist of a single person (Wright, 1995), and many people live together without being married. Gay men and lesbians form partnerships and sometimes adopt children. The face of the family in the United States is varied, providing a challenge to nurses to provide sensitive, competent care.

PSYCHIATRIC NURSING PRACTICE

In 1873, Linda Richards graduated from the New England Hospital for Women and Children in Boston. She went on to develop better nursing care in psychiatric hospitals and organized educational programs in state mental hospitals in Illinois. Richards is called the first American psychiatric nurse; she believed that "the mentally sick should be at least as well cared for as the physically sick" (Doona, 1984).

The first training of nurses to work with persons with mental illness was in 1882 at McLean Hospital in Waverly, Mass. The care was primarily custodial and focused on nutrition, hygiene, and activity. Nurses adapted medical-surgical principles to the care of psychiatric clients and treated them with tolerance and kindness. The role of psychiatric nurses expanded as somatic therapies for the treatment of mental disorders were developed. Treatments such as insulin shock therapy (1935), psychosurgery (1936), and electroconvulsive therapy (1937) required nurses to use their medical-surgical skills further.

The first psychiatric nursing textbook, *Nursing Mental Diseases* by Harriet Bailey, was published in 1920. In 1913, Johns Hopkins was the first school of nursing to include a course in psychiatric nursing in its curriculum. It was not until 1950 that the National League for Nursing, which accredits nursing programs, required schools to include an experience in psychiatric nursing to be accredited.

Psychiatric nursing practice was shaped by two early nursing theorists, Hildegard Peplau and June Mellow. Peplau published *Interpersonal Relations in Nursing* in 1952 and *Interpersonal Techniques: The Crux of Psychiatric Nursing* in 1962. Peplau described the therapeutic nurse-patient relationship with its phases and tasks and wrote extensively about anxiety (see Chap. 12). The interpersonal dimension that was crucial to her beliefs forms the foundations of practice today. Mellow's 1968 work *Nursing Therapy* described her approach of focusing on the client's psychosocial needs and strengths. Both Peplau and Mellow made substantial contributions to the practice of psychiatric nursing.

In 1973, the division of psychiatric and mental health practice of the American Nurses Association developed standards of care; they were revised in 1982 and 1994. **Standards of care** are authoritative statements by professional organizations that describe the responsibilities for which nurses are accountable. They are not legally binding unless they are incorporated into the state nurse practice act or state board rules and regulations. When legal problems or lawsuits arise, these professional standards are used to determine what is safe and acceptable practice and to assess the quality of care.

A two-part document, *Statement on Psychiatric-Mental Health Clinical Nursing Practice and Standards of Psychiatric-Mental Health Clinical Nursing Practice*, was jointly published in 1994 by the American Nurses Association, the American Psychiatric Nurses Association, the Association of Child and Adolescent Nurses Association, and the Society for Education and Research in Psychiatric-Mental Health Nursing. It outlines the areas of concern and standards of care for today's psychiatric-mental health nurse. The **phenomena of concern** describe the 12 areas of concern that mental health nurses focus on when caring for clients (Box 1-2). The standards of care include the phases of the nursing process, including specific types of interventions, for nurses in psychiatric settings, and standards for professional performance are outlined: quality of care, performance appraisal, education, collegiality, ethics, collaboration, research, and resource utilization (Box 1-3). Box 1-4 summarizes specific areas of practice and specific interventions for both basic and advanced nursing practice.

Box 1-2

➤ PSYCHIATRIC MENTAL HEALTH NURSING PHENOMENA OF CONCERN

Actual or potential mental health problems pertaining to:
- The maintenance of optimal health and well-being and the prevention of psychobiologic illness
- Self-care limitations or impaired functioning related to mental and emotional distress
- Deficits in the functioning of significant biologic, emotional, and cognitive symptoms
- Emotional stress or crisis components of illness, pain, and disability
- Self-concept changes, developmental issues, and life process changes
- Problems related to emotions such as anxiety, anger, sadness, loneliness, and grief
- Physical symptoms that occur along with altered psychological functioning
- Alterations in thinking, perceiving, symbolizing, communicating, and decision making
- Difficulties in relating to others
- Behaviors and mental states that indicate the client is a danger to self or others or has a severe disability
- Interpersonal, systemic, sociocultural, spiritual, or environmental circumstances or events that affect the mental or emotional well-being of the individual, family, or community
- Symptom management, side effects/toxicities associated with psychopharmacologic intervention, and other aspects of the treatment regimen

Box 1-3

➤ STANDARDS OF PSYCHIATRIC-MENTAL HEALTH CLINICAL NURSING PRACTICE

STANDARDS OF CARE

Standard I. Assessment
The psychiatric-mental health nurse collects client health data.

Standard II. Diagnosis
The psychiatric-mental health nurse analyzes the data in determining diagnoses.

Standard III. Outcome Identification
The psychiatric-mental health nurse identifies expected outcomes individualized to the client.

Standard IV. Planning
The psychiatric-mental health nurse develops a plan of care that prescribes interventions to attain expected outcomes.

Standard V. Implementation
The psychiatric-mental health nurse implements the interventions identified in the plan of care.

Standard Va. Counseling
The psychiatric-mental health nurse uses counseling interventions to assist clients in improving or regaining their previous coping abilities, fostering mental health, and preventing mental illness and disability.

Standard Vb. Milieu Therapy
The psychiatric-mental health nurse provides, structures, and maintains a therapeutic environment in collaboration with the client and other health care providers.

Standard Vc. Self-Care Activities
The psychiatric-mental health nurse structures interventions around the client's activities of daily living to foster self-care and mental and physical well-being.

Standard Vd. Psychobiologic Interventions
The psychiatric-mental health nurse uses knowledge of psychobiologic interventions and applies clinical skills to restore the client's health and prevent further disability.

Standard Ve. Health Teaching
The psychiatric-mental health nurse, through health teaching, assists clients in achieving satisfying, productive, and healthy patterns of living.

Standard Vf. Case Management
The psychiatric-mental health nurse provides case management to coordinate comprehensive health services and ensure continuity of care.

Standard Vg. Health Promotion and Maintenance
The psychiatric-mental health nurse employs strategies and interventions to promote and maintain mental health and prevent mental illness.
(Interventions Vh–Vj are advanced practice interventions and may be performed only by the certified specialist in psychiatric-mental health nursing.)

Standard VI. Evaluation
The psychiatric-mental health nurse evaluates the client's progress in attaining expected outcomes.

STANDARDS OF PROFESSIONAL PERFORMANCE

Standard I. Quality of Care
The psychiatric-mental health nurse systematically evaluates the quality of care and effectiveness of psychiatric-mental health nursing practice.

Standard II. Performance Appraisal
The psychiatric-mental health nurse evaluates his or her own psychiatric-mental health nursing practice in relation to professional practice standards and relevant statutes and regulations.

Standard III. Education
The psychiatric-mental health nurse acquires and maintains current knowledge in nursing practice.

Standard IV. Collegiality
The psychiatric-mental health nurse contributes to the professional development of peers, colleagues, and others.

Standard V. Ethics
The psychiatric-mental health nurse's decisions and actions on behalf of others are determined in an ethical manner.

Standard VI. Collaboration
The psychiatric-mental health nurse collaborates with the client, significant others, and health care providers in providing care.

Standard VII. Research
The psychiatric-mental health nurse contributes to nursing and mental health through the use of research.

Standard VIII. Resource Utilization
The psychiatric-mental health nurse considers factors related to safety, effectiveness, and cost in planning and delivering client care.

Box 1-4

▶ AREAS OF PRACTICE

BASIC-LEVEL FUNCTIONS

- Counseling
  Interventions and communication techniques
  Problem solving
  Crisis intervention
  Stress management
  Behavior modification
- Milieu therapy
  Maintain therapeutic environment
  Teach skills
  Encourage communication between clients and others
  Promote growth through role-modeling
- Self-care activities
  Encourage independence
  Increase self-esteem
  Improve function and health
- Psychobiologic interventions
  Administer medications
  Teaching
  Observations
- Health teaching
- Case management
- Health promotion and maintenance

ADVANCED-LEVEL FUNCTIONS

- Psychotherapy
- Prescriptive authority for drugs (in many states)
- Consultation
- Evaluation

STUDENT CONCERNS

Student nurses beginning their clinical experience in psychiatric-mental health nursing often have a variety of concerns. Psychiatric nursing seems very different, unlike any experience they have had previously. These concerns are normal and usually do not persist once the student has had initial contacts with clients.

Some common concerns and helpful hints for the beginning student are as follows:

- *What if I say the wrong thing?*

There is no one magic phrase that can solve a client's problems; likewise, there is no single thing a student can say that will make them significantly worse. Careful listening, showing genuine interest, and caring about the client are extremely important. If these elements are present, then if the student says something that sounds out of place, he or she can simply restate it by saying, "That didn't come out right. What I meant was . . ."

- *What will I be doing?*

In the mental health setting, many familiar tasks and responsibilities are minimal. There are no dressings to change or wounds to assess, and there are fewer diagnostic tests and procedures than in a busy medical-surgical setting. The idea of "just talking to people" may make the student feel as though he or she is not really doing anything. The student must deal with his or her own anxiety about approaching a stranger to talk about very sensitive and personal issues. Development of the therapeutic nurse–client relationship and trust takes times and patience.

- *What if no one will talk to me?*

Students sometimes fear that clients will reject them or refuse to have anything to do with a student nurse. Some clients may not want to talk or are reclusive, but they may show that same behavior with experienced staff; it should not be seen as a personal insult or failure on the part of the student. Generally, many people in emotional distress welcome the opportunity to have someone listen to them and show a genuine interest in them and their situation. Being available and willing to listen is often all it takes to begin a significant interaction with someone.

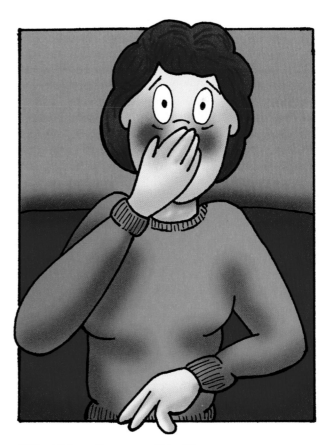

"What if I say the wrong thing?"

- *How will I handle bizarre or inappropriate behavior?*

The behavior and statements of some clients may be shocking or distressing to the student initially. It is important to monitor one's facial expressions and emotional responses so that clients do not feel rejected or ridiculed. The nursing instructor and staff are always available to assist the student in such situations. Students should never feel as if they will have to handle situations alone.

- *Is my physical safety in jeopardy?*

Often students have had little or no contact with seriously mentally ill persons. Media coverage of persons with mental illness who commit crimes is widespread, leaving the impression that most psychiatric clients are violent. Actually, clients hurt themselves more often than they harm others. Clients with a potential for violence are usually closely monitored by the staff for clues of an impending outburst. When physical aggression does occur, staff are specially trained to handle aggressive clients in a safe manner. The student should not become involved in the physical restraint of an aggressive client because he or she has not had the training and experience required. When talking to or approaching clients who are potentially aggressive, the student should sit in an open area rather than a closed room, provide plenty of space for the client, or request that the instructor or a staff person be present.

- *What if I encounter someone I know being treated on the unit?*

In any clinical setting, it is possible that a student nurse might see someone he or she knows, or a coworker. People often have additional fears because of the stigma that is still associated with seeking mental health treatment. It is essential in mental health that the client's identity and treatment be kept confidential. If the student recognizes someone he or she knows, the student should notify the instructor, who can decide how to handle the situation. It is usually best for the student (and sometimes the instructor or staff) to talk with the client and reassure him or her about confidentiality. The client should be reassured that the student will not read the client's record and will not be assigned to work with the client.

Students may discover that some of the problems, family dynamics, or life events of clients are similar to their own or those of their family. It can be a shock for students to discover that sometimes there are as many similarities between clients and staff as there are differences. There is no easy answer for this concern. Many people have stressful lives or abusive childhood experiences; some cope fairly successfully, and others are devastated emotionally. Although we know that coping skills are a key part of mental health, we do not always know what why some peo-

ple have serious emotional problems and others do not. Chapter 7 discusses these factors in more detail.

SELF-AWARENESS ISSUES

Self-awareness is the process by which the nurse gains recognition of his or her own feelings, beliefs, and attitudes. In nursing, being aware of one's feelings, thoughts, and values is a primary focus. Self-awareness is particularly important in mental health nursing. Everyone, including nurses and student nurses, has values, ideas, and beliefs that are a unique part of them and different from others. At times, the student's values and beliefs will conflict with those of the client or with the client's behavior. The nurse must learn to accept these differences among people and view the client as a worthwhile person regardless of his or her opinions and lifestyle. The student does not need to condone the client's views or behavior; he or she merely needs to accept it as different from his or her own and not let it interfere with care.

For example, a nurse who believes that abortion is wrong may be assigned to care for a client who has had an abortion. If the nurse is going to be of any help to the client, he or she must be able to separate his or her own beliefs about abortion from those of the client. The student must make sure personal feelings and beliefs do not interfere with or hinder the client's care.

Self-awareness can be accomplished through reflection, spending time consciously focusing on how one feels and what one values or believes. Although we all have values and beliefs, we may not have really spent time discovering how we feel or what we believe about certain issues, such as suicide or a client's refusal to take needed medications. The nurse needs to discover himself or herself and what he or she believes before trying to help others with different views.

Helpful Hints for Increasing Self-Awareness

- Keep a diary or journal that focuses on experiences and related feelings. Work on identifying feelings and the circumstances from which they arose. Review the diary or journal periodically to look for patterns or changes.
- Talk with someone you trust about your experiences and feelings. This might be a family member, friend, coworker, or nursing instructor. Discuss how he or she might feel in a similar situation, or ask how he or she deals with uncomfortable situations or feelings.
- Seek alternative points of view. Put yourself in the client's situation, and think about his or her feelings, thoughts, and actions.

INTERNET RESOURCES

Resource	Internet Address
▶ Department of Health and Human Services	http://www.dhhs.gov/
▶ World Health Organization	http://www.who.ch
▶ Nursing Net	http://www.nursingnet.org/
▶ National Alliance for the Mentally Ill	http://www.nami.org
▶ Center for the Study of the History of Nursing	http://www.upenn.edu/nursing/facres_history.html
▶ Men in American Nursing History	http://www.geocities.com/Athens/Forum/6011/index.html

• Do not be critical of yourself (or others) for having certain values or beliefs. Accept them as a part of yourself, or work to change those you wish to be different.

Critical Thinking

Questions

1. In your own words, describe mental health. Describe the characteristics, behavior, and abilities of someone who is mentally healthy.
2. When you think of mental illness, what images or ideas come to mind? Where do these ideas come from—movies, television, personal experience?
3. What personal characteristics do you have that indicate good mental health?

➤ KEY POINTS

• Mental health and mental illness are difficult to define and are influenced by one's culture and society.
• The World Health Organization defines health as a state of complete physical, mental, and social wellness, not merely the absence of disease or infirmity.
• Components of mental health include autonomy and independence, maximizing one's potential, tolerance of uncertainty, self-esteem, mastery of the environment, reality orientation, and stress management.

• There are many individual factors that influence mental health: biologic factors (sense of harmony in life, vitality, ability to find meaning in life, hardiness, spirituality, and positive attitude); interpersonal factors (effective communication, helping others, intimacy, and maintaining a balance of separateness and connectedness); and social/cultural factors (sense of community, access to resources, intolerance of violence, and support of diversity among people).
• Historically, mental illness was viewed as demonic possession, sin, or weakness, and people were punished accordingly.
• Today, mental illness is seen as a medical problem with symptoms causing dissatisfaction with one's characteristics, abilities, and accomplishments; ineffective or unsatisfying interpersonal relationships; dissatisfaction with one's place in the world; ineffective coping with life events; and lack of personal growth.
• Factors contributing to mental illness are biologic factors and anxiety, worries, and fears; ineffective communication; excessive dependence or withdrawal from relationships and loss of emotional control; and lack of resources, exposure to violence, homelessness, poverty, and discrimination.
• The DSM-IV is a taxonomy used to provide a standard nomenclature of mental disorders, define characteristics of disorders, and assist in identifying underlying causes of disorders.

- During the Renaissance, persons with mental illness were allowed to wander the streets if harmless or were thrown in prison if dangerous.
- In the 1790s, the concept of asylum as a safe, protected place was developed in Europe and was later brought to the United States.
- The period of scientific treatment began with Sigmund Freud and others who studied mental disorders and began treating patients.
- A significant advance in treating persons with mental illness was the development of psychotropic drugs in the early 1950s.
- The shift from institutional care to care in the community began in the 1960s, allowing many people to leave institutions for the first time in years.
- One result of deinstitutionalization is the "revolving door" of repetitive hospital admission without adequate community follow-up.
- It is estimated that 25% to 50% of the homeless population have a psychosis and 33% to 50% have substance abuse problems.
- The Department of Health and Human Services estimates that 51 million Americans have a diagnosable mental illness, but only one in four adults and one in three children receive treatment.
- The number of community mental health centers developed to treat deinstitutionalized persons has been inadequate.
- Community-based programs are the trend of the future, but they are underfunded and too few in number.
- Managed care, in an effort to contain costs, has resulted in withholding of services or approval of less expensive alternatives for mental health care.
- Mental health care is limited by days of service or dollar amounts; in contrast, insurance for medical illnesses rarely has such limitations.
- The population in the United States is becoming increasingly diverse in terms of culture, race, ethnicity, and family structure.
- Psychiatric nursing was recognized in the late 1800s, although it not required in nursing education programs until 1950.
- Psychiatric nursing practice has been profoundly influenced by Hildegard Peplau and June Mellow, who wrote about the nurse–patient relationship, anxiety, nurse therapy, and interpersonal nursing theory.
- The American Nurses Association has published standards of care that guide psychiatric-mental health nursing clinical practice.
- Common concerns of nursing students beginning a psychiatric clinical rotation include fear of saying the wrong thing, not knowing what to do, being rejected by clients, being threatened physically, recognizing someone they know as a client, and sharing similar problems or backgrounds with clients.
- Awareness of one's feelings, beliefs, attitudes, values, and thoughts, called self-awareness, is essential to the practice of psychiatric nursing.
- The goal of self-awareness is to know oneself so that one's values, attitudes, and beliefs are not projected to the client, interfering with nursing care. Self-awareness does not mean having to change one's values or beliefs, unless one desires to do so.
- Reflection, keeping a journal, talking with a trusted person, and trying to gain the client's perspective are methods that can be used to increase self-awareness.

REFERENCES

American Nurses Association (2000) *Scope and Standards of Psychiatric-Mental Health Nursing Practice.* Washington, DC: American Nurses Publishing, American Nurses Foundation/American Nurses Association.

Appleby, L., & Desai, P. N. (1993). Length of stay and recidivism in schizophrenia: A study of public psychiatric hospital patients. *American Journal of Psychiatry, 150*(1), 72–76.

Baly, M. (1982). A leading light. *Nursing Mirror, 155*(19), 49–51.

Department of Health and Human Services (1999). http:www.dhhs.gov/

Department of Health and Human Services. (2000). *Healthy People 2010.* Washington, DC: DHHS.

Doona, M. (1984). At least well cared for . . . Linda Richards and the mentally ill. *Image, 16*(2), 51–56.

Gollaher, D. (1995). *Voice for the mad: The life of Dorothea Dix.* New York: The Free Press.

Haugland, G., Siegel, C., Hopper, K., & Alexander, M. J. (1997). Mental illness among homeless individuals in a suburban county. *Psychiatric Services, 48*(4), 504–509.

International Association of Psychosocial Rehabilitation Services (IAPRS). (1990). *A national directory: Organizations providing psychosocial rehabilitation and related community support services in the United States.* Boston: Center for Psychiatric Rehabilitation, Boston University.

Johnson, B. S. (1997). *Psychiatric-mental health nursing: Adaptation and growth* (4th ed.). Philadelphia: Lippincott-Raven.

Keltner, N. L., Schwecke, L. H., & Bostrom, C. E. (1999). *Psychiatric nursing* (3rd ed.). St. Louis: Mosby, Inc.

Lamb, H. R., & Weinberger, L. E. (1998). Persons with severe mental illness in jails and prisons: A review. *Psychiatric Services, 49*(4), 483–492.

McMillan, I. (1997). Insight into Bedlam: One hospital's history. *Journal of Psychosocial Nursing, 3*(6), 28–34.

Mechanic, D. (1996). Key policy considerations for mental health in the managed care era. In R. Mandersheid

& M. Sonnenschein (Eds.). *Mental health, United States, 1996.* (DHHS Publication No. SMA 96-3098, pp. 1–16). Washington, DC: U. S. Government Printing Office.

Miller, P. E. (1996). Black Americans' and white Americans' views of the etiology and treatment of mental health problems. *Community Mental Health Journal, 32*(3), 235–241.

Randolph, F., Blasinsky, M., Leginski, W., Parker, L. B., & Goldman, H. H. (1997). Creating integrated service systems for homeless persons with mental illness: The ACCESS program. *Psychiatric Services, 48*(3), 369–373.

Ries, R. (1997). Advantages of separating the triage function from the emergency service. *Psychiatric Services, 48*(6), 755–756.

Rosenblatt, A. (1984). Concepts of the asylum in the care of the mentally ill. *Hospital and Community Psychiatry, 35,* 244–250.

Seaward, B. L. (1997). *Stand like mountains, flow like water.* Deerfield Beach, FL: Health Communications.

Torrey, E. F. (1997). The release of the mentally ill from institutions: A well-intentioned disaster. *Chronicle of Higher Education, 43*(40), B4.

Trudeau, M. E. (1993). Informed consent: The patient's right to decide. *Journal of Psychosocial Nursing & Mental Health Services, 31*(6), 9–12.

Wright, R. (1995). 20th century blues. *Time,* Aug. 28, 50–57.

ADDITIONAL READINGS

Rosenheck, R. (1997). Disability payments and chemical dependence: Conflicting values and uncertain effects. *Psychiatric Services, 48*(6), 789–791.

Spector, R. E. (2000). *Cultural diversity in illness and health* (5th ed.). Upper Saddle River, NJ: Prentice Hall Health.

Chapter Review

➤ MULTIPLE-CHOICE QUESTIONS

Select the best answer for each of the following questions.

1. Approximately how many Americans have a diagnosable mental illness?

    A. 26 million

    B. 42 million

    C. 51 million

    D. 83 million

2. The Department of Health and Human Services estimates that of the 750,000 homeless persons in the United States, the prevalence of psychosis is:

    A. Less than 23%

    B. 25% to 50%

    C. 51% to 75%

    D. More than 75%

3. Hospitals established by Dorothea Dix were designed to provide which of the following?

    A. Asylum

    B. Confinement

    C. Therapeutic milieu

    D. Public safety

4. Hildegard Peplau is best known for her writing about which of the following?

    A. Community-based care

    B. Humane treatment

    C. Psychopharmacology

    D. Therapeutic nurse–patient relationship.

5. How many adults in the United States who need mental health services actually receive care?

    A. 1 in 2

    B. 1 in 3

    C. 1 in 4

    D. 1 in 5

➤ TRUE-FALSE QUESTIONS

Identify each of the following statements as T (true) or F (false). Correct any false statements.

_____ 1. Asylums in the United States were built to confine mentally ill persons so the public would be protected.

_____ 2. Deinstitutionalization refers to the movement to decrease the population of patients in state hospitals.

_____ 3. Components of mental health include autonomy, tolerating uncertainty, self-esteem, and mastery of the environment.

_____ 4. Access to resources, intolerance of violence, and a sense of community are interpersonal factors influencing mental health.

_____ 5. Persons with mental illness have not been viewed as possessed by demons since the 1500s.

_____ 6. The period of enlightenment of the 1800s eliminated poor treatment for the mentally ill.

_____ 7. The period of scientific study began in the late 1800s with the work of Sigmund Freud.

_____

_____ 8. Treatment of mental illness with psychotropic drugs began in the 1950s.

_____

Indicate what type of information is recorded for each axis of the DSM-IV.

Axis I _____

Axis II _____

Axis III _____

Axis IV _____

Axis V _____

➤ SHORT-ANSWER QUESTIONS

1. Explain how the standards of practice developed by American Nurses Association are used.

2. Discuss three trends of mental health care in the United States.

3. Give an example of three different concerns of nursing students as they begin psychiatric nursing clinical experiences.

2

Neurobiologic Theories and Psycho-pharmacology

Learning Objectives

After reading this chapter, the student should be able to:

1. Describe the current neurobiologic research and theories that are the basis for current psychopharmacologic treatment of mental disorders.

2. Discuss the nurse's role in educating clients and families about current neurobiologic theories and medication management.

3. Discuss the categories of drugs used to treat mental illness and their mechanisms of action, side effects, and special nursing considerations.

4. Identify client responses that indicate treatment effectiveness.

5. Discuss common barriers to maintaining the medication regimen.

6. Develop a teaching plan for clients and families for implementation of the prescribed therapeutic regimen.

Key Terms

akathisia

anticholinergic effects

antidepressant drugs

antipsychotic drugs

anxiolytic drugs

computed tomography (CT)

depot injection

dopamine

dystonia

extrapyramidal symptoms (EPS)

epinephrine

efficacy

half-life

kindling process

limbic system

magnetic resonance imaging (MRI)

mood stabilizing drugs

neuroleptic malignant syndrome (NMS)

norepinephrine

neurotransmitter

positron emission tomography (PET)

potency

pseudoparkinsonism

psychoimmunology

psychopharmacology

psychotropic drugs

rebound

single photon emission computed tomography (SPECT)

serotonin

stimulant drugs

tardive dyskinesia

withdrawal

Although there is still much we do not know about what causes mental illness, science in the past 20 years has made great strides in helping us to understand how the brain works and in giving us possible causes of why some brains work differently from others. Such advances in neurobiologic research are constantly expanding the knowledge base in the field of psychiatry and are greatly affecting clinical practice. The psychiatric mental health nurse must have a basic understanding of how the brain functions and of the current theories regarding mental illness. This chapter includes an overview of the major anatomic structures of the nervous system and how it works—the neurotransmission process. In this chapter, we present the major current neurobiologic theories regarding what causes mental illness, including genetics and heredity, stress and the immune system, and infectious causes.

The use of medications to treat mental illness (**psychopharmacology**) has developed from these neurobiologic discoveries. These medications directly affect the central nervous system (CNS) and, subsequently, behavior, perceptions, thinking, and emotions. This chapter also discusses the five categories of drugs used to treat mental illness, including the role of the nurse, side effects, and client teaching. Although pharmacologic interventions are the most effective treatment for many psychiatric disorders, the success of treatment and the client's outcome are greatly enhanced by adjunctive therapies such as cognitive and behavioral therapy, family therapy, and psychotherapy. Chapter 3 discusses these psychosocial modalities.

THE NERVOUS SYSTEM AND HOW IT WORKS
Central Nervous System

The CNS is composed of the brain, the spinal cord, and associated nerves that control voluntary acts. Structurally, the brain is divided into the cerebrum, cerebellum, brain stem, and limbic system (Lewis, 2000). Figure 2-1 shows the locations of these structures.

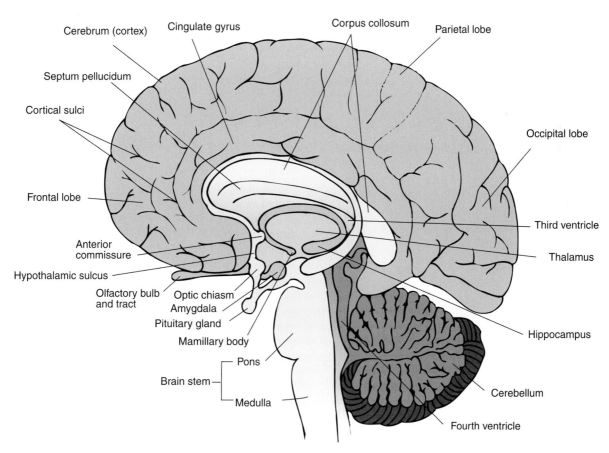

Figure 2-1. The limbic system.

CEREBRUM

The cerebrum is divided into two hemispheres, and except for the pineal gland, all lobes and structures are found in both halves of the brain. The corpus callosum is a pathway connecting the two hemispheres and coordinating their function. The left hemisphere of the brain controls the right side of the body and is the center for logical reasoning and analytic functions such as reading, writing, and mathematical tasks. The right hemisphere of the brain is the center for creative thinking, intuition, and artistic abilities and controls the left side of the body.

The cerebral hemispheres are each divided into four lobes: frontal, parietal, temporal, and occipital. Some of the functions of the lobes are distinct; others are integrated between the lobes. The frontal lobes control the organization of thought, body movement, memories, emotions, and moral behavior. The integration of all this information helps regulate arousal, focuses attention, and allows problem solving and decision making to occur. Abnormalities in the frontal lobes are associated with schizophrenia, attention deficit/hyperactivity disorder, and dementia.

The parietal lobes interpret sensations of taste and touch and assist in spatial orientation. The temporal lobes are centers for the sense of smell, hearing, memory, and the expression of emotions. The occipital lobes assist in coordinating language generation and visual interpretation, such as depth perception.

CEREBELLUM

The cerebellum is located below the cerebrum and is the center for coordination of movements and postural adjustments. The cerebellum receives and integrates information from all areas of the body, such as the muscles, joints, organs, and other components of the CNS. Research has shown that inhibited transmission of a neurotransmitter, dopamine, in this area is associated with the lack of smooth, coordinated movements in diseases such as Parkinson's disease and dementia.

BRAIN STEM

The brain stem includes the midbrain, pons, and medulla oblongata and the nuclei for cranial nerves 3 through 12. The medulla, located at the top of the spinal cord, contains vital centers for respiration and cardiovascular functions. Above the medulla and in front of the cerebrum, the pons bridges the gap both structurally and functionally, serving as a primary motor pathway. The midbrain includes most of the reticular activating system and the extrapyramidal system. The reticular activating system influences motor activity, sleep, consciousness, and awareness. The extrapyramidal system relays information about movement and coordination from the brain to the spinal nerves. The locus ceruleus is the area of the brain stem associated with stress, anxiety, and impulsive behavior.

LIMBIC SYSTEM

The **limbic system** is an area of the brain located above the brain stem that includes the thalamus, hypothalamus, hippocampus, and amygdala (although some sources differ on the structures included in this system). The thalamus regulates activity, sensation, and emotion. The hypothalamus is involved in temperature regulation, appetite control, endocrine function, sexual drive, and impulsive behavior associated with feelings of anger, rage, or excitement. The hippocampus and amygdala are involved in emotional arousal and memory. Disturbances in the limbic system have been implicated in a variety of mental illnesses, such as the memory loss seen in dementia or the poorly controlled emotions and impulses seen in psychotic or manic behavior.

Neurotransmitters

Approximately 100 billion brain cells form groups of neurons, or nerve cells, that are arranged in networks. These neurons communicate information with each other by sending electrochemical messages from neuron to neuron, a process called neurotransmission. These electrochemical messages pass from the dendrites (projections from the cell body), through the cell body, down the axon (long, extended structures), and across the gaps between cells (synapse) to the dendrite of the next neuron. In the nervous system, the electrochemical messages cross the gaps or synapses between neural cells by way of special chemical messengers called neurotransmitters.

Neurotransmitters are the chemical substances manufactured in the neuron that aid in the transmission of information throughout the body. They either excite or stimulate an action in the cells (excitatory) or inhibit or stop an action (inhibitory). These neurotransmitters fit into specific receptor cells embedded in the membrane of the dendrite, just like a certain key shape fits into a lock. After neurotransmitters are released into the synapse and relay the message to the receptor cells, they are either transported back from the synapse to the axon to be stored for later use (reuptake) or are metabolized and inactivated by enzymes, primarily monoamine oxidase (MAO) (Lewis, 2000) (Fig. 2-2).

These neurotransmitters are necessary in just the right proportions to relay messages across the

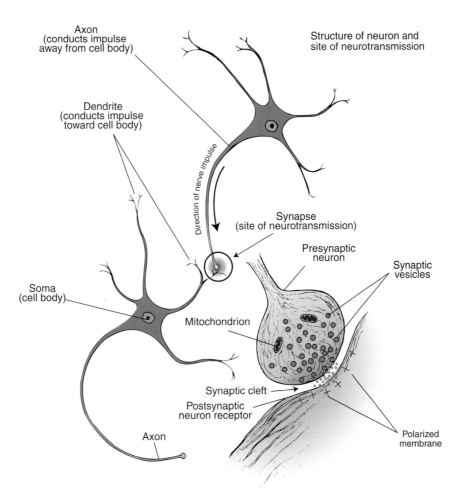

Figure 2-2. Structure of neuron and site of neurotransmission.

synapse. Studies are beginning to show that there is a difference in the amount of some neurotransmitters available in the brain of persons with certain mental disorders compared with persons with no signs of mental illness (Fig. 2-3).

Major neurotransmitters have been found to play a role in psychiatric illnesses as well as actions and side effects of psychotropic drugs. Table 2-1 lists the major types of neurotransmitters and their actions and effects. Dopamine and serotonin have received the most attention in terms of the study and treatment of psychiatric disorders (Tecott, 2000). The following is a discussion of the major neurotransmitters that have been associated with mental disorders.

DOPAMINE

Dopamine, a neurotransmitter located primarily in the brain stem, has been found to be involved in the control of complex movements, motivation, cognition, and regulation of emotional responses. Dopamine is generally excitatory and is synthesized from tyro-

sine, a dietary amino acid. Dopamine is implicated in schizophrenia and other psychoses, as well as movement disorders such as Parkinson's disease. Antipsychotic medications work by blocking dopamine receptors and reducing dopamine activity.

NOREPINEPHRINE

Norepinephrine, the most prevalent neurotransmitter in the nervous system, is located primarily in the brain stem and plays a role in changes in attention, learning and memory, sleep and wakefulness, and mood regulation. Norepinephrine and its derivative, **epinephrine**, are also known as noradrenaline and adrenaline, respectively. Excess norepinephrine has been implicated in a variety of anxiety disorders; deficits may affect memory loss, social withdrawal, and depression. Some antidepressants block the reuptake of norepinephrine, and others inhibit MAO from metabolizing it. Epinephrine has limited distribution in the brain but controls the fight-or-flight response in the peripheral nervous system.

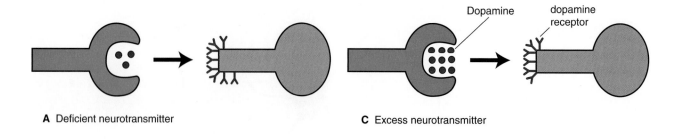

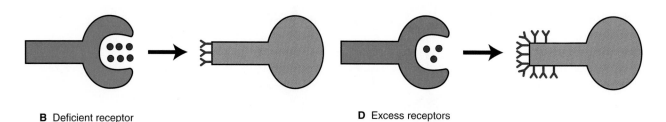

Figure 2-3. Abnormal neurotransmission causing some mental disorders because of excess transmission or excess responsiveness of receptors.

SEROTONIN

Serotonin is a neurotransmitter found only in the brain. Its function is mostly inhibitory, and it plays an important role in anxiety and mood disorders and schizophrenia. It has been found to play a role in the delusions, hallucinations, and withdrawn behavior seen in schizophrenia. Serotonin is derived from tryptophan, a dietary amino acid. Serotonin is involved in the control of food intake, sleep and wakefulness, temperature regulation, pain control, sexual behavior, and regulation of emotions. Some antidepressants block serotonin reuptake, thus leaving it available in the synapse for a longer time, which results in improved mood.

Table 2-1

MAJOR TYPES OF NEUROTRANSMITTERS

Type of Neurotransmitter	Mechanism of Action	Physiologic Effects
Dopamine	Excitatory	Controls complex movements, motivation, cognition; regulates emotional response
Norepinephrine (noradrenaline)	Excitatory	Changes in attention, learning and memory, sleep and wakefulness, mood
Epinephrine (adrenaline)	Excitatory	Fight-or-flight response
Serotonin	Inhibitory	Control of food intake, sleep and wakefulness, temperature regulation, pain control, sexual behaviors, regulation of emotions
Histamine	Neuromodulator	Alertness, control of gastric secretions, cardiac stimulation, peripheral allergic responses
Acetylcholine	Excitatory or inhibitory	Sleep and wakefulness cycle; signals muscles to become alert
Neuropeptides	Neuromodulators	Enhance, prolong, inhibit, or limit the effects of principal neurotransmitters
Glutamate	Excitatory	Neurotoxicity results if levels are too high
Gamma-aminobutyric acid (GABA)	Inhibitory	Modulates other neurotransmitters

HISTAMINE

The role of histamine in mental illness is under investigation. It is involved in producing peripheral allergic responses, control of gastric secretions, cardiac stimulation, and alertness. Some psychotropic drugs block histamine, resulting in weight gain, sedation, and hypotension.

ACETYLCHOLINE

Acetylcholine is a neurotransmitter found in the brain, spinal cord, and peripheral nervous system, particularly at the neuromuscular junction of skeletal muscle. It can be excitatory or inhibitory. It is synthesized from dietary choline found in red meat and vegetables and has been found to affect the sleep/wake cycle and signals muscles to become active. Studies have shown that persons with Alzheimer's disease have a decreased number of acetylcholine-secreting neurons, and persons with myasthenia gravis (a muscular disorder in which impulses fail to pass the myoneural junction, causing muscle weakness) have a reduced number of acetylcholine receptors.

GAMMA-AMINOBUTYRIC ACID (GABA)

GABA, an amino acid, is the major inhibitory neurotransmitter in the brain and has been found to modulate other neurotransmitter systems rather than providing a direct stimulus (Shank, Smith-Swintonky, & Twyman, 2000). Drugs that increase GABA function, such as benzodiazepines, are used to treat anxiety and induce sleep.

Glutamate is an excitatory amino acid that at high levels can have major neurotoxic effects. Glutamate has been implicated in the brain damage caused by stroke, hypoglycemia, sustained hypoxia or ischemia, and some degenerative diseases such as Huntington's or Alzheimer's disease.

BRAIN IMAGING TECHNIQUES

Previously, the brain could be studied only through surgery or autopsy. Several brain imaging techniques developed during the past 25 years now allow visualization of the brain structure and function. These techniques are useful for diagnosing some disorders of the brain and have helped correlate certain areas of the brain to specific functions. Brain imaging techniques are also useful in research to find the causes of mental disorders. Table 2-2 describes and compares these diagnostic tests.

Computed tomography (CT, also called computed axial tomography or CAT scan) is a procedure in which a precise x-ray beam takes cross-sectional images (slices) layer by layer. A computer reconstructs the images on a monitor and also stores the images on magnetic tape or film. CT can visualize the soft tissues of the brain and is used to diagnose tumors, effusions, and metastases and to determine the size of the ventricles of the brain. Some persons with schizophrenia have been shown to have enlarged ventricles; this is associated with a poorer prognosis and marked negative symptoms (see Chap. 13) (Fig. 2-4). The person undergoing a CT scan must lie motionless on a stretcher-like table for about 20 to 40 minutes as the stretcher is passed through a "ring" while the serial x-rays are taken.

In **magnetic resonance imaging** (MRI), a type of body scan, an energy field is created with a huge magnet and radio waves. The energy field is converted to a visual image or scan. MRI produces more tissue detail and contrast than CT and can show blood flow patterns and tissue changes such as areas of edema. It can also be used to measure the size and thickness of brain structures. Selemon and Goldman-Rakic (1995) found a 7% reduction in cortical thickness in persons with schizophrenia. The person undergoing a MRI must lie in a small, closed chamber and must remain motionless during the procedure, which takes about 45 minutes. Persons who feel claus-

Table 2-2

BRAIN IMAGING TECHNOLOGY

Procedure	Imaging Method	Results	Duration
Computed tomography (CT)	Serial x-rays of brain	Structural image	20–40 minutes
Magnetic resonance imaging (MRI)	Radio waves from brain detected from magnet	Structural image	45 minutes
Position emission tomography (PET)	Radioactive tracer injected into bloodstream and monitored as client performs activities	Functional	2–3 hours
Single photon emission computed tomography (SPECT)	Same as PET	Functional	1–2 hours

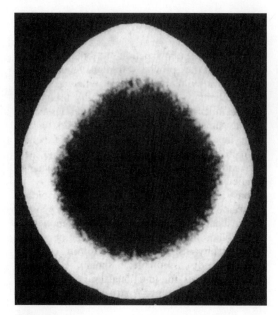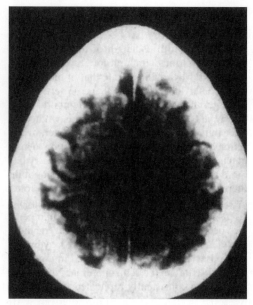

Figure 2-4. Example of computed tomography scan of brain of patient with schizophrenia compared to normal control.

trophobic or have increased anxiety may require sedation before the procedure. Persons with pacemakers or metal implants such as heart valves or orthopedic devices cannot undergo MRI.

More advanced imaging techniques, such as **positron emission tomography** (PET) and **single photon emission computed tomography** (SPECT), are also used to examine the function of the brain. Radioactive substances are injected into the blood and the flow of those substances in the brain is monitored as the client performs cognitive activities as instructed by the operator. PET uses the emission of two photons simultaneously; SPECT uses a single photon. PET provides better resolution, with sharper and clearer pictures. PET and SPECT are used for research but not for the diagnosis and treatment of persons with mental disorders (Karson & Renshaw, 2000; Malison & Innis, 2000) (Fig. 2-5). A PET scan takes about 2 to 3 hours; SPECT takes 1 to 2 hours. These scans have shown that persons with Alzheimer's disease have decreased glucose metabolism in the brain and decreased cerebral blood flow. Some persons with schizophrenia also demonstrate decreased cerebral blood flow. Figure 2-6 compares the images obtained from CAT, MRI, and PET scans (Fig. 2-6).

Limitations of Brain Imaging Techniques

Although imaging techniques such as PET and SPECT have helped bring about tremendous advances in the study of brain diseases, they have some limitations:

- The use of radioactive substances in PET and SPECT limits the number of times a person can undergo these tests. There is the risk that the client will have an allergic reaction to the substances. Some clients may find receiving intravenous doses of radioactive material frightening or unacceptable.

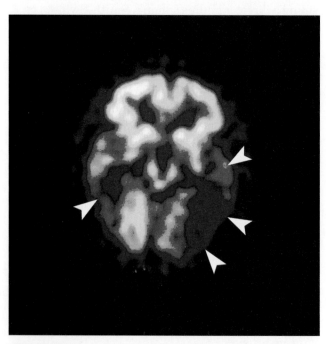

Figure 2-5. Example of axial (horizontal) PET scan of male patient with Alzheimer's disease, showing defects (arrowheads) in metabolism in the regions of cerebral cortex of brain.

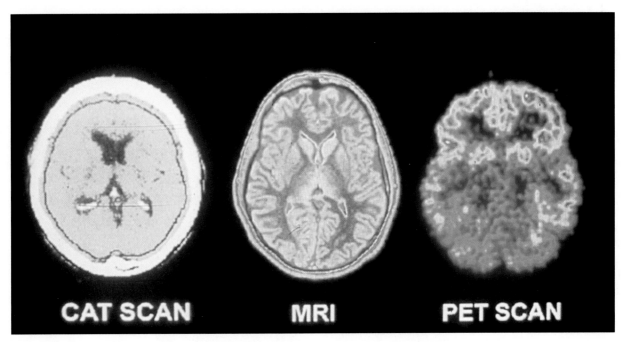

Figure 2-6. Comparison of computed tomography scan (*left*), magnetic resonance imaging scan (*center*), and positron emission tomography scan (*right*) (Chap. 7). (Courtesy of Monte S. Buchsbaum, MD, The Mount Sinai Medical Center and School of Medicine, New York, New York.)

- Imaging equipment is expensive to purchase and maintain, so availability can be limited. A PET camera costs about $2.5 million; a SPECT camera costs about $500,000.
- Some persons cannot tolerate these procedures because of fear or claustrophobia.
- Researchers are finding that many of the changes that occur in disorders such as schizophrenia are at the molecular and chemical level and cannot be detected with current imaging techniques (Karson & Renshaw, 2000; Malison & Innis, 2000).

GENETICS AND HEREDITY

Unlike many physical illnesses that have been found to be hereditary, such as cystic fibrosis, Huntington's disease, and Duchenne's muscular dystrophy, the origins of mental disorders do not seem to be that simple. Current theories and studies seem to indicate that several mental disorders may be linked to a specific gene or combination of genes, but the source is not solely genetic; nongenetic factors also play an important role.

To date, one of the most promising discoveries is the identification of two genes linked to Alzheimer's disease: chromosomes 14 and 21. Research is continuing in an attempt to find genetic links to other diseases, such as schizophrenia and mood disorders. This is the focus of ongoing research in the Human Genome Project, funded by the National Institute of Health and the Department of Energy in the United States. This international research project, started in 1988, is the largest research project of its kind. The goal is to identify all human DNA and the human characteristics and diseases it is related to (encoding). The researchers publish their results in the journal *Science*; further information can be obtained at www.nhgri.gov.

Three types of studies are commonly conducted to investigate the genetic basis of mental illness:

1. Twin studies are used to compare the rate of occurrence of certain mental illnesses or traits in both monozygotic or identical twins, who have an identical genetic makeup, and dizygotic or fraternal twins, who have a different genetic makeup. Fraternal twins have the same genetic similarities as nontwin siblings.
2. Adoption studies are used to determine a trait among biologic family members versus adoptive family members.
3. Family studies are used to compare whether a trait is more common among first-degree relatives (parents, siblings, or children) than among more distant relatives or the general population.

Although some genetic links have been found in certain mental disorders, studies have not shown that these illnesses are solely genetically linked. The debate continues about the influence of inherited traits versus the influence of the environment—the "nature versus nurture" debate. The influence of environmental or psychosocial factors is discussed in Chapter 3.

STRESS AND THE IMMUNE SYSTEM (PSYCHOIMMUNOLOGY)

Researchers are following many avenues to discover possible causes of mental illness. **Psychoimmunology**, a relatively new field of study, examines the effect of psychosocial stressors on the body's immune system. A compromised immune system could contribute to the development of a variety of illnesses, particularly in populations already genetically at risk. So far, efforts to link a specific stressor with a specific disease have been unsuccessful.

INFECTION AS A POSSIBLE CAUSE

Some researchers are focusing on infection as a cause of mental illness. Most studies involving viral theories have focused on schizophrenia, but so far none has provided specific or conclusive evidence. Theories that are being developed and tested include the existence of a virus that has an affinity for tissues of the CNS, the possibility that a virus may actually alter human genes, and maternal exposure to a virus during critical fetal development of the nervous system.

Susan Swedo, chief of pediatrics and developmental neuropsychiatry at the National Institutes of Mental Health, has studied the relation of *Streptococcus* bacteria and obsessive-compulsive disorder (OCD) in children. In a 1999 study of 28 children with OCD, Swedo replaced their blood plasma, which had high levels of *Streptococcus* antibodies, with healthy donor plasma. In 1 month, the incidence of tics had decreased by 50%, and other OCD symptoms had been reduced by 60% (Washington, 1999). Studies such as this sound promising in discovering a link between infection and mental illness.

THE NURSE'S ROLE IN RESEARCH AND EDUCATION

Amid all the reports of research in these areas of neurobiology, genetics, and heredity, the implications for clients and their families are still not clear or specific. Often reports in the media regarding new research and studies are confusing or poorly understood by clients and families. The nurse must help clients and families well informed about progress in these areas but must also help them distinguish between facts and hypotheses. The nurse can explain whether or how new research may affect a client's treatment or

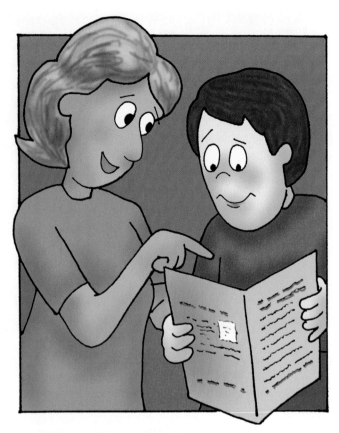

Keeping clients informed

prognosis. The nurse is a good resource for providing information and answering questions.

PSYCHOPHARMACOLOGY

Medication management is a crucial issue for many clients with mental disorders, and it greatly influences the outcomes of treatment. Several categories of drugs used to treat mental disorders (**psychotropic drugs**) will be discussed: antipsychotics, antidepressants, mood stabilizers, antianxiety drugs, and stimulants. It is important for the nurse to know how these drugs work, their side effects, contraindications, and interactions, and the nursing interventions required for helping clients manage medication regimens.

Several terms used in describing drugs and drug therapy are important for the nurse to know. **Efficacy** refers to the maximal therapeutic effect that can be achieved by a drug. **Potency** describes the amount of the drug needed to achieve that maximum effect. Drugs that have a low potency require higher dosages to achieve efficacy, whereas high-potency drugs achieve efficacy at lower dosages. **Half-life** is the amount of time it takes for half of the drug to be removed from the bloodstream. Drugs with a shorter half-life may need to be given three or four times a day, but drugs with a longer half-life may be given once a day. The amount of time needed for a drug to leave the body completely after it has been discontinued is about five times its half-life (Hyman, Arana, & Rosenbaum, 1995).

Principles That Guide Pharmacologic Treatment

The following are several principles to guide the use of medications in treating psychiatric disorders (Hyman, Arana, & Rosenbaum, 1995):

- A medication is selected based on its effect on the client's target symptoms, such as delusional thinking, panic attacks, or hallucinations. The effectiveness of the medication is evaluated in large part by its ability to diminish or eliminate the target symptoms.
- Many psychotropic drugs must be given in adequate dosages for a period of time before their full effect is realized. For example, tricyclic antidepressants can require 4 to 6 weeks to provide optimal therapeutic benefit.
- The dosage of medication is often adjusted to the lowest dosage effective for the client. Sometimes higher dosages may be needed to stabilize the client's target symptoms, and lower dosages can be used to sustain those effects over time.
- As a rule, elderly persons require lower dosages of a medication to produce therapeutic effects, and it may take longer for a drug to achieve its full therapeutic effect.
- Psychotropic medications are often decreased gradually (tapering) rather than abruptly discontinued. This is due to potential problems with **rebound** (temporary return of symptoms), recurrence of the original symptoms, or **withdrawal** (new symptoms resulting from discontinuation of the drug).
- Follow-up care is essential to ensure compliance with the medication regimen, to make needed adjustments in dosage, and to manage side effects.

Compliance with the medication regimen is often enhanced when the regimen is as simple as possible, in terms of both the number of medications prescribed and the number of daily doses.

Antipsychotic Drugs

Antipsychotic drugs, also known as neuroleptics, are used to treat the symptoms of psychosis, such as delusions and hallucinations. They work by blocking receptors of the neurotransmitter dopamine. They have been in clinical use since the 1950s. Anti-

psychotic drugs are the primary medical treatment for schizophrenia and are also used in psychotic episodes of acute mania, psychotic depression, and drug-induced psychosis. Persons with dementia who have psychotic symptoms sometimes respond to low dosages of antipsychotics. Short-term therapy with antipsychotics may be useful for transient psychotic symptoms, such as those seen in some persons with borderline personality disorder (Hyman, Arana, & Rosenbaum, 1995).

Table 2-3 lists available dosage forms, usual daily oral dosages, and extreme dosage ranges for typical and atypical antipsychotic drugs. The low end of the extreme range is typically used with children or elderly clients.

MECHANISM OF ACTION

The major action of all antipsychotics in the nervous system is to block receptors for the neurotransmitter dopamine; however, the therapeutic mechanism of action is only partially understood. Dopamine receptors are classified into subcategories (D1, D2, D3, D4, and D5), and D2, D3, and D4 have been associated with mental illness. The typical antipsychotic drugs are potent antagonists (blockers) of D2, D3, and D4. This makes them effective in treating target symptoms but also produces many extrapyramidal side effects (discussed below) because of the blocking of the D2 receptors. Newer, atypical antipsychotic drugs, such as clozapine (Clozaril), are relatively weak blockers of D2, which may account for the lower incidence of extrapyramidal side effects. In addition, atypical antipsychotics inhibit the reuptake of serotonin, as do some of the antidepressants, which makes them more effective in treating the depressive aspects of schizophrenia.

Two antipsychotics are available in **depot injection**, a time-release form of medication for maintenance therapy. The vehicle for these injections is sesame oil, so the medication is absorbed slowly over time; thus, less frequent administration is needed to maintain the desired therapeutic effects (Keltner, 1997). Fluphenazine (Prolixin) has a 7- to 28-day duration, and haloperidol (Haldol) has a duration of 4 weeks. Once the client's condition is stabilized with oral doses of these medications, administration by depot injection is required every 2 to 4 weeks to maintain the therapeutic effect.

SIDE EFFECTS

Extrapyramidal Side Effects. **Extrapyramidal symptoms** (EPS) are serious neurologic symptoms that are the major side effects of antipsychotic drugs. They include acute dystonia, pseudoparkinsonism,

Table 2-3

ANTIPSYCHOTIC DRUGS

Generic (Trade) Name	Forms	Daily Dosage*	Extreme Dosage Ranges*
TYPICAL ANTIPSYCHOTICS			
Phenothiazines			
Chlorpromazine (Thorazine)	T, L, INJ	200–1,600	25–2,000
Perphenazine (Trilafon)	T, L, INJ	16–32	4–64
Fluphenazine (Prolixin)	T, L, INJ	2.5–20	1–60
Thioridazine (Mellaril)	T, L	200–600	40–800
Mesoridazine (Serentil)	T, L, INJ	75–300	30–400
Trifluoperazine (Stelazine)	T, L, INJ	6–50	2–80
Thioxanthene			
Thiothixene (Navane)	C, L, INJ	6–30	6–60
Butyrophenones			
Haloperidol (Haldol)	T, L, INJ	2–20	1–100
Dibenzazepine			
Loxapine (Loxitane)	C, L, INJ	60–100	30–250
Dihydroindolone			
Molindone (Moban)	T, L	50–100	15–250
ATYPICAL ANTIPSYCHOTICS			
Clozapine (Clozaril)	T	150–500	75–700
Risperidone (Risperdol)	T	2–8	1–16
Olanzapine (Zyprexa)	T	5–15	5–20
Quetiapine (Seroquel)	T	300–600	200–750

* mg/day for oral doses only
T, tablet; C, capsule; L, liquid for oral use; INJ, injection for IM (usually prn) use.
Data from Hyman, S. E., Arana, G. W., & Rosenbaum, J. F. (1995). *Handbook of psychiatric drug therapy* (3d ed.). Boston: Little, Brown & Co., and Maxmen, Spratto, G. R. & Woods, A. L. (2000). *PDR Nurses' Drug Handbook*. Montvale, NJ: Medical Economics Company.

and akathisia. These neurologic side effects are often collectively referred to as EPS, although there is a distinction among the various reactions. One client can experience all the reactions in the same course of therapy, which makes it difficult to distinguish among the specific reactions. Blockade of D2 receptors in the midbrain region of the brain stem is responsible for the development of EPS.

Therapies for the neurologic side effects of acute dystonia, pseudoparkinsonism, and akathisia are similar and include lowering the dosage of the antipsychotic, changing to a different antipsychotic, or administering anticholinergic medication (Egan & Hyde, 2000).

Acute **dystonia** includes acute muscular rigidity and cramping, a stiff or thick tongue with difficulty swallowing, and in severe cases laryngospasm and respiratory difficulties. It is most likely to occur in the first week of treatment and in clients younger than 40, in males, and in those receiving high-potency drugs, such as haloperidol and thiothixene. Spasms or stiffness in muscle groups can produce **torticollis** (twisted head and neck), **opisthotonus** (tightness in the entire body with the head back and an arched neck), or **oculogyric crisis** (eyes rolled back in a locked position). Acute dystonic reactions can be painful and frightening for the client. Immediate

treatment with anticholinergic drugs, such as intramuscular benztropine mesylate (Cogentin) or intramuscular or intravenous diphenhydramine (Benadryl), usually brings rapid relief.

Table 2-4 lists the drugs used to treat EPS, along with routes and dosages. The addition of a regularly scheduled oral anticholinergic such as benztropine may allow the client to continue taking the antipsychotic drug with no further dystonia. Recurrent dystonic reactions would necessitate a lower dosage or a change in the antipsychotic drug.

Drug-induced parkinsonism, or **pseudoparkinsonism**, is often referred to by the generic label of EPS. Symptoms resemble those of Parkinson's disease and include a stiff, stooped posture; masklike facies; decreased arm swing; a shuffling, festinating gait (with small steps); cogwheel rigidity (ratchet-like movements of joints); drooling; tremor; bradycardia; and coarse pill-rolling movements of the thumb and fingers while at rest. Parkinsonism is treated by changing to an antipsychotic medication that has a lower incidence of EPS, or by adding an oral anticholinergic agent or amantadine.

Akathisia is reported by the client as an intense need to move about. The client appears restless or anxious and agitated, often with a rigid posture or gait and a lack of spontaneous gestures. This feeling

Table 2-4

DRUGS USED TO TREAT EXTRAPYRAMIDAL SIDE EFFECTS

Generic (Trade) Name	Oral Dosages (mg)	IM/IV Doses (mg)	Drug Class
Amantadine (Symmetrel)	100 bid or tid	–	Dopaminergic Agonist
Benztropine (Cogentin)	1–3 bid	1–2	Anticholinergic
Biperiden (Akineton)	2 tid–qid	2	Anticholinergic
Diazepam (Valium)	5 tid	5–10	Benzodiazepine
Diphenhydramine (Benadryl)	25–50 tid or qid	25–50	Antihistamine
Lorazepam (Ativan)	1–2 tid	–	Benzodiazepine
Procyclidine (Kemadrin)	2.5–5 tid	–	Anticholinergic
Propranolol (Inderal)	10–20 tid; up to 40 qid	–	Beta-blocker
Trihexaphenidyl (Artane)	2–5 tid	–	Anticholinergic

Data from Spratto, G. R. & Woods, A. L. (2000). *PDR Nurses' Drug Handbook.* Montvale, NJ: Medical Economics Company, and Bailey, K. P. (1998). *Psychotropic drug facts.* Philadelphia: Lippincott Williams & Wilkins.

of internal restlessness and the inability to sit still or rest often leads clients to discontinue their antipsychotic medication. Akathisia can be treated by a change in antipsychotic medication or the addition of an oral agent such as a beta-blocker, anticholinergic, or benzodiazepine.

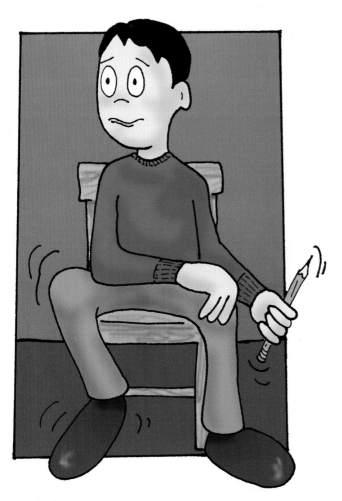

Akathisia

Neuroleptic Malignant Syndrome. **Neuroleptic malignant syndrome** (NMS) is a potentially fatal, idiosyncratic reaction to an antipsychotic (or neuroleptic) drug. Although the DSM-IV (1994) notes that the death rate from this syndrome in the literature has been reported at 10% to 20%, those figures may have been due to biased reporting; the reported rates are now decreasing. The major symptoms of NMS are rigidity, high fever, autonomic instability, such as unstable blood pressure, diaphoresis, and pallor, delirium, and elevated levels of enzymes, particularly CPK. Clients with NMS are usually confused and often mute; they may fluctuate from agitation to stupor. All antipsychotics seem to have the potential to cause NMS, but high dosages of high-potency drugs increase the risk. NMS most often occurs in the first 2 weeks of therapy or after an increase in dosage, but it can occur at any time.

Dehydration, poor nutrition, and concurrent medical illness all increase the risk for NMS. Treatment for NMS includes immediate discontinuance of all antipsychotic medications and the institution of supportive medical care, such as rehydration and hypothermia, until the client's physical condition stabilizes. After NMS, the decision to treat the client with other antipsychotic drugs requires full discussion between the client and the physician to weigh the relative risks against the potential benefits of therapy.

Tardive Dyskinesia. **Tardive dyskinesia** (TD), a syndrome of permanent, involuntary movements, is most commonly caused by the long-term use of typical antipsychotic drugs. At least 20% of persons treated with neuroleptics in the long term develop TD. The symptoms of TD include involuntary movements of the tongue, facial and neck muscles, upper and lower extremities, and truncal musculature. Tongue thrusting and protrusion, lip-smacking, blinking, grimacing, and other excessive, unnecessary facial movements are characteristic of TD. Once TD has developed, it is irreversible, although its progression can be arrested by decreasing or discontinuing the antipsychotic medication. Unfortunately, antipsychotic medications can mask the beginning symptoms of TD: that is, increased dosages of the antipsychotic medication will cause the initial symptoms to disappear temporarily. However, as the symptoms of TD worsen, they "break through" the effect of the antipsychotic drug.

One of the goals when administering antipsychotics is to prevent the occurrence of TD. This can be done by keeping maintenance dosages as low as possible, changing medications, and monitoring the client periodically for the initial signs of TD using a standardized assessment tool, such as the Abnormal Involuntary Movement Scale (see Chap. 13). Persons who have already developed signs of TD but still need to take an antipsychotic medication are often given clozapine, which has not yet been found to cause, or therefore worsen, TD (Egan & Hyde, 2000).

Anticholinergic Side Effects. **Anticholinergic side effects** often occur with the use of antipsychotics and include orthostatic hypotension, dry mouth, constipation, urinary hesitance or retention, blurred near vision, dry eyes, photophobia, nasal congestion, and decreased memory. These side effects usually decrease within 3 to 4 weeks but do not entirely remit. The client who is taking anticholinergic agents for EPS may have increased problems with anticholinergic side effects, but some nutritional or over-the-counter remedies can ease these symptoms (see below).

Other Side Effects. Antipsychotic drugs, with the exception of clozapine, also cause an increased blood prolactin level. Elevated prolactin may cause breast enlargement and tenderness in men and women, diminished libido and erectile and orgasmic dysfunction, menstrual irregularities, and an increased risk for breast cancer.

Clozapine produces fewer traditional side effects than most antipsychotic drugs, but it has the potentially fatal side effect of agranulocytosis. This develops suddenly and is characterized by fever, malaise, ulcerative sore throat, and leukopenia. This side effect may not be manifested immediately and can occur up to 24 weeks after the initiation of therapy. At present, persons taking clozapine in the United States have blood samples taken weekly to monitor the white blood cell count; they must present those results to their pharmacy to get the prescription refilled. The drug must be discontinued immediately if the white blood cell count drops by 50% or to less than 3,000 (Julien, 1998).

CLIENT TEACHING

Clients taking antipsychotic medication should be informed about the types of side effects that may occur and should be encouraged to report them to the physician instead of discontinuing the medication. The nurse should teach the client methods of managing or avoiding unpleasant side effects and maintaining the medication regimen (see Client Teaching & Medication Management: Antipsychotics). Drinking sugar-free fluids and eating sugar-free hard candy will ease dry mouth. Calorie-laden beverages and candy should be avoided because they promote dental caries, contribute to weight gain, and do little to relieve dry mouth. Constipation can be prevented or relieved by

---

▶ CLIENT TEACHING AND MEDICATION MANAGEMENT: ANTIPSYCHOTICS

- Drink sugar-free fluids and eat sugar-free hard candy to ease the anticholinergic effects of dry mouth.
- Avoid calorie-laden beverages and candy because they promote dental caries, contribute to weight gain, and do little to relieve dry mouth.
- Constipation can be prevented or relieved by increasing intake of water and bulk-forming foods in the diet and by exercising.
- Stool softeners are permissible, but laxatives should be avoided.
- Use sunscreen to prevent burning. Avoid long periods of time in the sun, and wear protective clothing. Photosensitivity can cause you to burn easily.
- Rising slowly from a lying or sitting position will prevent falls from orthostatic hypotension or dizziness due to a drop in blood pressure. Wait to walk until any dizziness has subsided.
- Monitor the amount of sleepiness or drowsiness you experience. Avoid driving a car or performing other potentially dangerous activities until your response time and reflexes seem normal.
- If you forget a dose of antipsychotic medication, take it if the dose is only 3 to 4 hours late. If the missed dose is more than 4 hours late or the next dose is due, omit the forgotten dose.
- If you have difficulty remembering your medication, use a chart to record doses when taken, or use a pill box labeled with dosage times and/or days of the week to help you remember when to take medication.

increasing water and bulk-forming foods in the diet and by exercising. Stool softeners are permissible, but laxatives should be avoided. The use of sunscreen is recommended, because photosensitivity can cause the client to burn easily.

Clients should monitor the amount of sleepiness or drowsiness they feel. They should avoid driving and performing other potentially dangerous activities until their response time and reflexes seem normal.

If the client forgets a dose of antipsychotic medication, he or she can take the missed dose if it is only 3 or 4 hours late. If the dose is more than 4 hours overdue, or the next dose is due, the forgotten dose can be omitted. Clients who have difficulty remembering to take their medication should be encouraged to use a chart and to record doses when taken, or to use a pill box that can be prefilled with accurate doses for the day or week.

Antidepressant Drugs

Antidepressant drugs are primarily used in the treatment of major depressive illness, panic disorder and other anxiety disorders, bipolar depression, and psychotic depression. Although the mechanism of action is not completely understood, antidepressants somehow interact with the two neurotransmitters, norepinephrine and serotonin, that regulate mood, arousal, attention, sensory processing, and appetite.

Antidepressants are divided into four groups:
- Tricyclic and the related cyclic antidepressants
- Selective serotonin reuptake inhibitors (SSRIs);
- Monoamine oxidase inhibitors (MAOIs)
- Other antidepressants, such as venlafaxine (Effexor), bupropion (Wellbutrin), trazodone (Desyrel), and nefazodone (Serzone).

Table 2-5 lists the dosage forms, usual daily dosages, and extreme dosage ranges.

The cyclic compounds became available in the 1950s and for years were the first choice of drugs to treat depression, even though they cause varying degrees of sedation, orthostatic hypotension (drop in blood pressure on rising), and anticholinergic side effects. In addition, cyclic antidepressants are potentially lethal if taken in an overdose.

During that same period of time, the MAOIs were discovered to have a positive effect on depressed persons. Although the MAOIs have a low incidence of

---

Table 2-5

ANTIDEPRESSANT DRUGS

Generic (Trade) Name	Forms	Usual Daily Dosages*	Extreme Dosage Ranges*
SELECTIVE SEROTONIN REUPTAKE INHIBITORS			
Fluoxetine (Prozac)	C, L	20	50–80
Fluvoxamine (Luvox)	T	150–200	50–300
Paroxetine (Paxil)	T	20	10–50
Sertraline (Zoloft)	T	100–150	50–200
CYCLIC COMPOUNDS			
Imipramine (Tofranil)	T, C, INJ	150–200	50–300
Desipramine (Norpramin)	T, C	150–200	50–300
Amitriptyline (Elavil)	T, INJ	150–200	50–300
Nortriptyline (Pamelor)	C, L	75–100	25–150
Doxepin (Sinequan)	C, L	150–200	25–300
Trimipramine (Surmontil)	C	150–200	50–300
Protriptyline (Vivactil)	T	15–40	10–60
Maprotiline (Ludiomil)	T	100–150	50–200
Amoxapine (Ascendin)	T	150–200	50–250
Clomipramine (Anafranil)	C, INJ	150–200	50–250
OTHER COMPOUNDS			
Bupropion (Wellbutrin)	T	200–300	100–450
Venlafaxine (Effexor)	T, C	75–225	75–375
Trazodone (Desyrel)	T	200–300	100–600
Nefazodone (Serzone)	T	300–600	100–600
Mirtazapine (Remeron)	T		
MONOAMINE OXIDASE INHIBITORS			
Phenelzine (Nardil)	T	45–60	15–90
Tranylcypromine (Parnate)	T	30–50	10–90
Isocarboxazid (Marplan)	T	20–40	10–60

*mg/day for oral dose
C, capsule; T, tablet; L, liquid; INJ, injection for IM use.
From Julien, R. M. (1998). *A primer of drug action* (8th ed.). New York: W. H. Freeman & Co.

sedation and anticholinergic effects, they must be used with extreme caution for several reasons:

1. A life-threatening side effect, hypertensive crisis, may occur if foods containing **tyramine** (an amino acid) are ingested while the client is taking MAOIs.
2. Because of the risk of potentially fatal drug interactions, MAOIs cannot be given in combination with other MAOIs, tricyclic antidepressants, or meperidine (Demerol), CNS depressants, many antihypertensives, or general anesthetics.

DRUG ALERT

OVERDOSE OF MAOI AND CYCLIC ANTIDEPRESSANTS

Both the cyclic compounds and MAOIs are potentially lethal when taken in overdose. Depressed or impulsive clients who are taking any antidepressants in these two categories may need to have prescriptions and refills in limited amounts to decrease this risk.

DRUG ALERT

MAOI DRUG INTERACTIONS

The following drugs can cause a potentially fatal drug interaction when taken with MAOI antidepressants:

Other MAOI antidepressants

SSRI antidepressants

Meperidine (Demerol)

Buspirone (BuSpar)

Dextromethorphan

General anesthetic

Keltner, N. L. & Folks, D. G. (1997). Psychotropic drugs (2nd ed.). St. Louis: Mosby–Year Book.

---

3. MAOIs are potentially lethal in overdose and pose a potential risk for depressed persons who may be considering suicide.

The SSRIs, first available in 1987 with the release of fluoxetine (Prozac), have replaced the cyclic drugs as the first choice in treating depression, because they are equal in efficacy and produce fewer troublesome side effects. The SSRIs and clomipramine are effective in the treatment of OCD as well.

PREFERRED DRUGS FOR CLIENTS AT HIGH RISK OF SUICIDE

Suicide is always a primary consideration when treating depressed persons. SSRIs, venlafaxine, nefazodone, trazodone, and bupropion are often a better choice for persons who are potentially suicidal or highly impulsive because they carry no risk of lethal overdose, in contrast to the cyclic compounds and the MAOIs. Evaluation of the risk for suicide must continue even after treatment with antidepressants is initiated. The client may feel more energized but may still have suicidal thoughts, increasing the likelihood of a suicide attempt. Also, because it often takes weeks before the medications have a full therapeutic effect, clients may become discouraged and tired of waiting to feel better, resulting in suicidal behavior.

DRUG ALERT

ANTIDEPRESSANTS AND SUICIDE RISK

Depressed clients who begin taking an antidepressant may have a continued or increased risk for suicide in the first few weeks of therapy. They may experience an increase in energy from the antidepressant but remain depressed. This increase in energy may make clients more likely to act on suicidal ideas and able to carry them out. Also, because antidepressants take several weeks to reach their peak effect, clients may become discouraged and act on suicidal ideas because they believe the medication is not helping them. For these reasons, it is extremely important to monitor the suicidal ideation of depressed clients until the risk has subsided.

MECHANISM OF ACTION

The precise mechanism by which antidepressants produce their therapeutic effects is not known, but much is known about their action on the CNS. The major interaction is with the monoamine neurotransmitter systems in the brain, particularly norepinephrine and serotonin. Both of these neurotransmitters are released throughout the brain and help to regulate arousal, vigilance, attention, mood, sensory processing, and appetite. Norepinephrine, serotonin, and dopamine are removed from the synapses after release by reuptake into presynaptic neurons. After reuptake, these three neurotransmitters are reloaded for subsequent release or metabolized by the enzyme MAO. The SSRIs block the reuptake of serotonin, the cyclic antidepressants and venlafaxine block the reuptake of norepinephrine primarily and serotonin to some degree, and the MAOIs interfere with enzyme metabolism. This is not the complete explanation, however: the blockade of serotonin and norepinephrine reuptake and the inhibition of MAO occur in a matter of hours, whereas antidepressants are rarely effective until 4 to 6 weeks. It is believed that the actions of these drugs are an "initiating event" and that the eventual therapeutic effectiveness results when neurons respond more slowly, making serotonin available at the synapses (Hyman, Arana, & Rosenbaum, 1995).

SIDE EFFECTS OF SSRIs

SSRIs have relatively few side effects compared with the cyclic compounds. Enhanced serotonin transmission can lead to several common side effects such as anxiety, agitation, akathisia (motor restlessness), nausea, insomnia, and sexual dysfunction, specifically diminished sexual drive or difficulty achieving an erection or orgasm. Nausea can usually be minimized by taking medications with food. Akathisia is usually treated with a beta-blocker, such as propranolol (Inderal), or a benzodiazepine. Insomnia may continue to be a problem, even if the medication is taken in the morning; a sedative-hypnotic or low-dosage trazodone may be needed.

Less common side effects include sedation (particularly with paroxetine [Paxil]), sweating, diarrhea, hand tremor, and headaches. Diarrhea and headaches can usually be managed with symptomatic treatment. Sweating and continued sedation most likely indicate the need for a change to another antidepressant.

SIDE EFFECTS OF CYCLIC ANTIDEPRESSANTS

Cyclic compounds have more side effects than do SSRIs and the newer, miscellaneous compounds. The individual medications in this category vary in terms of the intensity of side effects, but generally side effects fall into the same categories. The cyclic antidepressants block cholinergic receptors, resulting in **anticholinergic effects** such as dry mouth, constipation, urinary hesitancy or retention, dry nasal passages, and blurred near vision. More severe anticholinergic effects may occur, particularly in the elderly, such as agitation, delirium, and ileus. Other common side effects include orthostatic hypotension, sedation, weight gain, and tachycardia. Clients may develop tolerance to anticholinergic effects, but these

side effects are a common reasons that clients discontinue drug therapy. Sexual dysfunction is frequently reported by clients taking cyclic compounds, similar to problems experienced with SSRIs.

SIDE EFFECTS OF MAOIs

The most common side effects of MAOIs include daytime sedation, insomnia, weight gain, dry mouth, orthostatic hypotension, and sexual dysfunction. The sedation and insomnia are difficult to treat and may necessitate a change in medication. Of particular concern with MAOIs is the potential for a life-threatening hypertensive crisis if the client ingests food containing tyramine or takes sympathomimetic drugs. The symptoms of this crisis are severe hypertension, hyperpyrexia, tachycardia, diaphoresis, tremulousness, and cardiac arrhythmias. Drugs that may cause potentially fatal interactions with MAOIs include SSRIs, certain cyclic compounds, buspirone (BuSpar), dextromethorphan, and opiate derivatives such as meperidine. See the Drug Alert: MAOI Drug Interactions. The client must be able to follow a tyramine-free diet; Box 2-1 lists the foods to avoid.

DRUG INTERACTIONS

An uncommon but potentially serious drug interaction called serotonin or serotonergic syndrome can result from taking an MAOI and an SSRI at the same time. It can also occur if one of these drugs is taken too close to the end of therapy with the other. In other words, one drug must clear the person's system before therapy with the other is initiated. Symptoms include agitation, sweating, fever, tachycardia, hypotension, rigidity, hyperreflexia, and in extreme reactions even coma and death (Sternbach, 1991). These symptoms are similar to those seen with an SSRI overdose.

Box 2-1

➤ Foods (Containing Tyramine) to Avoid When Taking MAOIs

- No mature or aged cheeses or dishes made with cheese, such as lasagne or pizza. All cheese is considered aged except cottage cheese, cream cheese, ricotta cheese, and processed cheese slices.
- No aged meats such as pepperoni, salami, mortadella, summer sausage, beef logs, and similar products. Make sure meat and chicken are fresh and have been properly refrigerated.
- No Italian broad beans (fava) pods or banana peel. Banana pulp and all other fruits and vegetables are permitted.
- Avoid all tap beers and microbrewery beer. Drink no more than two cans or bottles of beer (including non-alcoholic beer) or 4 ounces of wine per day.
- No sauerkraut, soy sauce or soybean condiments, or marmite (concentrated yeast).

Adapted from Gardener, D. M., Shulman, K. I., Walker, S. E., & Tailor, S. A. N. (1996). The making of a user-friendly MAOI diet. Journal of Clinical Psychiatry, 57, 99–104.

SIDE EFFECTS OF OTHER ANTIDEPRESSANTS

Of the other or novel antidepressant medications, nefazodone, trazodone, and mirtazapine (Remeron) commonly cause sedation. Both nefazodone and trazodone commonly cause headaches. Nefazodone can also cause dry mouth and nausea. Bupropion and venlafaxine may cause loss of appetite, nausea, agitation, and insomnia. Venlafaxine may also cause dizziness, sweating, or sedation. Sexual dysfunction is much less common with the novel antidepressants, with one notable exception: trazodone can cause priapism (a sustained and painful erection that necessitates immediate treatment and discontinuation of the drug). Priapism may also result in impotence.

CLIENT TEACHING

SSRIs should be taken first thing in the morning, unless sedation is a problem; generally, paroxetine most often causes sedation. If a dose of an SSRI is forgotten, it can be taken up to 8 hours after the missed dose. Cyclic compounds should generally be taken at night in a single daily dose when possible to minimize side effects. If a dose of a cyclic compound is forgotten, it should be taken within 3 hours of the missed dose, or omitted for that day. Clients should exercise caution when driving or performing activities requiring sharp, alert reflexes until sedative effects can be determined.

Clients taking MAOIs need to be aware that a life-threatening hyperadrenergic crisis can occur if certain dietary restrictions are not observed. Clients should receive a written list of foods to avoid while taking MAOIs. Clients should be made aware of the risk of serious or even fatal drug interactions when taking MAOIs, and should be instructed not to take any additional medication, including over-the-counter preparations, without checking with the physician or pharmacist (Julien, 1998).

Client Teaching and Medication Management: Antidepressant Drugs summarizes client teaching points.

Mood Stabilizing Drugs

Mood stabilizing drugs are used to treat bipolar affective disorder by stabilizing the client's mood, avoiding or minimizing the highs and lows that characterize bipolar illness, and by treating acute episodes of mania. Lithium is the most established mood stabilizer; some anticonvulsant drugs, particularly carbamazepine (Tegretol) and valproic acid (Depakote, Depakene), are effective mood stabilizers. Other anticonvulsants, such as gabapentin (Neurontin) and lamotrigine (Lamictal), are being used on a trial basis for mood stabilization. Occasionally, clonazepam (Klonopin) is also used to treat acute mania. Clonazepam is included in the discussion of anti-anxiety agents.

MECHANISM OF ACTION

Although lithium has many neurobiologic effects, the mechanism of action that produces therapeutic effects in bipolar illness is poorly understood. Lithium normalizes the reuptake of certain neurotransmitters, such as serotonin, norepinephrine, acetylcholine, and

---

▶ CLIENT TEACHING AND MEDICATION MANAGEMENT: ANTIDEPRESSANT DRUGS

- Minimize nausea by taking medication with food.
- To reduce insomnia, take daily doses in the morning. If this is not effective, ask the physician if a medication for sleep is indicated. Do not use alcohol to induce sleep, because this will worsen insomnia.
- For diarrhea and headaches caused by the medication, take over-the-counter medications approved by the physician.
- Initial sedation effects generally lessen with time. If they persist, talk to the physician about modifying the dose or changing medications.
- For motor restlessness or hand tremor, ask the physician for a medication such as propranolol (Inderal) or a benzodiazepine.
- Use calorie-free beverages or sugar-free candy to relieve dry mouth. Avoid calorie-laden beverages, because they do not alleviate dry mouth and may add to weight gain.
- Try to eat a balanced diet to avoid excess weight gain. Exercise is also beneficial.
- Increase your intake of water and bulk-forming foods to prevent or relieve constipation. Stool softeners are permitted, but laxatives should be avoided.
- Do not drink alcohol while taking antidepressants.
- If problems with sexual drive or having an erection or orgasm occur, discuss them with the physician rather than altering or stopping medication. Other antidepressants may be appropriate.
- If you miss a dose of the drug, follow the directions given by your clinician.

dopamine. It also reduces the release of norepinephrine through competition with calcium. Lithium produces its effects intracellularly rather than within neuronal synapses, acting directly on G proteins and certain enzyme subsystems, such as cyclic adenosine monophosphates and phosphatidylinositol (Hyman, Arana, & Rosenbaum, 1995).

The mechanism of action for anticonvulsants is not clear as it relates to mood stabilization. Valproic acid is known to increase levels of the inhibitory neurotransmitter GABA. Both valproic acid and carbamazepine are thought to stabilize mood by inhibiting the **kindling process**. This can be described as the snowball-like effect seen when minor seizure activity seems to build up into more frequent and severe seizures. In seizure management, anticonvulsants raise the level of the threshold to prevent these minor seizures. It is suspected that this same kindling process may also occur in the development of full-blown mania, with stimulation by more frequent, minor episodes. This may explain why anticonvulsants are effective in the treatment and prevention of mania as well (Egan & Hyde, 2000).

DOSAGE

Lithium is available in tablets, capsules, liquid, and a sustained-released form, but no parenteral forms are available. The effective dosage of lithium is determined by monitoring serum lithium levels and assessing the client's clinical response to the drug. Daily dosages generally range from 900 to 3,600 mg; more importantly, the serum lithium level should be about 1.0 mEq/L. Serum lithium levels of less than 0.5 mEq/L are rarely therapeutic, and levels of more than 1.5 mEq/L are usually considered toxic. The lithium level should be monitored every 2 to 3 days while the therapeutic dosage is being determined, then weekly. When the client's condition is stable, the level may need to be checked once a month or less frequently (Hyman, Arana, & Rosenbaum, 1995; Julien, 1998).

Carbamazepine is available in liquid, tablet, and chewable tablet forms. Dosages usually range from 800 to 1,200 mg/day; the extreme dosage range is 200 to 2,000 mg/day. Valproic acid is available in liquid, tablet, and capsule forms and as sprinkles, with dosages ranging from 1,000 to 1,500 mg/day; the extreme dosage range is 750 to 3,000 mg/day. Serum drug levels, obtained 12 hours after the last dose of the medication, are monitored for therapeutic levels of both these anticonvulsants (Julien, 1998).

SIDE EFFECTS

Common side effects of lithium therapy include mild nausea or diarrhea, anorexia, fine hand tremor, polydipsia, polyuria, a metallic taste in the mouth, and fatigue or lethargy. Weight gain and acne are side effects that occur later in lithium therapy; both are distressing for clients. Taking the medication with food may help with nausea, and the use of propranolol often improves the fine tremor. Lethargy and weight gain are difficult to manage or minimize and frequently lead to noncompliance.

Toxic effects of lithium are severe diarrhea, vomiting, drowsiness, muscle weakness, and lack of coordination. Untreated, these symptoms worsen and can lead to renal failure, coma, and death. When toxic signs occur, the drug should be discontinued immediately. If lithium levels exceed 3.0 mEq/L, dialysis may be indicated.

Side effects of carbamazepine and valproic acid include drowsiness, sedation, dry mouth, and blurred vision. In addition, carbamazepine may cause rashes and orthostatic hypotension, and valproic acid may cause weight gain, alopecia, and hand tremor.

CLIENT TEACHING

For clients taking lithium and the anticonvulsants, it is important to monitor blood levels periodically. The time of the last dose must be accurate so that plasma levels can be checked 12 hours after the last dose has been taken. Taking these medications with meals will minimize nausea. Driving should not be attempted

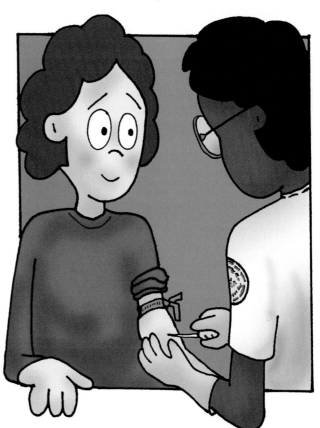

Periodic blood levels

> ## ▶ CLIENT TEACHING REGARDING MEDICATION MANAGEMENT: MOOD STABILIZING DRUGS
>
> - Have serum levels monitored periodically to ensure therapeutic levels of the medication.
> - Take the medication with food to minimize nausea.
> - For fine hand tremors, ask the physician to prescribe a beta-blocker such as propranolol (Inderal).
> - If lethargy (or tiredness, disinterest) is a problem as mood stabilizes, discuss this with the physician rather than stopping or reducing medication.
> - To help minimize weight gain, eat a balanced diet and get regular exercise. Expect some weight gain.
> - Minimize side effects of sedation or drowsiness from anticonvulsant medications by taking larger doses at bedtime and smaller doses during the day.
> - Use calorie-free beverages and sugar-free candy to relieve dry mouth. Avoid calorie-laden beverages, because they do not relieve dry mouth and stimulate more weight gain.
> - If you are taking lithium, keep water intake in a normal range and avoid heavy sweating, because this decreases serum lithium levels rapidly.

until dizziness, lethargy, fatigue, or blurred vision has subsided (Julien, 1998). Client Teaching Regarding Medication Management: Mood Stabilizing Drugs summarizes client teaching points.

Antianxiety Drugs (Anxiolytics)

Antianxiety drugs, or **anxiolytic drugs**, are used to treat anxiety and anxiety disorders, insomnia, OCD, depression, post-traumatic stress disorder, and alcohol withdrawal. Antianxiety drugs are among the most widely prescribed medications today. A wide variety of drugs from different classifications have been used in the treatment of anxiety and insomnia. Benzodiazepines have proved to be the most effective in relieving anxiety and are the drugs most frequently prescribed. Benzodiazepines may also be prescribed for their anticonvulsant and muscle relaxant effects. Buspirone is a nonbenzodiazepine that is often used for the relief of anxiety and therefore is included in this section. Other drugs that may be used to relieve anxiety such as propranolol, clonidine (Catapres), or hydroxyzine (Vistaril) are much less effective and are not included in this discussion.

DRUG ALERT

BENZODIAZEPINES

Benzodiazepines strongly enhance the effects of alcohol. Clients should not drink alcohol when taking benzodiazepines, or indeed any psychotropic drugs.

MECHANISM OF ACTION

Benzodiazepines mediate the actions of the amino acid GABA, the major inhibitory neurotransmitter in the brain. Because GABA receptor channels selectively admit the anion chloride into neurons, activation of GABA receptors hyperpolarizes neurons and thus is inhibitory. Benzodiazepines produce their effects by binding to a specific site on the GABA receptor. Buspirone is believed to exert its anxiolytic effect by acting as a partial agonist at serotonin receptors, decreasing serotonin turnover (Hyman, Arana, & Rosenbaum, 1995).

The benzodiazepines vary in terms of their half-life, the means by which they are metabolized, and their effectiveness in treating anxiety and insomnia. Table 2-6 lists dosages, half-lives, and speed of onset after a single dose. Drugs with a longer half-life require less frequent dosing and produce fewer rebound effects between doses; however, they can accumulate in the body and produce "next-day sedation" effects. Conversely, drugs with a shorter half-life do not accumulate in the body or cause next-day sedation, but they do have rebound effects and require more frequent dosing.

Temazepam (Restoril), triazolam (Halcion), and flurazepam (Dalmane) are most often prescribed for sleep rather than relief of anxiety. Diazepam (Valium), chlordiazepoxide (Librium), and clonazepam are often used to manage alcohol withdrawal, as well as being prescribed for relief of anxiety.

SIDE EFFECTS

Although not a side effect in the true sense, one of the chief problems encountered with the use of benzodiazepines is their tendency to cause physical dependence. Significant discontinuation symptoms occur when the drug is stopped that often resemble the original symptoms for which the client sought treatment. This is especially a problem for clients with long-term benzodiazepine use, such as those with panic disorder or generalized anxiety disorder. Psychological dependence on benzodiazepines is common: clients fear the return of anxiety symptoms or believe themselves incapable of handling anxiety without the drugs. This

Table 2-6

ANTIANXIETY (ANXIOLYTIC) DRUGS

Generic (Trade) Name	Daily Dosage Range	Half-Life (hours)	Speed of Onset
BENZODIAZEPINES			
Alprazolam (Xanax)	0.75–1.5	12–15	Intermediate
Chlordiazepoxide (Librium)	15–100	50–100	Intermediate
Clonazepam (Klonopin)	1.5–20	18–50	Intermediate
Chlorazepate (Tranxene)	15–60	30–200	Fast
Diazepam (Valium)	4–40	30–100	Very fast
Flurazepam (Dalmane)	15–30	47–100	Fast
Lorazepam (Ativan)	2–8	10–20	Moderately slow
Oxazepam (Serax)	30–120	3–21	Moderately slow
Temazepam (Restoril)	15–30	9.5–20	Moderately fast
Triazolam (Halcion)	0.25–0.5	2–4	Fast
NONBENZODIAZEPINES			
Buspirone (BuSpar)	15–30	3–11	Very slow

Data from Spratto, G. R. & Woods, A. L. (2000). *PDR Nurses' Drug Handbook.* Montvale, NJ: Medical Economics Company; and Julien, R. M. (1998). *A primer of drug action* (8th ed.). New York: W. H. Freeman & Co.

can lead to overuse or abuse of these drugs. Buspirone does not cause this type of physical dependence.

The side effects most commonly reported with benzodiazepines are those associated with CNS depression, such as drowsiness, sedation, poor coordination, and impairment of memory or clouded sensorium. When used for sleep, clients may complain of next-day sedation or a hangover effect. Clients often develop a tolerance to these symptoms, and they generally decrease in intensity. Common side effects from buspirone include dizziness, sedation, nausea, and headache (Hyman, Arana, & Rosenbaum, 1995).

Elderly clients may have more difficulty managing the effects of CNS depression. They may be more prone to falls from the effects on coordination and sedation. They may also have more pronounced memory deficits and may have problems with urinary incontinence, particularly at night.

CLIENT TEACHING

It is important for clients to know that antianxiety agents are aimed at relieving symptoms, such as anxiety or insomnia, but do not treat the underlying problems that cause the anxiety. Benzodiazepines strongly potentiate the effects of alcohol: one drink may have the effect of three drinks. Therefore, clients should not drink alcohol while taking benzodiazepines. Clients should be aware of decreased response time, slower reflexes, and possible sedative effects of these drugs when attempting activities such as driving or going to work.

Benzodiazepine withdrawal can be fatal: once a course of therapy has started, benzodiazepines should never be discontinued abruptly or without the supervision of the physician (Julien, 1998).

Client Teaching for Medication Management: Anxiolytics summarizes client teaching points.

Stimulants

Stimulant drugs, specifically amphetamines, were first used in the treatment of psychiatric disorders in the 1930s for their pronounced effects of CNS

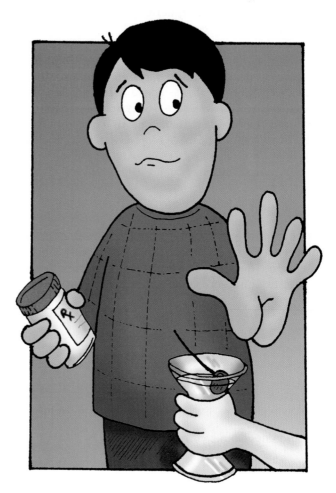

No alcohol with benzodiazepines

> ▶ CLIENT TEACHING FOR MEDICATION MANAGEMENT: ANXIOLYTICS
>
> • Take anxiolytic drugs only as prescribed. Do not increase the dosage or take extra doses even if your anxiety is increased without consulting the physician.
> • Do not stop taking benzodiazepines abruptly. Consult the physician.
> • Do not drive a car or engage in other potentially hazardous activities until reflexes and response time have returned to normal. Drowsiness and sedation usually decrease with time.
> • **Do not** drink alcoholic beverages while taking benzodiazepines, because they greatly enhance CNS depression.

stimulation. In the past, they were used to treat depression and obesity, but those uses are uncommon in current practice. Dextroamphetamine (Dexedrine) has been widely abused to produce a high or to remain awake for long periods of time. Today, the primary use of stimulants is for attention deficit/hyperactivity disorder (ADHD) in children and adolescents, residual attention deficit disorder in adults, and narcolepsy (attacks of unwanted but irresistible daytime sleepiness that disrupt the person's life).

The primary drugs used to treat ADHD are the CNS stimulants methylphenidate (Ritalin), pemoline (Cylert), and dextroamphetamine. Of these drugs, methylphenidate accounts for 90% of the medication given to children for ADHD (Julien, 1998). About 10% to 30% of persons with ADHD do not respond adequately to the stimulant medications and are considered treatment-resistant. These persons have been treated with antidepressants. Nortriptyline (Pamelor) produced the best results: about 76% of the persons studied reported a positive response. Fluoxetine and bupropion were not as effective as nortriptyline or the stimulant medications (Julien, 1998).

MECHANISM OF ACTION

Amphetamines and methylphenidate are often termed indirectly acting amines because they act by causing release of the neurotransmitters (norepinephrine, dopamine, and serotonin) from presynaptic nerve terminals, as opposed to having direct agonist effects on the postsynaptic receptors. They also block the reuptake of these neurotransmitters. Methylphenidate produces milder CNS stimulation than amphetamines; pemoline primarily affects dopamine and therefore has less effect on the sympathetic nervous system. It was originally thought that the use of methylphenidate and pemoline to treat ADHD in children produced the reverse effect of most stimulants—a calming or slowing of activity in the brain. However, this is not the case: stimulants do not have a calming effect on children who do not have ADHD.

DOSAGE

For the treatment of narcolepsy in adults, both dextroamphetamine and methylphenidate are given in divided doses totaling 20 to 200 mg/day. The higher dosages may be needed because adults with narcolepsy develop tolerance to the stimulants, requiring more medication to sustain improvement. Tolerance is not seen in persons with ADHD.

The dosages used to treat ADHD in children vary widely depending on the physician; the age, weight and behavior of the child; and the tolerance of the family for the child's behavior. Table 2-7 lists the usual dosage ranges for these stimulants. Arrangements must be made for the school nurse or another authorized adult to administer the stimulants to the child at school.

Table 2-7

STIMULANT DRUGS

Generic (Trade) Name	Dosage
Methylphenidate (Ritalin)	Adults: 20–200 mg/day, orally, in divided doses Children: 10–60 mg/day, orally, in 2–4 divided doses
Dextroamphetamine (Dexedrine)	Adults: 20–200 mg/day, orally, in divided doses Children: 5–40 mg/day, orally, in 2 or 3 divided doses
Pemoline (Cylert)	Children: 37.5–112.5 mg/day, orally, given once a day in the morning

Data from Spratto, G. R. & Woods, A. L. (2000). *PDR Nurses' Drug Handbook*. Montvale, NJ: Medical Economics Company; and Julien, R. M. (1998). *A primer of drug action* (8th ed.). New York: W. H. Freeman & Co.

SIDE EFFECTS

The most common side effects of stimulants are anorexia, weight loss, nausea, and irritability. Caffeine, sugar, and chocolate should be avoided because they may worsen these symptoms. Less common side effects include dizziness, dry mouth, blurred vision, and palpitations. The most common long-term problem with stimulants is the growth and weight suppression that occurs in some children. This can usually be prevented by taking "drug holidays" on weekends, holidays, or during summer vacation, which helps to restore normal eating and growth patterns.

CLIENT TEACHING

The potential for abuse exists with stimulants, but this is seldom a problem in children. Taking doses of stimulants after meals may minimize anorexia and nausea. Caffeine-free beverages are suggested; chocolate and excessive sugar should be avoided. Most important is to keep the medication out of the child's reach, because as little as a 10-day supply can be fatal. Client and Family Teaching for Medication Management: Stimulants summarizes teaching points for clients and families.

Disulfiram (Antabuse)

Disulfiram is a sensitizing agent that causes an adverse reaction when mixed with alcohol in the body. This agent's only use is as a deterrent to drinking alcohol in persons receiving treatment for alcoholism. It is useful for persons who are motivated to abstain from drinking and who are not impulsive. Five to ten minutes after someone who is taking disulfiram ingests alcohol, symptoms begin to appear: facial and body flushing from vasodilation, a throbbing headache, sweating, dry mouth, nausea, vomiting, dizziness, and weakness. In severe cases, there may be chest pain, dyspnea, severe hypotension, confusion, and even death. Symptoms progress rapidly and last from 30 minutes to 2 hours. Because disulfiram is metabolized by the liver, it is most effective in persons whose liver enzyme levels are within or close to normal range.

Disulfiram inhibits the enzyme aldehyde dehydrogenase, which is involved in the metabolism of ethanol. Acetaldehyde levels are then increased from 5 to 10 times higher than normal, resulting in the disulfiram–alcohol reaction. This reaction is potentiated by decreased levels of epinephrine and norepinephrine in the sympathetic nervous system caused by inhibition of dopamine beta-hydroxylase (Hyman, Arana, & Rosenbaum, 1995).

Education is extremely important for the client taking disulfiram. Many common products, such as shaving cream, aftershave lotion, cologne, and deodorant, and over-the-counter medications such as cough preparations contain alcohol; when used by the client taking disulfiram, these products can produce the same reaction as drinking alcohol. The client must read product labels carefully and select items that are alcohol-free.

Other side effects reported by persons taking disulfiram include fatigue, drowsiness, halitosis, tremor, or impotence. It can also interfere with the metabolism of other drugs the client is taking, such as phenytoin (Dilantin), isoniazid (INH), warfarin (Coumadin), barbiturates, and long-acting benzodiazepines such as diazepam and chlordiazepoxide.

CULTURAL CONSIDERATIONS

Studies have shown that persons of different ethnic backgrounds respond differently to certain drugs used to treat mental disorders. The nurse should be familiar with these cultural differences.

Studies have shown that African Americans respond more rapidly to antipsychotic medications and

---

▶ CLIENT AND FAMILY TEACHING FOR MEDICATION MANAGEMENT: STIMULANTS

- Never leave the supply of medication in a place the child can reach to avoid overdose or taking additional medication.
- Take the medication at meal time to minimize nausea and anorexia.
- Monitor the child's weight and height because growth suppression can be a long-term consequence of stimulant therapy. Not giving the drug on weekends or during the summer can help resume normal growth patterns.
- Try a dosage schedule that provides a dose of medication before beginning routine tasks of concentration such as nightly homework.
- Avoid beverages containing caffeine. Limit intake of chocolate, sugar, or any other substance that increases the child's activity level.
- Alleviate dry mouth with calorie-free beverages or sugar-free candy.
- Consult often with the school nurse or other person responsible for giving medications at school. Medications should be given in a manner that is not intrusive, nor should it draw undue attention to the child.

tricyclic antidepressants than Caucasians do. Also, African Americans have a greater risk of developing side effects from both these classes of drugs than do Caucasians (Lawson, 1996; Sramek & Pi, 1996). Asians metabolize antipsychotics and tricyclic antidepressants more slowly than do Caucasians and therefore require lower dosages to achieve the same effects (Ruiz et al., 1996). Hispanics also require lower dosages of antidepressants than do Caucasians to achieve the desired results (Kudzma, 1999).

Asians respond therapeutically to lower dosages of lithium than do Caucasians (Sramek & Pi, 1996). African Americans have higher blood levels of lithium than Caucasians when given the same dosage, and they also experience more side effects (Sramek & Pi, 1996). This suggests that African Americans require lower dosages of lithium than do Caucasians to produce desired effects (Lawson, 1996). See the section on cultural considerations in each disorder chapter for specific cultural differences associated with various drugs.

SELF-AWARENESS ISSUES

Nurses must examine their own beliefs and feelings about mental disorders as "illnesses" and the role of drugs in treating mental disorders. Some nurses may be skeptical about some mental disorders and may believe that clients could gain control of their lives if they would just put forth enough effort. Nurses who work with clients with mental disorders come to understand that many disorders are similar to chronic physical illnesses such as asthma or diabetes, which require lifelong medication to maintain health. Without proper medication management, clients with certain mental disorders, such as schizophrenia or bipolar affective disorder, cannot survive and cope with the world around them. The nurse must explain to the client and family that this is an illness that requires continuous medication management and follow-up, just like a chronic physical illness.

It is also important for the nurse to know about current biologic theories and treatments. Many clients and their families will have questions about reports in the news about research or discoveries. The nurse can help them distinguish between what is factual and what is experimental. Also, it is important to keep discoveries and theories in perspective.

Clients and families need more than factual information to deal with mental illness and its effect on their lives. Many clients do not understand the nature of their illness and ask, "Why is this happening to me?" They need simple but thorough explanations about the nature of the illness and how they can manage it. The nurse must learn to give out enough information about the illness while providing the care and support needed by all those confronted with mental illness.

Helpful Hints for the Nurse Working With Clients With Mental Illness

- Chronic mental illness has periods of remission and exacerbation, just like chronic physical illness. A recurrence of symptoms is not the client's fault, nor is it a failure of treatment or nursing care.

INTERNET RESOURCES

Resource	Internet Address
▶ Questions about FDA-approved drugs	http://www.DRUGINFO@CDER>FDA>GOV
▶ American Physiological Society	gopher://gopher.uth.tmc.edu:3300/1
▶ Clinical Pharmacology Online	http://www.cponline.gsm.com/
▶ Clinical trial finder	listserv@garcia.com
▶ Internet FDA	http://fda.gov/fdahomepage.html
▶ Research project relating to DNA & genetics and mental disorders	www.nhgri.gov

- Research regarding the neurobiologic causes of mental disorders is still in its infancy. Do not dismiss new ideas just because they may not yet help in the treatment of these illnesses.
- Often when clients stop taking medication or take medication improperly, it is not because they intend to; rather, it is the result of faulty thinking and reasoning, which is part of the illness.

Critical Thinking

Questions

1. It is possible to identify a gene associated with increased risk for the late onset of Alzheimer's disease. Should this test be available to anyone who requests it? Why or why not? What dilemmas might arise from having such knowledge?
2. What are the implications for nursing if it becomes possible to predict certain illnesses, such as schizophrenia, through the identification of genes responsible for or linked to the disease? Should this have an impact on whether people who carry such genes should have children? Who should make that decision, given the fact that many people with chronic mental illness depend on government programs for financial support?
3. Drug companies research and develop new drugs. Much more money and effort is expended to produce new drugs for common disorders rather than drugs needed to treat rare disorders such as Tourette syndrome (often called "orphan drugs"). What are the ethical and financial dilemmas associated with research designed to produce new drugs?

➤ KEY POINTS

- Neurobiologic research is constantly expanding our knowledge in the field of psychiatry and is significantly affecting clinical practice.
- The cerebrum is the center for coordination and integration of all information needed to interpret and respond to the environment.
- The cerebellum is the center for coordination of movements and postural adjustments.
- The brain stem contains centers that control cardiovascular and respiratory functions, sleep, consciousness, and impulses.
- The limbic system regulates body temperature, appetite, sensations, memory, and emotional arousal.
- Neurotransmitters are the chemical substances manufactured in the neuron that aid in the transmission of information from the brain throughout the body. Several important neurotransmitters, including dopamine, norepinephrine, serotonin, histamine, acetylcholine, GABA, and glutamate, have been found to play a role in mental disorders and are targets of pharmacologic treatment.
- Researchers continue to examine the role of genetics, heredity, and viruses in the development of mental illness.
- Pharmacologic treatment is based on the ability of medications to eliminate or minimize identified target symptoms.
- The following factors must be considered in the selection of medications to treat mental disorders: the efficacy, potency, and half-life of the drug; the age and race of the client; other medications being taken; and the side effects of the drugs.
- Antipsychotic drugs are the primary treatment for psychotic disorders such as schizophrenia, but they produce a host of side effects that may also require pharmacologic intervention. Neurologic side effects, which can be treated with anticholinergic medications, are called extrapyramidal symptoms and include acute dystonia, akathisia, and pseudoparkinsonism. Some of the more serious neurologic side effects include tardive dyskinesia (permanent involuntary movements) and neuroleptic malignant syndrome, which can be fatal.
- Because of the serious side effects of antipsychotic medications, clients must be well educated regarding their medications, medication compliance, and side effects. The regimen must be closely supervised by health care professionals.
- Antidepressant medications include cyclic compounds, SSRIs, MAOIs, and a group of newer drugs.
- Clients receiving MAOIs must be carefully instructed to avoid foods containing tyramine, because the combination produces a hypertensive crisis that can become life-threatening.
- The risk of suicide may increase as clients begin taking antidepressants. The medication may increase the client's energy while suicidal thoughts are still present, allowing the client to carry out a suicide plan.

- Lithium and selected anticonvulsants are used to stabilize mood, particularly in bipolar affective disorder.
- Serum lithium levels must be monitored regularly to ensure the level is in the therapeutic range and to avoid lithium toxicity. Symptoms of toxicity include severe diarrhea and vomiting, drowsiness, muscle weakness, and loss of coordination. Untreated, lithium toxicity leads to coma and death.
- Benzodiazepines are used to treat a wide variety of problems related to anxiety and insomnia. Alcohol should be avoided because it increases the effects of the benzodiazepines.
- The primary use of stimulants such as methylphenidate (Ritalin) is the treatment of children with attention deficit/hyperactivity disorder. Methylphenidate has been proven to be successful in allowing these children to slow down their activity and focus on the tasks at hand and their school work. Its exact mechanism of action is unknown.

REFERENCES

Egan, M. F., & Hyde, T. M. (2000). Schizophrenia: Neurobiology. In B. J. Sadock & V. A. Sadock (Eds.). *Comprehensive textbook of psychiatry, Vol. 1* (7th ed., pp. 1129–1147). Philadelphia: Lippincott Williams & Wilkins.

Hyman, S. E., Arana, G. W., & Rosenbaum, J. F. (1995). *Handbook of psychiatric drug therapy* (3rd ed.). Boston: Little, Brown & Co.

Julien, R. M. (1998). *A primer of drug action: A concise, nontechnical guide to the actions, uses and side effects of psychoactive drugs* (8th ed.). New York: W. H. Freeman & Co.

Karson, C. N., & Renshaw, P. F. (2000). Principles of neuroimaging: Resonance techniques. In B. J. Sadock & V. A. Sadock (Eds.). *Comprehensive textbook of psychiatry, Vol. 1* (7th ed., pp. 162–172). Philadelphia: Lippincott Williams & Wilkins.

Keltner, N. L. & Folks, D. G. (1997). *Psychotropic drugs* (2nd ed). St. Louis: Mosby—Year Book.

Kudzma, E. C. (1999). Culturally competent drug administration. *American Journal of Nursing, 99*(8), 46–52.

Lawson, W. B. (1996). The art and science of psychopharmacology of African Americans. *Mt. Sinai Journal of Medicine, 63*(5–6), 301–305.

Lewis, D. A. (2000). Functional neuroanatomy. In B. J. Sadock & V. A. Sadock (Eds.). *Comprehensive textbook of psychiatry, Vol. 1* (7th ed., pp. 3–31). Philadelphia: Lippincott Williams & Wilkins.

Malison, R. T., & Innis, R. B. (2000). Principles of neuroimaging: Radiotracer techniques. In B. J. Sadock & V. A. Sadock (Eds.). *Comprehensive textbook of psychiatry, Vol. 1* (7th ed., pp. 154–162). Philadelphia: Lippincott Williams & Wilkins.

Ruiz, S., Chu, P., Sramek, J. J., Rotavu, E., & Herrera, J. (1996). Neuroleptic dosing in Asian and Hispanic outpatients with schizophrenia. *Mt. Sinai Journal of Medicine, 63*(5-6), 306–309.

Selemon, L. D. & Goldman-Rakic, P. S. (1995). Prefrontal cortex. *American Journal of Psychiatry, 152*(1), 5.

Shank, R. P., Smith-Swintosky, V. L., & Twyman, R. E. (2000). Amino acid neurotransmitters. In B. J. Sadock & V. A. Sadock (Eds.). *Comprehensive textbook of psychiatry, Vol. 1* (7th ed., pp. 50–59). Philadelphia: Lippincott Williams & Wilkins.

Spratto, G. R. & Woods, A. L. (2000). *PDR: Nurses' Drug Handbook.* Montvale, NJ: Medical Economics Company.

Sramek, J. J., & Pi, E. H. (1996). Ethnicity and antidepressant response. *Mt. Sinai Journal of Medicine, 63*(5-6), 320–325.

Sternbach, H. (1991). The serotonin syndrome. *American Journal of Psychiatry, 148*(6), 705–712.

Tecott, L. H. (2000). Monoamine transmitters. In B. J. Sadock & V. A. Sadock (Eds.). *Comprehensive textbook of psychiatry, Vol. 1* (7th ed., pp. 41–50). Philadelphia: Lippincott Williams & Wilkins.

Washington, H. (1999). Infection connection. *Psychology Today, 4*, 43–44, 74–76.

ADDITIONAL READINGS

Bailey, K. P. (1998). *Psychotropic drug facts.* Philadelphia: Lippincott Williams & Wilkins.

Gardener, D. M., Shulman, K. I., Walker, S. E., & Tailor, S. A. N. (1996). The making of a user-friendly MAOI diet. *Journal of Clinical Psychiatry, 57*, 99–104.

Hsin-Tung, E., & Simpson, G. M. (2000). Medication-induced movement disorders. In B. J. Sadock & V. A. Sadock (Eds.). *Comprehensive textbook of psychiatry, Vol. 2* (7th ed., pp. 2265–2271). Philadelphia: Lippincott Williams & Wilkins.

Mathews, C. A., & Friemer, N. B. (2000). Genetic linkage analysis of the psychiatric disorders. In B. J. Sadock & V. A. Sadock (Eds.). *Comprehensive textbook of psychiatry, Vol. 1* (7th ed., pp. 184–198). Philadelphia: Lippincott Williams & Wilkins.

Snell, R. S. (1997). *Clinical neuroanatomy for medical students* (2nd ed.) Philadelphia: Lippincott-Raven.

Chapter Review

> ## ➤ MULTIPLE-CHOICE QUESTIONS

Select the best answer for each of the following questions.

1. The nurse is teaching a client taking an MAOI antidepressant about foods with tyramine that should be avoided. Which of the following statements would indicate that further teaching is needed?

   A. "I'm so glad I can have pizza as long as I don't order pepperoni."

   B. "I will be able to eat cottage cheese without worrying."

   C. "I will have to avoid drinking nonalcoholic beer."

   D. "I can eat green beans on this diet."

2. A client who has been depressed and suicidal started taking a tricyclic antidepressant 2 weeks ago and is now ready to leave the hospital to go home. Which of the following is a concern for the nurse as discharge plans are finalized?

   A. The client may need a prescription for diphenhydramine (Benadryl) to use for side effects.

   B. The nurse will evaluate the risk for suicide by overdose of the tricyclic antidepressant.

   C. The nurse will need to include teaching regarding the signs of neuroleptic malignant syndrome.

   D. The client will need regular lab work to monitor therapeutic drug levels.

3. The signs of lithium toxicity include which of the following?

   A. Sedation, fever, restlessness

   B. Psychomotor agitation, insomnia, increased thirst

   C. Elevated white blood cell count, sweating, confusion

   D. Severe vomiting, diarrhea, weakness

4. Which of the following is a concern for children taking stimulants for ADHD for several years?

   A. Dependence on the drug

   B. Insomnia

   C. Growth suppression

   D. Weight gain

5. The nurse is caring for a client with schizophrenia who is taking haloperidol (Haldol). The client complains of restlessness, cannot sit still, and has muscle stiffness. Of the following p.r.n. medications, which would the nurse administer?

   A. Haloperidol (Haldol) 5 mg p.o.

   B. Benztropine (Cogentin) 2 mg p.o.

   C. Propranolol (Inderal) 20 mg p.o.

   D. Trazodone 50 mg p.o.

> ## ➤ TRUE-FALSE QUESTIONS

Identify each of the following statements as T (true) or F (false). Correct any false statements.

_____ 1. The half-life of a drug refers to the amount of time it takes for the drug to become effective.

_____

_____ 2. The efficacy of a drug refers to the maximal therapeutic effect that can be achieved.

_____

_____ 3. High-potency drugs must be given in higher dosages to be effective.

_____

_____ 4. Antipsychotic drugs work by blocking the neurotransmitter dopamine.

_____

_____ 5. Excessive serotonin is responsible for the extrapyramidal side effects of anti-psychotic drugs.

_____ 6. Clients taking paroxetine (Paxil) may experience nausea or insomnia.

_____ 7. Clients taking citalopram (Celexa) should not receive a general anesthetic for surgery.

_____ 8. Tyramine in food interacts with MAOI antidepressants and produces a hypertensive crisis.

➤ FILL-IN-THE-BLANK QUESTIONS

Identify the drug classification for each of the following medications.

_____ 1. Clozapine (Clozaril)

_____ 2. Fluoxetine (Prozac)

_____ 3. Amitriptyline (Elavil)

_____ 4. Benztropine (Cogentin)

_____ 5. Methylphenidate (Ritalin)

_____ 6. Carbamazepine (Tegretol)

_____ 7. Clonazepam (Klonopin)

_____ 8. Quetiapine (Seroquel)

➤ SHORT-ANSWER QUESTIONS

1. Explain the rationale for tapering psychotropic medication doses before the drug is discontinued.

2. Describe the teaching needed for a client who is scheduled for positron emission tomography (PET).

3. Explain the kindling process as it relates to the manic episodes of bipolar affective disorder.

3

Psychosocial Theories and Therapy

Learning Objectives

After reading this chapter, the student should be able to:

1. Explain the basic beliefs and approaches of the following psychosocial theories: psychoanalytic, developmental, interpersonal, behavioral, and existential.

2. Describe the following psychosocial treatment modalities: individual psychotherapy, group psychotherapy, family therapy, behavior modification, systematic desensitization, token economy, self-help groups, support groups, education groups, cognitive therapy, milieu therapy, and psychiatric rehabilitation.

3. Identify the psychosocial theory on which each treatment strategy is based.

4. Identify how several of the theoretical perspectives have influenced current nursing practice.

Key Terms

behavior modification	parataxic mode
behaviorism	participant observer
client-centered therapy	positive reinforcement
closed group	prototaxic mode
countertransference	psychiatric rehabilitation
cognitive therapy	psychoanalysis
dream analysis	psychosocial interventions
education group	psychotherapy
ego	psychotherapy group
ego defense mechanisms	self-actualization
existentialism	self-help group
family therapy	subconscious
free association	superego
group therapy	support group
hierarchy of needs	syntaxic mode
humanism	systematic desensitization
id	therapeutic community or
individual psychotherapy	milieu
milieu therapy	therapeutic nurse–client
negative reinforcement	relationship
open group	transference
operant conditioning	

PSYCHOSOCIAL THEORIES

There are many theories that attempt to explain human behavior, health, and mental illness. Each suggests how normal development occurs based on the theorist's beliefs, assumptions, and view of the world. These theories suggest strategies that the clinician can use to work with clients. Many of the theories discussed in this chapter were not based on empirical or research evidence; rather, they evolved from individual experiences and might more appropriately be called conceptual models or frameworks.

Mental health treatment today has an eclectic approach, or one that incorporates concepts and strategies from a variety of sources. This chapter includes an overview of major psychosocial theories, highlights the ideas and concepts in current practice, and explains the various psychosocial treatment modalities. The psychosocial theories have produced many models that are used in individual therapy, groups, and treatment settings. The medical model of treatment is based on the neurobiologic theories discussed in Chapter 2.

Psychoanalytic Theorists

SIGMUND FREUD: THE FATHER OF PSYCHOANALYSIS

Psychoanalytic theory was developed by Sigmund Freud (1856–1939; Fig. 3-1) in the late 19th and early 20th centuries in Vienna, where Freud spent most of his life. Many other noted psychoanalysts and theorists have made contributions to this body of knowledge, but Freud is its undisputed founder. Many clinicians and theorists did not agree with much of Freud's psychoanalytic theory and later developed their own theories and styles of treatment.

Freud developed his initial ideas and explanations of human behavior from his experiences with a few clients, all women who displayed behaviors such as disturbances of sight and speech, inability to eat, and paralysis of limbs. These symptoms had no physiologic basis or cause and therefore were considered to be the "hysterical" or neurotic behavior of women. After many years of working with these women, Freud concluded that many of these problems resulted from childhood trauma, or failure to complete tasks of psychosexual development. Unmet needs and sexual feelings, as well as traumatic events, were repressed (driven from conscious awareness). Hysterical or neurotic behaviors resulted from these unresolved conflicts. These early experiences with female clients formed the basis for Freud's theories, beliefs, and psychoanalytic method of treatment.

Psychoanalytic theory supports the notion that all human behavior is caused and can be explained

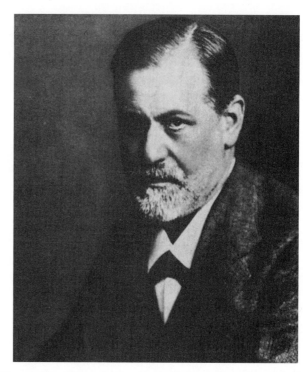

Figure 3-1. Sigmund Freud: the father of psychoanalysis.

(deterministic theory). Freud believed that much of human behavior is motivated by repressed sexual impulses and desires.

Personality Components: Id, Ego, and Superego. Freud conceptualized personality structure as having three components: id, ego, and superego. The **id** is the part of one's nature that reflects basic or innate desires, such as pleasure-seeking behavior, aggression, and sexual impulses. The id seeks instant gratification, causes impulsive, unthinking behavior, and has no regard for rules or social convention. The **superego** is the part of one's nature that reflects moral and ethical concepts, values, and parental and social expectations; therefore, it is in direct opposition to the id. The third component, the **ego**, is the balancing or mediating force between the id and the superego. The ego is thought to represent mature and adaptive behavior, which allows people to function successfully in the world. Anxiety was believed to result from the ego's attempts to balance the impulsive instincts of the id with the stringent rules of the superego. The cartoon demonstrates the relation between these personality structures.

Behavior Motivated by Subconscious Thoughts and Feelings. The human personality was believed to function at three levels of awareness: conscious, preconscious, and unconscious (Gabbard, 2000). Con-

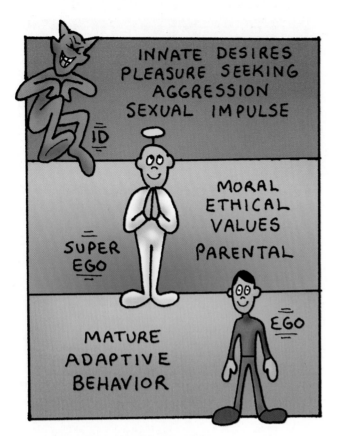

Freud's components of personality

scious refers to the perceptions, thoughts, and emotions that exist in the person's awareness, such as being aware of happy feelings or thinking about a loved one. Preconscious thoughts and emotions are not currently in the person's awareness, but they can be recalled with some effort—for example, an adult remembering what he or she did, thought, or felt as a child. The unconscious is the realm of thoughts and feelings that motivate a person, even though he or she is totally unaware of them. This would include most defense mechanisms and some instinctual drives or motivation. According to Freud's theories, the memory of traumatic events that are too painful for the person to remember are repressed into the unconscious.

Freud believed that much of what we do and say is motivated by our **subconscious** (below conscious level), thoughts or feelings that are in the preconscious or unconscious level of awareness. A "Freudian slip" is a term we commonly use to describe slips of the tongue—for example, saying, "You look portly today" to an overweight friend instead of, "You look pretty today." Freud believed these "slips" were not accidents or coincidence, but rather were indications of subconscious feelings or thoughts that accidentally emerged in casual day-to-day conversation.

Freud's Dream Analysis. Freud believed that a person's dreams reflected more of the subconscious and had significant meaning (Gabbard, 2000). **Dream analysis**, a primary method used in psychoanalysis, involved discussing a client's dreams to discover their true meaning and significance. Freud believed that dreams were significant because they revealed his or her subconscious thoughts and feelings, although sometimes the meaning was hidden or symbolic. For example, a client might report having recurrent, frightening dreams about snakes chasing her. Freud's interpretation might be that the woman feared intimacy with men; the snake would be viewed as a phallic symbol, representing the penis.

Another method used to gain access to subconscious thoughts and feelings is **free association**, in which the therapist tries to uncover the client's true thoughts and feelings by saying a word and asking the client to respond quickly with the first thing that comes to mind. Freud believed that such quick responses would be more likely to uncover subconscious or repressed thoughts or feelings.

Ego Defense Mechanisms. Freud believed the self or ego used **ego defense mechanisms**, methods of attempting to protect the self and cope with basic drives or emotionally painful thoughts, feelings, or events. Defense mechanisms are explained in Table 3-1. For example, a person who has been diagnosed with cancer and told he has 6 months to live but refuses to talk about his illness is using the defense mechanism of denial, or refusal to accept the reality of the situation. If a person dying of cancer exhibits continuously cheerful behavior, he could be using the defense mechanism of reaction formation to protect his emotions. Most of the defense mechanisms operate at the unconscious level of awareness, so people are not aware of what they are doing and often must be helped to see the reality.

Five Stages of Psychosexual Development. Freud's theory of childhood development was based on the belief that sexual energy, termed libido, was the driving force of human behavior. Children were thought to progress through five stages of psychosexual development: oral (birth to 18 months), anal (18 to 36 months), phallic/oedipal (3 to 5 years), latency (5 to 11 or 13 years), and genital (11 to 13 years). Table 3-2 describes these stages and the accompanying developmental tasks. Psychopathology results when a person has difficulty making the transition from one stage to the next, or when a person remains stalled at a particular stage or regresses to an earlier stage. Freud's open discussion of sexual impulses, particularly in children, was considered shocking at the time (Gabbard, 2000).

Transference and Countertransference. Freud developed the concept of transference and counter-

Table 3-1

EGO DEFENSE MECHANISMS

Compensation	Overachievement in one area to offset real or perceived deficiencies in another area.
	• Napoleon complex: diminutive man becoming emperor • Nurse with low self-esteem works double shifts so her supervisor will like her.
Conversion	Expression of an emotional conflict through the development of a physical symptom, usually sensorimotor in nature.
	• A teenager forbidden to see X-rated movies is tempted to do so by friends and develops blindness, and the teenager is unconcerned about the loss of sight.
Denial	Failure to acknowledge an unbearable condition; failure to admit the reality of a situation, or how one enables the problem to continue.
	• Diabetic eating chocolate candy • Spending money freely when broke • Waiting 3 days to seek help for severe abdominal pain
Displacement	Ventilation of intense feelings toward persons less threatening than the one who aroused those feelings.
	• A person who is mad at the boss yells at his or her spouse. • A child who is harassed by a bully at school mistreats a younger sibling.
Dissociation	Dealing with emotional conflict by a temporary alteration in consciousness or identity
	• Amnesia that prevents recall of yesterday's auto accident • An adult remembers nothing of childhood sexual abuse.
Fixation	Immobilization of a portion of the personality resulting from unsuccessful completion of tasks in a developmental stage.
	• Never learning to delay gratification • Lack of a clear sense of identity as an adult
Identification	Modeling actions and opinions of influential others, while searching for identity, or aspiring to reach a personal, social, or occupational goal
	• Nursing student becoming a critical care nurse since this is the specialty of an instructor she admires
Introjection	Accepting another person's attitudes, beliefs, and values as one's own
	• A person who dislikes guns becomes an avid hunter, just like a best friend
Projection	Unconscious blaming of unacceptable inclinations or thoughts on an external object
	• Man who has thought about same-gender sexual relationship, but never had one, beats a man who is gay • A person with many prejudices loudly identifies others as bigots
Rationalization	Excusing own behavior to avoid guilt, responsibility, conflict, anxiety, or loss of self-respect
	• Student blames failure on teacher being mean • Man says he beats his wife because she doesn't listen to him
Reaction Formation	Acting the opposite of what one thinks or feels
	• Woman who never wanted to have children becomes a super-mom • Person who despises the boss tells everyone what a great boss she is
Regression	Moving back to a previous developmental stage in order to feel safe or have needs met
	• Five-year-old asks for a bottle when new baby brother is being fed • Man pouts like a four-year-old if he is not the center of his girlfriend's attention
Repression	Excluding emotionally painful or anxiety-provoking thoughts and feelings from conscious awareness
	• Woman has no memory of the mugging she suffered yesterday • Woman has no memory before age 7 when she was removed from abusive parents
Resistance	Overt or covert antagonism toward remembering or processing anxiety-producing information
	• Nurse is too busy with tasks to spend time talking to a dying patient • Person attends court-ordered treatment for alcoholism, but refuses to participate
Sublimation	Substituting a socially acceptable activity for an impulse that is unacceptable
	• Person who has quit smoking sucks on hard candy when the urge to smoke arises • Person goes for a 15-minute walk when tempted to eat junk food
Substitution	Replacing the desired gratification with one that is more readily available
	• Woman who would like to have her own children opens a day care center

(continued)

Table 3-1

(Continued)

Suppression	Conscious exclusion of unacceptable thoughts and feelings from conscious awareness.
	• A student decides not to think about a parent's illness in order to study for a test.
	• A woman tells a friend she cannot think about her son's death right now.
Undoing	Exhibiting acceptable behavior to make up for or negate unacceptable behavior.
	• A person who cheats on a spouse brings the spouse a bouquet of roses.
	• A man who is ruthless in business donates large amounts of money to charity.

transference. **Transference** occurs when the client displaces onto the therapist attitudes and feelings that the client originally experienced in other relationships (Gabbard, 2000). Transference patterns occur automatically and unconsciously in the therapeutic relationship. For example, an adolescent female client working with a nurse who is about the same age as her parents might react to the nurse like she reacts to her parents. She might experience intense feelings of rebellion or make sarcastic remarks; these reactions are actually based on her experiences with her parents, not the nurse.

Countertransference occurs when the therapist displaces onto the client attitudes or feelings from his or her past. For example, a female nurse who has teenage children and who is experiencing extreme frustration with an adolescent client may respond by adopting a parental or chastising tone. The nurse is countertransfering her own attitudes and feelings toward her children onto the client. Nurses can deal with countertransference by examining their own feelings and responses, using self-awareness, and talking with colleagues.

CURRENT PSYCHOANALYTIC PRACTICE

Psychoanalysis focuses on discovering the causes of the client's unconscious and repressed thoughts, feelings, and conflicts believed to cause anxiety, and helping the client to gain insight into and to resolve these conflicts and anxieties. The analytic therapist uses the techniques of free association, dream analysis, and interpretation of behavior.

Psychoanalysis is still practiced today, but on a very limited basis. Analysis is lengthy, with weekly or more frequent sessions for several years. Psychoanalytic therapy is costly and is not covered by conventional health insurance programs; thus, it has become known as "therapy for the wealthy."

Table 3-2

FREUD'S DEVELOPMENTAL STAGES

Phase	Age	Focus
Oral	Birth to 18 months	Major site of tension and gratification is the mouth, lips, and tongue; includes biting and sucking activities.
		Id present at birth.
		Ego develops gradually from rudimentary structure present at birth.
Anal	18–36 months	Anus and surrounding area are major source of interest.
		Acquisition of voluntary sphincter control (toilet training)
Phallic/oedipal	3–5 years	Genital focus of interest, stimulation, and excitement
		Penis is organ of interest for both sexes.
		Masturbation is common.
		Penis envy (wish to possess penis) seen in girls; oedipal complex (wish to marry opposite-sex parent and be rid of same-sex parent) seen in boys and girls
Latency	5–11 or 13 years	Resolution of oedipal complex
		Sexual drive channeled into socially appropriate activities, such as school work and sports
		Formation of the superego
Genital	11–13 years	Final stage of psychosexual development
		Begins with puberty and the biologic capacity for orgasm; involves the capacity for true intimacy

Adapted from Gabbard, G. O. (2000). Theories of personality and psychopathology: Psychoanalysis.
In B. J. Sadock & V. A. Sadock (Eds.). *Comprehensive textbook of psychiatry*, Vol. 2 (7th ed., pp. 563–607).
Philadelphia, Lippincott Williams & Wilkins.

ERIK ERIKSON AND PSYCHOSOCIAL STAGES OF DEVELOPMENT

Erik Erikson (1902–1994) was a German-born psychoanalyst who extended Freud's work on personality development across the life span while focusing on social development as well as psychological development in the life stages. In 1950, Erikson published *Childhood and Society*, in which he described eight psychosocial stages of development. In each, the person must complete a life task that is essential to his or her well-being and mental health. These tasks allow the person to achieve life's virtues: hope, purpose, fidelity, love, caring, and wisdom. The stages, life tasks, and virtues are described in Table 3-3.

Erikson's eight psychosocial stages of development are still widely used in a variety of disciplines. In Erikson's view, psychosocial growth occurs in sequential phases, each stage dependent on completion of the previous stage and life task. For example, in the infant stage (birth to 18 months), trust versus mistrust, the baby must learn to develop basic trust (the positive outcome), such as trust that he or she will be fed and taken care of. The formation of trust is essential: mistrust, the negative outcome of this stage, will impair the person's development throughout his or her life.

Interpersonal Theorists

HARRY STACK SULLIVAN: INTERPERSONAL RELATIONSHIPS AND MILIEU THERAPY

Harry Stack Sullivan (1892–1949; Fig. 3-2) was an American psychiatrist who extended the theory of personality development to include the significance of interpersonal relationships. Sullivan believed that

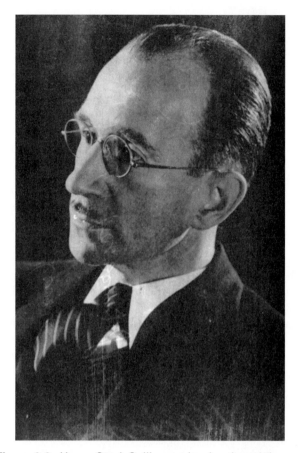

Figure 3-2. Henry Stack Sullivan, who developed the theory of the "therapeutic community or milieu," which regarded the interaction among patients as beneficial and emphasized the role of patient-to-patient interaction in treatment.

one's personality involved more than individual characteristics, particularly how one interacted with others. He thought that inadequate or unsatisfying relationships produced anxiety, which he saw as the

---

Table 3-3

ERIKSON'S STAGES OF PSYCHOSOCIAL DEVELOPMENT

Stage	Virtue	Task
Trust vs. mistrust (infant)	Hope	Viewing the world as safe and reliable, relationships as nurturing, stable, and dependable
Autonomy vs. shame and doubt (toddler)	Will	Achieving a sense of control and free will
Initiative vs. guilt (preschool)	Purpose	Beginning development of a conscience, learning to manage conflict and anxiety
Industry vs. inferiority (school age)	Competence	Emerging confidence in own abilities, taking pleasure in accomplishments
Identity vs. role confusion (adolescence)	Fidelity	Formulating a sense of self and belonging
Intimacy vs. isolation (young adult)	Love	Forming adult, loving relationships and meaningful attachments to others
Generativity vs. stagnation (middle adult)	Care	Being creative and productive, establishing the next generation
Ego integrity vs. despair (maturity)	Wisdom	Accepting responsibility for one's self and life

basis for all emotional problems (Sullivan, 1953). The importance and significance of interpersonal relationships in one's life was probably Sullivan's greatest contribution to the field of mental health.

Five Life Stages. Sullivan established five life stages of development (infancy, childhood, juvenile, preadolescence, and adolescence), each focusing on various interpersonal relationships (Table 3-4). Sullivan also described three developmental cognitive modes of experience and believed that mental disorders were related to the persistence of one of the early modes. The **prototaxic mode**, characteristic of infancy and childhood, involves brief unconnected experiences that have no relation to each other. Adults with schizophrenia exhibit persistent prototaxic experiences. The **parataxic mode** begins in early childhood as the child begins to connect experiences in sequence. The child may not make logical sense of the experiences and may see them as coincidence or chance events. The child seeks to relieve anxiety by repeating familiar experiences, although he or she may not understand what he or she is doing. Sullivan explained paranoid ideas and slips of the tongue as a person operating in the parataxic mode. In the **syntaxic mode**, which begins to appear in school-age children and becomes more predominant in preadolescence, the person begins to perceive himself or herself and the world within the context of the environment and can analyze experiences in a variety of settings. Maturity may be defined as predominance of the syntaxic mode (Sullivan, 1953).

Therapeutic Community or Milieu. Sullivan envisioned the goal of treatment as the establishment of satisfying interpersonal relationships. The therapist provides a corrective interpersonal relationship for the client. Sullivan coined the term **participant observer** for the therapist's role, meaning the therapist both participates in the relationship and observes the progress of the relationship.

Credit is also given to Sullivan for developing the first **therapeutic community** or **milieu** with young men with schizophrenia in 1929 (although that term was not used extensively until Maxwell Jones published *The Therapeutic Community* in 1953). In the concept of therapeutic community or milieu, the interaction among patients is seen as beneficial and the role of this patient-to-patient interaction is emphasized in treatment. Until this time, it

Table 3-4

SULLIVAN'S LIFE STAGES

Stage	Ages	Focus
Infancy	Birth to onset of language	Primary need for bodily contact and tenderness Prototaxic mode dominates (no relation between experiences) Primary zones are oral and anal. If needs are met, infant has sense of well-being; unmet needs lead to dread and anxiety.
Childhood	Language to 5 years	Parents viewed as source of praise and acceptance Shift to parataxic mode (experiences are connected in sequence to each other) Primary zone is anal. Gratification leads to positive self-esteem. Moderate anxiety leads to uncertainty and insecurity; severe anxiety results in self-defeating patterns of behavior.
Juvenile	5–8 years	Shift to the sytaxic mode begins (thinking about self and others based on analysis of experiences in a variety of situations). Opportunities for approval and acceptance of others Learn to negotiate own needs Severe anxiety may result in a need to control or restrictive, prejudicial attitudes.
Preadolescence	8–12 years	Move to genuine intimacy with friend of the same sex Move away from family as source of satisfaction in relationships Major shift to syntaxic mode Capacity for attachment, love, and collaboration emerges or fails to develop.
Adolescence	Puberty to adulthood	Lust is added to interpersonal equation. Need for special sharing relationship shifts to the opposite sex. New opportunities for social experimentation lead to the consolidation of self-esteem or self-ridicule. If the self-system is intact, areas of concern expand to include values, ideals, career decisions, and social concerns.

Adapted from Gabbard, G. O. (2000). Theories of personality and psychopathology: Psychoanalysis. In B. J. Sadock & V. A. Sadock (Eds.). *Comprehensive textbook of psychiatry*, Vol. 2 (7th ed., pp. 563–607). Philadelphia, Lippincott Williams & Wilkins.

was believed that the interaction between the patient and the psychiatrist was the one essential component to the patient's treatment. Sullivan and later Jones observed that interactions among patients in a safe, therapeutic setting provided great benefits to patients. The concept of **milieu therapy**, originally developed by Sullivan, involved patients' interactions with each other, practicing interpersonal relationship skills, giving each other feedback about behavior, and working cooperatively as a group to solve day-to-day problems.

Milieu therapy was regarded as one of the prime modes of treatment in the acute hospital setting. However, in today's health care environment, inpatient hospital stays are often too short for clients to develop meaningful relationships with each other. Therefore, the concept of milieu therapy receives little attention. Management of the milieu or environment is still a primary role for the nurse in terms of providing safety and protection for all clients and promoting social interaction.

HILDEGARD PEPLAU: THERAPEUTIC NURSE–PATIENT RELATIONSHIP

Hildegard Peplau (b. 1909; Fig. 3-3) is a nursing theorist and clinician who built on Sullivan's interpersonal theories and also saw the role of the nurse as a participant observer. Peplau developed the concept of the **therapeutic nurse–patient relationship**, which includes four phases: orientation, identification, exploitation, and resolution (Table 3-5). During these phases, the client accomplishes certain tasks and the relationship changes, which helps the healing process (Peplau, 1952).

1. The *orientation phase* is directed by the nurse and involves engaging the client in

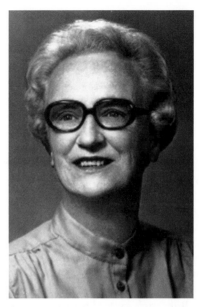

Figure 3-3. Hildegard Peplau, who developed the phases of the nurse–client therapeutic relationship, which has made great contributions to the foundation of nursing practice today.

treatment, providing explanations and information, and answering questions.
2. The *identification phase* begins when the client works interdependently with the nurse, expresses feelings, and begins to feel stronger.
3. In the *exploitation phase*, the client makes full use of the services offered.
4. In the *resolution phase*, the patient no longer needs professional services and gives up dependent behavior. The relationship ends.

Peplau's concept of the nurse–patient relationship, with tasks and behaviors characteristic of each

Table 3-5

PEPLAU'S STAGES AND TASKS OF RELATIONSHIPS

Stage	Tasks
Orientation	Clarification of patient's problems and needs Patient asks questions. Explanation of hospital routines and expectations Patient harnesses energy toward meeting problems. Patient's full participation is elicited.
Identification	Patient responds to persons he or she perceives as helpful. Patient feels stronger. Expression of feelings Interdependent work with the nurse Clarification of roles of both patient and nurse
Exploitation	Patient makes full use of available services. Goals such as going home and returning to work emerge. Patient's behaviors fluctuate between dependence and independence.
Resolution	Patient gives up dependent behavior. Services are no longer needed by patient. Patient assumes power to meet own needs, set new goals, and so forth.

Adapted from Peplau, H. (1952). *Interpersonal relations in nursing.* New York: G. P. Putnam's Sons.

stage, has been modified but remains in use today (see Chap. 5).

Roles of the Nurse in the Therapeutic Relationship.
Peplau also wrote about the roles of the nurse in the therapeutic relationship and how these roles helped meet the client's needs. The primary roles she identified were:

- *Stranger*: offering the client the same acceptance and courtesy that the nurse would to any stranger
- *Resource person*: providing specific answers to questions within a larger context
- *Teacher*: helping the client learn, formally or informally
- *Leader*: offering direction to the patient or group
- *Surrogate*: serving as a substitute for another, such as a parent or sibling
- *Counselor*: promoting experiences leading to health for the client, such as expression of feelings.

Peplau also believed there were many other roles a nurse could take on, such as consultant, tutor, safety agent, mediator, administrator, observer, and researcher. These were not defined in detail but were "left to the intelligence and imagination of the readers" (Peplau, 1952, p. 70).

Four Levels of Anxiety. Peplau defined anxiety as the initial response to a psychic threat. She described four levels of anxiety: mild, moderate, severe, and panic (Table 3-6). These serve as the foundation for working with clients with anxiety in a variety of contexts (see Chap. 12).

1. *Mild anxiety* is a positive state of heightened awareness and sharpened senses, allowing the person to learn new behaviors and solve problems. The person can take in all available stimuli (perceptual field).
2. *Moderate anxiety* involves a decreased perceptual field (focus on immediate task only); the person can learn new behavior or solve problems only with assistance. The person can be redirected to the task by another person.
3. *Severe anxiety* involves feelings of dread or terror. The person cannot be redirected to a task; he or she focuses only on scattered details and has physiologic symptoms of tachycardia, diaphoresis, and chest pain. Persons with severe anxiety often go to emergency rooms, believing they are having a heart attack.
4. *Panic anxiety* can involve loss of rational thought, delusions, hallucinations, and complete physical immobility and muteness. The

Table 3-6

ANXIETY LEVELS

Mild	Moderate	Severe	Panic
Sharpened senses	Selectively attentive	Perceptual field reduced to one detail or scattered details	Perceptual field reduced to focus on self
Increased motivation	Perceptual field limited to the immediate task	Cannot complete tasks	Cannot process environmental stimuli
Alert	Can be redirected	Cannot solve problems or learn effectively	Distorted perceptions
Enlarged perceptual field	Cannot connect thoughts or events independently	Behavior geared toward anxiety relief and is usually ineffective	Loss of rational thought
Can solve problems	Muscle tension	Feels awe, dread, horror	Personality disorganization
Learning is effective	Diaphoresis	Doesn't respond to redirection	Doesn't recognize danger
Restless	Pounding pulse	Severe headache	Possibly suicidal
GI "butterflies"	Headache	Nausea, vomiting, diarrhea	Delusions or hallucination possible
Sleepless	Dry mouth	Trembling	Can't communicate verbally
Irritable	Higher voice pitch	Rigid stance	Either cannot sit (may bolt and run) or totally mute and immobile
Hypersensitive to noise	Increased rate of speech	Vertigo	
	GI upset	Pale	
	Frequent urination	Tachycardia	
	Increased automatisms (nervous mannerisms)	Chest pain	
		Crying	
		Ritualistic (purposeless, repetitive) behavior	

Adapted from Peplau, H. (1952). *Interpersonal relations in nursing.* New York: G. P. Putnam's Sons.

person may bolt and run aimlessly, often exposing himself or herself to injury.

Humanistic Theories

Humanism represents a significant shift away from the psychoanalytic view of the individual as a neurotic, impulse-driven person with repressed psychic problems, and away from the focus on and examination of the client's past experiences. **Humanism** focuses on the positive qualities of the person, his or her capacity to change (human potential), and the promotion of self-esteem. Humanists do consider the person's past experiences, but they direct more attention toward the present and future.

ABRAHAM MASLOW: HIERARCHY OF NEEDS

Abraham Maslow (1921–1970) was an American psychologist who studied the needs or motivations of the individual. He differed from previous theorists in that he focused on the total person, not just one facet of the person, and emphasized health instead of simply illness and problems. Maslow (1954) formulated the **hierarchy of needs**, in which he used a pyramid arrangement to illustrate the basic drives or needs that motivate people. The most basic needs—the physiologic needs of food, water, sleep, shelter, sexual

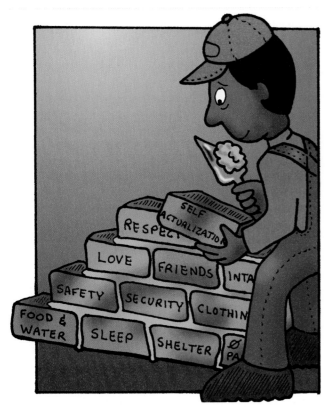

Building block arrangement of needs.

expression, and freedom from pain—must be met first. The second level involves safety and security needs, which include protection, security, and freedom from harm or threatened deprivation. The third level is love and belonging needs, which include enduring intimacy, friendship, and acceptance. The fourth level involves esteem needs, which include the need for self-respect and esteem from others. The highest level is self-actualization, the need for beauty, truth, and justice.

Maslow hypothesized that the basic needs at the bottom of the pyramid would dominate the person's behavior until those needs were met, at which time the next level of needs would become dominant. For example, if needs for food and shelter are not met, they become the overriding concern in life: the hungry person risks danger and social ostracism to find food.

Maslow used the term **self-actualization** to describe a person who has achieved all the needs of the hierarchy and has developed his or her fullest potential in life. Few people ever become fully self-actualized.

Maslow's theory explains individual differences in terms of a person's motivation, which is not necessarily stable throughout the lifetime. Traumatic life circumstances or compromised health can cause the person to regress to a lower level of motivation. For example, if a 35-year-old woman who is functioning at the "love and belonging" level discovers she has cancer, she may regress to the "safety" level to undergo treatment for the cancer and preserve her own safety and health. This theory helps nurses understand how clients' motivations and behavior change when life crises occur (see Chap. 7).

CARL ROGERS: CLIENT-CENTERED THERAPY

Carl Rogers (1902–1987) was a humanistic American psychologist who focused on the therapeutic relationship and developed a new method of client-centered therapy. Rogers was one of the first to use the term "client" rather than "patient." **Client-centered therapy** focused on the role of the client, rather than the therapist, as the key to the healing process. Rogers believed that everyone experiences the world differently and knows his or her own experience best (Rogers, 1961). According to Rogers, clients do "the work of healing," and within a supportive and nurturing client–therapist relationship, clients can cure themselves. Clients are in the best position to know their own experiences and make sense of them, to regain their self-esteem, and to progress toward self-actualization.

The therapist takes a person-centered approach, a supportive role, rather than a directive or expert role. Rogers viewed the client as the expert on his or her life. The therapist must promote the client's self-esteem as much as possible. This includes three central concepts identified by Rogers:

- *Unconditional positive regard*, a nonjudgmental caring for the client that is not dependent on the client's behavior
- *Genuineness* or realness, or congruence between what the therapist feels and says to the client
- *Empathetic understanding*, in which the therapist senses the feelings and personal meaning from the client and communicates this understanding to the client.

Unconditional positive regard promotes the client's self-esteem and decreases his or her need for defensive behavior. As the client's self-acceptance grows, the natural self-actualization process can continue.

Rogers also believed that it is our basic nature to become self-actualized or to move toward self-improvement and constructive change. We are all born with a positive self-regard and a natural inclination to become self-actualized. If relationships with others are supportive and nurturing, the person retains feelings of self-worth and progresses toward self-actualization, which is healthy. However, if the person encounters repeated conflicts with others or is in relationships that are not supportive, he or she loses self-esteem, becomes defensive, and is no longer inclined toward self-actualization; this is not healthy.

Behavioral Theories

Behaviorism as a school of psychology grew out of a reaction to introspection models that focused on the contents and operations of the mind. **Behaviorism** is a school of psychology that focuses on observable behaviors and what one can do externally to bring about behavior changes. It does not attempt to explain how the mind works.

Behaviorists believe that behavior can be changed by a system of rewards and punishments. For adults, receiving a paycheck on a regular basis is a constant positive reinforcer. The paycheck is a continuous positive reinforcer and is one of the reasons people continue to go to work every day and try to go a good job. It helps motivate positive behavior in the workplace. If someone stops receiving a paycheck, he or she is most likely to stop working.

If a motorist consistently speeds (negative behavior) and does not get caught, he or she is likely to continue to speed. If the driver receives a speeding ticket (a negative reinforcer), he or she is likely to slow down. However, if the motorist does not get caught for speeding for the next 4 weeks (negative reinforcer is removed), he or she is likely to resume speeding again.

IVAN PAVLOV: CLASSICAL CONDITIONING

Laboratory experiments with dogs provided the basis for the development of Ivan Pavlov's theory of classical conditioning: behavior can be changed by conditioning with external or environmental conditions or stimuli. His experiment with dogs involved his observation that dogs naturally began to salivate (response) when they saw or smelled food (stimulus). Pavlov (1849–1936) set out to change this salivating response or behavior by conditioning. He would ring a bell (new stimulus) and then produce the food, and the dogs would salivate (the desired response). Pavlov repeated this ringing of the bell along with the presentation of food many times. Eventually, he could ring the bell and the dogs would salivate without seeing or smelling food. The dogs had been "conditioned" or had learned a new response—to salivate when they heard the bell. Their behavior had been modified through classical conditioning or a conditioned response.

B. F. SKINNER: OPERANT CONDITIONING

One of the most influential behaviorists was B. F. Skinner (1904–1990), an American psychologist. He developed the theory of **operant conditioning**, which says that behavior is learned from one's history or past experiences, particularly from experiences that were repeatedly reinforced. Although some criticize his theories for not taking into account the role that thoughts, feelings, or needs play in motivating behavior, his work has provided several important principles that are still used today. Skinner did not deny the existence of feelings and needs in motivation, but he viewed behavior as only that which could be observed, studied, and learned or unlearned. He maintained that if the behavior could be changed, then so too could the accompanying thoughts or feelings. Changing the behavior was what was important.

The following principles of operant conditioning described by Skinner (1974) form the basis for behavior techniques in use today:

1. All behavior is learned.
2. There are consequences that result from behavior—broadly speaking, reward and punishment.
3. Behavior that is rewarded with reinforcers tends to recur.
4. Positive reinforcers that follow a behavior increase the likelihood that the behavior will recur.
5. Negative reinforcers that are removed after a behavior increase the likelihood that the behavior will recur.
6. Continuous reinforcement (a reward every time the behavior occurs) is the fastest way to increase that behavior, but the behavior will not last long after the reward ceases.

7. Random, intermittent reinforcement (a reward for the desired behavior once in a while) is slower to produce an increase in behavior, but the behavior continues after the reward ceases.

These behavioral principles of rewarding or reinforcing behaviors are used to help people change their behavior in a therapy known as behavior modification. **Behavior modification** is a method of attempting to strengthen a desired behavior or response by reinforcement, either positive or negative. For example, if the desired behavior is assertiveness, whenever the client uses assertiveness skills in a communication group, the group leader provides positive reinforcement by giving the client attention and positive feedback. **Negative reinforcement** involves removing a stimulus immediately after a behavior occurs so that the behavior is more likely to occur again. For example, if a client becomes anxious when waiting to talk in a group, he or she may volunteer to speak first to avoid the anxiety.

In a group home setting, operant principles may come into play in a **token economy**, a way to get residents involved in performing activities of daily living. A chart of desired behaviors, such as getting up on time, taking a shower, and getting dressed, is kept for each resident. Each day, the chart is marked when the desired behavior occurs. At the end of the day or the week, the resident gets a reward or token for each time each of the desired behaviors occurred. The tokens can be redeemed for items such as snacks, TV time, or a relaxed curfew.

Conditioned responses, such as fears or phobias, can be treated with behavioral techniques. **Systematic desensitization** can be used to help clients overcome irrational fears and anxiety associated with a phobia. The client is asked to make a list of situations involving the phobic object, from the least anxiety-provoking to the most anxiety-provoking. The client learns and practices relaxation techniques to decrease and manage anxiety. The client then is exposed to the least anxiety-provoking situation, using the relaxation techniques to manage the resulting anxiety. The client is gradually exposed to more and more anxiety-provoking situations until he or she can manage the most anxiety-provoking situation.

Behavioral techniques can be used for a variety of different problems. In the treatment of anorexia nervosa, the goal is weight gain. A behavioral contract between the client and therapist or physician is initiated when treatment begins. Initially, the client has little unsupervised time and is restricted to the hospital unit. The contract may specify that if the client gains a certain amount of weight, such as 0.2 kg/day, in return he or she will get increased amounts of unsupervised time or time off the unit, as long as the weight gain progresses (Agras, 1995).

Existential Theories

Existential theorists believe that behavioral deviations occur when a person is out of touch with himself or herself or the environment. The person who is alienated from himself or herself is lonely and sad and feels helpless. Lack of self-awareness, coupled with harsh self-criticism, prevents the person from participating in satisfying relationships. The person is not free to choose from all possible alternatives because of self-imposed restrictions. Existential theorists believe the person is avoiding personal responsibility and giving in to the wishes or demands of others.

All existential therapies have the goal of returning the person to an authentic sense of self. Personal responsibility for one's self, feelings, behaviors, and choices is emphasized. The person is encouraged to live fully in the present and to look forward to the future. Carl Rogers is sometimes grouped with existential therapists. Table 3-7 summarizes existential therapies.

COGNITIVE THERAPY

Many existential therapists use **cognitive therapy**, which focuses on immediate thought processing—how

---

Table 3-7

EXISTENTIAL THERAPIES

Therapy	Therapist	Therapeutic Process
Rational emotive therapy	Albert Ellis	A cognitive therapy using confrontation of "irrational beliefs" that prevent the individual from accepting responsibility for self and behavior
Logotherapy	Viktor E. Frankl	A therapy designed to help individuals assume personal responsibility. The search for meaning (*logos*) in life is a central theme.
Gestalt therapy	Frederick S. Perls	A therapy focusing on the identification of feelings in the here and now, which leads to self-acceptance
Reality therapy	William Glasser	Therapeutic focus is need for identity through responsible behavior. Individuals are challenged to examine ways in which their behavior thwarts their attempts to achieve life goals.

a person perceives or interprets his or her experience and determines how he or she feels and behaves. For example, if a person interprets a situation as dangerous, he or she experiences anxiety and tries to escape. Basic emotions of sadness, elation, anxiety, and anger are reactions to perceptions of loss, gain, danger, and wrongdoing by others (Beck & Rush, 1995).

RATIONAL EMOTIVE THERAPY

Albert Ellis, founder of rational emotive therapy, identified 11 "irrational beliefs" that people use to make themselves unhappy. An example of an irrational belief is, "If I love someone, he or she must love me back just as much." Ellis claimed that continuing to believe this patently untrue statement will make the person utterly unhappy, but he or she will blame it on the person who does not return his or her love. Ellis also believes that people have "automatic thoughts" that cause them unhappiness in certain situations. He used the ABC technique to help people identify these automatic thoughts: *A* is the activating stimulus or event, *C* is the excessive inappropriate response, and *B* is the blank in the person's mind that he or she must fill in by identifying the automatic thought.

VIKTOR FRANKL AND LOGOTHERAPY

Victor Frankl based his beliefs on his observations of people in concentration camps in Germany in World War II. His curiosity about why some survived and others did not led him to conclude that survivors were able to find meaning in their life, even under miserable conditions. Hence, the search for meaning (*logos*) is the central theme in logotherapy.

GESTALT THERAPY

Gestalt therapy, founded by Frederick "Fritz" Perls, emphasizes identifying the persons's feelings and thoughts in the here and now. Perls believed that self-awareness leads to self-acceptance and responsibility for one's own thoughts and feelings.

REALITY THERAPY

William Glasser devised an approach called reality therapy that focuses on the person's behavior and how that behavior keeps him or her from achieving life goals. He developed this approach while working with persons with delinquent behavior, unsuccessful school performance, and emotional problems. He believed that persons who were unsuccessful often blame their problems on other people, the system, or society. He believed they needed to find their own identity through responsible behavior. In reality therapy, clients are challenged to examine ways in which their own behavior thwarts their attempts to achieve life goals.

CULTURAL CONSIDERATIONS

The major psychosocial theorists were white and born in Europe or the United States, as were many of the people they treated. What they considered normal or typical may not apply equally well to persons with different racial, ethnic, or cultural backgrounds.

TREATMENT MODALITIES

Benefits of Community Mental Health Treatment

Mental health treatment has been affected by recent changes in health care and reimbursement, as have all areas of medicine, nursing, and related health disciplines (see Chap. 4). Inpatient treatment is often the last, rather than the first, mode of treatment for mental illness. Current treatment reflects the belief that it is more beneficial and certainly more cost-effective for clients to remain in the community and receive outpatient treatment whenever possible. The client can often continue to work and can stay connected with family, friends, and other support systems while participating in therapy. Outpatient therapy also takes into account that a person's personality or behavior patterns, such as coping skills, styles of communication, and level of self-esteem, gradually develop over the course of a lifetime and cannot be changed in a relatively short inpatient course of treatment. Hospital admission is indicated when the person is severely depressed and suicidal, severely psychotic, experiencing alcohol or drug withdrawal, or exhibiting behaviors that require close supervision in a safe supportive environment.

This section briefly describes the treatment modalities currently used in both inpatient and outpatient settings.

Individual Psychotherapy

Individual psychotherapy is a method of bringing about change in a person by exploring his or her feelings, attitudes, thinking, and behavior. It involves a one-to-one relationship between the therapist and the client. People generally seek this kind of therapy based on their desire to understand themselves and their behavior, to make personal changes, to improve interpersonal relationships, or to get relief from emotional pain or unhappiness. The relationship between the client and the therapist proceeds through stages similar to those of the nurse–client relationship: introduction, working, and termination. Cost-containment measures mandated by health maintenance organizations and other insurers may necessitate moving into the working phase rapidly so the client can get the maximum benefit possible from therapy.

The therapist–client relationship is key to the success of this type of therapy. The client and the therapist must be compatible for therapy to be effective. Therapists vary in their formal credentials, experience, and model of practice. Selecting a therapist is extremely important in terms of successful outcomes for the client. The client must select a therapist whose theoretical beliefs and style of therapy are congruent with the client's needs and expectations of therapy. The client may also have to try different therapists to find a good match.

A therapist's style of therapy is strongly influenced by his or her theoretical beliefs (discussed earlier in this chapter). For example, a therapist grounded in interpersonal theories emphasizes relationships, whereas an existential therapist focuses on the client's self-responsibility.

The nurse or other health care provider who is familiar with the client may be in a position to recommend a therapist or a choice of therapists. He or she may also help the client understand what different therapists have to offer.

The client should select a therapist carefully and should ask about the therapist's treatment approach and area of specialization. State laws regulate the practice and licensing of therapists; thus, from state to state the qualifications to practice psychotherapy, the requirements for licensure, or even the need for

a license can vary. A few therapists have little or no formal education, credentials, or experience but still practice entirely within the legal limits of their state. Legal credentials can be verified with the state licensing board, found in the state government listings in the local phone book. The Better Business Bureau can inform consumers whether a particular therapist has been reported to them for investigation. Calling the local mental health services agency or contacting the primary care provider is another way for a client to check on the credentials and ethical practices of a therapist.

Group Therapy

In **group therapy**, clients participate in sessions with a group of people. The members share a common purpose and are expected to contribute to the group to benefit others and receive benefit from others in return. Group rules are established that must be observed by all members. These rules vary according to the type of group. Being a member of a group allows the client to learn new ways of looking at a problem or ways of coping or solving problems and also helps him or her learn important interpersonal skills. For example, by interacting with other members, clients often receive feedback on how others perceive and react to them and their behavior. This is extremely important information for many clients with mental disorders, who often have difficulty with interpersonal skills.

The therapeutic results of group therapy (Yalom, 1995) include:

- Gaining new information or learning
- Gaining inspiration or hope
- Interacting with others
- Feeling acceptance and belonging
- Becoming aware that one is not alone and that others share the same problems
- Gaining insight into one's problems and behaviors and how they affect others
- Giving of oneself for the benefit of others (altruism).

Therapy groups vary, with different purposes, degrees of formality, and structures. Our discussion will include psychotherapy groups, family therapy, education groups, support groups, and self-help groups.

Psychotherapy Groups

The goal of a **psychotherapy group** is for members to learn about their behavior and to make positive changes in their behavior by interacting and communicating with others as a member of a group. Groups may be organized around a specific medical diagnosis, such as depression, or a particular issue, such as improving interpersonal skills or managing anxiety. Group techniques and processes are used to help group members learn about their behavior with

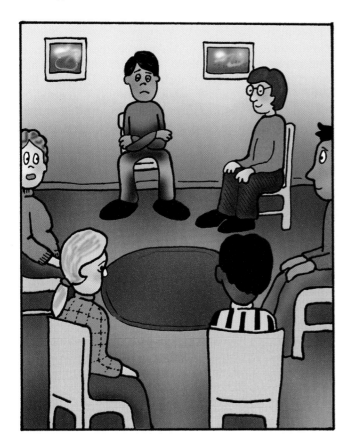

Group therapy

other people and how it relates to core personality traits. Members also learn that they have responsibilities to others and can help other members achieve their goals (Alonso, 2000).

Psychotherapy groups are often formal in structure, with one or two therapists as the group leaders. One of the tasks of the group leader or the entire group is to establish the rules for the group. These rules deal with confidentiality, punctuality, attendance, and social contact between members outside of group time.

There are two types of groups: open groups and closed groups. **Open groups** are ongoing and run indefinitely, allowing members to join or leave the group as they need to. **Closed groups** are structured to keep the same members in the group for a specified number of sessions. If the group is closed, the members decide how to handle members who wish to leave the group and the possible addition of new group members (Yalom, 1995).

Family Therapy

Family therapy is a form of group therapy in which the client and his or her family members participate. The goals include understanding how family dynamics contribute to the client's psychopathology, mobilizing the family's inherent strengths and functional resources, restructuring maladaptive family behavioral styles, and strengthening family problem-solving behaviors (Steinglass, 1995). Family therapy can be used both to assess and treat various psychiatric disorders. Although one family member is usually identified initially as the one who has problems and needs help, it often becomes evident through the therapeutic process that other family members also have emotional problems and difficulties.

Education Groups

The goal of an **education group** is to provide information to members on a specific issue—for instance, stress management, medication management, or assertiveness training. The group leader has expertise in the subject area and may be a nurse, therapist, or other health professional. Education groups are usually scheduled for a specific number of sessions and retain the same members for the duration of the group. Typically, information is presented by the leader, and then members can ask questions or practice new techniques.

In a medication management group, the leader may discuss medication regimens and possible side effects, may screen clients for side effects, and in some instances may actually administer the medication (for instance, depot injections of haloperidol [Haldol] or fluphenazine [Prolixin]).

Support Groups

Support groups are organized to help members who share a common problem cope with the problem. The group leader explores members' thoughts and feelings and creates an atmosphere of acceptance so that members feel comfortable expressing themselves. Support groups often provide a safe place for group members to express their feelings of frustration, boredom, or unhappiness and also to discuss common problems and potential solutions. Rules for support groups differ from those in psychotherapy in that members are allowed—in fact, encouraged—to contact each other or socialize outside the sessions. Confidentiality may be a rule for some groups; this is decided by the members. Support groups tend to be open groups in which members can join or leave as their needs dictate.

Common support groups include those for cancer or stroke victims, persons with AIDS, and family members of someone who has committed suicide. One national support group, Mothers Against Drunk Driving (MADD), is for family members of someone killed in a car accident caused by a drunk driver.

Self-Help Groups

In a **self-help group**, members share a common experience, but the group is not a formal or structured therapy group. Although some self-help groups are organized by a professional, many are run by members and often do not have a formally identified leader. Various self-help groups are available. Some are locally organized and announce their meetings in local newspapers. Other groups are nationally organized, such as Alcoholics Anonymous, Parents Without Partners, Gamblers Anonymous, or Al-Anon (a group for spouses and partners of alcoholics), and have national headquarters and Internet websites (see Internet Resources).

Most self-help groups have a rule of confidentiality: whoever is seen at a meeting or what is said at the meetings cannot be divulged to others or discussed outside the group. In many 12-step programs, such as Alcoholics Anonymous and Gamblers Anonymous, people use only their first names, so their identity is not divulged (although in some settings, group members do know each other's names).

Psychiatric Rehabilitation

Psychiatric rehabilitation involves providing services to persons with severe and persistent mental illness to help them to live in the community. These programs are often called community support services or community support programs. Psychiatric rehabilitation focuses on the client's strengths, not just his or her illness. The client is an active participant in program planning. The programs are designed to help the client manage the illness and symptoms, gain access to needed services, and live successfully in the community.

Clients are assisted with activities of daily living such as transportation, shopping, food preparation, money management, and hygiene. Social support and interpersonal relationships are recognized as a primary need for successful community living. Opportunities for socialization are provided, such as drop-in centers, places clients can go to be with others in a safe, supportive environment. Vocational referral, training, job coaching, and support are available for clients who want to seek and maintain employment. Community support programs also provide education about the client's illness and treatment and help the client obtain health care when needed.

THE NURSE AND PSYCHOSOCIAL INTERVENTIONS

Intervention is a crucial component of the nursing process. **Psychosocial interventions** are nursing activities that enhance the client's social and psychological functioning and improve social skills, interpersonal relationships, and communication. Nurses often use psychosocial interventions to help meet clients' needs and achieve outcomes in all practice settings, not just mental health. For example, a medical-surgical nurse might need to use interventions that incorporate behavioral principles, such as setting limits with manipulative behavior or giving positive feedback.

For example, a diabetic client tells the nurse, *"I promise to have just one bite of cake. Please! It's my grandson's birthday cake"* (manipulative behavior). The nurse might use behavioral limit-setting by saying, *"I can't give you permission to eat the cake. Your blood sugar will go up if you do, and your insulin can't be adjusted properly."* When a client first attempts to change a colostomy bag but needs some assistance, the nurse might say, *"You gave it a good effort. You were able to complete the task with a little assistance"* (giving positive feedback).

Understanding the theories and treatment modalities presented in this chapter can help the nurse select appropriate and effective intervention strategies. In later chapters dealing with particular mental disorders or problems, specific psychosocial interventions are described that the nurse might use.

SELF-AWARENESS ISSUES

The nurse must examine his or her beliefs about the theories of psychosocial development and realize that a variety of treatment approaches are available. Different treatments may work for different clients: no one single approach works for everyone. Sometimes the nurse's personal opinions may not agree with those of the client, but the nurse must make sure that those beliefs do not inadvertently affect the therapeutic process. For example, an overweight client may be working on accepting herself as being overweight rather than trying to lose weight, but the nurse thinks the client really just needs to lose weight. The nurse's responsibility is to support the client's needs and goals, not promote the nurse's own ideas about what the client should do. Hence, the nurse must support the client's decision to work on self-acceptance. For the nurse who believes that being overweight is simply a lack of will power, it might be difficult to support a client's participation in a self-help weight-loss group, such as Overeaters Anonymous, that emphasizes overeating as a disease and accepting oneself.

The following are helpful tips for nurses regarding psychosocial theories and treatment:

- No one theory explains all human behavior. No one approach will work with all clients.
- Becoming familiar with the variety of psychosocial approaches toward working

with clients will increase the nurse's effectiveness in promoting the client's health and well-being.

- The client's feelings and perceptions about his or her situation are the most influential factors in determining his or her response to therapeutic interventions, rather than what the nurse believes the client should do.

Critical Thinking

Questions

1. Can sound parenting and nurturing in a loving environment overcome a genetic or biologic predisposition to mental illness?
2. Can children raised in a hostile environment without parental love, support, and consistency avoid mental health problems as adults? If so, how, or what factors could help a person overcome a neglected or traumatic childhood?

➤ KEY POINTS

- Psychosocial theories help to explain human behavior—both mental health and mental illness. There are several types of psychosocial theories, including psychoanalytic theories, interpersonal theories, humanistic theories, behavioral theories, and existential theories.
- Psychoanalysis was developed by Sigmund Freud, who believed the personality was made up of three components: the id, the ego, and the superego.
- Freud believed that human behavior is motivated by repressed sexual impulses and desires, and that childhood development was based on sexual energy (libido) as the driving force.
- Psychoanalysis is practiced today on a limited basis because of the lengthy nature and high cost of the treatment. Treatment can often take years of weekly sessions, which focus on exploring the depths of the client's psyche and feelings and analyzing dreams for hidden meanings.
- Erik Erikson's theories focused on both social and psychological development across the life span. He proposed eight stages of psychosocial development, each including a developmental task and a virtue to be achieved (hope, will, purpose, fidelity, love, caring, and wisdom). Erikson's theories remain in wide use today.
- Harry Stack Sullivan's theories focused on development in terms of interpersonal relationships. He viewed the therapist's role (termed participant observer) as key to the client's treatment.
- Hildegard Peplau is a nursing theorist whose theories formed much of the foundation of modern nursing practice, including the therapeutic nurse–patient relationship, the role of the nurse in the relationship, and the four anxiety levels.
- Abraham Maslow developed a hierarchy of needs, stating that people were motivated by progressive levels of needs; each level must be satisfied before the person can progress to the next level. The levels begin with physiologic needs, then safety and security needs, belonging needs, esteem needs, and finally self-actualization needs.
- Carl Rogers developed client-centered therapy, in which the therapist plays a supportive role, demonstrating unconditional positive regard, genuineness, and empathetic understanding to the client.
- Behaviorism focuses on the client's observable performance and behaviors and external influences that can bring about behavior changes, rather than focusing on feelings and thoughts.
- Ivan Pavlov's experiments with dogs led to the theory of classical conditioning, which concludes that behavior can be changed by conditioning with external or environmental conditions or stimuli.
- Systematic desensitization is an example of conditioning in which a person who has an excessive fear of something, such as frogs or snakes, is conditioned into not fearing the object after being progressively exposed to it in a relaxed and controlled environment.
- B. F. Skinner is a behaviorist who developed the theory of operant conditioning, in which people are motivated to learn behavior or change behavior with a system of rewards or reinforcement.
- Behaviorists believe that behavior can be changed through a system of rewards or punishments, such as token economy.
- Existential theorists believe that problems result when the person is out of touch with the self or the environment. The person has self-imposed restrictions, criticizes himself or herself harshly, and does not participate in satisfying interpersonal relationships.
- Founders of existentialism include Albert Ellis (rational emotive therapy), Viktor Frankl (logotherapy), Frederick Perls

(gestalt therapy), and William Glasser (reality therapy).

- All existential therapies have the goals of returning the person to an authentic sense of self, emphasizing personal responsibility for oneself and one's feelings, behavior, and choices.
- Cognitive therapy is based on the premise that how a person thinks about or interprets life experiences determines how he or she will feel or behave. It seeks to help the person change how he or she thinks about things to bring about an improvement in mood and behavior.
- Treatment for mental disorders and emotional problems can include one or more of the following: individual psychotherapy, group psychotherapy, family therapy, psychiatric rehabilitation, self-help groups, support groups, and education groups, and other psychosocial interventions, such as setting limits or giving positive feedback.
- An understanding of psychosocial theories and treatment modalities can help the nurse select appropriate and effective intervention strategies to use with clients.

REFERENCES

Agras, W. S. (1995). Behavior therapy. In H. I. Kaplan & B. J. Sadock (Eds.). *Comprehensive textbook of psychiatry, Vol. 2* (6th ed., pp. 1877–1806). Philadelphia: J. B. Lippincott.

Alonso, A. (2000). Group psychotherapy, combined individual and group therapy. In B. J. Sadock & V. A. Sadock (Eds.). *Comprehensive textbook of psychiatry, Vol. 2* (7th ed., pp. 2146–2157). Philadelphia: Lippincott Williams & Wilkins.

Beck, A. T., & Rush, A. J. (1995). Cognitive therapy. In H. I. Kaplan & B. J. Sadock (Eds.). *Comprehensive textbook of psychiatry, Vol. 2* (6th ed., pp. 1847–1856.) Philadelphia: J. B. Lippincott.

Ellis, A. (1989). *Inside rational emotive therapy.* San Diego: Academic Press.

Erikson, E. H. (1963). *Childhood and society* (2d ed.). New York: Norton.

Gabbard, G. O. (2000). Theories of personality and psychopathology: Psychoanalysis. In B. J. Sadock & V. A. Sadock (Eds.). *Comprehensive textbook of psychiatry, Vol. 2* (7th ed., pp. 563–607). Philadelphia: Lippincott Williams & Wilkins.

Maslow, A. H. (1954). *Motivation and personality.* New York: Harper & Row.

Peplau, H. (1952). *Interpersonal relations in nursing.* New York: G. P. Putnam's Sons.

Rogers, C. R. (1961). *On becoming a person: A therapist's view of psychotherapy.* Boston: Houghton Mifflin.

Skinner, B. F. (1974). *About behaviorism.* New York: Alfred A. Knopf, Inc.

Steinglass, P. (1995). Family therapy. In H. I. Kaplan & B. J. Sadock (Eds.). *Comprehensive textbook of psychiatry, Vol. 2* (6th ed., pp 1838–1846). Philadelphia: J. B. Lippincott.

Sullivan, H. S. (1953). *The interpersonal theory of psychiatry.* New York: Norton.

Yalom, I. D. (1995). *The theory and practice of group psychotherapy.* New York: Basic Books.

ADDITIONAL READINGS

Beck, A. T. (1976). *Cognitive therapy and the emotional disorders.* New York: The New American Library, Inc.

Berne, E. (1964). *Games people play.* New York: Grove Press.

Caplan, G. (1964). *Principles of preventive psychiatry.* New York: Basic Books.

Crain, W. C. (1980). *Theories of development: Concepts and application.* Englewood Cliffs, NJ: Prentice-Hall, Inc.

Frankl, V. E. (1959). *Man's search for meaning: An introduction to logotherapy.* New York: The Beacon Press.

Glasser, W. (1965). *Reality therapy: A new approach to psychiatry.* New York: Harper & Row.

Miller, P. H. (1983). *Theories of developmental psychology.* San Francisco: W. H. Freeman & Co.

Millon, T. (Ed.). (1967). *Theories of psychopathology.* Philadelphia: W. B. Saunders.

Perls, F. S., Hefferline, R. F., & Goodman, P. (1951). *Gestalt therapy: Excitement and growth in the human personality.* New York: Dell Publishing Co., Inc.

Schultz, J. M., & Videbeck, S. D. (1998). *Lippincott's manual of psychiatric nursing care plan* (5th ed.). Philadelphia: Lippincott-Raven.

Sugarman, L. (1986). *Life-span development: Concepts, theories and interventions.* London: Methuen & Co., Ltd.

Szasz, T. (1961). *The myth of mental illness.* New York: Hoeber-Harper.

Viscott, D. (1996). *Emotional resilience: Simple truths for dealing with the unfinished business of your past.* New York: Harmony Books.

Chapter Review

➤ MULTIPLE-CHOICE QUESTIONS

Select the best answer for each of the following questions.

1. Which of the following theorists believed that a corrective interpersonal relationship with the therapist was the primary mode of treatment?

   A. Sigmund Freud

   B. William Glasser

   C. Hildegard Peplau

   D. Harry Stack Sullivan

2. Dream analysis and free association are techniques for which of the following?

   A. Client-centered therapy

   B. Gestalt therapy

   C. Logotherapy

   D. Psychoanalysis

3. Four levels of anxiety were described by:

   A. Erik Erikson

   B. Sigmund Freud

   C. Hildegard Peplau

   D. Carl Rogers

4. Correcting how one thinks about the world and oneself is the focus of:

   A. Behaviorism

   B. Cognitive therapy

   C. Psychoanalysis

   D. Reality therapy

5. The personality structures of id, ego, and super-ego were described by:

   A. Sigmund Freud

   B. Hildegard Peplau

   C. Frederick Perls

   D. Harry Stack Sullivan

➤ TRUE-FALSE QUESTIONS

Identify each of the following statements as T (true) or F (false). Correct any false statements.

_____ 1. Sigmund Freud described three cognitive modes: prototaxic, parataxic, and syntaxic.

_____ 2. Psychiatric rehabilitation focuses on treating persons with medications.

_____ 3. Hildegard Peplau described the therapeutic nurse–patient relationship and its stages.

_____ 4. Repressed sexual energy as the driving force in personality development was conceived by Harry Stack Sullivan.

_____ 5. Transference refers to the feelings a nurse might develop toward a client.

_____ 6. The nursing role of teacher involves being a substitute for another, such as a parent.

_____ 7. Unconditional positive regard means the client is accepted without regard for his or her behavior.

_____

_____ 8. Behaviorists believe that behavior results from disturbed interpersonal relationships.

_____

➤ FILL-IN-THE-BLANK QUESTIONS

Write the name of the appropriate theorist beside the statement or theory. Names may be used more than once.

_____ 1. The client is the key to his or her own healing.

_____ 2. Social as well as psychological factors influence development.

_____ 3. Behavior change occurs by conditioning with environmental stimuli.

_____ 4. People make themselves unhappy by clinging to irrational beliefs.

_____ 5. Behavior is learned from past experience that is reinforcing.

_____ 6. Client-centered therapy

_____ 7. Gestalt therapy

_____ 8. Hierarchy of needs

_____ 9. Logotherapy

_____ 10. Rational emotive therapy

_____ 11. Reality therapy.

➤ SHORT-ANSWER QUESTIONS

Describe each of the following types of groups, and give an example.

1. Group psychotherapy

2. Education group

3. Support group

4. Self-help group

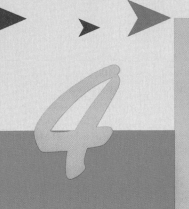

Treatment Settings and Therapeutic Programs

4

Learning Objectives

After reading this chapter, the student should be able to:

1. Discuss traditional treatment settings.

2. Describe different types of residential treatment settings and the services they provide.

3. Describe community treatment programs that provide services to persons with mental illness.

4. Identify barriers to effective treatment for homeless persons with mental illness.

5. Discuss the issues related to persons with mental illness in the criminal justice system.

6. Describe the roles of members of a multidisciplinary team.

7. Identify the different roles of the nurse in varied treatment settings and programs.

Key Terms

ACCESS demonstration project

assertive community treatment

case management

clubhouse model

criminalization of mental illness

evolving consumer household

multidisciplinary team

PACED model

partial hospitalization program

residential treatment setting

Mental health care has undergone profound changes in the past 50 years. Before the 1950s, humane treatment in large institutions was the best available strategy for persons with chronic and persistent mental illness. In the 1950s, psychotropic medications offered the first hope of treating the symptoms of mental illnesses. Large state facilities were filled with patients, many of whom stayed for months or years. In the 1970s, patients' rights decisions and changes in commitment laws led to deinstitutionalization and a new era of treatment (McGihon, 1999). People with mental illness could no longer be held indefinitely in institutions, and treatment in the "least restrictive environment" became a right of patients. This led to the emptying of large state hospitals with the belief that treatment in the community would replace much of state hospital inpatient care. However, adequate funding for community programs and treatment has not kept pace with the need for such programs (see Chap. 1).

Today, persons with mental illness are found in a variety of settings. Some are not in touch with needed treatment services at all and may find themselves homeless or in jail. This chapter describes the range of treatment settings that are available for persons with mental illness and the psychiatric rehabilitation programs that have been developed to meet the needs of persons with mental illness. The challenges of integrating persons with mental illness into the community are discussed in both of these sections. Two populations of people receiving inadequate treatment, those who are homeless or in jail, are also addressed. In addition, the multidisciplinary team, including the role of the nurse as a member of this team, is described. Finally, psychosocial nursing in public health and home care is discussed briefly.

TREATMENT SETTINGS

Inpatient Hospital Treatment

In the 1980s, inpatient psychiatric care was still a primary mode of treatment for persons with mental illness (McGihon, 1999). A typical psychiatric unit emphasized "talk therapy," or one-on-one interactions with staff, and milieu therapy, meaning the total environment and its effect on the client's treatment. Individual and group interactions focused on building trust, self-disclosure by patients to staff and each other, and active participation in groups. Effective milieu therapy required longer lengths of stay because the more stabilized patients helped provide structure and support for newly admitted, more acute patients (McGihon, 1999).

In the 1990s, the economics of health care began to change dramatically, and the length of stay decreased to just a few days. Most Americans are now insured under some form of managed care, which has changed inpatient treatment significantly. Managed care exerts cost-control measures such as recertification of admissions, utilization review, and case management (Mitchell & Reaghard, 1996). The growth of managed care has been associated with a declining number of admissions, shorter lengths of stay, reduced reimbursement, and increased acuity of inpatients (Brett et al., 1997). Therefore, clients are sicker when they are admitted and do not stay as long in the hospital.

THE PACED MODEL

McGihon (1999) maintains that inpatient hospital units need to change their approach to inpatient care if they are to be effective (that is, if they are to meet the clients' needs given the constraints on admission and length of stay). She believes that many units are still trying to function according to the milieu therapy approach, which is no longer practical or effective for inpatients. Today, inpatient units must provide rapid assessment, stabilization of symptoms, and discharge planning, and they must accomplish these goals quickly. To meet these goals, McGihon has proposed the **PACED model**, a patient-centered, multidisciplinary approach to a brief stay (Box 4-1).

Box 4-1

➤ The PACED Model for Inpatient Psychiatric Treatment

Patient-centered
Assessment and stabilization of symptoms, brought about by brief interventions, medication, and testing done in a timely manner
Case management, beginning at admission, formulating short-term treatment goals and planning follow-up care
Evaluation of outcomes
Discharge planning and follow-up within an integrated system of health care delivery

---

McGihon, N. N. (1999). Psychiatric nursing for the 21st century: The PACED model. Journal of Psychosocial Nursing, 37(10), 22–27.

Pacing treatment is one of the important concepts of this model. Clinicians must learn to help clients recognize symptoms, identify coping skills, and choose discharge supports. Once the client is safe and stable, long-term issues can be identified for the client to pursue in outpatient therapy. Box 4-2 gives appropriate treatment objectives for an inpatient stay. **Case management** is another crucial concept in this model. The case manager, most often a nurse or social worker, follows the patient from admission to discharge and serves as a liaison to community resources, home care, and third-party payers.

DISCHARGE PLANNING

The PACED model of care is not the only one that recognizes the importance of discharge planning. Gantt et al. (1999) wrote that "as the focus of inpatient psychiatric care shifts to an emphasis on quick resolution of acute symptoms, and rapid transfer to stepdown, less costly treatment interventions, the role of discharge planning has become even more central" (p. 2). Environmental supports, such as housing and transportation, and access to community resources and services are crucial to successful discharge planning. In fact, the adequacy of these discharge plans was a better predictor of the length of time the person could remain in the community than clinical indicators such as psychiatric diagnosis (Caton & Gralnick, 1987).

Impediments to successful discharge planning include alcohol and drug abuse, criminal or violent behavior, noncompliance with medication, and suicidal ideation (Gantt et al., 1999). In other words, optimal housing is often not available to persons with a recent history of drug or alcohol abuse or a criminal history. Also, persons who still had suicidal ideas or had a history of noncompliance with medication were ineligible for some treatment programs or services. The study found that persons with these impediments to successful discharge planning often had a marginal discharge plan in place because optimal

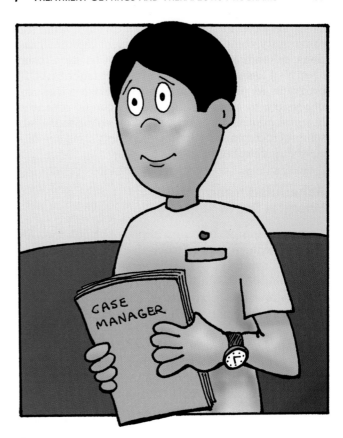

Case manager

services or plans were not available to them. Consequently, people discharged with marginal plans were readmitted more quickly and more frequently than those who had better discharge plans.

Creating successful discharge plans that offer optimal services and housing is essential if persons with mental illness are to be integrated into the community. Gibson (1999) wrote that a holistic approach to reintegrating persons into the community is the only way that repeated hospital admissions can be avoided and that quality of life for clients can be improved. She maintains that community programs after discharge from the hospital should emphasize social services, day treatment, and housing programs.

Box 4-2

➤ PATIENT OBJECTIVES FOR INPATIENT TREATMENT IN THE PACED MODEL

The patient will:
- Identify three ways to manage current symptoms
- Identify three relapse triggers and ways to avoid them
- Establish a timeline for addressing underlying or long-term issues safely in outpatient therapy
- Become knowledgeable about recommended medication and decide with the provider on a course of treatment
- Select three resources in the community that will help maintain recovery after discharge
- Establish contacts with those resources and make appointments for first 2 weeks of follow-up care.

McGihon, N. N. (1999). Psychiatric nursing for the 21st century: The PACED model. Journal of Psychiatric Nursing, 37(10), 22–27.

These services must be geared toward survival in the community, compliance with treatment recommendations, rehabilitation, and independent living. Gibson identified **assertive community treatment** (ACT) programs as providing most of the services that are necessary to stop the revolving door of repeated hospital admissions, punctuated by unsuccessful attempts at community living. ACT programs are discussed in detail later in this chapter.

Scheduled Intermittent Hospital Stays

A unique approach to providing inpatient care for persons who seek it is scheduled, intermittent inpatient hospital stays (Dilonardo et al., 1998). A study conducted in a Veterans Administration hospital followed two groups of persons with severe and persistent mental illness who were frequently admitted to the hospital. One group had predetermined, scheduled admissions to the inpatient unit over a period of 2 years; the other group used hospital admission during crises, as they had been doing. At the end of the 2 years, the number of hospital stays for the two groups was similar, but there were remarkable differences: the group with scheduled admissions had higher self-esteem, greater feelings of control over their lives, and fewer negative symptoms and physical symptoms than the other group. The authors suggested that the group with crisis admission perceived coming to the hospital as a failure, whereas the scheduled admissions group saw admission as successful implementation of their treatment plan. The authors believe that inpatient care is important in the continuum of services, and that scheduled admissions might be an alternative way to deliver inpatient care to those who continue to need it.

Partial Hospitalization Programs

Partial hospitalization programs (PHP) are designed to help clients make a gradual transition from being an inpatient to living independently and to prevent repeat admissions (Pittman et al., 1990). In day treatment programs, clients return home at night; evening programs are just the reverse. The services offered vary from one program to another, but most include groups for building communication and social skills, problem solving, medication monitoring or management, and education. Individual sessions are available in some PHPs, as well as vocational assistance and occupational and recreation therapy.

Each client has an individualized treatment plan and goals, which are developed with the client, the case manager, and other members of the treatment team. Eight broad categories of goals usually addressed in PHPs (Swearingen, 1987) are:
- Stabilizing psychiatric symptoms
- Monitoring drug effectiveness
- Stabilizing living environment
- Improving activities of daily living
- Learning to structure time
- Developing social skills
- Obtaining meaningful work, paid employment, or a volunteer position
- Providing follow-up of any health concerns.

Clients in PHPs may complete the program after an inpatient hospital stay, which is usually too short to address anything other than stabilization of symptoms and medication effectiveness. Other clients may come to a PHP to treat problems earlier, thus avoiding a costly and unwanted hospital stay. Others may make the transition from a PHP to longer-term outpatient therapy. Wilberg et al. (1999) reported that completion of a day treatment program was effective in stabilizing symptoms and improving daily functioning, and it encouraged poorly functioning clients with personality disorders to participate in outpatient therapy. Pittman et al. (1990) found that day treatment for clients with severe and persistent mental illness prevented hospital admission and improved the quality of clients' lives with respect to socialization, structure, and support.

Residential Settings

Persons with mental illness may live in community **residential treatment settings** that vary according to structure, level of supervision, and services provided. Some settings are designed as transitional housing, with the expectation that residents will progress to more independent living. Other residential programs serve clients for as long as the need exists, sometimes for years. Board and care homes often provide a room, bathroom and laundry facilities, and one common meal a day. Adult foster homes may care for one to three clients in a family-like atmosphere, including meals and social activities with the family. Halfway houses usually serve as a temporary placement that provides support as the client prepares for independence. Group homes house six to ten residents who take turns cooking meals and share household chores under the supervision of one or two staff persons. Independent living programs are often housed in an apartment complex, where clients share an apartment. Staff are available for crisis intervention, transportation, assistance with daily living tasks, and sometimes drug monitoring. In addition to on-site staff, many residential settings provide case management services for clients and put them in touch with other programs (e.g., vocational rehabilitation, medical, dental, and psychiatric care, or psychosocial rehabilitation programs or services) as needed.

Boydell et al. (1999) found that a client's living environment affected his or her level of functioning, rate of reinstitutionalization, and the length of time he or she could remain in the community setting. In fact, the living environment was more predictive of the client's success than were the characteristics of his or her illness. A client who had a poor living environment in the community would leave the community or would be readmitted to the hospital. This study showed the need for finding quality living situations for clients, an often difficult task. Boydell et al. found that many clients found themselves living in crime-ridden or commercial, rather than residential, areas.

Frequently, residents oppose plans to establish a group home or residential facility in their neighborhood. They argue that having a group home will decrease their property values, and they may believe that persons with mental illness are violent, act bizarrely in public, or will be a menace to their children. These people have strongly ingrained stereotypes and a great deal of misinformation. Local residents must be given the facts so that safe, affordable, and desirable housing can be established for persons needing residential care.

Evolving Consumer Households

The **evolving consumer household** (ECH) is a group living situation in which the residents will make the transition from a traditional group home to a residence where they fulfill their own responsibilities and function without on-site supervision from paid staff (Ware, 1999). This concept was developed as part of the Boston McKinney Research Demonstration Project in the early 1990s, sponsored by the National Institute of Mental Health. One of the problems with housing for persons with mental illness is that they may have to move many times, from one type of setting to another, as their independence increases. This continual moving necessitates readjustment in each setting, making it difficult for clients to sustain their gains in independence. Because the ECH is a permanent living arrangement, the problem of relocation is eliminated.

During the demonstration project, it was found that poverty among persons with mental illness was a significant barrier to maintaining housing. This barrier is seldom addressed in psychiatric rehabilitation (Ware & Goldfinger, 1997). Residents often rely on government entitlements, such as Social Security insurance (SSI) or Social Security disability insurance (SSDI), for their income, which averages $400 to $450 per month. Although many clients express the desire to work, many cannot do so consistently. Even

with vocational services, jobs tend to be unskilled and part-time, resulting in income that is inadequate to maintain independent living. In addition, the SSI system is often a disincentive to making the transition to paid employment: the client would have to trade a reliable source of income and much-needed health insurance for a poorly paying, relatively insecure job that is unlikely to include fringe benefits (Ware & Goldfinger, 1997). The authors believed that poverty among persons with mental illness must be addressed both in psychiatric rehabilitation programs and at the societal level to remove this barrier to independent living and self-sufficiency.

PSYCHIATRIC REHABILITATION PROGRAMS

Psychiatric rehabilitation, sometimes called psychosocial rehabilitation, refers to services designed to promote the recovery process for persons with mental illness (Box 4-3). This recovery goes beyond symptom control and medication management to include personal growth, reintegration into the community, empowerment, increased independence, and improved quality of life (Wilbur & Arns, 1998). Community support programs and services provide psychiatric rehabilitation to varying degrees, often depending on the resources and funding available for such programs. Some programs focus primarily on reducing hospital readmissions through symptom control and medication management, whereas others include social and recreation services. There are not enough programs available nationwide to meet the needs of persons with mental illness.

Box 4-3

> ## GOALS OF PSYCHIATRIC REHABILITATION

- Recovery from mental illness
- Personal growth
- Quality of life
- Community reintegration
- Empowerment
- Increased independence
- Decreased hospital admissions
- Improved social functioning
- Improved vocational functioning
- Continuous treatment
- Increased involvement in treatment decisions.

Adapted from Wilbur, S., & Arns, P. (1998). Psychosocial rehabilitation nurses. Journal of Psychosocial Nursing, 36(4), 33–41; and Hughes, W. C. (1999). Managed care, meet community support. Health & Social Work, 24(2), 103–110.

Hughes (1999) stated that the likelihood of achieving even minimal treatment goals is unlikely without a broad array of psychosocial, vocational, and housing services, even though these services are typically not included under the "medically necessary" services that are funded under managed care. He identified ten reasons why community support should be included in comprehensive services for persons with mental illness (Box 4-4).

Psychiatric rehabilitation has improved client outcomes by providing community support services to decrease hospital readmission rates and increase community integration (Mallik et al., 1998). At the same time, managed care has reduced the "medically necessary" services that will be funded. For example, because skills training was found to be successful in assisting clients in the community, managed care organizations defined psychiatric rehabilitation as *only* skills training and did not fund other aspects of rehabilitation, such as socialization or environmental supports. Clients and providers identified poverty, lack of jobs, and inadequate vocational skills as barriers to community integration, but because these barriers were not included in the "medically necessary" definition of psychiatric rehabilitation by managed care, services to overcome these barriers were not funded (Mallik et al., 1998).

Clubhouse Model

In 1948, Fountain House pioneered the **clubhouse model** of community-based rehabilitation in New York City. Currently, more than 350 such clubhouses have been established worldwide (Aquila et al., 1999). Fountain House is an "intentional community" based on the belief that men and women from serious and persistent psychiatric disability can and will achieve normal life goals when given opportunity, time, support, and fellowship. The essence of membership in the clubhouse is based on the four guaranteed rights of members: a place to come to, meaningful work, meaningful relationships, and a place to return to (lifetime membership).

The clubhouse provides members with many opportunities, including daytime work activities focused on the care, maintenance, and productivity of

---

Box 4-4

➤ TEN REASONS TO INCLUDE COMMUNITY SUPPORT IN EVERY BEHAVIORAL HEALTH PLAN

1. **Decreased hospitalization means lower cost of care.** Clients who have access to more intensive support are less likely to decompensate to a point where they require inpatient hospitalization.
2. **Normalization.** Clients respond favorably to community interactions that are more "normal" and not directly treatment-related, such as pursuing a hobby or joining the YMCA or YWCA with the help of their community support worker.
3. **Linkage to resources.** Community support workers can identify and access resources for the client when he or she may be unable to do so.
4. **Effective advocacy.** Community support workers can confront individuals or institutions in a professional manner to resolve any attempts to prevent a client from reaching goals.
5. **Improved quality of life.** Because clients often survive on SSI benefits, they need assistance to access such services as food pantries, energy grants, and weatherization programs to help make ends meet.
6. **Respite for natural caregivers.** Community support workers can arrange doctor's appointments and lab work, pick up drugs, and monitor compliance with medications to alleviate the stress of these tasks on the client's caregiver. They also can provide direct support and information to caregivers to make their tasks easier.
7. **Consolidated funding.** Services in the community are often provided and funded by a variety of programs and agencies. Community support workers can advocate for the enhancement of community support services and improved, adequate funding of these services.
8. **Equalization of a two-tiered system.** Private sector mental health care is often limited when the illness is persistent and severe. Consequently, clients revert to care provided through public funds. All payers, public or private, could benefit from community support programs to promote wellness and manage crises or serious mental illness.
9. **Flexibility.** Community support employs a variety of persons at different skill levels to provide assistance with everything from daily activities to psychiatric care, depending on the needs of the client.
10. **Continuum of care.** Community support provides the opportunity for clients to move along a continuum of services without repeated transfers to different programs with unfamiliar staff.

Hughes, W. C. (1999). Managed care, meet community support. Health & Social Work, 24 *(2), 103–110.*

the clubhouse; evening, weekend, and holiday leisure activities; transitional and independent employment support and efforts; and housing options. Members are encouraged and assisted to use psychiatric services, usually local clinics or private practitioners.

The clubhouse model recognizes the physician–patient relationship as a key to successful treatment and rehabilitation while acknowledging that brief encounters that focus on symptom management are not sufficient to promote rehabilitation efforts. The "rehabilitation alliance" refers to the network of relationships that needs to develop over time to support people with psychiatric disabilities. This alliance includes the client, family and friends, clinicians, and even landlords, employers, and neighbors. The rehabilitation alliance needs community support, opportunities for success, coordination of service providers, and involvement of the member so that a positive focus on life goals, strengths, creativity, and hope can be maintained as the member pursues recovery. The clubhouse model exists to promote the rehabilitation alliance as a positive force in the member's life.

The clubhouse focus is on health, not illness. Taking prescribed drugs, for example, is not a condition of participation in the clubhouse. The member, not the staff, must ultimately make decisions about treatment, such as whether hospital admission is needed. Clubhouse staff support members, help them obtain needed assistance, and most of all allow them to make the decisions that ultimately affect them in all aspects of their lives. This approach to psychiatric

rehabilitation is the cornerstone and the strength of the clubhouse model.

Assertive Community Treatment

One of the most effective approaches to community-based treatment for persons with mental illness is assertive community treatment (ACT) (Box 4-5). Marx, Test, and Stein conceived this idea in 1973 in Madison, Wisconsin, while working at Mendota State Hospital. They believed that skills training, support, and teaching should be done in the community, where it was needed, rather than in the hospital. Their program was first known as the Madison model, then "training in community living," and finally assertive community treatment or the program for assertive treatment. The mobile outreach and continuous treatment programs of today all have their roots in the Madison model (Hughes, 1999).

An ACT program has a problem-solving orientation; staff members attend to specific life issues, no matter how mundane. Most services are provided directly rather than relying on referrals to other programs or agencies, and they take place in the client's home or community, not in an office. The ACT services are also intense; three or more face-to-face contacts with clients are tailored to meet clients' needs. The team approach allows all staff to be equally familiar with all clients, so clients do not have to wait for an assigned person. ACT programs also make a long-term commitment to clients, providing services

---

Box 4-5

> ## COMPONENTS OF AN ACT PROGRAM

- Having a multidisciplinary team that includes a psychiatrist, psychiatric-mental health nurse, vocational rehabilitation specialist, and a social worker for each 100 clients (low staff–client ratio)
- Identifying a fixed point of responsibility for clients with a primary provider of services
- Ameliorating or eliminating the debilitating symptoms of mental illness
- Improving client functioning in adult social and employment roles and activities
- Decreasing the family's burden of care by providing opportunities for clients to learn skills in real-life situations
- Implementing an individualized, ongoing treatment program defined by client's needs
- Involving all needed support systems for holistic treatment of clients
- Promoting mental health through the use of a vast array of resources and treatment modalities
- Emphasizing and promoting client independence
- Using daily team meetings to discuss strategies to improve the care of clients
- Providing services 24 hours a day that would include respite care to deflect unnecessary hospitalization and crisis intervention to prevent destabilization with unnecessary emergency department visits
- Client outcomes are measured on the following aspects: symptomatology; social, psychological, and familial functioning; gainful employment; client independence; client empowerment; use of ancillary services; client, family, and societal satisfaction; hospital use; agency use; rehospitalization; quality of life; and costs.

De Cangas, J. (1997). Characteristics of assertive case management systems. http://www.mohan.com/services.html

for as long as the need persists, with no time constraints (McGrew et al., 1996). When participants were asked which components of ACT were most satisfying to them, they identified staff availability, home visits, and help with everyday problems (McGrew et al., 1996).

Fekete et al. (1998) studied the effectiveness of ACT programs in rural areas; ACT programs was developed and had flourished in urban settings. Services are more limited and fragmented in rural areas and are more difficult to obtain than in cities. Fekete et al. noted that although 20% of the U.S. population is rural, 33% of the poor population is rural. Therefore, rural areas have less money to fund services. Further, in rural areas there is a greater social stigma about mental illness and a higher percentage of negative attitudes about public service programs. The study found that ACT programs were successful in rural areas and resulted in fewer hospital admissions, greater housing stability, an improved quality of life, and improved psychiatric symptoms. This success occurred even though certain modifications of traditional ACT programs were required, such as two-person teams, fewer and shorter contacts with clients, and minimal participation from some disciplines.

SPECIAL POPULATIONS OF PERSONS WITH MENTAL ILLNESS

Homeless

Homeless persons with mental illness have been the focus of recent studies. For this population, shelters, rehabilitation programs, and prisons may serve as a makeshift alternative to inpatient care or supportive housing (Haugland et al., 1997). The marginal existence of this population is worsened by frequent shifts between the street, programs, and institutions. Compared with homeless persons without mental illness, the mentally ill homeless are homeless longer, spend more time in shelters, have less family contact, spend more time in jail, and face greater barriers to employment (Haugland et al., 1997). For this population, professionals supercede families as the primary source of help.

Providing housing alone does not significantly alter the prognosis (Dickey et al., 1996). In a study conducted in Boston, homeless persons with mental illness were given permanent housing in a apartment or an ECH, access to mental health treatment, and specialized social services. There was no difference in the housing stability of the two groups based on the type of residence. Both groups significantly increased their housing stability and use of mental health treatment services. Similarly, Shern et al. (1997) followed

896 homeless mentally ill adults in four major cities. By providing stable community housing, community support, and rehabilitation services, 78% of the participants were housed stably at the 12- to 24-month final follow-up. The success of projects such as these suggest that it is possible to make significant differences in the lives of mentally ill homeless by providing active psychiatric rehabilitation services along with housing alternatives.

The **Access to Community Care and Effective Services and Support (ACCESS) Demonstration Project** was initiated in 1994 by the Center for Mental Health Services to assess whether more integrated systems of service delivery enhance the quality of life of homeless people with serious mental disabilities through the use of services and outreach. ACCESS was a 5-year demonstration program with locations in 18 communities of 15 U.S. cities, representing most geographic areas of the continental United States (Chinman et al., 1999). Each site provides outreach and intensive case management to 100 homeless people with severe mental illnesses every year.

Participants in the first 2 years of the ACCESS demonstration project were surveyed to determine whether they had formed a relationship with their assigned case manager and what, if any, differences they experienced in terms of homelessness, symptom management, and use of substances. A total of 2,798 participants completed the survey process. Only 48% reported having a relationship or personal connection with their case manager, underscoring the difficulty in establishing a therapeutic relationship with the homeless mentally ill. Clients reporting such a relationship described more social support, received more public support and education, were less psychotic, were homeless fewer days, and were intoxicated fewer days than participants who reported having no relationship with their assigned case manager. Although it is difficult to engage this population in a therapeutic relationship, results are positive when that relationship is established. More reports from the ACCESS demonstration project will be forthcoming in future years.

Prisoners

Clinical studies suggest that 6% to 15% of persons in city and county jails and 10% to 15% of persons in state prisons have severe mental illness (Lamb & Weinberger, 1998). These offenders generally have acute and chronic mental illness and poor functioning, and many are homeless. Factors cited as reasons why mentally ill persons are placed in the criminal justice system include deinstitutionalization, more rigid cri-

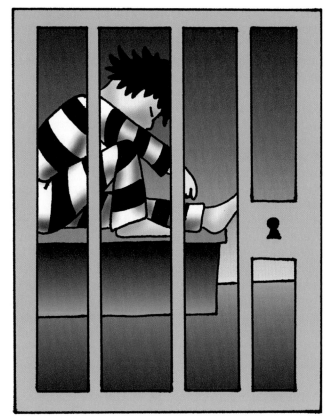

City and county jails

ment had been obtained, some persons with mental illness may not have engaged in criminal activity.

The public concern about the potential danger of persons with mental illness is fueled by the media attention that surrounds any violent criminal act committed by a mentally ill person. Although it is true that persons with major mental illnesses who do not take prescribed medication are more likely to be violent (Lamb & Weinberger, 1998), most persons with mental illness do not represent a significant danger to others. However, this does not keep citizens from clinging to stereotypes of the mentally ill as people to be feared, avoided, and institutionalized. If such persons cannot be confined in a mental hospital for any period, there seems to be public support for arresting and incarcerating them as an alternative.

Persons with mental illness who are in the criminal justice system face several barriers to successful community reintegration, according to Roskes et al. (1999) (Box 4-6).

Lamb and Weinberger (1998) made several recommendations to prevent or alleviate the urgent problem of mentally ill persons in the criminal justice system:

- Provide a mental health consultation to police in the field to provide mental health treatment, rather than incarceration, for those who need it
- Provide formal training of police officers to help them recognize mental illness and to improve their attitudes toward mentally ill persons
- Perform careful screening of incoming prisoners to provide treatment, including medication, when needed
- Encourage the diversion of mentally ill persons who have committed minor offenses to the mental health system

teria for civil commitment, lack of adequate community support, and the attitudes of police and society (Lamb & Weinberger, 1998). The phrase **criminalization of mental illness** refers to the practice of arresting and prosecuting mentally ill offenders, even for misdemeanors, at a rate four times that of the general population in an effort to contain them in some type of institution where they might receive needed treatment. The authors noted that if needed treat-

---

Box 4-6

▶ BARRIERS TO SUCCESSFUL COMMUNITY REINTEGRATION

- **Double stigma:** Individuals are stigmatized as being "cons" as well as enduring the stigma of mental illness.
- **Lack of family or social support:** Offenders are often estranged from family members even more so than clients with mental illness who are not in jail, and they have few or no friends to provide social support.
- **Comorbidity:** Substance abuse is a problem for most of the mentally ill offenders in the program sponsored by the authors, and 50% have severe chronic or subacute medical illnesses.
- **Adjustment problems:** Many offenders report difficulty readjusting to living in the community after a prison term, including a lack of support in the community.
- **Boundary issues:** Offenders often view any person, including psychiatrists or other health professionals, as being an extension of correctional staff. This makes trust very difficult.

Roskes, E., Feldman, R., Arrington, S., & Leisher, M. (1999). A model program for the treatment of mentally ill offenders in the community. Community Mental Health Journal, 35(5), 461–475.

- Implement assertive case management (ACT programs) to provide outreach services in the community
- Provide social control interventions, such as outpatient commitment, court-ordered treatment, psychiatric conservatorship, or 24-hour structured care, as conditions of probation for persons who do not voluntarily accept treatment or services
- Ensure involvement of, and support for, families
- Provide appropriate mental health treatment.

Some programs for mentally ill persons who have committed crimes have been successful. Kravitz and Kelly (1999) described a mandatory forensic outpatient program for mentally ill offenders who were found not guilty by reason of insanity. Since they enrolled in the program, 47% were admitted to the hospital at least once, and 19% were rearrested or had committed a new crime. With respect to psychiatric stability, only 24% were in full remission, and 68% showed at least one indicator of difficulty reintegrating into the community. The authors suggested that although successful outcomes often include decreased hospital admission rates, inpatient care may be a positive outcome for this population.

Johnson and Hickey (1999) studied the criminal justice involvement of offenders with mental illness who participated in a clubhouse-type psychosocial rehabilitation program. The extent of criminal justice involvement diminished but was not completely eliminated for clubhouse participants. They had fewer arrests and incarcerations than they had before psychosocial rehabilitation. In some cases, the reduction in criminal justice involvement did not continue long after clubhouse participation ended. The study has positive implications for involving offenders with mental illness in ongoing psychosocial rehabilitation as a way to decrease involvement in the criminal justice system.

Roskes et al. (1999) proposed a model of working with mentally ill offenders that calls for a collaborative working relationship between a community mental health center and a probation office. On release from incarceration, each offender is assigned to a parole officer and a psychiatrist, who work with the offender to avoid rearrest or parole violation and to obtain needed mental health services. Their results were anecdotal in nature, but they had success in diverting many long-term offenders from the criminal justice system and into mental health services.

MULTIDISCIPLINARY TEAM

Regardless of the treatment setting, rehabilitation program, or population, a **multidisciplinary team** approach is most useful in dealing with the multi-faceted problems of persons with mental illness. Different members of the team have expertise in specific areas, and by collaborating they can meet clients' needs more effectively. Members of the multidisciplinary (or interdisciplinary) team include the psychiatrist, psychologist, psychiatric nurse, psychiatric social worker, occupational therapist, recreation therapist, and vocational rehabilitation specialist. Their primary roles are described in Box 4-7. Not all settings have a full-time member from each discipline on their team; the programs and services the team offers determine its composition in any setting.

The role of the case manager has become increasingly important with the proliferation of managed care and the variety of services needed by clients. However, there is no standard formal educational program to become a case manager, and people from many different backgrounds may fill this role. In some settings, a social worker or psychiatric nurse may be the case manager. In other settings, persons who work in psychosocial rehabilitation settings may take on the role of case manager with a baccalaureate degree in a related field, such as psychology, or by virtue of their experience and demonstrated skills.

As clients' needs become more varied and complex, the psychiatric nurse is in an ideal position to fulfill the role of case manager. In 1994, the American Nurses Association stated that the psychiatric nurse can assess, monitor, and refer clients for general medical problems, as well as psychiatric problems; administer drugs; monitor for drug side effects; provide drug and patient and family health education; and monitor for general medical disorders that have psychological and physiologic components. Registered nurses bring unique nursing knowledge and skills to the multidisciplinary team (Wilbur & Arns, 1998).

PSYCHOSOCIAL NURSING IN PUBLIC HEALTH AND HOME CARE

Psychosocial nursing is an important area of public health nursing practice (Collins & Diego, 2000) and home care. Public health nurses working in the community provide mental health prevention services to reduce risks to the mental health of persons, families, and communities. Examples include primary prevention, such as stress management education; secondary prevention, such as early identification of potential mental health problems; and tertiary prevention, such as monitoring and coordinating rehabilitation services for the mentally ill.

The clinical practice of public health and home care nurses includes caring for clients and families with issues such as substance abuse, domestic violence, child abuse, grief, and depression. In addition,

> Box 4-7

> ➤ MULTIDISCIPLINARY TEAM PRIMARY ROLES

- **Psychiatrist:** Certification of a physician in psychiatry by the American Board of Psychiatry and Neurology requires a 3-year residency, 2 years of clinical practice, and completion of an examination. The primary function of the psychiatrist is diagnosis of mental disorders and prescription of medical treatments.
- **Psychologist:** The clinical psychologist has a doctorate (Ph.D.) in clinical psychology and is prepared to practice therapy, conduct research, and interpret psychological tests. Psychologists may also participate in the design of therapy programs for groups of individuals.
- **Psychiatric nurse:** The registered nurse gains experience in working with psychiatric clients after graduation from an accredited program of nursing and completion of the licensure examination. The nurse has a solid foundation in health promotion, illness prevention, and rehabilitation in all areas, allowing him or her to view the client holistically. The nurse is also an essential team member in evaluating the effectiveness of medical treatment, particularly medications. Registered nurses who obtain a master's degree in mental health may be certified as clinical specialists or licensed as advanced practitioners, depending on individual state nurse practice acts. Advanced practice nurses are certified to prescribe drugs in many states.
- **Psychiatric social worker:** Most psychiatric social workers are prepared at the master's level, and they are licensed in some states. Social workers may practice therapy and often have the primary responsibility for working with families, community support, and referral.
- **Occupational therapist:** Occupational therapists may have an associate degree (certified occupational therapy assistant) or a baccalaureate degree (certified occupational therapist). Occupational therapy focuses on the functional abilities of the client and ways to improve client functioning, such as working with arts and crafts and focusing on psychomotor skills.
- **Recreation therapist:** Many recreation therapists complete a baccalaureate degree, but in some instances persons with experience fulfill these roles. The recreation therapist helps the client to achieve a balance of work and play in his or her life and provides activities that promote constructive use of leisure or unstructured time.
- **Vocational rehabilitation specialist:** Vocational rehabilitation includes determining clients' interests and abilities and matching them with vocational choices. Clients are also assisted in job-seeking and job-retention skills, as well as pursuit of further education if that is needed and desired. Vocational rehabilitation specialists can be prepared at the baccalaureate or master's level and may have different levels of autonomy and program supervision based on their education.

public health nurses care for children in schools and teach health-related subjects to community groups and agencies. Mental health services provided by public health and home care nurses can reduce the suffering that many people experience as a result of physical disease, mental disorders, social and emotional disadvantages, and other vulnerabilities.

SELF-AWARENESS ISSUES

Psychiatric-mental health nursing is evolving as changes continue to occur in health care. The focus is shifting from traditional hospital-based goals of symptom and medication management to more client-centered goals, which include improved quality of life and recovery from mental illness. Therefore, the nurse must also expand his or her repertoire of skills and abilities to assist clients in their efforts. These challenges may overwhelm the nurse at times, and he or she may feel underprepared or ill equipped to meet them.

Mental health services are moving into some nontraditional settings, such as jails and homeless shelters. As nursing roles expand in these alternative settings, the nurse does not have the array of backup services found in a hospital or clinic, such as on-site physicians and colleagues, medical services, and so forth. This requires the nurse to practice in a more autonomous and independent manner, which can be unsettling.

Empowering clients to make their own decisions about treatment is an essential part of full recovery. This differs from the model of the psychiatrist or treatment team as the authority on what is the best course for the client to follow. It is a challenge for the nurse to be supportive to the client when the nurse believes the client has made choices that are less than ideal.

The nurse may experience frustration when working with mentally ill adults who are homeless, incarcerated, or both. Typically, these clients are difficult to engage in a therapeutic relationship and may present great challenges to the nurse. The nurse may feel rejected by clients who do not engage readily in a relationship, or the nurse may feel inadequate in attempts to engage these clients.

Helpful Hints for the Nurse Working with Clients in Expanded, Community-Based Settings

- The client can make mistakes, survive them, and learn from them. This is a part of normal life for everyone, and it is not the nurse's role to protect clients from such experiences.
- The nurse will not always have the answer to solve a client's problems or resolve a difficult situation.
- As clients move toward recovery, they need support to make decisions and follow a course of action, even if the nurse thinks the client is making decisions that are not likely to be successful.
- Working with clients in community settings is a more collaborative relationship than the traditional role of caring for the client. The nurse may be more familiar and comfortable with the latter.

➤ KEY POINTS

- Persons with mental illness are found in a variety of settings, and some are not in touch with needed services at all.
- Shortened inpatient hospital stays necessitate changes in the ways hospitals deliver services to clients.
- The PACED model of inpatient care is a client-centered approach that uses a multidisciplinary approach to brief hospital stays.

The model includes rapid assessment, stabilization of symptoms, and discharge planning.

- Adequate discharge planning is a good indicator of how successful the client's community placement will be.
- Impediments to successful discharge planning include alcohol and drug abuse, criminal or violent behavior, noncompliance with medications, and suicidal ideation.
- Partial hospitalization programs, or day and evening treatment programs, are designed to help clients make a gradual transition from the hospital to community life and to prevent repeat admission.
- Partial hospitalization programs usually address the client's psychiatric symptoms, medication use, living environment, activities of daily living, leisure time, social skills, work, and health concerns.
- Community residential settings vary in terms of structure, level of supervision, and services provided. Some residential settings are transitional, with the expectation that clients will progress to independent living; others serve the client for as long as he or she needs.
- Types of residential settings include board and care homes, adult foster homes, halfway houses, group homes, and independent living programs.

INTERNET RESOURCES

Resource	Internet Address
▶ National Rehabilitation Information Center	http://www.naric.com/naric
▶ National Association for Home Care	http://www.nahc.org/
▶ Center for Mental Health Services	http://www.samhsa.gov/cmhs.htm
▶ Knowledge Exchange Network	http://www.mentalhealth.org/
▶ Homeless Handbook	http://www.infoxchange.net.au/hhb
▶ Homes for the Homeless	http://www.opendoor.com/hfh/
▶ National Law Center on Homelessness and Poverty	http://www.nlchp.org/

Critical Thinking

1. Discuss the role of the nurse in advocating for social or legislative policy changes needed to provide psychiatric rehabilitation services for clients in all settings.
2. When are programs for special populations, such as mentally ill adults who are offenders or homeless, considered successful?
3. What is an acceptable target for recidivism among the mentally ill offender population?
4. Is finding stable housing for 50% of homeless clients a sign of a successful program?

- A client's ability to remain in the community is closely related to the quality and adequacy of his or her living environment.
- The evolving consumer household is a group living situation in which the residents will make the transition from a traditional group home to a residence where they fulfill their own responsibilities and function without on-site supervision from paid staff.
- Poverty among persons with mental illness is a significant barrier to maintaining housing in the community and is seldom addressed in psychiatric rehabilitation.
- Psychiatric rehabilitation refers to services designed to promote the recovery process for clients with mental illness. This recovery goes beyond symptom control and medication management to include personal growth, reintegration into the community, empowerment, increased independence, and improved quality of life.
- The likelihood of achieving even minimal treatment goals is unlikely without a broad array of psychosocial, vocational, and housing services, even though these services are not typically included as "medically necessary" services that are funded under managed care.
- The clubhouse model of psychosocial rehabilitation is an intentional community based on the belief that men and women with mental illness can and will achieve normal life goals when provided time, opportunity, support, and fellowship.
- Assertive community treatment is one of the most effective approaches to community-based treatment. It includes 24-hour-a-day services, low staff–client ratios, in-home or community services, intense and frequent contact, and unlimited length of service.
- Psychiatric rehabilitation services such as ACT must be provided along with stable housing to produce positive outcomes for mentally ill adults who are homeless.
- Adults with mental illness may be placed in the criminal justice system more frequently due to deinstitutionalization, rigid criteria for civil commitment, lack of adequate support, and the attitudes of police and society.
- Barriers to community reintegration for mentally ill persons who have been incarcerated include double stigma, lack of family or social support, comorbidity, adjustment problems, and boundary issues.
- Recommendations to address the problem of mentally ill persons in the criminal justice system include mental health field consultation and formal education for police, screening of new prisoners, diversion to mental health for minor offenses, ACT programs, provision of treatment and family support, and social control interventions such as outpatient commitment, court-ordered treatment, psychiatric conservatorship, or 24-hour structured care as a condition of release.
- The multidisciplinary team includes the psychiatrist, psychologist, psychiatric nurse, psychiatric social worker, occupational therapist, recreation therapist, and vocational rehabilitation specialist.
- The psychiatric nurse is in an ideal position to fulfill the role of case manager. The nurse can assess, monitor, and refer clients for general medical and psychiatric problems; administer drugs; monitor for drug side effects; provide drug and patient and family health education; and monitor for general medical disorders that have psychological and physiologic components.
- Psychosocial nursing is an important area of public health nursing practice and home care.
- The nurse may feel overwhelmed by challenges as mental health services move into alternative settings such as jails and homeless shelters.
- Empowering clients to pursue full recovery requires a collaborative working relationship with the client, rather than the traditional approach of caring for the client.

REFERENCES

Aquila, R., Santos, G. Malamud, T. J., & McCrory, D. (1999). The rehabilitation alliance in practice: The clubhouse connection. *Psychiatric Rehabilitation Journal, 23*(1), 19–23.

Boydell, K. M., Gladstone, B. M., Crawford, E., & Trainor, J. (1999). Making do on the outside: Everyday life in the neighborhoods of people with psychiatric disabilities. *Psychiatric Rehabilitation Journal, 23*(1), 11–17.

Brett, J., Bueno, M., Royal, N., & Kendall-Sengin, K. (1997). Integrating utilization management, discharge planning, and nursing case management into the outcomes management role. *Journal of Nursing Administration, 27*(2), 37–45.

Caton, C., & Gralnick, A. (1987). A review of issues surrounding length of psychiatric hospitalization. *Hospital and Community Psychiatry, 38*, 858–863.

Chinman, M. J., Rosenheck, R., & Lam, J. A. (1999). The development of relationships between people who are homeless and have a mental disability and their case managers. *Psychiatric Rehabilitation Journal, 23*(1), 47–55.

Collins, A. M., & Diego, L. (2000). Mental health promotion and protection. *Journal of Psychosocial Nursing, 38*(1), 27–32.

De Cangas, J. (1997). Characteristics of assertive case management systems. (Lakehead University). *http://www.mohan.com/services.html*

Dickey, B., Gonzalez, O., Latimer, E., Powers, K., Schutt, R., & Goldfinger, S. (1996). Use of mental health services by formerly homeless adults residing in group and independent housing. *Psychiatric Services, 47*(2), 152–158.

Dilonardo, J. D., Connely, C. E., Gurel, L., Kendrick, K., & Deutsch, S. I. (1998). Scheduled intermittent hospitalization for psychiatric patients. *Psychiatric Services, 49*(4), 504–509.

Fekete, D. M., Bond, G. R., McDonel, E. C., Salyers, M., Chen, A., & Miller, L. (1998). Rural assertive community treatment: A field experiment. *Psychiatric Rehabilitation Journal, 21*(4), 371–379.

Gantt, A. B., Cohen, N. L., & Saintz, A. (1999). Impediments to the discharge planning effort for psychiatric inpatients. *Social Work in Health Care, 29*(1), 1–14.

Gibson, D. M. (1999). Reduced hospitalizations and reintegration of persons with mental illness into community living: A holistic approach. *Journal of Psychosocial Nursing, 37*(11), 20–25.

Haugland, G., Siegel, C., Hopper, K., & Alexander, M. J. (1997). Mental illness among homeless individuals in a suburban county. *Psychiatric Services, 48*(4), 504–509.

Hughes, W. C. (1999). Managed care, meet community support: Ten reasons to include direct support services in every behavioral health plan. *Health & Social Work, 24*(2), 103–110.

Johnson, J., & Hickey, S. (1999). Arrests and incarcerations after psychosocial program involvement: Clubhouse vs. jailhouse. *Psychiatric Rehabilitation Journal, 23*(1), 66–69.

Kravitz, H. M., & Kelly, J. (1999). An outpatient psychiatry program for offenders found not guilty by reason of insanity. *Psychiatric Services, 50*(12), 1597–1605.

Lamb, H. R., & Weinberger, L. E. (1998). Persons with severe mental illness in jails and prisons: A review. *Psychiatric Services, 49*(4), 483–492.

Mallik, K., Reeves, R. J., & Dellario, D. J. (1998). Barriers to community integration for people with severe and persistent psychiatric disabilities. *Psychiatric Rehabilitation Journal, 22*(2), 175–180.

McGihon, N. N. (1999). Psychiatric nursing for the 21st century: The PACED model. *Journal of Psychosocial Nursing, 37*(10), 22–27.

McGrew, J. H., Wilson, R. G., & Bond, G. R. (1996). Client perspectives on helpful ingredients of assertive community treatment. *Psychiatric Rehabilitation Journal, 19*(3), 13–21.

Mitchell, A., & Reaghard, D. (1996). Managed care and psychiatric-mental health nursing services: Implications for practice. *Issues in Mental Health Nursing, 17*(1), 1–9.

Pittman, D. C., Parson, R., & Peterson, R. W. (1990). Easing the way: A multifaceted approach to day treatment. *Journal of Psychosocial Nursing, 28*(11), 6–11.

Roskes, E., Feldman, R., Arrington, S., & Leisher, M. (1999). A model program for the treatment of mentally ill offenders in the community. *Community Mental Health Journal, 35*(5), 461–475.

Shern, D. L., Felton, C. J., Hough, R. L., Lehman, A. F., Goldfinger, S., Valencia, E., Dennis, D., Straw, R., Wood, P. A. (1997). Housing outcomes for homeless adults with mental illness: Results from the second-round McKinney program. *Psychiatric Services, 48*(2), 239–241.

Swearingen, L. (1987). Transitional day treatment: An individualized goal-oriented approach. *Archives of Psychiatric Nursing, I*(2), 104–110.

Ware, N. C. (1999). Evolving consumer households. *Psychiatric Rehabilitation Journal, 23*(1), 3–10.

Ware, N. C., & Goldfinger, S. (1997). Poverty and rehabilitation in severe psychiatric disorders. *Psychiatric Rehabilitation Journal, 21*(1), 3–9.

Wilberg, T., Urnes, O., Friis, S., Irion, T., Pedersen, G., & Karterud, S. (1999). One-year follow-up of day treatment for poorly functioning patients with personality disorders. *Psychiatric Services, 50*(10), 1326–1330.

Wilbur, S., & Arns, P. (1998). Psychosocial rehabilitation nurses: Taking our place on the multidisciplinary team. *Journal of Psychosocial Nursing, 36*(4), 33–41.

Chapter Review

> ## MULTIPLE-CHOICE QUESTIONS

Select the best answer for each of the following questions.

1. All of the following are characteristics of ACT except:

   A. Services are provided in the home or community.

   B. Services are provided by the client's case manager.

   C. There are no time limitations on ACT services.

   D. All needed support systems are involved in ACT

2. Research has shown that scheduled, intermittent hospital admissions result in which of the following?

   A. Decreased number of inpatient hospital stays

   B. Increased sense of control for the client

   C. Feelings of failure when hospitalized

   D. Shorter hospital stays

3. The PACED model for inpatient psychiatric care focuses on all of the following except:

   A. Brief interventions

   B. Case management

   C. Discharge planning

   D. Independent living skills

4. How many persons in the state prison population have severe mental illness?

   A. Less than 5%

   B. 10% to 15%

   C. 25% to 30%

   D. More than 45%

5. Which of the following interventions is an example of primary prevention implemented by a public health nurse?

   A. Reporting suspected child abuse

   B. Monitoring compliance with medications for a client with schizophrenia

   C. Teaching effective problem-solving skills to high school students

   D. Helping a client apply for disability benefits

> ## TRUE-FALSE QUESTIONS

Identify each of the following statements as T (true) or F (false). Correct any false statements.

_____ 1. The ACCESS demonstration project is designed to provide increased access to mental health services for homebound clients.

_____ 2. Criminalization of mental illness refers to the fact that mentally ill persons who commit misdemeanors often end up in jail rather than in facilities for mental health treatment.

_____ 3. Poverty is a factor that perpetuates homelessness among persons with mental illness.

_____ 4. Managed care provides funding for all aspects of successful psychiatric rehabilitation programs.

_____ 5. A client's past history of alcohol abuse or violence is an impediment to optimal discharge planning.

_____ 6. The purpose of psychiatric rehabilitation programs is to stabilize the client's psychiatric symptoms.

_____

_____ 7. A client's success at community integration is greatly affected by his or her psychiatric diagnosis.

_____

_____ 8. Partial hospitalization programs can help clients make the transition from an inpatient setting into the community.

_____

➤ FILL-IN-THE-BLANK QUESTIONS

Identify the multidisciplinary team member responsible for the functions listed below.

_____ Works with families, community supports, and referrals

_____ Focuses on functional abilities and work with arts and crafts

_____ Makes diagnoses and prescribes treatment

_____ Emphasizes job-seeking and job-retention skills.

➤ SHORT-ANSWER QUESTIONS

1. Identify three barriers to community reintegration faced by mentally ill offenders.

2. Discuss the concept of evolving consumer households.

3. List factors that have caused an increased number of persons with mental illness to be detained in jails.

Building the Nurse–
Client Relationship

5 Therapeutic Relationships

Learning Objectives

After reading this chapter, the student should be able to:

1. Describe and implement the phases of the nurse–client relationship as outlined by Hildegard Peplau.
2. Describe the importance of self-awareness and therapeutic use of self in the nurse–client relationship.
3. Explain the importance of values, beliefs, and attitudes in the development of the nurse–client relationship.
4. Define Carper's four patterns of knowing, and give examples of each.
5. Describe the differences between social, intimate, and therapeutic relationships.
6. Identify self-awareness issues that can enhance or hinder the nurse–client relationship.
7. Describe how the nurse uses the necessary components involved in building and enhancing the nurse–client relationship (congruence, genuine interest, empathy, acceptance, and positive regard).
8. Explain the negative behaviors that can hinder or diminish the nurse–client relationship.
9. Explain the various possible roles of the nurse as teacher, caregiver, advocate, and parent surrogate in the nurse–client relationship.

Key Terms

acceptance

advocacy

attitudes

beliefs

congruence

countertransference

empathy

exploitation

genuine interest

intimate relationship

orientation phase

patterns of knowing

positive regard

preconception

problem identification

self-awareness

social relationship

termination or resolution phase

therapeutic relationship

transference

unknowing

values

working phase

The ability to establish therapeutic relationships with clients is one of the most important skills a nurse can develop. This relationship, although important in any nursing speciality, is especially important to the success of interventions with psychiatric clients. The therapeutic relationship and the communication within that relationship serve as the underpinning for treatment and success. The client's psychiatric disorder probably has components such as paranoia, low self-esteem, or anxiety, so establishing trust is a challenge.

In this chapter, we will examine the elements involved in establishing a therapeutic nurse–client relationship, such as trust, acceptance, genuine interest, and positive regard, and the nurse's interpersonal skills and self-awareness, which are crucial components in establishing appropriate relationships with clients. We will also examine the tasks that should be accomplished in each phase of the nurse–client relationship and the techniques the nurse can use to help accomplish these tasks. We will also discuss each of the therapeutic roles of the nurse (teacher, caregiver, advocate, and parent surrogate).

COMPONENTS OF A THERAPEUTIC RELATIONSHIP

Many factors can enhance the nurse–client relationship, and it is the nurse's responsibility to develop these factors. These factors will also promote communication and enhance relationships in all aspects of the nurse's life.

Trust

The nurse–client relationship requires trust. Trust is built when the client feels confidence in the nurse and the nurse's presence conveys confidence, integrity, and reliability. Trust is built in a relationship when one feels confident that the other person will be consistent in his or her words and actions and can be relied on to do what he or she says. Some behaviors the nurse can exhibit to help build the client's trust include being friendly, caring, inter-

---

Box 5-1

▶ TRUSTING BEHAVIORS

Trust is built in the nurse–client relationship when the nurse exhibits the following behaviors:
- Friendly
- Caring
- Interest
- Understanding
- Consistent
- Treats the client as a human being
- Suggests without telling
- Approachability
- Listening
- Keeps promises
- Provides schedules of activities
- Honesty

---

ested, understanding, and consistent; keeping promises; and listening to and being honest with the client (Box 5-1).

Congruence occurs when words and actions match—for example, if the nurse says to the client, "I have to leave now to go to clinical conference, but I will be back at 2 pm," and the nurse does indeed return at 2 pm to see the client. The nurse needs to exhibit congruent behaviors to build trust with the client. Trust is eroded when a client sees inconsistency between what the nurse says and does. Inconsistent or incongruent behaviors include making verbal commitments and not following through on them. For example, the nurse tells the client she will work with him every Tuesday at 10 am, but the very next week she has a conflict with her conference schedule and does not show up.

Another instance in which incongruent behaviors can occur is when the nurse's voice or body language is not consistent with the words being spoken. For example, an angry client confronts a nurse and accuses her of not liking her. The nurse responds by saying, "Of course I like you, Sally! I am here to help you." But as these words are being spoken, the

---

CLINICAL VIGNETTE: THERAPEUTIC RELATIONSHIPS

The group of 12 nursing students have arrived for their first day on the psychiatric unit. They are apprehensive, not sure what to expect, and are standing in a row just inside the locked doors. They are not at all sure how to react to these clients and fearful of what to say at the first meeting. Suddenly, they hear one of the clients shout; "I'll take the chubby one on the end." Feelings of embarrassment and anger start to well up in Lisa, who is standing at the end of the line of students and who is already self-conscious about her weight. And so, these students' nurse–client relationships have just begun—not quite in the best or textbook circumstances, but nevertheless they had begun.

nurse is backing away from the client and looking over her shoulder: the verbal and nonverbal components of the message do not match.

When working with a client with psychiatric problems, some of the symptoms of the disorder may make trust even more difficult to establish. For example, a client with depression has little psychic energy to listen or comprehend what the nurse is saying. Likewise, a client with panic disorder often has too much anxiety to focus on the nurse's communication. Although clients with mental disorders often give incongruent messages because of their illness, the nurse must continue to provide consistent, congruent messages in return. Examining one's own behavior and doing one's best to make it clear, simple, and congruent help create trust between the nurse and the client.

Many clients with psychiatric problems exhibit concrete thinking that focuses on their immediate concerns or feelings rather than subtle concerns. For example, if a client mentions that it is getting dark outside, the nurse should address the immediate concern and turn on the light rather than asking if or why the client is frightened.

Genuine Interest

When the nurse is comfortable with himself or herself, aware of his or her strengths and limitations, and clearly focused, the client will perceive a genuine person showing **genuine interest**. Even persons with mental illness can detect when someone is exhibiting dishonest or artificial behavior, such as asking the client a question and then not waiting for the answer, talking over the client, or assuring the client everything will be all right. The nurse should be open and honest and display congruent behavior. Sometimes the nurse, by responding with truth and honesty, may not provide the best professional response. The nurse may chose to disclose to the client a personal experience related to the client's current concerns. This develops trust and allows the client to see the nurse as a real person with perhaps similar concerns or problems, and it may stimulate the client to reveal more information to the nurse. This self-disclosure, revealing personal information about oneself (e.g., biographical data, personal ideas, thoughts, or feelings), can enhance openness and honesty. However, the nurse must not shift emphasis to the nurse's problems rather than the client's.

Empathy

Empathy is the ability of the nurse to perceive the meanings and feelings of the client and to communicate that understanding to the client. It is often con-

sidered one of the essential skills a nurse can develop. Being able to put himself or herself in the client's shoes does not mean the nurse has had the same exact experiences. However, by listening and sensing the importance of the situation to the client, the nurse can imagine the client's feelings about this experience. Both the client and the nurse give a "gift of self" when empathy occurs—the client by feeling safe enough to share the feelings, and the nurse by listening closely and purely enough to understand. Empathy has been shown to have a positive impact on client outcomes. Clients tend to feel better about themselves and feel more understood when the nurse is empathetic.

Several therapeutic communication techniques, such as reflection, restatement, and clarification, help the nurse send empathetic messages to the client. For example, the client says, *"I'm so confused! My son just visited and said he wants to know where the safety deposit box key is."* Using reflection, the nurse responds, *"You're confused because your son asked for the safety deposit key?"* The nurse who wanted to use clarification would respond, *"Are you confused about the purpose of your son's visit?"* From these empathetic moments, a bond can be established to serve as the foundation for the nurse–client relationship. More examples of therapeutic communication techniques can be found in Chapter 6.

The nurse needs to understand the difference between empathy and sympathy (feelings of concern or compassion shown by one for another). By expressing sympathy, the nurse may project his or her own

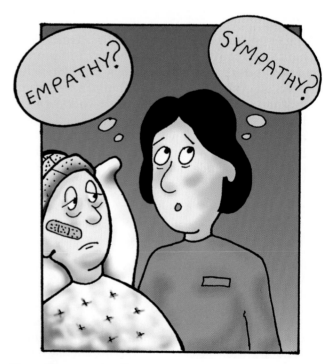

Empathy vs. sympathy

feelings onto the client, thus preventing the client from continuing to express his or her feelings. In the above example, the nurse using sympathy would have responded, "I know how confusing sons can be. My son confuses me, too, and I know how bad that makes you feel." The nurse's feelings of sadness or even pity may influence the relationship and hinder the nurse's abilities to focus on the client's needs. Sympathy often causes the emphasis to shift to the nurse's feelings, hindering the nurse's ability to view the client's needs objectively.

Acceptance

The nurse who does not get upset or respond negatively to a client's outbursts, anger, or acting out conveys **acceptance** to the client. Avoiding judgments of the person, no matter what the behavior, is acceptance. This does not mean acceptance of inappropriate behavior, but acceptance of the person as worthy. The nurse must set boundaries for behavior in the nurse–client relationship. By being clear and firm, but without anger or judgment, the nurse allows the client to feel intact while still conveying that the behavior is unacceptable. For example, a client puts his arm around the nurse's waist. An appropriate response would be for the nurse to remove his hand and say, *"John, do not place your hand on me. We are working on your relationship with your girlfriend, and that does not require you to touch me. Now, let's continue."* An inappropriate response would be, *"John, stop that! What's gotten into you? I am leaving, and maybe I'll return tomorrow."* Leaving and threatening not to return punishes the client and does not clearly address the behavior.

Positive Regard

The nurse who appreciates the client as a unique, worthwhile human being will be able to respect the client regardless of the client's behavior, background, or lifestyle. This unconditional, nonjudgmental attitude is known as **positive regard** and implies respect. The client often has little self-respect because of past experiences with others. When the nurse conveys respect by calling the client by name, spending time with the client, and listening and responding in an open manner, the client understands that he or she is respected. The nurse conveys this positive regard by taking the client's ideas and preferences into account when planning care. This shows the client that the nurse believes the client has achievement potential. The nurse uses presence or "attending," which is using nonverbal and verbal communication techniques to let the client know the nurse is giving the client full attention. Leaning toward the client and maintaining eye contact, being relaxed, and having arms resting at sides are nonverbal techniques that provide an atmosphere of presence. In verbal communication, the nurse must avoid making value judgments about the client's behavior.

Self-Awareness and Therapeutic Use of Self

The nurse must first know himself or herself before he or she can begin to understand others. This process of developing an understanding of one's own values, beliefs, thoughts, feelings, attitudes, motivations, prejudices, strengths, and limitations and how one's thoughts and behaviors affect others is called **self-awareness**. Self-awareness allows the nurse to observe, pay attention to, and understand the subtle responses and reactions of clients when interacting with them.

Values are abstract standards that give a person a sense of what is right and wrong and establish a code of conduct for living. Sample values include hard work, honesty, sincerity, and being clean and orderly. For the nurse to understand himself or herself and his or her personal values, the values clarification process is helpful.

The values clarification process has three steps: choosing, prizing, and acting. Choosing is when the

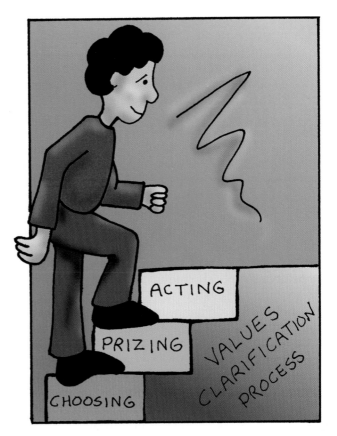

Values clarification process

person considers a range of possibilities and freely chooses a value that feels right. Prizing is when the person considers the value, cherishes it, and publicly attaches the value to himself or herself. Acting is when the person puts the value into action. For example, an orderly student has been assigned a roommate who leaves clothes and food all over their room. At first the orderly student is not sure why she is hesitant to return to the room and why she feels tense around her roommate. As she examines the situation, she realizes that they view use of personal space differently (choosing). Next, she discusses her conflict and choices with her adviser and friends (prizing) and decides to negotiate with her roommate for a compromise (acting).

Beliefs are ideas that one holds to be true—for example, "all old people are hard of hearing," "if the sun is shining it will be a good day," or "peas should be planted on St. Patrick's Day." Some beliefs have objective evidence to substantiate them; others are irrational beliefs that one believes regardless of existing empirical evidence to the contrary. If we believe in evolution, we have accepted the evidence that supports the evolution of life. Many people harbor irrational beliefs about cultures different from their own. These irrational beliefs may be fed by others' comments or simply fear of the unknown.

Attitudes are general feelings or a frame of reference around which a person organizes knowledge about the world. Attitudes such as hopeful, optimistic, pessimistic, positive, and negative color how we look at the world and people. A positive mental attitude occurs when a person chooses to put a positive spin on an experience, comment, or judgment. For example, the person ahead of you in line at the grocery store pays with change, slowly counting it out. A person with a positive attitude would be thankful for the extra minutes and would begin to use them to do deep-breathing exercises and relax. Having a negative attitude colors how we look at the world and others around us. For example, a person who had an unpleasant experience with a rude waiter may develop a negative attitude toward all waiters. Such a negative attitude might cause the person to behave impolitely and unpleasantly with every waiter he or she deals with.

Beliefs and attitudes should be re-evaluated and readjusted periodically as one gains more experience and wisdom. Gaining self-awareness allows the nurse to accept values, attitudes, and beliefs of others that may be different from his or her own. A person who does not assess personal attitudes and beliefs may hold a prejudice (hostile attitude) toward a group of people because of preconceived ideas or stereotypical images of that group. For example,

Sally comes from a white, Protestant, middle-class environment. Until beginning nursing school in an multicultural urban environment, she had little experience with cultures other than her own. She came with an ethnocentric attitude, believing that her culture was superior to any other. Once she became friends with students from Mexico and Kenya, she began to realize that each culture has its own beauty and style, and each was as important as the other. By letting her new experiences and friends become part of how she sees the world, Sally has revised her beliefs and attitudes and has expanded her understanding of people and the world (Box 5-2).

By developing self-awareness and beginning to understand his or her own personality and attitudes, the nurse can begin to use aspects of his or her personality, experiences, values, feelings, intelligence, needs, coping skills, and perceptions to establish relationships with clients. This is called **therapeutic use of self**. For a more detailed discussion of therapeutic use of self, see Chapter 6. Nurses should become aware of their own beliefs and thoughts regarding various cultural groups by asking the questions in Box 5-3.

PATTERNS OF KNOWING

Nurse theorist Hildegard Peplau (1952) identified preconceptions as a roadblock to the formation of an authentic relationship. **Preconceptions**, or ways one person expects another to behave or speak, often prevent people from getting to know each other. Preconceptions and different or conflicting personal beliefs and values may prevent the nurse from developing a therapeutic relationship with a client. Here is an example of preconceptions that interfere with a therapeutic relationship. Mr. Lopez, a client, has the preconceived, stereotypical idea that all male nurses are homosexual and refuses to have Samuel, a male nurse, take care of him. Samuel has a preconceived, stereotypical notion that all Hispanics use switchblades, so he is relieved that Mr. Lopez has refused to work with him. Both men are missing the opportunity to work together and perhaps do some important work together because of incorrect preconceptions.

Carper (1978) identified four **patterns of knowing** in nursing: empirical knowing (derived from the science of nursing), personal knowing (derived from life experiences), ethical knowing (derived from moral knowledge of nursing), and aesthetic knowing (derived from the art of nursing). These patterns provide the nurse with a clear method of observing and understanding every client interaction. Understanding where knowledge comes from and how it affects

Box 5-2

> **VALUES CLARIFICATION EXERCISE**

VALUES CLARIFICATION

Your values are your ideas about what is most important to you in your life—what you want to live by and live for. They are the silent forces behind many of your actions and decisions. The goal of "values clarification" is for their influence to become fully conscious, for you to explore and honestly acknowledge what you truly value at this time in your life. You can be more self-directed and effective when you know which values you really choose to keep and live by as an adult, and which ones will get priority over others. Identify your values first, and then rank your top three or five.

- Being with people
- Being loved
- Being married
- Having a special partner
- Having companionship
- Loving someone
- Taking care of others
- Having someone's help
- Having a close family
- Having good friends
- Being liked
- Being popular
- Getting someone's approval
- Being appreciated
- Being treated fairly
- Being admired

- Being independent
- Being courageous
- Having things in control
- Having self-control
- Being emotionally stable
- Having self-acceptance
- Having pride or dignity
- Being well organized
- Being competent
- Learning and knowing a lot
- Achieving highly
- Being productively busy
- Having enjoyable work
- Having an important position
- Making money

- Striving for perfection
- Making a contribution to the world
- Fighting injustice
- Living ethically
- Being a good parent (or child)
- Being a spiritual person
- Having a relationship with God
- Having peace and quiet
- Making a home
- Preserving your roots
- Having financial security
- Holding on to what you have
- Being safe physically
- Being free from pain

- Not getting taken advantage of
- Having it easy
- Being comfortable
- Avoiding boredom
- Having fun
- Enjoying sensual pleasures
- Looking good
- Being physically fit
- Being healthy
- Having prized possessions
- Being a creative person
- Having deep feelings
- Growing as a person
- Living fully
- "Smelling the flowers"
- Having a purpose

By Joyce Sichel. From Bernard, M. E., & Wolfe, J. L. (Eds.) (2000). The RET resource book for practitioners. *New York: Albert Ellis Institute.*

our behavior helps the nurse become more self-aware (Table 5-1). Munhall (1993) added another pattern that she called **unknowing**: for the nurse to admit she does not know the client or the client's subjective world opens the way for a truly authentic encounter. The nurse in a state of unknowing is open to seeing and hearing the client's views without imposing any of his or her values or viewpoints. In psychiatric nursing, where negative preconceptions on the nurse's part can adversely affect the therapeutic relationship, it is important to work on developing this openness and acceptance toward the client.

TYPES OF RELATIONSHIPS

Each nurse–client relationship is unique because of the unique combination of individuals involved. Although the relationships may differ, the types of relationships may be categorized into three major types: social, intimate, and therapeutic.

Social

A **social relationship** is primarily initiated for the purpose of friendship, socialization, companionship, and accomplishment of a task. The communication is usually centered around sharing ideas, feelings, and experiences and meets the basic needs of people to interact together. Roles may shift during social interactions, and communication is often superficial. Outcomes of this kind of relationship are rarely assessed. In a social relationship, advice is often given and basic needs are met. When a nurse greets a client and chats about the weather or a sports event or engages in small talk or socializing, this is a social interaction. This is acceptable in nursing, but for the nurse–client relationship to accomplish the goals

Box 5-3

➤ CULTURAL AWARENESS QUESTIONS

Acknowledging Your Cultural Heritage

- What ethnic group, socioeconomic class, religion, age group, and community do you belong to?
- What experiences have you had with people from ethnic groups, socioeconomic classes, religions, age groups, or communities different from your own?
- What were those experiences like? How did you feel about them?
- When you were growing up what did your parents and significant others say about people who were different from your family?
- What about your ethnic group, socioeconomic class, religion, age, or community do you find embarrassing or wish you could change? Why?
- What sociocultural factors in your background might contribute to being rejected by members of other cultures?
- What personal qualities do you have that will help you establish interpersonal relationships with persons from other cultural groups? What personal qualities may be detrimental?

Hutchinson, R. (1986). Ethnicity and urban recreations: Whites, blacks, and Hispanics in Chicago's public parks. Journal of Leisure Research, 19(3), 205–222.

Table 5-1

CARPER'S PATTERNS OF NURSING KNOWLEDGE

Pattern	Example
Empirical knowing (obtained from the science of nursing)	Client with panic disorder begins to have an attack. Panic attack will raise pulse rate.
Personal knowing (obtained from life experience)	Client's face shows the panic.
Ethical knowing (obtained from the moral knowledge of nursing)	Although the nurse's shift has ended, she remains with the client.
Aesthetic knowing (obtained from the art of nursing)	Although the client shows outward signals now, the nurse has sensed previously the client's jumpiness and subtle differences in the client's demeanor and behavior.

Carper, B. (1978). Fundamental patterns of knowing in nursing. *Advances in Nursing Sciences, 13–23.*

that have been decided on, social interaction must be limited. If the relationship becomes more social than therapeutic, serious work that moves the client forward will not be done.

Intimate Relationship

A healthy **intimate relationship** involves two people who are emotionally committed to each other and are both concerned about having their needs met and helping each other do so. The relationship may include sexual or emotional intimacy as well as sharing of mutual goals. Evaluation of the interaction may be ongoing or not. The intimate relationship has no place in the nurse–client interaction.

Therapeutic Relationship

The **therapeutic relationship** differs from the social or intimate relationship in many ways because it is focused on the needs, experiences, feelings, and ideas of the client. The areas to be worked on are agreed on, and the outcomes are continually evaluated. The nurse uses communication skills, personal strengths, and understanding of human behavior to interact with the client. In the therapeutic relationship, the parameters are clear: the focus is the client's needs, not the nurse's. The nurse should not be concerned whether the client likes him or her or even is grateful to the nurse. This is a signal that the nurse

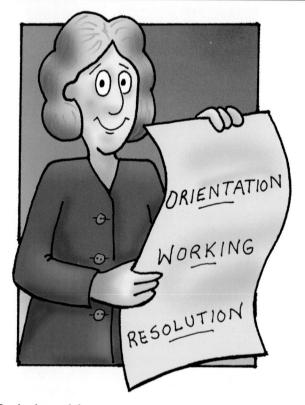

Peplau's model

is focusing on his or her own need to be liked or needed. The nurse must guard against allowing the therapeutic relationship to slip into a more social relationship. The nurse must constantly focus on the client's needs, not his or her own.

The nurse's level of self-awareness can either benefit or hamper the therapeutic relationship. For example, if the nurse is nervous around the client, the relationship is more apt to stay social because superficiality is safer. If the nurse is aware of his or her fears, they can be discussed and allayed by the instructor, paving the way for a more therapeutic relationship to develop.

ESTABLISHING THE THERAPEUTIC RELATIONSHIP

The nurse who has self-confidence rooted in self-awareness is ready to establish appropriate therapeutic relationships with clients. Because personal growth is ongoing throughout a lifetime, the nurse cannot expect to have complete self-knowledge, but awareness of his or her strengths and limitations at any particular moment is a good start.

Phases

Peplau has studied and written about the interpersonal processes and the phases of the nurse–client relationship for the past 35 years. Her work has provided the nursing profession with a model that can be used to understand and document progress with interpersonal interactions. Peplau's model (1952) has three phases: orientation, working, and resolution or termination (Table 5-2). In real life, these phases are not that clear-cut; they overlap and interlock.

ORIENTATION

The **orientation phase** begins when the nurse and client meet and ends when the client begins to identify problems to examine. During the orientation phase, the nurse establishes roles, the purpose of meeting, and the parameters of subsequent meetings, identifies the client's problems, and clarifies expectations.

Before meeting the client, the nurse has important work to do. The nurse reads background materials available on the client, becomes familiar with any medications the client is taking, gathers necessary paperwork, and arranges for a quiet, private, comfortable setting. This is a time for self-assessment. The nurse should consider his or her personal strengths and limitations in working with this client. Are there any areas that might signal difficulty because of past experiences? For example, if this client is a spouse bat-

terer and the nurse's father was also, the nurse needs to think over the situation: How does it make him or her feel? What memories are brought up, and can he or she work with the client without them interfering? The nurse must examine preconceptions about the client and ensure that he or she can put them aside and get to know the real person. The nurse must come to each client without preconceptions or prejudices. It may be useful for the nurse to discuss all potential problem areas with the instructor.

During the orientation phase, the nurse begins to build trust with the client. It is the nurse's responsibility to establish a therapeutic environment that fosters trust and understanding (Table 5-3). Appropriate information about the nurse should be shared at this time: name, reason for being on the unit, and level of schooling—for example, "Hello, James. My name is Miss Ames and I will be your nurse for the next 6 Tuesdays. I am a senior nursing student at the University of Mississippi."

The nurse needs to listen closely to the client's history, perceptions, and misconceptions. The nurse needs to overcome nervousness and convey feelings of warmth, expertise, and understanding. If the relationship gets off to a positive start, it is more likely to be successful and to meet established goals (Forchuk, 1994a,b).

At the first meeting, the client may be distrustful if previous relationships with nurses have been unsatisfactory. The client may use rambling speech, acting out, or exaggeration of episodes as ploys to avoid discussing the real problems. It may take several sessions until the client believes the nurse can be trusted.

Nurse–Client Contracts. Although many clients have had prior experiences in the mental health system, it is important for the nurse once again to outline the nurse and client responsibilities. At the outset, these responsibilities should be agreed on in an informal or verbal contract. In some instances a formal or written contract may be used. If a written contract has been necessary in the past with the client or if the client "forgets" the agreed-on verbal contract, a written contract may be appropriate.

The contract should state:

- Time, place, and length of sessions
- When the sessions will terminate
- Who will be involved in the treatment plan (family members? health team members?)
- Client responsibilities (arrive on time, end on time)
- Nurse's responsibilities (arrive on time, end on time, maintain confidentiality at all times, evaluate progress with client, document sessions).

Table 5-2

PHASES OF THE NURSE–CLIENT RELATIONSHIP

Orientation	Working		Resolution
	Identification	**Exploitation**	
CLIENT			
• Seeks assistance • Conveys needs • Asks questions • Shares pre-conceptions and expectations of nurse due to past experience	• Participates in identifying problems • Begins to be aware of time • Responds to help • Identifies with nurse • Recognizes nurse as a person • Explores feelings • Fluctuates dependence, independence, and inter-dependence in relation-ship with nurse • Increases focal attention • Changes appearance (for better or worse) • Understands continuity between sessions (process and content) • Testing maneuvers decrease	• Makes full use of services • Identifies new goals • Attempts to attain new goals • Rapid shifts in behavior: dependent, independent • Exploitative behavior • Self-directing • Develops skill in inter-personal relationships and problem-solving • Displays changes in manner of communication (more open, flexible)	• Abandons old needs • Aspires to new goals • Becomes independent of helping person • Applies new problem-solving skills • Maintains changes in style of communication and interaction • Shows positive changes in view of self • Integrates illness • Exhibits ability to stand alone
NURSE			
• Responds to client • Gives parameters of meetings • Explains roles • Gathers data • Helps client identify problem • Helps client plan use of community resources and services • Reduces anxiety and tension • Practices active listening • Focuses client's energies • Clarifies pre-conceptions and expectations of nurse	• Maintains separate identity • Exhibits ability to edit speech or control focal attention • Shows unconditional acceptance • Helps express needs, feelings • Assesses and adjusts to needs • Provides information • Provides experiences that diminish feelings of helplessness • Does not allow anxiety to overwhelm client • Helps client focus on cues • Helps client develop responses to cues • Uses word stimuli	• Continues assessment • Meets needs as they emerge • Understands reason for shifts in behavior • Initiates rehabilitative plans • Reduces anxiety • Identifies positive factors • Helps plan for total needs • Facilitates forward move-ment of personality • Deals with therapeutic impasse	• Sustains relationship as long as client feels necessary • Promotes family inter-action to assist with goal planning • Teaches preventive measures • Uses community agencies • Teaches self-care • Terminates nurse–patient relationship

Adapted from Forchuck, C., & Brown, B. (1989). Establishing a nurse–client relationship. *Journal of Psycho-social Nursing, 27*(2), 30–34.

Table 5-3

COMMUNICATION DURING THE PHASES OF THE NURSE–CLIENT RELATIONSHIP

Phase of Relationship	Sample Conversation	Communication Skill
Orientation	**Nurse:** "Hello, Mr. O'Hare. I am Sally Fourth, a nursing student from Orange County Community College. I will be coming to the hospital for the next 6 Mondays. I would like to meet with you each time I am here to help support you as you work on your treatment goals."	Establishing trust; placing boundaries on the relationship and first mention of termination in 6 weeks
Orientation	**Nurse:** "Mr. O'Hare, we will meet every Monday from June 1 to July 15 at 11 a.m. in conference room #2. We can use that time to work on your feelings of loss since the death of your twin sister."	Establishing specifics of the relationship time, date, place, and duration of meetings (can be written as a formal contract or stated as an informal contract)
Orientation	**Nurse:** "Mr. O'Hare, it is important that I tell you I will be sharing some of what we talk about with my instructor, peers, and staff at clinical conference. I will not be sharing any information with your wife or children without your permission. If I feel a piece of information may be helpful, I will ask you first if I may share it with your wife."	Establishing confidentiality
Working	**Client:** "Nurse, I miss my sister Eileen so much." **Nurse:** "Mr. O'Hare, how long have you been without your sister?"	Gathering data
Working	**Client:** "Without my twin, I am not half the person I was." **Nurse:** "Mr. O'Hare, let's look at the strengths you have."	Promoting self-esteem
Working	**Client:** "Oh, why talk about me. I'm nothing without my twin." **Nurse:** "Mr. O'Hare, you are a person in your own right. I believe working together we can identify strengths you have. Will you try with me?"	Overcoming resistance
Termination	**Nurse:** "Well, Mr. O'Hare, as you know I only have one week left to meet with you." **Client:** "I am going to miss you. I feel better when you are here." **Nurse:** "I will miss you also, Mr. O'Hare."	Sharing of the termination experience with the client demonstrates the partnership and the caring of the relationship.

Confidentiality. Adult clients can decide which family members, if any, may be involved in treatment and may have access to clinical information. Ideally, the persons close to the client and responsible for his or her care would be involved. However, the client must decide who will be included. For the client to feel safe, the boundaries must be clear. Information about who will have access to client assessment data and progress evaluations must be clearly stated to the client. The client should be told that the mental health team shares appropriate information among themselves to provide consistent care, and that only with the client's permission can a family member be included. If the client has an appointed guardian, that person can review client information and make treatment decisions that are in the client's best interest. For a child, the parent or appointed guardian is allowed access to information and can make treatment decisions as outlined by the health care team.

Chapter 6 offers more information on confidentiality.

WORKING

The **working phase** of the nurse–client relationship is usually divided into two subphases: **problem identification**, when the client identifies the issues or concerns causing problems, and **exploitation**, when the nurse guides the client to examine feelings and responses and to develop better coping skills and a more positive self-image, encouraging behavior change and developing independence. The trust established between the nurse and the client at this point allows the problems to be examined and worked on within the security of the relationship. The client must feel that the nurse will not turn away or be upset when experiences, issues, behaviors, and problems are revealed. Sometimes the client will use outrageous stories or acting-out behaviors to test the nurse. Testing behavior challenges the nurse to stay focused and not to react and get off track. Often when the client becomes uncomfortable with getting too close to the truth, these testing behaviors will be used to avoid the subject. The nurse may respond by saying, "It seems as if we have hit a spot that is uncomfortable for you. Would you like to let it go for now?" This statement focuses on the issue at hand and diverts attention from the testing behavior.

The nurse must remember that it is the client who examines and explores problem situations and relationships. The nurse must be nonjudgmental and refrain from giving advice, instead allowing the client to analyze situations. The nurse can guide the client to observe patterns of behavior and whether the expected response occurs. For example, Mrs. O'Shea suffers from depression. She continues to whine to the nurse about the lack of concern her children show toward her. With Nurse Jones' assistance, she explores how she communicates with her children and discovers that her approach is usually highly critical and needy. Mrs. O'Shea begins to realize that her behavior plays a part in driving her children away. With Nurse Jones, she begins to explore how she might change her methods of communication.

The specific tasks of the working phase include:
- Maintaining the relationship
- Gathering more data
- Exploring perceptions of reality
- Developing positive coping mechanisms
- Promoting a positive self-concept
- Encouraging verbalization of feelings
- Facilitating behavior change
- Working through resistance
- Evaluating progress and redefining goals as appropriate
- Providing opportunities for the client to practice new behaviors
- Promoting independence.

As the nurse and client work together, it is common for the client unconsciously to transfer to the nurse feelings he or she has for significant people in his or her life. This is called **transference**. For example, if the client has had negative experiences with authority figures, such as his father or teachers or principals, he may display similar reactions of negativity and resistance to the nurse, who is also viewed as an authority. A similar process can occur when the nurse responds to the client based on personal unconscious needs and conflicts; this is called **countertransference**. For example, if the nurse is the youngest in her family and often felt as if no one listened to her when she was a child, she may respond with anger to a client who does not listen or resists her help. Again, self-awareness is important so that the nurse can identify when transference and

countertransference might occur. By being aware of such "hot spots," the nurse has a better chance of responding appropriately rather than letting old unresolved conflicts interfere with the relationship.

TERMINATION

The **termination phase**, also known as the **resolution phase**, is the final stage in the nurse–client relationship. It begins when the problems are resolved, and it ends when the relationship is ended. Both nurse and client often have feelings about the ending of the relationship; the client especially may feel the termination as an impending loss. Often clients may try to avoid termination by acting angry or as if the problem has not been resolved. The nurse can acknowledge the client's feelings of anger and assure the client that this is a normal response to ending a relationship. If the client tries to reopen and discuss old resolved issues, the nurse must avoid feeling as if the sessions were unsuccessful; instead, he or she should identify the client's stalling maneuvers and refocus the client on newly learned behaviors and skills to handle the problem. It is appropriate to tell the client that the nurse enjoyed the time spent with the client and will remember him or her, but it is inappropriate for the nurse to agree to see the client outside of the therapeutic relationship.

Nurse Jones comes to see Mrs. O'Shea for the last time. Mrs. O'Shea is weeping quietly.

Mrs. O'Shea: *"Oh, Ms. Jones, you have been so helpful to me. I just know I will go back to my old self without you here to help me."*

Nurse Jones: *"Mrs. O'Shea, I think we've had a very productive time together. You have learned so many new ways to help you in having a better relationship with your children, and I know you will go home and be able to use those skills. When you come back for your follow-up visit, I will want to hear all about how things have changed at home."*

AVOIDING BEHAVIORS THAT DIMINISH THE THERAPEUTIC RELATIONSHIP

The nurse has power over the client by virtue of his or her professional role. That power can be abused if excessive familiarity or an intimate relationship occurs, or if confidentiality is breached.

Inappropriate Boundaries

All staff, both new and veteran, are at risk for allowing a therapeutic relationship to expand into an inappropriate relationship. Self-awareness is extremely important: the nurse who is in touch with his or her own feelings and aware of his or her impact on others can help maintain the boundaries of the professional relationship. Professional boundaries need to be maintained for the best therapeutic outcomes to occur. It is the nurse's responsibility to define the boundaries of the relationship clearly in the orientation phase and to ensure that those boundaries are maintained throughout the relationship. The nurse must act in a warm and empathetic manner but must not try to be friends with the client. Social interactions that continue beyond the first few minutes of a meeting allow the conversation to stay on the surface. This lack of focus on the problems that have been agreed on for discussion erodes the professional relationship.

If a client is attracted to a nurse or vice versa, it is up to the nurse to maintain professional boundaries. Accepting gifts or giving a client one's home address or phone number would be considered a breach of ethical conduct. Nurses must continually assess themselves and ensure that their feelings are kept in check and focused on the client's interests and needs. Nurses can assess their behavior by using the Nursing Boundary Index in Table 5-4.

Feelings of Sympathy and Encouraging Client Dependency

The nurse must not let feelings of empathy turn into sympathy for the client. Unlike the therapeutic use of empathy, the nurse who feels sorry for the client often tries to compensate by trying to please the client. When the nurse's behavior moves into a sympathy mode, the client finds it easier to manipulate the nurse's feelings. This discourages the client from exploring his or her problems, thoughts, and feelings, discourages client growth, and often leads to client dependency.

The client may make increased requests of the nurse for help and assistance or may regress and act as if he or she cannot carry out tasks previously done. These can be signals that the nurse has been "overdoing" for the client and may be contributing to the client's dependency. Clients often test the nurse to see how much the nurse is willing to do. If the client cooperates only when the nurse is in attendance and will not carry out agreed-on behavior in the nurse's absence, the client has become too dependent. In any of these instances, the nurse needs to reassess his or her professional behavior and refocus on the client's needs and therapeutic goals.

Table 5-4

Nursing Boundary Index

Please rate yourself according to the frequency that the following statements reflect your behavior, thoughts, or feelings within the past 2 years while providing patient care.

1. Have you ever received any feedback about your behavior being overly intrusive with patients or their families?	Never	Rarely	Sometimes	Often
2. Do you ever have difficulty setting limits with patients?	Never	Rarely	Sometimes	Often
3. Do you arrive early or stay late to be with your patient for a longer period of time?	Never	Rarely	Sometimes	Often
4. Do you ever find yourself relating to patients or peers as you might a family member?	Never	Rarely	Sometimes	Often
5. Have you ever acted on sexual feelings you have for a patient?	Never	Rarely	Sometimes	Often
6. Do you feel that you are the only one who understands the patient?	Never	Rarely	Sometimes	Often
7. Have you ever received feedback that you get "too involved" with patients or families?	Never	Rarely	Sometimes	Often
8. Do you derive conscious satisfaction from patients' praise, appreciation, or affection?	Never	Rarely	Sometimes	Often
9. Do you ever feel that other staff members are too critical of "your" patient?	Never	Rarely	Sometimes	Often
10. Do you ever feel that other staff members are jealous of your relationship with a patient?	Never	Rarely	Sometimes	Often
11. Have you ever tried to "match-make" a patient with one of your friends?	Never	Rarely	Sometimes	Often
12. Do you find it difficult to handle patients' unreasonable requests for assistance, verbal abuse, or sexual language?	Never	Rarely	Sometimes	Often

Any item that is responded to with a "sometimes" or "often" should alert the nurse to a possible area of vulnerability. If the item is responded to with a "rarely," the nurse should determine if it was an isolated event or a possible pattern of behavior.

Pilette, P., Berck, C., & Achber, L. (1995). Therapeutic management. *Journal of Psychosocial Nursing, 33*(1), 45.

Nonacceptance and Avoidance

The nurse–client relationship can be jeopardized if the nurse finds the client's behavior unacceptable or distasteful and allows those feelings to show by avoiding the client or making verbal responses or facial expressions of annoyance or turning away from the client. The nurse should be aware of the client's behavior and background before beginning the relationship; if any conflicts are raised, the nurse needs to explore these with a colleague. If the nurse is aware of a prejudice that would place the client in an unfavorable light, such issues need to be explored. Sometimes by talking about and confronting these feelings, the nurse can accept the client and not let a prejudice hinder the relationship. However, if the nurse cannot resolve such negative feelings, he or she should consider requesting another assignment. It is the nurse's responsibility to treat each client with acceptance and positive regard, regardless of the client's history. Part of the nurse's responsibility is to continue to become more self-aware and to confront and resolve any prejudices that threaten to hinder the nurse–client relationship (Box 5-4).

THERAPEUTIC ROLES OF THE NURSE IN A RELATIONSHIP

As in any other nursing relationship, the nurse often uses a variety of roles to provide the client with needed care. The nurse understands the importance of assuming the role that is appropriate for the work being done with the client.

Teacher

During the working phase of the nurse–client relationship, the nurse may teach the client new methods of coping and solving problems and may provide information about the medication regimen and available community resources. The teacher role is inherent in most aspects of client care. To be a good teacher, the nurse must feel confident about the knowledge he or she has and must know the limitations of that knowledge base. The nurse should be familiar with the resources in the health care setting and the community and on the Internet that can provide needed information for clients. The nurse must be honest about what information he or she can provide and when and where to refer clients for further information. This behavior and honesty builds client trust.

Caregiver

If the client requires traditional nursing care, the nurse can establish and develop a therapeutic relationship while performing physical care procedures. The need for touch while performing physical care may need to be explained to the client, depending on his or her understanding of boundaries (see Chap. 6), because the client may confuse physical care with intimacy and sexual interest. This can erode the therapeutic relationship. The nurse needs to keep in mind the boundaries and parameters of the relationship that have been established and must repeat the goals that were established together at the beginning of the relationship.

Advocate

In the advocate role, the nurse informs the client and then supports him or her in whatever decision he or she makes (Kohnke, 1982). However, in psychiatric-mental health nursing, advocacy is a bit different because of the nature of the client's illness: the nurse cannot support a client's decision to hurt himself or herself or another person. **Advocacy** is defined as the process of "acting in the patient's behalf by

---

Box 5-4

> POSSIBLE WARNINGS OR SIGNALS OF ABUSE OF THE NURSE–CLIENT RELATIONSHIP

- Secrets, reluctance to talk about practice
- Sudden increase in phone calls between nurse and client
- Changes in unit atmosphere–for example, a tension between staff and clients
- More acting out on unit that is hard to explain
- Nurse making more exceptions for the client than normal
- Increased rivalries between patients
- Change in the nurse's body language, dress, or appearance (if there is no other satisfactory explanation)
- Having hunches or instincts that something is not as it should be

Adapted from Gallop, R. (1998). Abuse of power in the nurse–client relationship. Nursing Standard, 12*(37), 43–47.*

INTERNET RESOURCES

Resource	Internet Address
▶ **Countertransference and the therapeutic relationship**	http://psychematters.com/papers/hinshelwood.htm
▶ **Analysis: difficult relationship**	http://www.nursing.ouhsc.edu/N3034/Unit3/Module2/Activity2_Analysis.htm
▶ **Hildegard Peplau home page**	http://www.uwo.ca/nursing/homepg/peplau.html
▶ **Boundaries and countertransference in treatment**	http://www.abbington.com/cpi/6900.html

ensuring privacy and modesty, promoting informed consent, preventing unnecessary examinations and procedures, and guaranteeing freedom from sexual abuse and exploitation by a health professional or authority figure" (Boyd & Nihart, 1998, p. 817). For example, if a physician begins to examine a client without closing the curtains and the nurse steps in and properly drapes the client and closes the curtains, the nurse has just acted as the client's advocate. Being an advocate has risks. In the previous example, the physician may be embarrassed and angry and make a comment to the nurse. The nurse needs to stay focused on the appropriateness of his or her behavior and not be intimidated. To take on the advocate role, nurses need to be open-minded and have a broad understanding of people, society, and the social order (Kohnke, 1982).

Parent Surrogate

When a client exhibits childlike behavior or when a nurse is required to provide personal care such as feeding or bathing, the nurse is often tempted to take on the parental role, as evidenced in choice of words and nonverbal communication. The nurse may begin to sound authoritative, with an attitude of "I know what's best for you." Often the client responds by acting more childlike and stubborn. Neither one realizes they have fallen from adult–adult communication to parent–child communication. It is easy for the nurse in such circumstances to be viewed as a parent surrogate by the client. In such situations, the nurse must be clear and firm and set limits or reiterate the limits that have been previously set. By retaining an open, easygoing, nonjudgmental attitude, the nurse

can continue to nurture the client while establishing boundaries. The nurse must ensure that the relationship remains therapeutic and does not become social or intimate (Box 5-5).

SELF-AWARENESS ISSUES

Self-awareness is a crucial factor in establishing a therapeutic nurse–client relationship. For example, a nurse who has a prejudice against people from a certain culture or religion and is not consciously aware of it may have difficulty relating to a client from that culture or religion. If the nurse is aware of the prejudice and acknowledges it and is open to reassess it, the relationship has a better chance of being authentic. If the nurse has certain beliefs and attitudes that he or she will not change, it may be best for another nurse to care for the client. Examining one's own strengths and weaknesses helps one gain a strong sense of self. Understanding oneself helps one understand and accept others who may have different ideas and values. The nurse must continue on a path of self-discovery to become more self-aware and more effective in caring for clients.

Helpful Hints for the Student Learning to Build a Therapeutic Relationship

- Attend workshops on values clarification, beliefs, and attitudes to help you assess and learn about yourself.
- Keep a journal of thoughts, feelings, and lessons learned to provide insight into yourself.

Box 5-5

> ## METHODS TO AVOID INAPPROPRIATE RELATIONSHIPS BETWEEN NURSES AND CLIENTS

- Realize that all staff, whether male or female, junior or senior, and from all disciplines, are at risk of over-involvement and loss of boundaries—not just front-line staff.
- Assume that this will occur. Supervisors should recognize potential problem clients and regularly raise the issue of sexual feelings or boundary loss with staff.
- Provide opportunities for staff to discuss their dilemmas and effective ways of dealing with them.
- Develop orientation programs to include how to set limits, how to recognize clues that the relationship is losing boundaries, what the institution expects of the professional, a clear understanding of consequences, case studies, developing skills for maintaining boundaries, and recommended reading.
- Provide resources for confidential and nonjudgmental assistance.
- Hold regular meetings to discuss inappropriate relationships and feelings toward clients.
- Provide senior staff to lead groups and model effective therapeutic interventions with difficult clients.
- Use clinical vignettes for training.
- Use situations that reflect not only sexual dilemmas, but also other problems over use of authority.

___

Adapted from Gallop, R. (1998). Abuse of power in the nurse–client relationship. Nursing Standard, 12(37), 43–47.

- Participate in group discussions on self-growth at the local library or women's health center to aid self-understanding.
- Develop a continually changing care plan for self-growth.
- Read books on topics that support the strengths you have identified and help develop your areas of weakness.

Critical Thinking

Questions

1. For the next several client interactions, evaluate your responses as social, intimate, or therapeutic.
2. Discuss the relationship-building behaviors you would use with a client that is very distrustful of the health care system.
3. Complete the boundary index in Table 5-4. What do your answers tell you about your own behavior that could enhance nurse–client relationships? What do your answers tell you about your own behavior that could diminish nurse–client relationships?
4. Complete the values clarification exercise in Box 5-4. How might the information gleaned from this exercise help you as you establish nurse–client relationships?
5. For the next several client interactions, document the phases and development of the nurse–client relationship. Evaluate the techniques you are using that enhance or diminish the relationship.

> ## KEY POINTS

- There are three types of relationships: social, intimate, and therapeutic. The nurse–client relationship should be a therapeutic relationship, not social or intimate.
- Building trust is of utmost importance in allowing the nurse–client relationship to begin and develop.
- Factors that enhance the nurse–client relationship include congruence, genuine interest, empathy, acceptance, and positive regard.
- Self-awareness is crucial in the therapeutic relationship. The nurse's values, beliefs, and attitudes all come into play as a nurse and a client form a relationship.
- To be effective, nurses need to clarify their own values.
- Carper identified four patterns of knowing: empirical, aesthetic, personal, and ethical.
- Munhall established the pattern of unknowing as an openness that the nurse brings to the relationship that prevents preconceptions from clouding the nurse's view of the client.
- The phases of the nurse–client relationship—orientation, working (with subphases of problem identification and exploitation), and termination or resolution—were developed by nurse theorist Hildegard Peplau in 1952. They are ongoing and overlapping.
- The orientation phase begins when the nurse and client meet and ends when the client begins to identify problems to examine.

- Tasks of the working phase include maintaining the relationship, gathering more data, exploring perceptions of reality, developing positive coping mechanisms, promoting a positive self-concept, encouraging verbalization of feelings that facilitate behavior change, working through resistance, evaluating progress and redefining goals as appropriate, providing opportunities for the client to practice new behaviors, and promoting independence.
- Termination begins when the problems are resolved and ends with the termination of the relationship.
- Factors that diminish the nurse–client relationship include loss of boundaries or unclear boundaries, intimacy, and abuse of power.
- Therapeutic roles of the nurse in the nurse–client relationship include teacher, caregiver, advocate, and parent surrogate.

REFERENCES

Bernard, M. E., & Wolfe, J. L. (Eds.) (1993). *The RET resource book for practitioners.* New York: Institute for Rational-Emotive Therapy.

Carper, B. (1978). Fundamental patterns of knowing in nursing. *Advances in Nursing Science,* 13–23.

Forchuk, C. (1994*a*). Preconceptions in the nurse–client relationship. *Journal of Psychiatric and Mental Health Nursing, 1,* 145–149.

Forchuk, C. (1994*b*). The orientation phase of the nurse–client relationship: Testing Peplau's theory. *Journal of Advanced Nursing, 20,* 532–537.

Forchuk, C., & Brown, B. (1989). Establishing a nurse–client relationship. *Journal of Psychosocial Nursing, 27*(2), 30–34.

Gallop, R. (1998). Abuse of power in the nurse–client relationship. *Nursing Standard, 12*(37), 43–47.

Kohnke, M. F. (1982). Advocacy: What is it? *Nursing and Health Care, 3*(6), 314–318.

Munhall, P. (1993). Unknowing: Toward another pattern of knowing in nursing. *Nursing Outlook, 41*(3), 125–128.

Peplau, H. E. (1952). *Interpersonal relations in nursing.* New York: J. P. Putnam's Sons.

Pilette, P., Berck, C., & Achber, L. (1995). Therapeutic management. *Journal of Psychosocial Nursing, 33*(12), 45.

ADDITIONAL READINGS

Beeber, L. (1998). Treating depression through the therapeutic nurse–client relationship. *Nursing Clinics of North America, 33*(1), 153–172.

Boyd, M. A., & Nihart, M. A. (1998). *Psychiatric nursing: Contemporary practice.* Philadelphia: Lippincott Williams & Wilkins.

Forchuk, C. (1995). Development of nurse–client relationships: What helps? *Journal of the American Psychiatric Nurses Association, 1*(5), 146–153.

Forchuk, C. (1995). Uniqueness within the nurse–client relationship. *Archives of Psychiatric Nursing, 9*(1), 34–39.

Forchuk, C., Westwell, J., Martin, M., Azzapardi, W. B., Kosterewa-Tolman, D., & Hux, M. (1998). Factors influencing movement of chronic psychiatric patients from the orientation to the working phase of the nurse-client relationship on an inpatient unit. *Perspectives in Psychiatric Care, 34*(1), 36–44.

Schafer, P. (1997). When a client develops an attraction: Successful resolution versus boundary violation. *Journal of Psychiatric and Mental Health Nursing, 4,* 203–211.

Chapter Review

➤ MULTIPLE-CHOICE QUESTIONS

Select the best answer for each of the following questions.

1. Building trust is important in.
   A. The orientation phase of the relationship
   B. The problem identification subphase of the relationship
   C. All phases of the relationship
   D. The exploitation subphase of the relationship

2. Abstract standards that provide a person with his or her code of conduct are:
   A. Values
   B. Attitudes
   C. Beliefs
   D. Personal philosophy

3. Ideas that one holds as true are.
   A. Values
   B. Attitudes
   C. Beliefs
   D. Personal philosophy

4. The emotional frame of reference by which one sees the world is created by:
   A. Values
   B. Attitudes
   C. Beliefs
   D. Personal philosophy

➤ TRUE-FALSE QUESTIONS

Identify each of the following statements as T (true) or F (false). Correct any false statements.

_____ 1. Empathy and sympathy are different words for the same emotion.
_____

_____ 2. Unlike in the past, it is considered acceptable today for the nurse to give the client his or her home address.
_____

_____ 3. Unknowing is when a nurse has to admit, "I don't know."
_____

_____ 4. When the nurse willingly accepts a wanted gift from the client, the relationship had moved from therapeutic to intimate.
_____

➤ FILL-IN-THE-BLANK QUESTIONS

Identify the pattern of knowing as described by Carper.

_____ The client's medication regimen is reviewed by the nurse.

_____ The nurse notices that the client is in a dark, cluttered room, knows the importance of environment, and begins to open the drapes.

_____ The nurse's grandmother also suffered from dementia, so she is not surprised by the client's behavior.

_____ As report is given, the nurse realizes client confidentiality has been breached.

1. Give a dialogue example of each of the following:

   Congruence

   Positive regard

   Acceptance

2. For each of the following client statements, write a response the nurse might make and the rationale for each.

Client: "I don't believe my doctor really went to medical school."

Client: "I thought you said you were going to be here for 8 weeks, not 6!"

> **CLINICAL EXAMPLE**

Mr. V., age 56, emigrated to the United States 25 years ago. He has seen many groups of student nurses come and go on his unit. He looks over the newest group and picks out the nurse he wants. "I'll take the cute little thing over there," he announces to the instructor and students. He sidles up to the chosen student and puts his arm around her. You are the one he has chosen. Create a dialogue that indicates an orientation phase with evidence of trust-building and relationship-enhancing behaviors for working with this client.

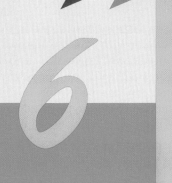

Therapeutic Communication

Learning Objectives

After reading this chapter, the student should be able to:

1. List the goals of therapeutic communication.

2. Identify and use verbal communication skills.

3. Identify nonverbal communication skills such as interpreting facial expressions, body language, vocal cues, and eye contact and understanding levels of meaning and context.

4. Describe how cultural differences and spirituality can affect therapeutic communication.

5. Explain the importance of confidentiality, self-disclosure and privacy, and boundaries in therapeutic communication.

6. Start a therapeutic communication, use therapeutic communication techniques to get the client's story, and formulate a client-centered goal of communication.

7. Identify your own type of nonverbal communication, thoughts, feelings, and needs.

8. Record a therapeutic communication using an Interpersonal Process Analysis format.

Key Terms

abstract messages
active listening
active observation
body language
circumstantiality
cliché
client-centered goal
closed body positions
communication
concrete message
confidentiality
congruent message
connecting islands
   of information
consensual validation
content
context
contract
cues (overt and covert)
culture
depth listening
directive role
distance zones

duty to warn
eye contact
incongruent message
intimate zone
metaphors
mottoes
nondirective role
nonverbal communication
personal zone
pressured speech
process
proverbs
proxemics
public zone
religion
social zone
spirituality
surface listening
symbolism
therapeutic communication
underlying needs
verbal communication

Communication is the process people use to exchange information. Messages are simultaneously sent and received on two levels: verbally, through the use of words, and nonverbally, by behaviors that accompany the words (Balzer-Riley, 1996).

Verbal communication consists of the words a person uses to speak to one or more listeners. Words are symbols used to identify the objects and concepts being discussed. The order and the meaning of these symbols are created by placing the words into phrases and sentences, which are understandable to both speaker and listener.

Nonverbal communication is the behavior that accompanies verbal content, such as body actions, eye and facial expressions, tone of voice, speed and hesitations in speech, grunts and groans, and distance from the listener. Nonverbal communication can indicate the speaker's thoughts, feelings, needs, and values, which are acted out mostly on an unconscious level.

Content is verbal communication, the literal words that are spoken by a person. **Process** denotes all nonverbal messages used by the speaker to give meaning and context to the message. **Context** is the environment in which a communication takes place and can include the time and the physical, emotional, social, and cultural environment (Weaver, 1996). Context includes the circumstances or parts that clarify the meaning of the content of the message.

The process component of communication requires the listener to observe the behaviors and sounds that accent the words and to interpret the speaker's nonverbal behaviors to assess whether the behaviors agree or disagree with the verbal content. A **congruent message** is given when content and process agree. For example, a client says, "I think you are the best nurse in the world," and this compliment is accompanied by a sincere gaze, an appreciative smile, and a warm tone of voice. The process validates the content as being true. But when the content and process disagree—when what the speaker says and what he or she does not agree—the speaker is giving an **incongruent message**. For example, if the client says, "I think you are the best nurse in the world" but has a rigid posture, clenched fists, an agitated and frowning facial expression and snarls the words through clenched teeth, this is an incongruent message. The process or observed behavior invalidates what the speaker says (content).

Nonverbal process represents a more accurate message than the verbal content. "Yeah, I copied your paper and handed it in as my own," is readily believable when the speaker has a slumped posture, a resigned tone of voice, downcast eyes, and a shameful facial expression, because the content and process are congruent. The same sentence said in an incredulous tone of voice and with raised eyebrows, a piercing gaze, an insulted facial expression, and hands on hips, showing outraged body language, invalidates the words (incongruent message) and really means, "How dare you accuse me of anything so vile?"

WHAT IS THERAPEUTIC COMMUNICATION?

Therapeutic communication is an interpersonal interaction between the nurse and client during which the nurse focuses on the specific needs of the client to promote an effective exchange of information between the nurse and the client. Skill in the use of therapeutic communication techniques helps the nurse understand and empathize with the client's experience. All nurses need therapeutic communication skills to apply nursing process and meet standards of care for their clients.

Therapeutic communication is used to accomplish many goals, including the following:
* Establish a therapeutic nurse–client relationship
* Identify the most important client concern at that moment in time (the client-centered goal)
* Assess the client's perception of the problem, as the event unfolded over a period of time. This includes detailed actions (behavior and messages) of the people involved; thoughts about the situation, others, and oneself related to the situation; and feelings about the situation, others, and oneself.
* Recognize the client's underlying needs
* Guide the client toward identifying pathways to a satisfying and socially acceptable solution.

THERAPEUTIC USE OF SELF

During therapeutic communication, nurses use themselves as a therapeutic tool to establish a therapeutic relationship with a client, to help the client grow, change, and heal. Using one's humanity—personality, experiences, values, feelings, intelligence, needs, coping skills, and perceptions—to help a client grow and change is called the therapeutic use of self (Northouse & Northouse, 1998). Peplau (1952), who described this therapeutic use of self in the nurse–client relationship, believed that nurses must have a clear understanding of themselves to promote their clients' growth and to avoid limiting clients' choices to those valued by the nurse.

Self-awareness means an understanding of one's personality, emotions, sensitivity, motivations, ethics, philosophy of life, physical and social image, and capacities (Campbell, 1980). The greater the nurse's understanding of his or her own feelings and responses, the better he or she can communicate with and understand others.

The nurse's personal actions arise out of conscious and unconscious responses, which are formed by one's life experiences and educational, spiritual, and cultural values. Nurses tend to use many automatic responses or behaviors just because that is the way things were done in the past. They need to examine such accepted ways of doing tasks and evaluate how they help or hinder the therapeutic relationship. For example, nurses were previously taught to be stiff and efficient. This got tasks done but did not allow the nurse to share himself or herself and may have prevented the development of an effective therapeutic relationship.

One tool that is useful in learning more about oneself is the Johari window (Luft, 1970), which creates a "word portrait" of a person in four areas and indicates how well a person knows himself or herself and communicates with others. The four areas evaluated are:

- Quadrant 1: Open/public self: qualities one knows about oneself and others also know
- Quadrant 2: Blind/unaware self: qualities known only to others
- Quadrant 3: Hidden/private self: qualities known only to oneself
- Quadrant 4: Unknown: an empty quadrant to symbolize qualities as yet undiscovered by oneself or others.

In creating a Johari window, the first step is to appraise one's own qualities by creating a list of those qualities: one's values, attitudes, feelings, strengths, behaviors, accomplishments, needs, desires, and thoughts. The second step is to find out how others perceive you by interviewing others and asking them to identify qualities they see in you, both positive or negative. To learn from this exercise, the opinions given must be honest; there must be no sanctions taken against those who list negative qualities. The third step is to compare lists and assign qualities to the appropriate quadrant.

If quadrant 1 is the longest list, this indicates the person is open to others; a smaller quadrant 1 means the person shares little about himself or herself with others. If quadrants 1 and 3 are both small, the person demonstrates little insight. Any change in one quadrant will be reflected by changes in other quadrants. The goal is to work toward moving qualities from quadrants 2, 3, and 4 into quad-

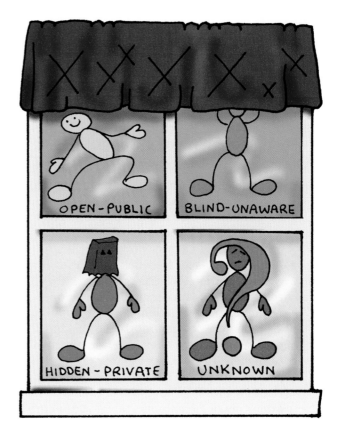

Johari window

rant 1 (qualities know to oneself and others), which indicates the person is gaining self-knowledge and awareness. See the figure for an example of a Johari window.

SELF-AWARENESS ISSUES

Therapeutic communication is the primary vehicle used to apply the nursing process in mental health settings. The nurse's skill in therapeutic communication influences the effectiveness of many interventions. Therefore, the nurse must evaluate and improve his or her communication skills on an ongoing basis. When the nurse examines his or her personal beliefs, attitudes, and values as they relate to communication, he or she is gaining awareness of the factors influencing communication. Gaining awareness of how one communicates is the first step toward improving communication.

The nurse will experience many different emotional reactions to clients, such as sadness, anger, frustration, or discomfort. The nurse must reflect on these experiences to determine how emotional responses affect both verbal and nonverbal communication. When working with clients from different cultural or ethnic backgrounds, the nurse needs to know or find out what communication styles are comfortable for the client in terms of eye contact, touch, proximity, and so forth. The nurse can then adapt his or her communication style in ways that will be beneficial to the nurse–client relationship.

Helpful Hints for Working on Therapeutic Communication Skills

- Remember that nonverbal communication is just as important as the words you speak. Be mindful of your facial expression, body posture, and other nonverbal aspects of communication as you work with clients.
- Ask colleagues for feedback about your communication style. Ask them how they communicate with clients in difficult or uncomfortable situations.
- Examine your communication by asking questions such as, "How do I relate to men? to women? to authority figures? to elderly persons? to people from cultures different than my own?" "What types of clients or situations make me uncomfortable? sad? angry? frustrated?" Use these self-assessment data to improve your communication skills.

ESSENTIAL COMPONENTS OF THERAPEUTIC COMMUNICATION

Establishing a therapeutic relationship is one of the most important responsibilities of the nurse when working with clients. Communication is the means by which a therapeutic relationship is initiated, maintained, and terminated. (The therapeutic relationship is discussed in depth in Chap. 5). Confidentiality, self-disclosure, privacy and respect for boundaries, and active listening skills are essential components of a therapeutic relationship

Confidentiality

Confidentiality means respecting the client's right to keep private any information about his or her mental and physical health and related care. Confidentiality means allowing only those dealing with the client's care to have access to the information divulged by the client. Only under precisely defined conditions can third parties have access to this information; for example, many states require that staff report suspected child and elder abuse.

The nurse must be alert if a client asks him or her to keep a secret, because this information may relate to the client's harming himself or herself or others. Avoid any promises to keep secrets. If the nurse has

promised not to tell before hearing the message, he or she could be jeopardizing the client's trust. In most cases, even when the nurse refuses to agree to keep information secret, the client will continue to relate issues anyway. The following is an example of a good response to a client who is suicidal but requests secrecy:

Client: *"I am going to jump off the 14th floor of my apartment building tonight, but please don't tell anyone."*

Nurse: *"I cannot keep such a promise, especially if it has to do with your safety. I sense you are feeling frightened. The staff and I will help you stay safe."*

The nurse who hears a homicidal threat must report this to the nursing supervisor and attending physician so that both the police and the intended victim can be notified of this threat. The *Tarasoff vs. Regents of the University of California* (1976) decision releases professionals from privileged communication with their clients and requires them to notify intended victims and police of the homicidal threat. This is called **duty to warn**.

The nurse documents the client's problems with planned interventions. The client must understand that the nurse will collect data about him or her that helps in making a diagnosis, planning health care, including medications, and protecting the client's civil rights. The client needs to know the limits of confidentiality of the nurse–client interactions and how this information will be used and shared with professionals involved in client care.

Self-Disclosure

Self-disclosure means revealing personal information about oneself to clients, such as biographical information and personal ideas, thoughts, and feelings (Deering, 1999). Conventional wisdom held that nurses should share only their name, marital status, and number of children, and perhaps should give a general idea about their residence, such as "I live in Ocean County." However, it is now believed that more self-disclosure can create greater rapport between the nurse and client (Deering, 1999). Self-disclosure can be used to convey support, educate clients, demonstrate that a client's anxiety is normal, and even facilitate emotional healing (Deering, 1999).

Nurses should remember these therapeutic goals of self-disclosure and use it to help the client feel more comfortable and more willing to share thoughts and feelings. Sharing may help the client gain insight about his or her situation or encourage him or her to resolve his or her concerns. It should not be used to meet the nurse's needs.

When using self-disclosure, consider cultural factors. For example, if the client is from a culture that is stoic and noncommunicative, self-disclosure may be deemed inappropriate. Keep self-disclosure brief and comfortable, respect the client's privacy by making sure the discussion takes place out of the earshot of others, and understand that each experience is different. The nurse must monitor his or her own comfort level. If the nurse has unresolved feelings about the issue, he or she should not share personal experiences.

Disclosing personal information can be harmful and inappropriate for a client, so the nurse must give it careful thought. If the client does not seem ready to deal with the issue, or the conversation is purely social, it is not a good time to disclose information about oneself (Hancock, 1998).

Privacy and Respecting Boundaries

Privacy is desirable but not always possible in therapeutic communications. An interview room is optimal. Privacy is often difficult to achieve in a semi-private room, when the two clients are immobilized. In such cases, the following can promote privacy:
- Talking softly
- Drawing the curtain between roommates
- Turning on the TV to muffle the conversation.

With mobile clients, a walk down the hall to a more private spot is helpful.

Proxemics is the study of distance zones between people when they communicate with one another. People feel more comfortable with smaller distances when communicating with someone they know rather than strangers (Northouse & Northouse, 1998). For Americans and Canadians, there are generally four **distance zones**:
- **Intimate zone** (0″ to 18″ between people): This amount of space is comfortable for parents with young children or people with the mutual desire for personal contact, or for whispering a message. Invasion of this intimate zone by anyone else is threatening and produces anxiety.
- **Personal zone** (18″ to 36″): This is the comfortable distance between family and friends talking.
- **Social zone** (4 to 12 feet): This is an acceptable distance for communication in social, work, and business settings.
- **Public zone** (12 to 25 feet): This is an acceptable distance between a speaker and an audience, small groups, and other informal functions (Hall, 1963).

People from some cultures (eg, Hispanic, Mediterranean, East Indian, Asian, or Middle Eastern) feel more comfortable with less than 4 to 12 feet of space while talking. The nurse of European American or African American heritage may feel uncomfortable with clients from these cultures who stand closer when talking. Conversely, the nurse may be perceived as remote and indifferent by clients from these cultural backgrounds (Andrews & Boyle, 1999).

Both the client and the nurse can feel threatened if one invades the other's personal or intimate zone, and this can result in tension, irritability, fidgeting, or even flight. When the nurse must invade the intimate or personal zone, he or she should always ask the client's permission. For example, if a nurse performing an assessment in a community setting needs to take the client's blood pressure, he or she should say, "Mr. Eichinger, to take your blood pressure I will wrap this cuff around your arm and listen with my stethoscope. Is this acceptable to you?" Permission should be asked in a yes/no format so the client's response is clear. This is one of the few times when yes/no questions are appropriate.

The therapeutic communication interaction is most comfortable when the nurse and client are 3 to 6 feet apart. If a client invades the nurse's intimate space (0″ to 18″), the nurse should set limits in a gradual manner, depending on the number of times the client has used this maneuver and the safety of the situation.

Touch

As intimacy increases, the need for distance decreases. Knapp (1980) identified five types of touch.
- Functional-professional touch is used in examinations or procedures, such as when the nurse touches a client to assess skin turgor or a masseuse performs a massage.
- Social-polite touch is used in greeting, such as a handshake, the "air kisses" some women use for greeting acquaintances, or a gentle hand to guide someone in the correct direction.
- Friendship-warmth touch involves a hug in greeting, an arm thrown around the shoulder of a good friend, or the back-slapping some men use to greet friends and relatives.
- Love-intimacy touch involves tight hugs and kisses between lovers or close relatives.
- Sexual-arousal touch is used by lovers.

Touching a client can be comforting and supportive when it is welcome and permitted. The nurse should observe the client for cues that show whether touch is desired or indicated. For example, holding the hand of a sobbing mother whose child is ill is appropriate and therapeutic, but if the mother pulls her hand away, that is a signal to the nurse that she feels uncomfortable being touched. Many older clients

Saying he wanted to discuss his wife's condition, a man accompanied the nurse down the narrow hallway of his house but did not move away when they reached the parlor. He was 12″ away from the nurse. The nurse was uncomfortable with his closeness, but she did not perceive any physical threat from him. Because this was the first visit to this home, the nurse indicated two easy chairs and said, "Let's sit over here, Mr. Barrett" (offering collaboration). If sitting down were not an option and Mr. Barrett moved in to compensate for the nurse's backing up, the nurse could neutrally say, "I feel uncomfortable when anyone invades my personal space, Mr. Barrett. Please back up at least 12 inches" (setting limits). In this message, the nurse has taken the blame instead of shaming the other person and has gently given an order for a specific distance to be kept between herself and Mr. Barrett. If Mr. Barrett were to move closer to the nurse again, the

nurse would note the behavior and ask the client about it—for example, "You have moved in again very close to me, Mr. Barrett. What is that about?" (encouraging evaluation). The use of an open-ended question provides an opportunity for the client to address his behavior. He may have difficulty hearing the nurse, may want to keep this discussion confidential so his wife will not hear it, may come from a culture in which 12″ is an appropriate distance for a conversation, or may be using his closeness as a manipulative behavior (ensure attention, threat, or sexual invitation). After discussing Mr. Barrett's response and understanding that he can hear adequately, the nurse can add, "We can speak just fine from two or three feet apart, Mr. Barrett. Otherwise, I will leave or we can continue this discussion in your wife's room," (setting limits). If Mr. Barrett again moves closer, the nurse will leave or move to the wife's room to continue the interview.

who have lost their spouses feel comforted by being touched and even enjoy a simple pat on the back.

Although touch can be comforting and therapeutic, it is an invasion of intimate and personal space. Some clients with mental illness have difficulty understanding the concept of personal boundaries or

knowing when touch is or is not appropriate. Consequently, most psychiatric inpatient, outpatient, and ambulatory care units have policies against clients touching one another or staff. Unless staff need to get close to a client to perform some nursing care, staff members should serve as role models and refrain from invading clients' personal and intimate spaces. When a staff member is going to touch a client while performing nursing care, the staff member must verbally prepare the client before starting the procedure. A paranoid client may interpret being touched as a threat and may attempt to protect himself or herself by striking the staff person.

Active Listening and Observation

To receive the sender's simultaneous messages, the nurse must use active listening and active observation of the sender's nonverbal actions. **Active listening** means refraining from other internal mind activities and concentrating exclusively on what the client is saying. **Active observation** means observing the speaker's nonverbal actions as he or she communicates.

Peplau (1952) used observation as the first step in the therapeutic interaction. The nurse observes the client's behavior and guides him or her in giving detailed descriptions of behavior. The nurse also documents these details. To help the client develop insight into his or her interpersonal skills, the nurse analyzes the information obtained, determines the underlying needs that relate to the behavior, and connects islands of information (makes links between various sections of the conversation).

Four types of touch. A—Functional-professional touch; B—Social-polite touch; C—Friendship-warmth touch; D—Love-intimacy touch.

CLINICAL VIGNETTE: PREPARING CLIENT WHEN INVADING PERSONAL SPACE

Thomas Joseph Luciano, 89, has chronic organic brain disorder and is being cared for in his home by his three widowed daughters. Thomas is fearful when approached by strangers and has been known to strike out and hurt caregivers hired when one or more of his daughters were ill. He recently had an abscess in his left thigh incised and drained. The nurse visiting today has to remove the old gauze, irrigate the wound, and repack it with iodoform gauze. On entering his room, the nurse stands just inside and to the right or left of the doorway (to avoid blocking the exit) and says, "Hello, Mr. Luciano. I am Gail Hecox, your nurse." When he looks at her, she sits in a chair near the door and adds, "I am here to change the bandage on your left leg. Will you let me do this?" Mr. Luciano looks frightened and shakes his head. Gail relaxes in her chair and begins to engage in chit-chat about the weather. After a few minutes, Mr. Luciano appears less anxious, and the nurse again asks him if it is all right for her to approach him and change his dressing. She asks one of his daughters to stand next to Mr. Luciano as she changes the dressing to comfort him. His daughter says, "Dad, it will be all right. I'm right here with you." Mr. Luciano nods his head in agreement.

A common misconception by students learning the art of therapeutic communication is that they must always be ready with a question to ask the instant the client has finished speaking. Hence, they are constantly trying to think ahead regarding the next question rather than actively listening to what the client is saying. The result can be that the nurse does not understand the client's concerns, and the conversation is vague, superficial, and frustrating to both participants. When a superficial conversation occurs, the nurse may complain that the client is not cooperating, is saying the same thing over and over, or is not taking responsibility for getting better. However, superficiality is usually the result of the nurse's failure to listen to the cues in the client's responses and asking the same question over and over. The nurse does not get details and works from own assumptions rather than the client's true situation.

While listening to a client's story, it is almost impossible for the nurse not to make assumptions. A person's life experiences, knowledge base, values, and prejudices often color the interpretation of a message. In therapeutic communication, the nurse must ask numerous specific questions to get the real story from the client's perspective, to help answer questions and clarify assumptions, and to develop empathy with the client. Empathy is the ability to place oneself into the experience of another for a moment in time. Empathy is developed by gathering as much information about an issue directly from the client so that the nurse avoids interjecting his or her personal experiences and interpretation of the situation. The nurse asks as many questions as it takes to gain a clear understanding of the client's perceptions of an event or issue.

Active listening and observation help the nurse to:
- Recognize the issue the client has identified as the topic of importance at that moment

- Ask questions related to the specific topic
- Use open-ended therapeutic communication techniques to prompt the client to continue with his or her perception of the issue
- Identify cues or signals in the content and process of the message so that the nurse can proceed with data collection
- Understand the client's perception of the issue and hear the client's story instead of leaping to conclusions
- Interpret and respond to the message in an objective manner (Boyd and Nihart, 1998).

VERBAL COMMUNICATION SKILLS

Using Concrete Messages

Use words that are as clear as possible when speaking to the client so the message can be understood. Anxious people lose cognitive processing skills—the higher the anxiety, the less ability to process concepts—so concrete messages are important for accurate information exchange. In a **concrete message**, the words are explicit and need no interpretation; nouns are used instead of pronouns—for example, "What health symptoms were the reason you came to the hospital today, Mr. Liu?" or, "Where did you put the new box of gauze dressings that was delivered this afternoon?" Concrete questions are clear, direct, and easy to understand. They elicit more accurate responses and avoid the need to go back and rephrase unclear questions, which interrupts the flow of a therapeutic interaction.

Abstract messages, in contrast, are unclear patterns of words, often containing figures of speech, that are difficult to interpret. They require the listener to interpret what is being asked. For example, a nurse who wants to know why a client was admitted to the unit asks, "How did you get here?" This is an abstract message: the terms "how" and "here" are vague. An anxious client might not be aware of where he or she is and reply, "Where am I?" or might interpret this as a question about how he or she was conveyed to the hospital and respond, "The ambulance brought me." Clients who are anxious, those from different cultures, those who are cognitively impaired, or those with some mental disorders often function at a concrete level of comprehension and have difficulty answering abstract questions. The nurse must be sure that statements and questions are clear and concrete. Box 6-1 gives examples of concrete (clear) and abstract (unclear) messages.

Therapeutic Communication Techniques

There are several therapeutic communication techniques the nurse can use to help the client feel relaxed and accepted, ready to examine the problem and focus on the primary issue. Table 6-1 lists these techniques and gives examples. In contrast, there are many nontherapeutic techniques that should be avoided (Box 6-2).

Interpreting Signals or Cues

To understand what a client means, the nurse watches and listens carefully for cues. **Cues** are verbal or nonverbal messages that signal key words or issues for the client. Finding cues is a function of active listening. They can be buried in what a client says or can be acted out in the process of communication. Often cue words introduced by the client can help the nurse to know what to ask next, or how to respond to the client. The nurse builds his or her responses on

these cue words or concepts. Understanding this can relieve pressure on students who are worried and anxious about what question to ask next (Box 6-3).

If a client has difficulty attending to a conversation and drifts off into a rambling discussion or a flight of ideas, the nurse listens carefully for a **theme**, a topic around which the client's words are composed. Using this theme, the nurse can assess the nonverbal behaviors accompanying the client's words and build responses based on these cues. The following are examples of identifying themes. The underlined words are themes and cues to help the nurse formulate further communication.

Theme of sadness:

Client: *"Oh, hi, nurse."* (<u>face is sad</u>, <u>eyes look teary</u>; <u>voice is low</u>, <u>with little inflection</u>)

Nurse: *"You seem sad today, Mrs. Venezia."*

Client: *"Yes, it is the <u>anniversary</u> of my husband's death."*

Nurse: *"<u>How long ago</u> did your husband die?"* (Or the nurse can go with the other cue.)

Nurse: *"Tell me about your <u>husband's death</u>, Mrs. Venezia."*

Theme of loss of control:

Client: *"I had an accident this morning, a fender bender. I'm OK. I lost my wallet and I have to go to the bank to cover a check I wrote last night. I can't get in contact with my husband at work. <u>I don't know where to start.</u>"*

Nurse: *"I sense you feel out of control."* (translating into feelings)

There are many word patterns clients may use to cue the listener to the intent of the speaker's words. **Overt cues** are clear statements of intent, such as, "I want to die." This is a clear message that the client is thinking of suicide or self-harm. **Covert cues** are vague or hidden messages that need interpretation and follow-up—for example, if a client says, "There is nothing that can help me." The nurse is unsure, but it sounds as if the client might be saying he feels so hopeless and helpless that he plans to commit suicide. The nurse can follow up on this covert cue to clarify the client's intent and to protect the client. Most suicidal people are ambivalent about whether to live or die and often admit their plan when directly asked about it. When the nurse suspects self-harm or suicide, a yes/no question is used to get a clear response

Theme of hopelessness and suicidal ideation:

Client: *"Life is hard. I want it to be done. There is no rest. Sleep, sleep is good . . . forever."*

Nurse: *"I hear you saying things seem hopeless. I wonder if you are planning to kill yourself."* (verbalizing the implied)

(text continues on page 118)

Box 6-1

▶ CONCRETE VERSUS ABSTRACT MESSAGES

Abstract (unclear) message: "Get the stuff from him."

Concrete (clear) message: "Between 5 and 6 pm, Art will be home, so you can pick up the software he's going to give us."

Abstract (unclear) message: "You'll have to get it now."

Concrete (clear) message: "For you to administer medications tomorrow, you'll have to understand how to calculate dosages by the end of today's class."

Table 6-1

THERAPEUTIC COMMUNICATION TECHNIQUES

Therapeutic Communication Technique	Examples of Technique
Accepting—indicating that nurse has heard and is willing to hear what client has to say	Nurse: "Yes." Nodding. "I follow what you said." "It is OK to tell me."
Assessing relationship—exploring client's relationship with another person. Asking client to describe relationship between self and others is a helpful way to gather information.	Client: "I went home with Joan." Nurse: "Tell me about you and Joan."
Broad openings—using open-ended questions that provide opportunity for client to introduce topic	"What's new?" "What are you thinking about?" "What's been happening in your life?" "How has life been treating you?"
Consensual validation—two or more people achieving agreement of interpretation of an event, behavior, or issue	Client: "The atmosphere here is scary." Nurse: "Yes, it is like being in a dark cellar." Client: "My sister passed last year." Nurse: "Give me your definition of the word 'passed'." or "Help me understand what 'passed' means." Nurse: "You had said you were worried about your visit from your wife after the way you had behaved before admission. I did see you holding hands during your visit. How did things go?"
Encouraging comparison—helping client understand by looking at similarities and differences. Create exhaustive list of similarities, then differences.	"Tell me about another time you had a similar experience." "What's one way I look like your daughter?" "What's another way I look like your daughter?" "What's one way I look different from your daughter?"
Encouraging description of perceptions—Having client describe his or her view of an event or experience.	"Describe this fear of driving over bridges." "Tell me when you feel anxious." "Start at the beginning and describe what happened." "You threatened to hit John. What's that about?" "You're smiling, but I sense you're very angry at me."
Encouraging evaluation—asking client to appraise the quality of his or her experiences (discuss one at a time)	"What are your thoughts about the way you asked Joe not to wear your coat anymore?" "What are your feelings in regard to Mark's behavior when he said he was angry?" "What have you learned from this experience?"
Focusing—concentrating on a single, important point	Client: "This world is rotten." Nurse: "What's one thing that is rotten about this world?" Client: "I hate all doctors." Nurse: "Who is one doctor you hate?" Client: "Everyone hates me." Nurse: "Who is one person who has told you he or she hates you?"
Formulating a plan of action—planning appropriate resolution of a problem in graded steps. Always use nouns instead of pronouns to clarify who is involved.	"Next time you argue with Donna, what is one way you can handle your anger, in an appropriate manner?" "How can you tell Terry you are upset that he ignored you, without hitting him?"
General leads—encouraging continuation	"And then. . . ?" "Continue." "Tell me about the accident."
Giving recognition—objective acknowledgment	"Hello, Mr. Thomas." "I notice you've combed your hair." "You walked the length of the hall."
Humor—harmless humor can help reduce mild to moderate anxiety, gives perspective on life events, and reduces social distance. Client must not be hurt by this humor.	Client: "My husband says I am too emotional about having diabetes and I could take some lessons from Mr. Spock on *Star Trek*, who never gets upset." Nurse: "I'm not sure pointed ears are in this year, so let's look at one of your concerns about having diabetes."

(continued)

Table 6-1

(Continued)

Therapeutic Communication Technique	Examples of Technique
Making observations—verbalizing what nurse sees in client's appearance and behaviors.	"You seem upset." "I sense you feel alone right now." "I notice that you're biting your lip."
Offering self—introducing self and identifying relationship	"Hello, my name is Mark Taylor. I'm a student nurse from OCC." "I'll stay here with you for a while." "I have a half-hour to spend with you."
Placing event in time or sequence—assessing time frame and sequence of an event over time	"What seemed to lead up to. . . ?" "When did this happen?" "Then what happened?" "When did John say this?" "What did you say?" "What did he say or do?" "How did you respond?"
Presenting Reality—giving a realistic explanation of what the client sees or hears	"That sound was a car backfiring." "I see no one else in the yard." "I understand you think you hear music from the angels, but what I hear is the clock chiming 2 p.m."
Reflecting—directing client actions, thoughts, and feelings back to client.	Client: "Do you think I should tell the doctor about . . . ?" Nurse: "What would you *like* to do?" or "What are your thoughts about telling the doctor about . . .?" Client: "My sister spends all my money and then has the nerve to ask for more." Nurse: "Ask for more?"
Restating—repeating the chief issues expressed	Client: "I'm scared. My mother died when she was 36 in the operating room. I'm only 35! I don't want it to happen to me." Nurse: "You fear you might die in the operating room?" or "You're afraid this might happen to you?"
Seeking clarification—trying to clear up confusion about events or people. Use nouns or proper nouns instead of pronouns used by the client. Keep asking specific questions until the information is completely understood.	Client: "He'll get here soon to take them to her house." Nurse: "Who is coming?" Client: "Kay will come to take them." Nurse: "Who will Kay take with her when she goes?" Client: "She will take Cody and Miles." Nurse: "Where will Kay take Cody and Miles?" Client: "To Melissa's house." Nurse: "So Kay will take Cody and Miles to Melissa's house, right?" Other examples of clarifying questions: "Who is one person on staff here who yells at you?" "Who are 'they'?" "I'm not sure that I understand how you think you are God." "I'm unclear about how you think the governor of New Jersey appointed you as the chief of New Jersey Secret Service."
Silence—absence of verbal communication provides time for the client to put actions, thoughts, or feelings into words and slows pace of interaction. Gives client time to develop insights. Silence is helpful when client seems to be considering whether to share additional information. Client may need this unspoken "permission" to take the time to share this information. Conversely, client anxiety may be increased by silence and client might blurt out the issue to fill the silence.	
Suggestion collaboration—offering to work together with the client	"Perhaps you and I can discuss what thoughts, behaviors, or feelings increase your anxiety."

(continued)

Table 6-1

(Continued)

Therapeutic Communication Technique	Examples of Technique
Summarizing—organizing key issues that have been discussed	"You've said that . . ." "During this half-hour, you and I have discussed . . ."
Theme identification—identifying recurring issues or problems	"I've noticed that in all of the relationships you have discussed, you've been hurt or rejected when you mention marriage. What do you think this is about?" "You have mentioned having no one, staying home every weekend, the phone not ringing. I sense you are lonely."
Translating into feelings—attempting to verbalize client's feelings expressed only indirectly	Client: "I'm dead." Nurse: "Lifeless?" Client: "I'm all by myself in this world." Nurse: "I sense your feeling is one of loneliness."
Verbalizing the implied—voicing what has been suggested or hinted at	Client: "I can't talk to you or to anyone. It's a waste of time." Nurse: "I sense you feel that no one understands."
Voicing doubt—gently questioning the reality of the client's perceptions	"How can it be that you think you get pregnant and deliver babies in 5 days when it takes around 280 days for this to happen for other women?" "That's unusual." "Where did you get the idea you were Allah?"

Adapted from Hayes, J. S., & Larsen, K. (1963). *Interactions with patients.* Macmillan Press.

Box 6-2

➤ NONTHERAPEUTIC COMMUNICATION TECHNIQUES

Advising—telling the patient what to do or how to solve problems
Nontherapeutic response: "I think you should . . ." "If I were you, I'd . . ."
Therapeutic Response: "Let's put our heads together and see how to solve this problem" or "What have you already done to try to resolve this situation?"

Agreeing—indicating agreement with client
Nontherapeutic responses: "That's right." "I agree."
Therapeutic responses: "What did you think of Fran yelling at you?" or "What part of this argument did you think was right?"

Approval—sanctioning the patient's ideas or behavior
Nontherapeutic response:
"You were good to have done that."
"I'm glad that you. . . "
Therapeutic response:
"Tell me how you think you performed when you told Lucy you were sorry for hurting her feelings."
"What do you see as the best part of giving a present to Denise?"

Belittling feelings expressed—misjudging the degree of the client's discomfort
Nontherapeutic response: "Everybody gets down into the dumps." "I've felt that way sometimes."
Therapeutic response: "Tell me about being down in the dumps." "You have the right to your own feelings."

Challenging—demanding proof
Nontherapeutic response: "But how can you have cancer when all your tests are negative?" "Why?"
Therapeutic response: "I hear you saying you are still concerned that you have cancer. Tell me about that." "What went into your choice to break the window?"

Defending—attempting to protect someone or something from verbal attack
Nontherapeutic response: "No one here would lie to you." "Miss _____ is a very capable nurse."
Therapeutic response: "Who is one person you think lied to you?" "I can't speak for Miss _____, but I see you are upset. Tell me your concerns."

Destructive humor—any humor that belittles, implies guilt or incompetence, continually refocuses client on topic selected by nurse, or is met with client displeasure

Continued

Box 6-2

➤ NONTHERAPEUTIC COMMUNICATION TECHNIQUES—cont'd

Disagreeing—opposing the client's ideas
  Nontherapeutic responses: "That's wrong."
    "I don't believe that."
  Therapeutic responses: "What do you think
    would happen to you if you jumped off the
    roof?" "Where did you get the idea you were
    President Clinton?"

Disapproving—denouncing the client's actions,
  thoughts, feelings, or needs
  Nontherapeutic responses: "It is silly to think
    people want to hurt you." "You're crazy." "You
    hate to hear the truth."
  Therapeutic responses: "Who is one person you
    believe wants to hurt you?" "You seem upset."
    "What is the most difficult concern you have
    about your job?"

Egocentric focus—occurs in two ways: 1) nurse
  enjoys being center of attention and answering
  questions about self and winds up being interviewed by the client; 2) nurse is focused on thinking what to ask next instead of actively processing
  client's message.
  Nurse: "Tell me about yourself."
  Client: "What is to tell. What about you?"
  Nontherapeutic response by nurse: "My girl-
    friend and I love to go camping. We have been
    to 36 states so far. We dance and make stained
    glass, too."
  Therapeutic response: "What is one of your
    hobbies?"

Indicating the existence of an external source—
  attributing to a source outside the patient
  Nontherapeutic response: "What causes you to
    feel that way?" "What makes you say that?"
  Therapeutic responses: "Tell me about feeling
    sad." Where did you get the idea. . . ."

Interpreting—seeking to make conscious that
  which is unconscious
  Nontherapeutic response: "What you really
    mean is . . ." "Unconsciously you're saying . . ."
  Therapeutic responses: "Your conversation re-
    volves around Sam's getting the scholarship.
    What do you think this is about?"

Introducing an unrelated topic—changing the subject.
  Client: "I wish I were dead."
  Nontherapeutic response: "Did you have
    visitors?"
  Therapeutic responses: "Tell me about wishing
    you were dead." "What is going on that you
    wish to be dead?" "Are you planning to commit
    suicide?"

Judging—rejecting the client's actions, thoughts,
  or feelings because they do not agree with your
  moral code or life choices.

Nontherapeutic responses: "How can you consider
  divorce when you have four children?" "How can
  having a baby fix your relationship when you're
  not even married?" "That's not living by the
  Golden Rule." "Get a life." "Shape up." "You need
  to start a new relationship."
Therapeutic responses: "What is one reason you
  are considering divorce?" "What is one way you
  believe having a baby would save your relationship?" "How do you see yourself handling this
  problem?"

Literal response—dealing with abstract symbols or
  metaphors in a concrete manner
  Client: "My head is going around and around."
  Nurse's nontherapeutic response: "You're lying
    perfectly still."
  Therapeutic response: "You might be dizzy. When
    did this start?"
  or
  Client: "My head is full of snakes."
  Nurse's nontherapeutic response: "Snakes can't
    live there."
  Therapeutic response: "Sounds like you have many
    thoughts squirming around there.
    What is the most difficult thought?"

Making stereotyped comments—offering meaning-
  less clichés when client is sad or upset
  Nontherapeutic nurse responses: "He'll be a vege-
    table." "Tomorrow brings sunshine." "It's all for
    the best."
  Therapeutic responses: "Three tests have revealed
    no brain activity. This means his brain has
    stopped working and he is being kept alive by the
    ventilator." "Put your sadness into words." "Tell
    me thing you'll miss the most about your
    brother."

Probing—persistent questioning of the client or ask-
  ing about unrelated topics
  Client: "And so my wife and I split up."
  Nontherapeutic response: "Now tell me about
    your mother."
  Therapeutic response: "Tell me about you and
    your wife splitting up."

Reassuring—trying to make the client feel better su-
  perficially and not to worry or be anxious
  Nontherapeutic responses: "Don't worry about
    your test results. They'll be alright." "You'll be
    fine and home soon."
  Therapeutic responses: "Tell me your greatest con-
    cern at this moment." "Put your anxiety into
    words to help me understand."

Rejecting—an angry or punitive response to client's
  action, thoughts, or feelings

Continued

Box 6-2

➤ NONTHERAPEUTIC COMMUNICATION TECHNIQUES—cont'd

Nontherapeutic responses: "You don't need to call your mother at midnight." "Don't ever let me hear you are thinking about running away again."

Therapeutic responses: "What's going on that you feel like running away?" "Your mom says she gets frightened when you call her at night. Tell me what you are experiencing so we can work together on helping you to wait till the morning to call Mom."

Requesting an explanation—demanding the rationale for an action, thought, or feeling

Nontherapeutic responses: "Why can't you sleep?" "Why do you feel this way?"

Therapeutic responses: "What do you think is going on that you are unable to sleep?" "What is one thing your mother does that 'drives you up the wall'?"

Testing—appraising the patient's degree of insight or knowledge unrelated to topic

Nontherapeutic responses: "What are you here in the hospital for?" "What day is this?"

Therapeutic responses: "We have been talking about your disagreement with your son and how he is ungrateful. What have you learned about yourself in relation to this disagreement?"

Using denial—refusing to admit that a problem exists. Closes off avenue for discussion.

Client: "I'm dead."

Nontherapeutic response: "You can't mean that."

Therapeutic responses: "What is one aspect of yourself that has withered and died?" "What is going on that you say you are dead?"

Value statements—judging the actions or feelings of clients and implying they are good or bad; making biased statements

Nontherapeutic responses: "That was good of you to pour the coffee." "Scary movies upset everyone." "That must make you feel horrible to hear your mother does not want you back home."

Therapeutic responses: "I see you poured the coffee. Thank you." "What upset you about this scary movie?" "What was your first response to hearing your mom did not want you to move back home?"

Volatile verbiage—harsh, negative, and often judgmental words, causing client to feel increased anxiety and shame

Nontherapeutic responses: "That was a pretty hostile answer." "You took the battering-ram approach."

Therapeutic responses: "I could hear you were upset when you answered. Tell me about that." "What was your feeling just before you broke the door to your mom's house?"

"Yes/no" questions—allows client to give one-word, dead-end responses that show no thoughts or emotions

Nontherapeutic questions: "Will you take your medicine?" "Are you going out?" "Can you ask for more help?" "Do you worry a lot?"

Therapeutic questions: "When will you be taking your medicine?" "Where are you going now?" "Whom could you ask to help you with this situation?" "What causes you to worry?"

Adapted from Hays, J. S., & Larson, K. (1963). Interactions with parents. *New York: Macmillan.*

Box 6-3

➤ FORMULATING QUESTIONS FROM CLIENT'S COVERT CUES

Client: "None of us ever believed that John walked away from a burning house with the possibility of people inside."

NURSE'S POSSIBLE RESPONSES:

"Who are the people you refer to when you say 'none of us'?" (seeking clarification)

"What did you, specifically, believe about this situation with John?" (focusing)

"Where did you get the idea that someone, possibly John, walked away from a burning house?" (encouraging description of perceptions)

"Describe what you know about this house that burned." (encouraging description of perceptions)

"How do you know there were possibly people inside of this burning house?" (focusing)

Client: "I had a boyfriend when I was young."

NURSE'S POSSIBLE RESPONSES:

"Had, Miss Kelly?" (reflection)

"Tell me about you and your boyfriend when you were young." (encouraging description)

"How old were you when you had this boyfriend?" (placing events in time or sequence)

Other word patterns that need further clarification for meaning include metaphors, proverbs, clichés, symbolism, and mottoes. When these figures of speech are used, the nurse must follow up with questions to clarify what the client is trying to say.

A **metaphor** is used to describe an object or situation by comparing it to something else familiar.

Client: *"My son's bedroom looks like a bomb went off."*

Nurse: *"You're saying your son is not very neat."* (verbalizing the implied)

Client: *"My mind is like mashed potatoes."*

Nurse: *"I sense you find it difficult to put thoughts together."* (translating into feelings)

Client: *"You're mixing apples and oranges."*

Nurse: *"Where did you get the idea that I'm talking about two different issues when I compare your anger at your boss to your coming home and abusing your wife?"* (seeking clarification)

Proverbs are old, accepted sayings.

Client: *"Where there's smoke, there's fire."*

Nurse: *"We have been discussing your belief that your wife is having an affair because you have had 12 hang-up calls this past week. Help me understand how you arrived at the conclusion that these hang-ups indicate your wife's being unfaithful."* (summarizing and seeking clarification)

A **cliché** is a trite phrase such as, "she has more guts than brains." This implies that the speaker thinks this woman is not smart or acts before thinking, or has no common sense. The nurse can clarify what is meant by saying, "Give me one example of how you see Mary as having more guts than brains" (focusing).

Symbolism is using one object to represent another, such as, "Sally is smart as a whip," which means that Sally is sharp and incisive. The nurse can clarify by asking, "Give me one example of how you see Sally as being smart as a whip" (focusing).

Mottos are slogans that people live by. The nurse must clarify the client's meaning: "You have said *Semper Fi* [the Marine Corps motto meaning "forever loyal"] at least five times in the past 5 minutes, but you say you have had two children by women other than your wife in the 2 years of your marriage. Who are you being faithful to?" (presenting reality).

Table 6-2 provides further definitions and examples of these word patterns.

NONVERBAL COMMUNICATION SKILLS

Nonverbal communication (behavior that is acted out by a person while he or she is delivering verbal

---

Table 6-2

COMMUNICATION PATTERNS

Communication Patterns	Nurse's Response to Help Clarify
Metaphor—applying a descriptive term to an object or action. "I love her to death." "Life is a battlefield."	"How does death relate to loving this woman?" (encouraging comparison) "What is one way you see yourself at war?" (focusing) "With whom are you at war?" (seeking clarification)
Overt cue—clearly stated message. "I want to die."	"Are you planning to commit suicide?" (consensual validation) "How do you see death as your only option?" (encouraging evaluation)
Covert cue—vague or hidden message. "This is more than I can bear."	"I sense you feel hopeless." (translating into feelings) "What is one issue you find unbearable?" (focusing)
Proverb—brief, true saying "People who live in glass houses shouldn't throw stones."	"Who do you believe is criticizing you but has problems similar to yours?" (encouraging description of perceptions)
Clichè—trite phrase "Have a good day."	"What events qualify for a 'good' day?" (encouraging evaluation)
Symbolism—using one object to represent another. "My brain is full of dynamite." "She has legs of steel."	"I sense you feel out of control. What is going on in your life?"(translating into feelings/encouraging description of perceptions) "Sounds as if you want to explode. I am a good listener." (translating into feelings/offering self)
Motto—slogan to live by "Be happy!" "Beware of gift horses."	"What is one thing you have to be happy about?" (Discuss this thoroughly, then help client create a list of other "happy" life issues, discussing each. When this list is complete, start on list of issues that are unhappy in the client's life, discussing each.) (encouraging comparison) "Who is one person you believe is trying to harm you?" (focusing)
Theme—recurrent topic "Once I saw a boy kill a cat. . . my dog was killed by a car. . . my cousin died of cancer." (theme: death or termination)	"How is this theme of death related to what is happening to you at this point in time?" (encouraging comparison)

content) includes facial expression, eye contact, silence, vocal prompts such as "uh huh," space, time, boundaries, and body movements. Nonverbal communication is as important, if not more so, than verbal communication. It is estimated that 45% of meaning is transmitted by words and by paralinguistic cues such as tone of voice, and 55% by body cues. Often the speaker verbalizes what he or she thinks the listener wants to hear; thus, nonverbal communication is deemed more accurate. Nonverbal communication involves the unconscious mind acting out emotions related to the verbal content, the situation, the environment, and the relationship between the speaker and the listener.

Knapp and Hall (1992) listed the ways in which nonverbal messages accompany verbal messages:
- Accent: flashing eyes, hand movements
- Complement: quizzical looks, nodding
- Contradict: rolling eyes to demonstrate that the meaning is the opposite of what is being said
- Regulate: taking a deep breath to demonstrate readiness to speak, using "and uh" to signal the wish to continue speaking
- Repeat: using nonverbal behaviors to augment the verbal message, such as shrugging after saying "Who knows?"
- Substitute: culturally determined body movements that stand in for words, such as pumping the arm up and down with a closed fist to indicate success.

Interpreting Facial Expressions

The human face produces the most visible, complex, and sometimes confusing nonverbal messages (Weaver, 1996). Facial movements connect with words to illustrate meaning; this connection demonstrates the speaker's internal dialogue (Arnold & Boggs, 1995; Schrank, 1998). Facial expressions can be categorized into expressive, impassive, and confusing:
- An expressive face advertises the person's moment-by-moment thoughts, feelings, and needs, or may "leak" expressions even when the person does not want to show expression.
- An impassive face is frozen into an emotionless, deadpan expression, similar to a mask.
- A confusing face has an expression that is the opposite of what the person wants to convey; has only one expression for all occasions, such as cranky, bored, or saucy; or occurs on a person who believes he or she is acting out a specific expression for the receiver to understand but actually is not (Cormier et al., 1997; Northouse & Northouse, 1998).

Facial expressions can often affect the listener's response. Strong emotional facial expressions can persuade the listener to believe the message. For example, by appearing perplexed and confused, a client could manipulate the nurse into staying longer than scheduled. Facial expressions such as happy, sad, concerned, concentrating, embarrassed, regal, impudent, and angry usually have the same meaning across cultures, but the nurse should identify the facial expression and ask the client to validate the nurse's interpretation of the expression—for instance, "You're smiling, but I sense you are very angry" (Schrank, 1998).

Frowns, smiles, puzzlement, agreement, serenity, relief, fear, surprise, and anger are common facial communication signals. Looking away, not meeting the client's eyes, and yawning indicate the listener is disinterested, lying, or bored. To ensure the accuracy of information, the nurse identifies the nonverbal communication and checks its congruency with the content (van Servellen, 1997). An example is, "Christian, you said you took your medicine today, yet you frowned as you were speaking. I sense you are unsure whether or not you took today's dose" (verbalizing the implied).

Interpreting Body Language

There should be no physical barriers between the nurse and client during therapeutic communication. Tables, desks, or even the back of a chair are barriers to communication and demonstrate the nurse's need to be protected or separated from the client.

Body language (gestures, posture, movements, and body position) is a nonverbal form of communication. **Closed body positions**, such as crossed legs or arms, indicate the listener is threatened by the interaction and is defensive. The nurse who sits with legs crossed at the knees signals that he or she is rejecting the interaction with the client and guarding a potential invasion of the lower body. Sitting with arms folded across the chest is another closed position that indicates defensiveness and nonacceptance. A better, more accepting body position is to sit facing the client with both feet on the floor, with knees parallel, hands at the side of the body, and legs uncrossed or crossed only at the ankle. This is an open posture that demonstrates unconditional positive regard, trusting, caring, and acceptance. The nurse indicates interest in and acceptance of the client by facing and slightly leaning toward him or her while maintaining nonthreatening eye contact.

Hand gestures add meaning to the content. A slight lift of the hand from the arm of a chair can punctuate or strengthen the meaning of the words. Hand gestures may include creating a circle with the

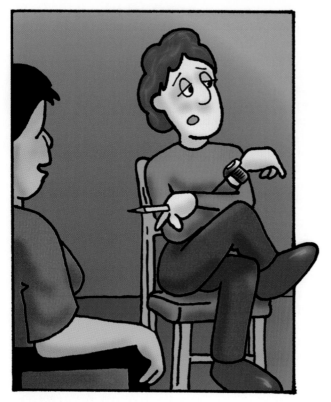

Closed body position

index fingers and thumbs of each hand to illustrate the size of an object, or acting out erasing a blackboard to demonstrate the speaker's wish to take back words that are inaccurate or painful to the listener. Flicking the wrist while making a statement indi-

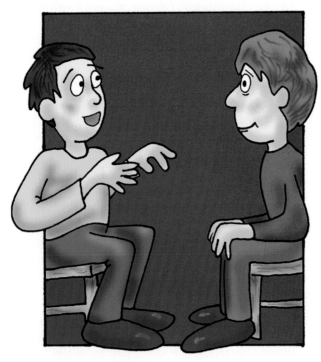

Accepting body position

cates that the person is being sarcastic and does not mean what was said: "Sure, I'll work 4 hours overtime without being paid."

Interpreting Vocal Cues

Vocal cues are nonverbal sound signals that are transmitted along with the content. The voice volume, tone, pitch, intensity, emphasis, speed, and pauses augment the sender's message. Volume, the loudness of the voice, can indicate anger, fear, happiness, or deafness. Tone can indicate whether someone is relaxed, agitated, or bored. Pitch varies from shrill and high to low and threatening. Intensity is the power, severity, and strength behind the words, indicating the importance of the message. Emphasis refers to accents on words or phrases that highlight the subject or give insight on the topic. Speed is number of words spoken per minute. Pauses also add significance to the message, often adding emphasis or feeling.

The high-pitched, rapid delivery of a message indicates anxiety. The use of extraneous words, with long-winded descriptions, is called **circumstantiality**. Circumstantiality can indicate the client is confused about what is important to the story or is spinning an untrue story (Morley et al., 1967). A client who delivers a monologue using intense, uninterrupted words, ignoring anyone else's attempt to enter into the conversation, is said to be using **pressured speech**. Pressured speech usually indicates the speaker is anxious or believes what he or she has to say is more important than what anyone else has to say. Slow, hesitant responses can indicate that the person is depressed, is confused and searching for the correct words, is having difficulty finding the right words to describe an incident, or is reminiscing. A pompous delivery style could mean the speaker is arrogant and has an inflated opinion of himself or herself, or it could mean he or she is insecure and tries to cover up his or her low self-image by speaking in a pretentious, arrogant manner. The nurse must use assessment to determine the causes of certain speech patterns.

Interpreting Eye Contact

The eyes have been called the mirror of the soul, because they often reflect our emotions. Messages given by the eyes include humor, lust, rejection, interest, puzzlement, hatred, happiness, sadness, horror, warning, and pleading. **Eye contact**, looking into the other person's eyes during communication, is used to assess the other person and the environment and to indicate whose turn it is to speak; it is increased while listening but decreased while speaking (Northouse & Northouse, 1998).

Eye positioning is a way to assess the predominant mode of processing information in a person. Bandler and Grinder (1982) developed a neurolinguistic model from theory in linguistics, neurophysiology, psychology, cybernetics, and psychiatry, observing that eye positioning can indicate how one's brain works. Those who look up and to the right while thinking are visual learners (learn best by seeing things). Auditory learners (those who learn best by what they hear) scan the environment from side to side. Kinesthetic learners (those who learn best by doing) gaze down at their dominant hand. Humans can learn through all three of these methods, but one of the three is the dominant method a person uses to process information or to think. Unless the nurse is aware of such normal eye positioning, he or she might misinterpret these as signs of disinterest or irritation.

UNDERSTANDING LEVELS OF MEANING

Few messages in social and therapeutic communication have only one level of meaning; there can be many layers of need transmitted in one message (deVito, 1991). The nurse must try to discover these other levels of meaning in the client's words rather than hearing only the literal words spoken. The ability to do this requires surface and depth listening. **Surface listening** means hearing the concrete message. **Depth listening** requires posing several interpretations of the message, then gathering detailed information to validate or invalidate each assumption. To interpret a client's message, the nurse examines the underlying needs of the client's words and actions. **Underlying needs** are those unspoken and often unconscious things a person wants that create the anxiety that promotes the person's behavior.

It is sometimes easier for clients to act out their emotions than to organize their thoughts and feelings into words to describe feelings and needs. For example, people who outwardly appear as dominating and strong personalities and often manipulate and criticize others in reality often have a low self-esteem and feel insecure. Their true feelings are not verbalized but are acted out in their actions toward others. Insecurity and low self-esteem often translate into jealousy and mistrust of others and attempts to feel more important and strong by dominating or criticizing others.

UNDERSTANDING CONTEXT

Understanding the context of a communication is extremely important in interpreting the meaning of a message. For example, if a client says "I collapsed," she may mean she fainted or felt weak and had to sit down, or she could mean she was tired and went to bed. To clarify these terms and view them in the context of the action, the nurse could say something like, *"Start at the beginning with where you were, how this incident started, and who was present"* or *"Describe where you were and what you were doing just before this episode where you collapsed"* (placing events in time and sequence).

Understanding the context of a situation gives the nurse more information and reduces the risk of assumptions and biases. Think of the difference in meaning of "I am going to kill you!" when stated in two different contexts: said in anger during an argument, and said when one friend discovers another is planning a surprise party for him or her.

To clarify the context of a situation, the nurse must gather information from verbal and nonverbal sources and integrate it with the client's spiritual

CLINICAL VIGNETTE: INTERPRETING BEHAVIORS

Nancy is in a 10-week women's health and relaxation group being led by a community health nurse. Nancy tells extensive stories to illustrate the issues being discussed. While many of Nancy's stories have been helpful, she has started trying to outtalk others who choose to share personal experiences and acts as if her experiences were more important than those of others. Once she gets started talking, it is difficult for others to add anything. She wants to be the center of attention all the time in the group. At first the others were pleasant to Nancy, but after 3 weeks, they begin to roll their eyes, sigh or grimace in disgust, and talk to each other when Nancy begins one of her stories.

Finally, the nurse took Nancy aside in a private conference and told Nancy that they appreciated her sharing all her experiences, but she needed to let others have a chance. She took this as an insult and replied, "No one has ever told me I talked too much before." Later, in another private session with the nurse, Nancy confided that she felt like no one really liked her much. She did not have many close friends. She thought if she could answer a lot of questions, tell some good stories, and entertain everyone, the others in the group would like her more.

and culturally relevant issues. To help the nurse understand the context of a message, he or she should ask focused, open-ended questions about:

- The identity of participants
- The participants' moods, attitudes, and relationships
- What happened before the incident began
- How the incident started, progressed, and ended
- Where the incident occurred
- How the participants behaved, in a timewise progression.

UNDERSTANDING SPIRITUALITY

The American Nurses Association code for nurses (1985) states that nurses must ensure human dignity for all clients regardless of differences in culture, economic status, ethnic origin, nationality, politics, race, religion, role, and sexual orientation. The spiritual well-being of a client is as important as the psychosocial and physical components of nursing care.

Spirituality is a client's belief about life, health, illness, death, and one's relationship to the universe (Gary & Kavanagh, 1991). Spirituality differs from religion: **religion** is an organized system of beliefs about one or more all-powerful, all-knowing powers that govern the universe and offer guidelines for living in harmony with the universe and others (Andrews & Boyle, 1999). Spiritual and religious beliefs are usually supported by others who share these beliefs and follow the same rules and rituals for daily living. Spirituality and religion often provide comfort and hope to people and can greatly affect a person's health and health care practices.

The nurse must first assess his or her own spiritual and religious beliefs. Religion and spirituality are highly subjective issues and can be vastly different from person to person. The nurse must remain objective and nonjudgmental regarding the client's beliefs and must not allow them to alter nursing care. The nurse must assess the client's spiritual and religious needs and guard against imposing his or her own on the client. The nurse must ensure that the client is not ignored or ridiculed because his or her beliefs and values differ from those of the staff (Burgess, 1997).

As the therapeutic relationship develops, the nurse must be aware of and respect the client's religious and spiritual beliefs. Ignoring or being judgmental will quickly erode trust and could stall the relationship. For example, a nurse working with a Native American client finds him looking up at the sky and talking to "Grandmother Moon." If she did not realize that his spirituality embodies all things with spirit, including the sun, moon, earth, and trees, she could misinterpret his actions as inappropriate.

Chapter 7 gives a more detailed discussion on spirituality.

CULTURAL CONSIDERATIONS

Culture is all of the socially learned behaviors, values, beliefs, and customs transmitted down to each generation by people. The rules about the way in which communication should be conducted vary because they arise from the culture's social relationship patterns (Kreps & Kunimoto, 1994). Each culture has its own rules governing verbal and nonverbal communication. For example, in Western cultures, the handshake is a nonverbal greeting used primarily by men, often to size up or judge someone just met. For women, a polite "hello" is an accepted form of greeting. In some Asian cultures, bowing is the accepted form of greeting and departing and a method of designating social status.

Because of these differences, cultural assessment is necessary when establishing a therapeutic relationship. The nurse must assess the client's emotional expression, beliefs, values, and behaviors; modes of emotional expression; and views about mental health and illness.

When caring for persons from other cultures who do not speak English, it is necessary to have a qualified translator who is skilled at obtaining accurate data. He or she should be able to translate technical words into another language while retaining the original intent of the message and without injecting his or her own biases into the message. The nurse is responsible for knowing how to contact a translator, whether the setting is inpatient or outpatient or in the community.

The nurse must understand the differences in how various cultures communicate. It helps to see how a person from another culture acts and speaks toward others. Americans and many European cultures are individualistic cultures that value self-reliance and independence, and focusing on individual goals and achievements. Other cultures, such as Chinese and Korean, are collectivistic cultures in which members value the group and obligations are to the security of the group. Persons from these cultures are more private and guarded when speaking to members outside the group and sometimes may even ignore outsiders until they are formally introduced to the group.

Cultural Differences in Speech Patterns and Habits

In individualistic cultures, it is desirable to speak in low-context language—clear language with enough repetition to help the listener understand what is being said. In contrast, persons from collectivistic cultures use high-context language, which assumes that the listener has a great deal of knowledge and needs little or no details and explanation. Giving too much explanation and details actually is insulting to the listener. There is more emphasis on promoting the good relationship between the speaker and listener and support of the group than on what is being said.

These cultural differences in communication patterns can cause problems for the nurse unless he or she is aware of them. For example, nurses from a Western Europe culture often give detailed instructions to the client regarding care and ask the client to repeat these details without much personal interchange. Such detailed and impersonal communication would offend the client from a collectivistic culture, who would feel insulted by the nurse's assumption that he or knows nothing and by the fact that the information was delivered without taking time to reinforce the relationship. The client might believe that the nurse does not genuinely care about him or her but only wants to complete the assigned task. The same misunderstanding can occur if an Asian nurse is teaching someone from a Western culture: because of Asian cultural customs, the nurse might not give enough detail and information. This cultural pattern of giving only minimal information might be one reason Westerners often perceive Asians as difficult to understand.

Although it is important to accommodate the values and views of each cultural group, cultural stereotyping is not useful—for example, assuming that all Asians honor and care for their aged and that all Latino men are macho.

Cultural Differences in Styles of Speech and Expression

Each culture and ethnic group has different styles of communication. Some cultures have strict rules governing verbal communication between the genders, and culture plays an important role in the manner in which a message is delivered. An Arab American will deliver important information in an intensely vigorous and high-volume manner. Clicking of the tongue by a Pakistani indicates disagreement.

Asians are much quieter in speech, because shouting or raising one's voice implies loss of control. Asian Americans will address someone passing by in the same volume as someone face-to-face. Silence also indicates respect for an elder's message or the need to have some time to think about the message. Asian Americans are discouraged from expressing anger because harmony in relationships is more highly valued than personal emotions (Andrews & Boyle, 1999).

Some cultures, such as Northern European and Native Americans, are more stoic and demonstrate less emotion than cultures from the Mediterranean area, such as Greece and Italy, where emotions are expected to be repeatedly verbalized and demonstrated. Many Hispanic Americans may nod the head or express agreement with a speaker's viewpoints and requests, even if they do not agree. This is a cultural expression of tact and courtesy. They may not verbalize any disapproval or disagreement but will not comply with the request. For example, the nurse may schedule a return appointment that the client cannot make, but the client will nod rather than disagree with the nurse.

Gestures can have different interpretations in other cultures. For example, forming a circle with the thumb and index finger means "OK" or "success" for most Americans, but to some South Americans, especially Brazilians, this is a demeaning sexual gesture (Wilson & Kneisl, 1996). A thumbs-up gesture in the United States means "all right," but in Japan it symbolizes the number 5, and it is sometimes used as a rude gesture by Australians (Schrank, 1998). Pointing with the index finger to single out a person from a group or gesturing with the index finger to indicate "follow me" is acceptable to most Americans but is considered an insult by Arab Americans.

Cultural Differences Regarding Eye Contact

In American culture, eye contact with short periods of looking away indicates interest, but a continual gaze is considered uncomfortable, threatening, and invasive (Andrews & Boyle, 1999). In other cultures (Native American, some Hispanic, African Americans, Appalachians, Indochinese, and Asian Americans), it is unacceptable to establish eye contact when talking; to do so is a sign of disrespect. These cultures teach children to look down as a sign of respect for the other person. African Americans may avoid eye contact when listening but use eye contact when speaking.

Direct eye contact between the genders is discouraged in Muslim cultures. Modesty is shown by downcast eyes; women look into only their husband's eyes. Hasidic Jewish men avoid eye contact with women. They may turn their heads in the opposite direction when speaking to or walking around a woman, or move to another seat to avoid eye contact with a woman who selects a seat nearby.

Nurses must be careful not to insult clients by using behaviors, such as direct eye contact, that are offensive to their culture. Rather than misinterpreting the client's nonverbal behaviors by assuming the client is uninterested, noncompliant, or insulting, ask the client to clarify which mode of eye contact is comfortable for him or her (Andrews & Boyle, 1999).

Cultural Differences in Touch

Touch practices vary by culture. Some men from India or Cambodia shake hands with other men, but not women. Touch is important to Egyptians, who freely touch members of the same gender. South Koreans consider touch by strangers an insult and unacceptable between the genders. North Koreans are comfortable with touch of the same gender. Touching the head of Cambodians is offensive because it is considered the center of life.

Touch is encouraged in Mexico, where touching a child neutralizes the "evil eye." In the Philippines, a bit of saliva on a finger is used to make the sign of the cross on the child's head to ward off the "evil eye." In many Arabic countries, such as Morocco and Saudi Arabia, men walk hand in hand and use extended handshakes (Geissler, 1998).

The best way to know which form of touch is appropriate for a client from a different culture is to ask. The nurse could say, "Please help me learn about your culture so we can be comfortable with one another. How would you like to be addressed, and what touch is acceptable to you?" Also, the nurse can prepare the client for the functional-professional touch required during each episode of care: "I will wrap this material around your arm to take your blood pressure. Is this all right with you?" or "You will have many procedures that require someone to touch you. Would you feel more comfortable with a male or a female nurse touching you?"

Cultural Differences in Concept of Time

The concept of time can be very different for various cultures. Time orientation of Native Americans, Hispanics, and Arabic cultures is global rather than linear, so people from these cultures are more relaxed in their perception of time than European Americans, who have high regard for scheduled linear time. Therefore, a 12:30 pm appointment for a person from Brazil or Mexico can be casually translated to mean "sometime in the afternoon." A nurse from a European American heritage might have difficulty understanding this different view of time.

Many of these cultures are present-oriented rather than future-oriented, so little attention may be paid to advice on diet, exercise, and other health practices that affect future health status (e.g., a diabetic diet to lessen the chance of blindness and kidney failure in a diabetic, or a low-fat and low-cholesterol diet and a moderate exercise program to avoid future cardiac problems in someone with an elevated cholesterol level) (Geissler, 1998).

Cultural Differences in Health and Health Care

In some groups, such as Native Americans, health is viewed as harmony within nature and natural forces. Other cultures view health as a balance between opposite forces, such as the Hispanic concept of hot and cold (*caliente/frio*) and the Asian concept of female and male forces (*yin/yang*). Foods and medicine are also divided into *yin* or *yang* forces; hence, treatments for certain illnesses or disorders are supposed to add either *yin* or *yang* to achieve balance between these forces in the body. Colds, tension, and gastrointestinal problems are believed to be caused by an overabundance of *yin* (female) force, whereas fever and dehydration indicate too much *yang* (male) force. In Asia as well as in some Arabic cultures, it is considered unacceptable to admit to anxiety or depression, so clients from those cultures may complain of body aches and pains rather than talking about their emotional problems (Andrews & Boyle, 1999).

THE THERAPEUTIC COMMUNICATION SESSION
Goals

The nurse uses all the therapeutic communication techniques and skills described above to help achieve the following goals:

- Establish rapport with the client, being empathetic, genuine, caring, and unconditionally accepting of the client regardless of his or her behavior or beliefs
- Actively listen to the client to identify the issues of concern and to formulate a client-generated, client-centered goal for the conversation
- Gain an in-depth understanding of the client's perception of the issue, and foster empathy in the nurse–client relationship
- Explore the client's thoughts and feelings related to each aspect of the issue
- Assess the client's issue in the context of his or her cultural and spiritual needs
- Uphold ethical principles and ensure confidentiality
- Believe the client is capable of growth and change

- Guide the client to develop new skills in problem-solving
- Promote the client's evaluation of solutions.

Preparing for the Session

There are several ways that the nurse can promote active listening during the session:

1. Sit facing the client. Face-to-face interaction permits each participant to read the other's facial expression. Many clients have better comprehension when they lip-read as the words are spoken. Sitting down sends the message that the nurse is prepared to spend time talking with the client.
2. Establish moderate eye contact, not staring, with the client. This demonstrates interest and can convey warmth and understanding.
3. Remove as many barriers as possible between the nurse and client, including tables or chairs. This allows each participant to observe the other's body language and promotes communication. Sit about 3 to 4 feet from the client, a comfortable distance. Do not straddle a chair, with the back of the chair between the client and the nurse. The only exception to this rule is the presence of a bed tray, which may hold tissues, water, or food (mealtime is often a good time for the client to talk with the nurse).
4. Lean the upper body toward the client and keep arms and legs uncrossed. Leaning forward indicates, "I really want to hear what you are saying." As noted above, when legs are crossed at the knees or arms are crossed over the chest, this indicates that the nurse may be trying to guard himself or herself from the client, and the client may perceive the nurse is uncomfortable.

Introduction and Establishing a Contract

Introducing oneself and establishing a contract for the relationship is an appropriate start for therapeutic communication. The nurse should introduce himself or herself using both first and last names. This is courteous and gives the client the opportunity to choose which form of address is comfortable. Some clients feel more comfortable addressing staff by first name only; others may choose to use the staff member's last name. When the nurse introduces himself or herself using a first name only, this could indicate a lack of respect, or trust or fear about disclosing his or her last name.

A **contract** for the relationship includes outlining the care the nurse will be giving the client, the times the nurse will be with the client, and acceptance of these conditions by the client.

> **Nurse:** *"Hello, Mr. Kirk. My name is Alex McNelis. I'm a student nurse from Ocean County College, and I will be caring for you today from 7 a.m. to 3 p.m. Right now I have a few minutes, and I see you are dressed and ready for the day. I would like to spend some time talking with you if this is a convenient time."* (giving recognition and introducing self, setting limits of contract)

After the introduction is made and the contract is established, the nurse can engage in small talk to break the ice and help the nurse and client get acquainted. This few minutes of relaxed, social chit-chat helps the client feel more comfortable with the nurse. Then the nurse can use a broad opening question to guide the client toward identifying the major topic of concern. The nurse should not ask the client what he or she wants to talk about immediately after the introduction and contract. This abruptly puts the responsibility on the client to select a subject to discuss and could make the client feel pressured and anxious, which is detrimental to the therapeutic relationship.

Broad opening questions are helpful to begin the therapeutic communication session, but the nurse should carefully phrase this broad opening so that the client relates his or her emotional issues and feelings rather than launching into complaints about the hospital or hospital personnel. The following is a good example of how to begin the therapeutic communication:

> **Nurse:** *"Hello, Mrs. Nagy. My name is Donna Gail and I am your nurse today and tomorrow from 7 a.m. to 3 p.m."* (introduction of self, establishing limits of relationship)
>
> **Client:** *"Hi, Donna."*
>
> **Nurse:** *"The rain today has been a welcome relief from the heat of the past few days."*
>
> **Client:** *"Really? It's hard to tell what it's doing outside. Still seems hot in here to me."*
>
> **Nurse:** *In my experience, taking time out of life to be hospitalized (or ill) creates disruption in people's lives. What is your greatest concern at this moment?"* (broad opening)

Finding Client-Centered Goals

The nurse does not select the topic to be discussed; it is the client who identifies the problem he or she wants to talk about. The nurse uses active listening skills to identify the topic of concern. Thorough investigation using many finely focused questions helps the nurse understand the client's experience. The goal is identified by the client and gathering information about this topic is focused on the client. The nurse acts as a guide in this conversation. The therapeutic communication centers on achieving the goal in the time limits of the conversation.

The following are examples of client-centered goals:

- Client will discuss her concerns about her 16-year-old daughter not answering the phone each time the client has called at varied hours during the past 2 days of her hospital stay.
- Client will describe difficulty looking at husband's amputated foot.
- Client will share her distress about son's drug abuse.
- Client will identify the scariest issues to her about being a single parent.

The nurse generally assumes a **nondirective role** in therapeutic communication, using broad openings and open-ended questions to collect information and help the client to identify and discuss the topic of concern. The client does most of the talking. The nurse steers the client through his or her story from beginning to end, clarifying issues and relationships. When the client is suicidal or in a crisis, the nurse uses a **directive role**, asking direct, yes/no questions and using problem-solving to help the client to develop new coping mechanisms. The problem-solving process is discussed later in this chapter.

The following is an example of a therapeutic communication sequence to help develop the client-centered goal:

Nurse: *"Hello, Mrs. Rogers. I am Marge Bamford and I will be your nurse from now until 7 p.m. today and tomorrow."* (establishing a contract)

Client: *"I hope this will be a better hospitalization than my last one, 10 years ago."*

Nurse: *"Tell me one thing what was not good about your hospitalization 10 years ago, Mrs. Rogers."* (focusing; identified client-centered goal: Mrs. Rogers will describe issues related to her dissatisfaction with her hospitalization 10 years ago)

Client: *"I had emergency abdominal surgery. I was supposed to be having a hysterectomy and woke up with a colostomy bag on my abdomen."*

Nurse: *"A colostomy bag?"* (reflecting)

Client: *"Yes. I remember waking up, seeing that I was in ICU and running my hands over my abdomen. I felt the colostomy bag and couldn't believe this was what it was. I'm a registered nurse, so I know colostomy bags, but how could I have one? So I asked a nurse, 'What is this on my abdomen?'"*

Nurse: *"Then what happened?"* (placing event in sequence)

Client: *"The nurse said, 'Hasn't your doctor talked to you?' I said, 'No. I just recovered from anesthesia. I am asking you.' So she just smiled and walked away from me. I laid there thinking the surgeon must have found cancer in me and it must be pretty bad to have had a colostomy. I drifted in and out of sleep all that night, but every time I was awake, the colostomy bag was the first thing I reached for to find out if it was still there."*

Nurse: *"Cancer?"* (reflecting)

Client: *"Yes. Cancer kills my family members. So I figured it was my turn to have cancer, with this genetic history."*

Nurse: *"What had you wanted the nurse to tell you?"* (focusing)

Client: *"The reason I was in ICU with a colostomy bag on my side."*

Nurse: *"What was the reason for ICU and the colostomy bag?"* (seeking clarification)

Client: *"Diverticular disease, with previous ruptured diverticula that had adhered to other bowel, uterus, tubes, and ovaries. The gynecologists started surgery doing a hysterectomy only to find the current peritonitis and old adhesions, so they had to get a team of surgeons to deal with the bowel, and surgery lasted 7 hours. I had a hysterectomy and a temporary colostomy to rest the distal bowel. Two months later, the surgeon reanastomosed the bowel."*

Nurse: *"How long did it take for you to find out about your surgery?"* (placing events in time)

Client: *"Seems like it was forever, but it was the next night the surgeon made rounds and told me the saga, including the wonderful news that I did not have cancer. It was a rough 24 hours."*

Nurse: *"What was the roughest part about this experience?"* (focusing)

Client: *"A few things, actually. Thinking I had cancer decades younger than the rest of my family, and staff being afraid to take care of me. You see, I've been a nurse for 25 years and it seemed like all the nurses on staff were afraid to care for me because I guess they thought I would be evaluating their performance all the time."*

In some communications, there is no problem to solve: the client only wants to share his or her story with an interested listener. Often just sharing a distressing event can allow the client to vent thoughts and emotions that he or she has been carrying around. It serves as a way to lighten the emotional load and release feelings without a need to alter the situation—as in the example above. Other times, the client may need to reminisce and share pleasant memories of past events. Elderly clients often find great solace in reminiscing about events in their life, such as weddings, graduations, and their grandchildren's activities.

How to Phrase Questions

The manner in which questions are phrased is important. Open-ended questions elicit information; yes/no questions do not and put the burden of conversation on the nurse (which is not where it belongs). The nurse asks specific questions designed to take the client step by step through the issue, from beginning to end, by asking specific questions of "who, what, when, where, and how" rather than "why." The nurse must differentiate between thoughts and feelings, stay focused on the client's story, and ask for clarification. The nurse uses active listening to build questions based on the cues the client has given in his or her responses.

In English, the word "feel" is frequently substituted for "think." Emotions differ from the cognitive process of thinking, so using the appropriate term is important. For example, "What do you feel about that test?" is a vague question that could get several types of answers. A more specific question would be, "How well do you think you did on the test?" The nurse should ask, "What did you think about . . . ?" when discussing cognitive issues and "How did you feel about . . . ?" when trying to elicit the client's emotions and feelings. Box 6-4 lists "feeling" words that are commonly used to express or describe emotions. The following are examples of different responses that could be given to questions using "think" and "feel":

Nurse: *"What did you think about your daughter's role in her automobile accident?"*
Client: *"I believe she is just not a careful driver. She drives too fast."*
Nurse: *"How did you feel when you heard about your daughter's automobile accident?"*
Client: *"Relieved that neither she nor anyone else was injured."*

Staying Focused: "Getting the Story"

Using active listening skills, asking many open-ended questions, and building on the client's responses will help the nurse obtain a complete description of an issue or an event and help the nurse to understand the client's experience. Some clients do not have the skill or patience to describe how an event unfolded over time without assistance from the nurse. Clients tend to recount the beginning and the end of a story, leaving out crucial information about their own behavior. The nurse can help the client tell the story by asking specific step-by-step, moment-by-moment questions.

When a client is anxious and has difficulty communicating, the nurse can ask only about the actions of the people involved in the situation and how the events occurred. It is best to do this in a step-by-step sequence, asking the client to go back to the time and place before the incident began and to explain how the incident started, who was involved, what each person did and said, how the incident developed over time, and how the incident ended.

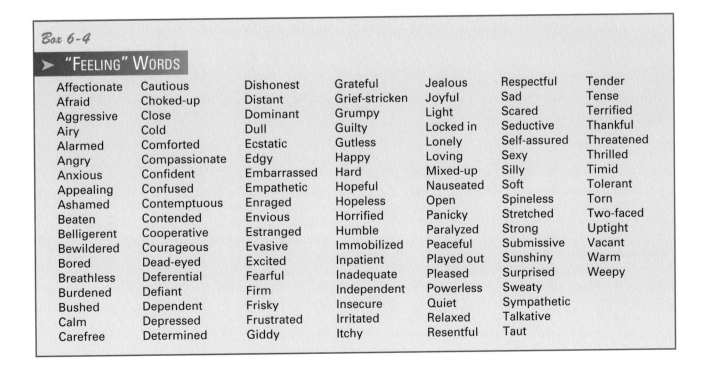

Box 6-4

➤ "FEELING" WORDS

Affectionate	Cautious	Dishonest	Grateful	Jealous	Respectful	Tender
Afraid	Choked-up	Distant	Grief-stricken	Joyful	Sad	Tense
Aggressive	Close	Dominant	Grumpy	Light	Scared	Terrified
Airy	Cold	Dull	Guilty	Locked in	Seductive	Thankful
Alarmed	Comforted	Ecstatic	Gutless	Lonely	Self-assured	Threatened
Angry	Compassionate	Edgy	Happy	Loving	Sexy	Thrilled
Anxious	Confident	Embarrassed	Hard	Mixed-up	Silly	Timid
Appealing	Confused	Empathetic	Hopeful	Nauseated	Soft	Tolerant
Ashamed	Contemptuous	Enraged	Hopeless	Open	Spineless	Torn
Beaten	Contended	Envious	Horrified	Panicky	Stretched	Two-faced
Belligerent	Cooperative	Estranged	Humble	Paralyzed	Strong	Uptight
Bewildered	Courageous	Evasive	Immobilized	Peaceful	Submissive	Vacant
Bored	Dead-eyed	Excited	Inpatient	Played out	Sunshiny	Warm
Breathless	Deferential	Fearful	Inadequate	Pleased	Surprised	Weepy
Burdened	Defiant	Firm	Independent	Powerless	Sweaty	
Bushed	Dependent	Frisky	Insecure	Quiet	Sympathetic	
Calm	Depressed	Frustrated	Irritated	Relaxed	Talkative	
Carefree	Determined	Giddy	Itchy	Resentful	Taut	

It is helpful to break the story into smaller segments and discuss each segment in depth. Once the situation has been described to the nurse's satisfaction and the nurse has a clear understanding, all vague issues have been clarified, and all questions have been answered, then the nurse should ask the client to go back and label his or her thoughts and feelings related to each aspect of the incident.

The following is an example of staying focused to get the story:

Client: *"Running your own business is tough."*

Nurse: *"What is one tough thing about running your own business?"* (focusing)

Client: *"Have I told you about my trip to Italy?"*

Nurse: *"Not yet, but let's get back to one thing that is difficult about running your own business."* (focusing)

ASKING FOR CLARIFICATION

Nurses often believe they should always be able to understand what the client is saying and make connections between statements, but often this is not the case: the client's thoughts and communications may be unclear. The nurse should never assume that he or she understands; rather, the nurse should ask for clarification if there is doubt. Asking for clarification to confirm the nurse's understanding of what the client intends to convey is paramount to accurate data collection.

If the nurse needs more information or clarification on a previously discussed issue, he or she may need to go back to that issue. The nurse may also need to ask questions in some areas to clarify information. The nurse can then use the therapeutic technique of **consensual validation**, which means repeating his or her understanding of the event just described by the client to see whether their perceptions agree. It is important to go back and clarify rather than working on assumptions.

The following is an example of clarifying and focusing techniques:

Client: *"I saw it coming. No one else had a clue this would happen."*

Nurse: *"What was it that you saw coming?"* (seeking clarification)

Client: *"We were doing well, and then the floor dropped out from under us. There was little anyone could do but hope for the best."*

Nurse: *"Help me understand by describing what 'doing well' refers to."* (seeking clarification)

"Who are the 'we' you refer to?" (focusing)

"Tell me about you and _____." (Assessing relationship)

"How did the floor drop out from under you?" (encouraging description of perceptions)

"What did you hope would happen when you 'hoped for the best'?" (encouraging evaluation)

CONNECTING ISLANDS OF INFORMATION

If a client moves from one topic to the next without demonstrating how the topics are related, the nurse needs to ask how these two topics are connected. This technique is known as **connecting islands of information**. The nurse must use active listening to grasp potentially related information.

Client: *"I came home from work and found no one home. My sister has a lot to offer to the new college that hired her."*

Nurse: *"How does your finding no one home after work relate to your sister's having a lot to offer to the new college that hired her?"* (connecting islands of information)

Client: *"Oh, I had forgotten my wife and daughter were going to the airport to pick up my sister from her job interview. We were all excited because my sister was hired on the spot during her interview, and we were all going to help her move to Boston."*

CLIENT'S AVOIDANCE OF THE ANXIETY-PRODUCING TOPIC

Sometimes clients begin discussing a topic of minimal importance because it is less threatening than the issue that is increasing the client's anxiety. The client is discussing a topic but seems to be focused elsewhere. Active listening and observing changes in the intensity of the nonverbal process help give the nurse a sense of what is going on. There are many options that can help the nurse determine which topic is more important:

1. Ask the client which issue is more important at this time.
2. Go with the new topic because the client has given nonverbal messages that this is the issue that needs to be discussed.
3. Reflect the client's behavior signaling there is a more important issue to be discussed.
4. Mentally file the other topic away for later exploration.
5. Ignore the new topic, because it seems the client is trying to avoid the original topic.

The following example shows how the nurse can try to identify which issue is most important to the client:

Client: *"I don't know whether it is better to tell or not tell my husband that I won't be able to work anymore. He gets so upset whenever he hears bad news. He has an ulcer, and bad news seems to set off a new bout of ulcer bleeding and pain."*

Nurse: *"Which is the most difficult issue for you to confront right now, your bad news or your husband's ulcer?"*

The nurse should avoid asking questions about feelings before getting a thorough description of the situation. Clients have more difficulty describing feelings than actions, and asking first about feelings can preclude getting detailed information about the situation.

In the following example, the nurse fails to use active listening and asks an unrelated question that sidetracks the client from relating his story:

Client: *"Well, here I am in the hospital."*

Nurse: *"How did you get here?"*

Client: *"The police brought me. I was just standing on the corner of Morris and Bernard, and the cops stopped and brought me here."*

Nurse: *"How do you like it here?"* (unrelated question that disrupts the client's story)

IDENTIFYING PARTICIPANTS AND RELATIONSHIPS

While discussing the situation, the nurse needs to get the first names of all participants to ensure that both nurse and client know which person is being discussed. The nurse then asks the client to describe his or her relationship to each person. For example, "Tell me about you and Donna," will elicit information about the relationship. Other ways to assess the client's perception of a person is to ask, "Paint a word picture of Terry" or "Give me a thumbnail sketch of your relationship with Bill."

Box 6-5 gives a sample dialogue in which the nurse guides the client to "get the story" using active listening techniques and building questions based on the client's responses, asking one question at a time, and giving adequate time for the client to respond.

Box 6-5

▶ EFFECTIVE THERAPEUTIC DIALOGUE: GETTING THE CLIENT'S STORY AND PROBLEM-SOLVING

Client (C): "Well, here I am in the hospital." A chagrined smile.

Nurse (N): "What was going on that you had to be hospitalized?" **(encouraging description of perceptions).** Turn toward client with interested demeanor.

C: "I was just standing on the corner of Morris and Bernard, and the cops stopped and brought me in here." Shrugs, looks as if he is not interested in continuing conversation because he is glancing away.

N: "What were you doing while you were standing on the corner of Morris and Bernard?" **(focusing)** Interested; tilt head slightly left to let the client know I want to hear his story. Sitting with hands resting on lap and legs uncrossed. Facing him at an angle.

C: "Nothing." Client has a blank look on his face. His eyes dart to a point beyond my head.

N: "Who was with you on this corner of Morris and Bernard?" **(focusing)** Said gently so as not to challenge him.

C: "My friend." Eyes still looking beyond my head but seems now to be focused on some place to help him think. Allowing a few moments of silence so he can gather his thoughts.

N: "Which friend?" **(focusing)** Used a gentle tone of voice and nodded to encourage him to share his story.

C: "Robert." Clipped tone of voice.

N: Allows a few moments so he doesn't feel pressured:"Tell me about you and Robert." Voice is soft and looking at him. **(assessing relationship)**

C: "There's nothing much to tell. I just met him that day on the corner." Shrugs and looks down at floor about 1½ feet in front of his feet.

N: "Just met him that day on the corner?" **(reflecting)** Gently puzzled tone of voice, scrunch my eyebrows a little.

C: "Yeah, he sold me some crack." His voice is stronger, looks up at me to see my reaction when he says "crack." He grasps the arm of his chair.

N: "What did you do with the crack?" **(focusing)** Do not change expression to demonstrate acceptance and genuine interest.

C: "What do you think? It was good stuff. I used it. Robert showed me how." He has a small grin, as if he has made a joke. His hands still grasp the arms of his chair.

N: "What was going on that you chose to use crack?" **(encouraging description of perceptions)** Tilt head to the left, very slight quizzical expression with eyebrows raised with eye contact.

C: "I was bored." He looks down at floor again, with a disgusted frown on his face.

N: "Bored?" **(reflecting)**

C: "Well, not really." Long pause. "I had a fight with someone in the boarding house." Lowers his voice and shifts body.

N: "With whom did you fight at the boarding house?" **(placing event in sequence)** I shift my body also, cross ankles, loosen up a bit more, and look at him once again.

C: "Clarissa." Dreamy look to face, slight smile at reminiscence, looking beyond my head again.

N: "Who is Clarissa?" **(assessing relationship).** Eyes widen, slight smile, showing interest, look down, then glance at him.

Continued

Box 6-5

➤ EFFECTIVE THERAPEUTIC DIALOGUE:—cont'd

C: "This girl who lives in the boarding house. I used to like her." Looks directly at me, leans forward, sassy smile, lifts right arm to punctuate last sentence.

N: "Used to?" (reflecting) Gently, with eye contact.

C: "Yeah! 'Til that day. She called me a baby." Voice ends with kind of a shamed tone. Distressed with his behavior. Looks down, shoulders slump.

N: "What did you say to Clarissa when she called you a baby?" (placing event in sequence) Tilt my cheek onto the fingers of my right hand, lean on right elbow, look ready to listen.

C: "Nothing. I ran away." Voice is soft, still has a shamed tone.

N: "What did you think running away would do?" (encouraging evaluation) I matched his soft tone without the shamed element.

C: "Well, everyone laughed when she called me a baby." Eyes narrow, face tightens, hands curl into fists. Crosses leg away from me.

N: "Who is everyone?" (focusing) Keeping voice accepting and gentle.

C: "Two other guys from the boarding house. They all laughed. So I ran out of the house." Knuckles clenched. Right fist hits armrest. Legs tensed.

N: "Then what did you do?" (placing event in sequence) Gently, objectively, acceptingly.

C: "I walked on the beach." Rubs face with both hands. Legs still crossed.

N: "What were you thinking as you walked on the beach?" (encouraging evaluation) Again, I wait a few beats before talking to give him time to relive the experience.

C: "I was thinking how I'd show them. I'd show them I'm not a baby." Holds hands on temples, shakes head from side to side.

N: "Them?" (seeking clarification) Slightly raise eyebrows.

C: "Yeah. Clarissa, Comanche, and . . . uh . . . oh yeah, Joe. I'd really show them." Bends top of body over knees, then shifts back in chair, sits up, and looks at me with an intense look as if he had a goal in mind.

N: "So what did you do?" (placing event in sequence) Punctuate the question by raising my right hand about 2" from armrest.

C: "I went to this corner and brought crack." Still has intense look of reliving action. Crosses leg toward me. Leans toward the right, then looks at me as if to gauge my reaction again.

N: "I am not sure how buying crack relates to your being upset because someone called you a baby." (connecting islands of information) Accepting tone of voice, slight eyebrow raise, tried for a deadpan expression.

C: "Well, you see, Clarissa called me a baby because she asked me for some drugs, you know, like grass or coke . . . and I said I didn't do none of that stuff and she shouldn't either. So she laughed and called me a baby." Body relaxes into his story, uses arms and hands to punctuate explanation.

N: "So you bought this crack and then what happened? (placing event in sequence) Said without any visual or verbal sanction. Tilt my head toward client.

C: "I used it. It was my first time and I don't ever plan to use it again!" Shakes head several times as he emphasizes the word "ever." Voice firm. Then sighs.

N: "What happened when you used the crack?" (encouraging description of perceptions) Accepting, interested, shift in seat a little to listen more.

C: "Weird stuff, man. I soared up to heaven . . . then fell down in the middle of the road." Uses hands to illustrate soaring and falling.

N: "Fell in the road?" (reflecting)

C: "Yeah, man, I thought I was dying. My heart just about raced out of my chest and I got weak and couldn't walk." Clutched chest, harried look on face, shrinks up in chair, voice softens and slows.

N: "Then what happened?" (placing event in sequence)

C: "I woke up in the medical center . . . A few days later they transferred me here to this behavioral health hospital. I've been here before, you see." Sounds relieved, long pauses between sentences. Looked at me to see if I understand/accept.

N: "Let's go back to when you ran out of the boarding house and walked on the beach. How did you decide on using crack when you had never used it before?" (encouraging evaluation) Accepting look on face.

C: "Well, you see, I thought I could show them." Patient, reasonable tone. Body open and relaxed. Looks like lecturing professor in his armchair.

N: "Show what to whom?" (seeking clarification) Soft tone of voice.

C: "Show Clarissa, Comanche, and Joe I was a man." Emphatically said, raised right arm from chair and beat it against chest when he said "man".

N: "How do you think doing crack makes you a man?" (encouraging evaluation) Nonchallenging tone to soften the message and not make it into an argument.

C: "I don't know. I mean I know it doesn't. Those drugs are killers. It almost killed me. The doctor said I could have died." Starts out softly, moves to exasperated tone of voice, rubs right temple with right hand.

N: "What have you learned about using crack to show you're a man?" (encouraging evaluation) Gently, with slight shrug of shoulders to ask question.

C: "It doesn't work. I thought I could be a man by doing crack. Boy, was I wrong. What a dope I was." Shaking head and looking as if he were still processing this.

N: "How do you think that you can show people you're a man?" (guiding a plan of action) Patiently, softly.

C: "I don't know." Looks helpless.

Continued

Box 6-5

➤ EFFECTIVE THERAPEUTIC DIALOGUE:—cont'd

N: "Well, who do you know that you consider to be a man?" **(guiding a plan of action)** Thoughtful, exploring tone.

C: "My old man." Said after a pause and looking off into far space, then nodding.

N: "Your father?" **(seeking clarification)** Acceptingly.

C: "Yeah, my father." Face lights up with answer he has devised.

N: "What behavior does your father demonstrate that identifies him as a 'man'?" **(encouraging evaluation)** Tilt head, open eyes more.

C: "He's tough." Emphatically said.

N: "What is one way you think your father is tough?" **(encouraging evaluation)** Slowly, as if thinking out loud.

C: "He'd never let anyone call him a baby. He'd punch their lights out." Again emphatically.

N: "You think punching someone's lights out proves manhood?" **(encouraging evaluation)** Softly and gently asking, nonjudgmental.

C: "Yeah, like _____." Mentions name of sports celebrity who was arrested.

N: "He was jailed as a rapist. How do you think that relates to being a man?" **(encouraging comparison)** Gently asking him to help me understand this.

C: "Not much, I guess." Rubs chin, shrugs shoulders.

N: "Let's get back to your father. Tell me about one time you saw him punch out someone's lights." **(focusing)**

C: "Well, I don't recall." Rubbing chin, looking up.

N: "You're saying you've not seen your father punch someone." **(consensual validation)** Nod as I understand better.

C: "Naw, he wouldn't do that. He's a church deacon, but you know, one look at him and everyone respected him." Proudly sits up, shoulders back. Satisfied smile.

N: Waited for him to enjoy this moment. "What's one way your father behaved that he got everyone's respect?" **(encouraging evaluation)**

C: "I don't know." Shoulders slump, voice leaden.

N: "Well, tell me how he walked." **(encouraging evaluation)** Encouraging, positive tone that implies I know he can do this.

C: "Oh, he walked tall—you know, like a cowboy walking into the sunset." Shoulders lift, sits erect, chin up.

N: "How did your father talk?" **(encouraging evaluation)** Interested tone but not sure if this is concrete enough for him to answer.

C: "What do you mean?" Puzzled tone.

N: "Oh, his tone of voice, loudness, even the way his face matched his words." **(encouraging evaluation)** Embarrassed I was not clearer before.

C: Face lights up with understanding. "Oh, that. Well, he spoke like he knew what he was talking about, and he acted like he knew what he was talking about." More erect posture.

N: "What can you learn from your father's behavior in terms of sending the message to people that you are a man?" **(encouraging evaluation)** Provide time for him to respond.

C: "Walk tall and look like I know what I'm talking about." Swings arm as if he were marching. Smiling.

N: "If a similar situation happened to you, such as the one where Clarissa called you a baby, how might you handle this differently?" **(formulating plan of action)** Open eyes slightly more and give encouraging look, waiting for his response.

C: "Well, I could pull myself up tall and say, 'Hey, pretty lady, you've got it wrong. Just look at how you're acting.' (Seems to be doing a fine movie cowboy imitation). "Then I'd turn and walk off. Yeah, that would work." Looking off to distance, smiling to self.

Guiding the Client in Problem-Solving and Empowering the Client to Change

Many therapeutic situations involve problem-solving. The nurse is not expected to be an expert or to tell the client what to do to fix his or her problem. Rather, the nurse should help the client to explore possibilities and find solutions to his or her problem. Often, just helping the client discuss and explore his or her perceptions of a problem stimulates potential solutions in the client's mind. The nurse should introduce the concept of problem-solving and offer himself or herself in this process.

Virginia Satir (1967) explained how important the client's participation is to finding effective and meaningful solutions to problems. If someone else tells the client how to solve his or her problems and does not allow the client to participate and develop problem-solving skills and paths for change, the client may fear growth and change. The nurse who gives advice or directions about the way to fix a problem does not allow the client to play a role in the process and implies that the client is less than competent. This process makes the client feel helpless and not in control and lowers self-esteem. The client may even resist the directives in an attempt to regain a sense of control.

When a client is more involved in the problem-solving process, he or she is more likely to follow through on the solutions. The nurse who guides the client to solve his or her own problems helps the client to develop new coping strategies, maintains or increases the client's self-esteem, and demonstrates the belief that the client is capable of change. These goals encourage the client to expand his or her repertoire of skills and to feel competent, and feeling effective and in control is a comfortable state for any client.

Problem-solving is frequently used in crisis intervention but is equally effective for general use. The problem-solving process is used when the client has difficulty finding ways to fix the problem or when working with a group of people whose divergent viewpoints hinder finding solutions. It involves several steps:

1. Identify the problem.
2. Brainstorm.
3. Group potential interventions.
4. Select the best three interventions.
5. Plan for implementation.
6. Implement the intervention.
7. Evaluate the situation (McGhee, 1998).

Identifying the problem involves engaging the client in therapeutic communication. The client tells the nurse the problem and what he or she has tried to do to fix the problem: ·

Nurse: *"I see you frowning. What is going on?"*

Client: *"I've tried to get my husband more involved with the children, other than yelling at them when he comes in from work, but I've had little success, even with me here in bed instead of being out there with the kids."*

Nurse: *"What have you tried that has not worked?"*

Client: *"Before my surgery, I tried to involve him in their homework. My husband is a math whiz. Then I tried TV time together, but the kids like cartoons and he wants to watch stuff about history, natural science, or travel."*

Nurse: *"How have you involved your husband in this plan for him to get more involved with the children?"*

Client: *"Uh, I haven't. I mean, he always says he wants to spend more quality time with the kids, but he doesn't. Do you mean it would be better for him to decide how he wants to do this—I mean, spend quality time with the kids?"*

Nurse: *"Sure, starting with what his definition of quality time is."*

Client: *"He'll be here tomorrow, when you come to change my dressing. Do you think you can give us some direction about talking about this?"*

Nurse: *"Yes. I have 20 minutes scheduled for your visit, and we can start as I am changing your dressing. I'll tell you and your husband how to problem-solve in case you need more time to reach some conclusions. Then, of course I'll be visiting you the following day, so we can discuss how this worked out."*

In the brainstorming stage, the nurse and client collaborate to create a list of all potential solutions that come to mind, without labeling them as good ideas or bad ideas. Judging potential solutions during the brainstorming phase may inhibit the client from suggesting ideas. Creativity is encouraged in the brainstorming phase, and all ideas or solutions are accepted.

In the grouping of potential interventions stage, each solution is reviewed and assigned to one of three categories: workable, possibly workable, or not workable now. From the workable category, the plan that is deemed best is selected and becomes plan A. The next-best solutions become plans B and C and are set aside for future use if needed.

In planning of implementation, the nurse and client plan how plan A will be implemented. Items necessary for the intervention are gathered, and the time and place of the intervention are set. The nurse can use role-playing to increase the client's skill and comfort in carrying out the intervention. The intervention is fine-tuned in this stage.

After the plan is implemented, the intervention is evaluated by the nurse and client. If plan A was successful, the results are discussed and learning occurs. If plan A was unsuccessful, the plan is reviewed to see whether it is still a good idea and needs to be repeated or repeated with modifications, or whether plan B should be implemented.

In some situations, the nurse must take a more directive role and offer clear suggestions for solutions, particularly when the client is in crisis or is suicidal. The nurse assumes an authoritative demeanor, giving directions to the client until the client's anxiety level is manageable and the problem-solving process can ensue. Further information on the nurse's role in crisis and suicide is given in Chapter 14.

DOCUMENTING THERAPEUTIC COMMUNICATION: THE INTERPERSONAL PROCESS ANALYSIS

Therapeutic communication occurs between two people, the nurse and the client, and reflects the personality of each. The Interpersonal Process Analysis (IPA) takes into consideration not only the thoughts and feelings of the client but also those of the nurse (nurse's self-awareness). The purpose of the IPA is to document communication with the client to assess the client's behavior, thoughts, feelings, and needs and to document the nurse's self-awareness. This tool helps the nurse discover the client-centered goal of the interaction. Unlike the nursing process goal, where the client outcome is to fix the problem, the IPA goal is short-term, to be accomplished in the time frame of the therapeutic communication, and is related only to that specific communication. The goal is stated in measurable terms, using action verbs—for example, Mr. Anderson will verbalize concerns about his responsibility to raise his grandson.

The IPA has a beginning, a middle, and an end. The beginning stage (orientation) includes broad openings the nurse uses to encourage the client to select a topic, and identification of the goal. The middle stage (working) reflects the use of focused therapeutic communication techniques to gain a comprehensive picture of the situation and its associated thoughts, feelings, needs, and relationships. The end stage includes the temporary or permanent termination of the nurse–client relationship.

Cover Page

Several formats can be used to record therapeutic communication between the nurse and client. The following format covers the components of the therapeutic communication that are most important to record. As the student nurse gains skill in therapeutic communication, the components become a mental checklist as the interpersonal process ensues. At this point, written documentation in the following format helps the student develop a framework to accomplish this vital nursing intervention.

The written framework of an IPA starts with a cover page that contains the client-centered goal of the interaction, the developmental theorist the nurse chooses to use to describe the client's developmental status, and the assessment of the client's developmental stage (Box 6-6).

Interaction and Interpretation

The interaction between the client and nurse is recorded as close to verbatim as possible and includes nonverbal process communications. Practice sessions between two student nurses (one student playing the nurse and the other playing the client) can be videotaped so verbatim transcriptions can be written. This enables the "nurse" to assess his or her success in active listening; picking up on cues; setting a client-identified, client-centered goal; using open-ended techniques with numerous finely focused questions to gather in-depth data from the client, get the client's perception of the incident from start to end, and assess the relationships between participants; and guid-

---

Box 6-6

➤ INTERPERSONAL PROCESS ANALYSIS (IPA) COVER PAGE

STUDENT:

DATE: _____

CLIENT INITIALS: _____

CLIENT AGE: _____

DEVELOPMENTAL STAGE
(Use stages of any theorist—for instance, Havinghurst, Erickson, Piaget, Freud, Sullivan)
1. Identify the theorist.
2. Label the developmental stage of the client.
   If the theorist used polar labels for each stage, such as generativity vs. isolation, underline which pole you believe the client is in.
3. Describe all the tools and tasks of this developmental stage:
   a. Those the client has achieved
   b. Those (if any) the client has not mastered/achieved. (If there are many unmet tasks, perhaps the client is in an earlier developmental stage than you believe him or her to be.)
4. Assess whether the client's developmental stage and chronologic age concur.
5. If the client's chronologic age and developmental stage do **not** concur:
   a. According to client's age, identify in which developmental stage the client should be.
   b. Discuss the tools and tasks of this stage and document the ways in which you believe the client has never developed or has lost tools and tasks through the advent of his or her anxiety or mental illness, and identify the developmental stage you believe the client demonstrates.

Goal of Interaction (Client-Centered Goal):
The IPA goal is a short-term goal and is related only to that particular communication. Often, just discussing the client's issue becomes the goal of the interaction. The goal is to be stated in measurable terms, using action verbs.

Example of goal: Mr. A. will verbalize concerns about his responsibility to raise his grandson.

ing the client to generate solutions. Videotaping also enables the students to spot nonverbal behaviors that help and hinder the therapeutic communication process.

The nurse analyzes and interprets each nurse–client interaction. The nurse identifies the specific therapeutic communication technique used, the rationale for using that technique, thoughts and feelings about himself or herself and the client at that moment in time, and his or her own needs during the interaction. If the intervention used was nontherapeutic, the nurse would specify a more therapeutic intervention (Box 6-7). The description of the interaction includes both the nurse's and the client's verbal and nonverbal messages and relevant information about the environment, such as noise, heat, light, presence of other people, and where each person was positioned.

Evaluation

The IPA concludes with the nurse's self-evaluation (Box 6-8). There is also a peer evaluation tool that can be used to assess other students' videotaped practice IPAs (Box 6-9). Both tools help the student identify areas of growth in therapeutic communication skill and areas needing more practice.

COMMUNITY-BASED CARE

As community care for persons with physical and mental health problems continues to expand, the nurse's role expands as well. Nurses may become the major caregiver and resource person for increasingly high-risk clients treated in the home and for the client's family and will become more responsible for primary prevention in wellness and health maintenance. Therapeutic communication techniques and skills are essential to successful management of clients in the community.

Caring for the elderly in the family unit and in communities today is a major nursing concern and responsibility. It is important to assess the relationships of family members, identifying their areas of agreement and conflict, which can greatly affect the care of clients. To be responsive to the needs of these clients and their families for support and caring, the nurse must be able to communicate and relate to clients and establish a therapeutic relationship.

When practicing in the community, the nurse needs self-awareness and knowledge about the cultural differences discussed in this chapter. When the nurse enters the home of a client, the nurse is the outsider and must learn to negotiate the cultural

---

Box 6-7

➤ INTERPERSONAL PROCESS ANALYSIS (IPA) SCROLL FORMAT

Document for each nurse–client interaction:

INTERACTION

Nurse:
Content in quotation
Process: nonverbals and metacommunication.
Client:
Content in quotation
Process: nonverbals and metacommunication.
Information about the milieu.

INTERPRETATION

After each nurse–client interaction:
State your interpretation of what was taking place:

1. Technique: the specific interpersonal technique used
2. Rationale: the therapeutic value of using this technique, not merely a definition of the technique
3. Thoughts: Discuss your thoughts and impressions about yourself and the client, as well as what you believe to be going on between you. Examine your past experiences to see how they affect your present thoughts and impressions at this moment in time during this IPA.
4. Feelings: Describe your feelings and/or gut reactions at that point in time during the interaction. This includes feelings about yourself and the client. Examine your past experiences to see how they affect your feelings at this moment in this IPA.
5. Needs: Speculate on your needs at that moment and indicate whether they were met or unmet as they occur.
6. Corrections: If you used a nontherapeutic technique in this specific interaction, write what would have been more appropriate to say.

Box 6-8

➤ SELF-EVALUATION OF INTERPERSONAL PROCESS ANALYSIS (IPA)

This is the final portion of a transcribed IPA. The nurse answers the following questions about the interview:

1. To what extent were the goals for this interview realized?
2. What other goals emerged?
3. What factors helped or hindered goal achievement?
4. a. Did I allow the client to freely express the way things seem to him or her?
   b. Did I push the client too much?
5. a. Did I use myself as a facilitator in helping him or her explore his or her own space?
   b. How effective was I in getting the specific details of the client's story?
6. a. Did I use open-ended communication techniques?
   b. Which nontherapeutic communication techniques did I use?
7. Was my attitude one that allowed the client to get closer to his or her own feelings?
8. a. Did I really listen, or was I busy getting an answer ready?
   b. Did I unintentionally change the topic or the focus of the topic?
9. a. Was the client afraid or hesitant to express himself or herself?
   b. What did I do to relieve those feelings?
10. a. What themes were expressed by the client?
    b. Did I pick up on themes, symbols, metaphors?
11. a. When was the client most comfortable during the interview?
    b. When was he or she uncomfortable during the interview?
12. a. When was I most comfortable during the interview?
    b. When was I uncomfortable during the interview?

Adapted from Hein, E. C. (1980). Communication in nursing practice, *2nd ed. (pp. 77–78)*. Boston: Little, Brown & Co.

Critical Thinking

Questions

1. Use therapeutic techniques in your next several client or peer interactions, and evaluate the difference between the use of focused, open-ended techniques as opposed to closed questions.
2. As a staff nurse in a hospital, you have spent the past 15 minutes listening to your 64-year-old client describe her distress over her husband's decision to move back to his hometown 600 miles away as soon as she is better. She wants to stay where they currently live, because their children and friends are nearby. She says she has no clue why he wants to move back: he no longer has relatives or even old friends in his hometown.
   a. List the questions you would ask her to get the additional information necessary to clarify this issue in your mind.
   b. Making sure you do not attempt to fix her problem for her, how would you encourage this client to problem-solve?
3. Explain why the nurse's attempt to solve the client's problem is less effective than guiding the client to identify his or her own ways to resolve the issue.
4. What is the rationale for getting detailed information about a topic?
5. A client on the orthopedic unit who has a broken pelvis has been talking incessantly about his former girlfriend, who no longer wants him around. One day he tells you he has decided to kill her when he gets out of the hospital, and he has a gun to do it.
   a. What is your legal and ethical responsibility, knowing this information?
   b. How is the issue of confidentiality affected by the threats this client has made?
6. Assess your own spiritual values and needs and those of a client, and compare them to see whether they are alike or different.
7. Create your own Johari window.

context of each family, understanding their beliefs, customs, and practices and not judging them according to his or her own. Asking the family for help in learning about their culture demonstrates the nurse's unconditional positive regard and genuineness. Families from other cultural backgrounds often respect nurses and health care professionals and are quite patient and forgiving of the cultural mistakes nurses might make as they learn different customs and behaviors.

Another reason the nurse needs to understand the health care practices of various cultures is to make sure these practices do not hinder or alter the prescribed therapeutic regimens. Some cultural heal-

ing practices and remedies and even dietary practices may alter the client's immune system and may enhance or interfere with prescribed medications.

The nurse in community care is a member of the health care team and must learn to deal with not only the client and family but also other health care providers who are involved in the client's care, such as physicians, physical therapists, psychologists, and home health aides. Dealing with several people at one time, rather than just the client, becomes the standard in community care. Self-awareness and sensitivity to the beliefs, behaviors, and feelings of others are paramount to the successful care of clients in the community setting.

Box 6-9

➤ PEER EVALUATION TOOL FOR VIDEOTAPED PRACTICE OF INTERPERSONAL PROCESS ANALYSIS (IPA)

Directions: Circle one of the four descriptions for each of the 11 categories.
Add scores on the bottom of each column and total. Enter total score on bottom left cell.
Client identified goal of therapeutic communication:

	4	3	2	1
1. Goal of IPA recognized	Accurately	Adequately	Minimally	Not recognized
2. Goal reached	Thoroughly	Adequately	Minimally	Not reached
3. Emergent goal	Connected to goal	Deferred to later	Ignored or not heard	Confused issue
4. Open-ended techniques	Almost always	Half the time	Less than half of the time	Rarely
5. Time for client responses	Almost always	Adequate	Minimal	Rare
6. Nontherapeutic techniques	Rarely	Occasionally	Many	Predominantly
7. In-depth exploration of client issues	Almost always	Adequate	Superficial	Ignored client issue
8. Interested, genuine demeanor	Almost always	Adequate	Distracted	Not interested
9. Active listener	Picked up on each cue	Attended to many cues	Dealt with some cues	Ignored cues
10. Problem resolution	Guided client to self-resolution	Initiated client problem resolution	Tried to fix client's problem	No attempt at problem resolution
11. Assessed context of issues	Almost always	Adequately	Sometimes	Rarely
Sub Total: _____	_____ × 4 = _____	_____ × 3 = _____	_____ × 2 = _____	_____ × 1 = _____

TOTAL SCORE _____   Interpretation of score:

_____ × 4 = _____   34 to 44   Excellent therapeutic communication skills
_____ × 3 = _____   23 to 33   Adequate
_____ × 2 = _____   12 to 22   Minimal: practice more
_____ × 1 = _____   11 Need to practice therapeutic communication skills.

INTERNET RESOURCES

Resource	Internet Address
▶ Therapeutic games and activities	http://home.att.net/~recroom
▶ Communication skills	http://www.personal.u-net.com/osl/m263.htm
▶ Psychology of listening and communicating	http://www.allaboutcounseling.com/listening.htm
▶ BOLA: The Johari window	http://sol.brunel.ac.uk.~jarvis/bola.communications/johari.html
▶ On being assertive	http://www.exxnet.com/resources/assert.htm
▶ Team communication	http://www.yorkteam.com/teamc.htm

➤ KEY POINTS

- Communication is the process people use to exchange information through verbal and nonverbal messages.
- Communication is composed of both the literal words or content and all the nonverbal messages (behavior, thoughts, feelings, needs, values) that accompany the words called process. To communicate effectively, the nurse must be skilled at interpreting both content and process.
- Therapeutic communication is an interpersonal interaction in which the nurse uses the self to focus on the client's emotional issues, establish a therapeutic relationship, identify client issues, discern the most important topic at that time, and guide the client toward identifying his or her own solutions to problems.
- The nurse should use open-ended therapeutic communication techniques to elicit information from the client unless there is suspected suicide ideation or thoughts of self-harm; in that case, direct, yes/no questions are appropriate.
- The crucial components of therapeutic communication are confidentiality, privacy and respect for boundaries, self-disclosure, and active listening skills.
- Using one's humanity (personality, experiences, values, feelings, intelligence, needs,

coping skills, and perceptions) to help a client grow and change is called the therapeutic use of self.
- Self-awareness is an understanding of one's personality, emotions, sensitivity, motivations, ethics, philosophy of life, physical and social image, and capacities. The greater the nurse's understanding of his or her own feelings and responses, the better the nurse can communicate and understand others.
- Active listening involves concentrating on the client's words and behaviors to comprehend his or her message, and listening and watching for cues so that the nurse can respond and formulate questions.
- Metaphors, cues, proverbs, clichés, symbolism, mottoes, and themes are word patterns that signal the intent of the speaker's words.
- Verbal messages need to be clear and concrete rather than vague and abstract. Abstract messages requiring the client to make assumptions can be misleading and confusing. The nurse needs to clarify any areas of confusion so that he or she does not make assumptions based on his or her own experience.
- Nonverbal communication includes facial expressions, body language, eye contact, proxemics (environmental distance), touch, and vocal cues. All of these are important in understanding the speaker's message.

- Cultural differences can greatly affect the therapeutic communication process. The nurse must understand these differences in specific cultures so that he or she can communicate with those of various cultures and meet their health care needs.

- Spirituality and religion can greatly affect a client's health and health care. These beliefs vary widely among people and are highly subjective issues that must be assessed and understood by the nurse. The nurse must be careful not to impose his or her beliefs on the client or allow differences to erode trust.

- Understanding the context is important to the accuracy of the message. The nurse must understand all the details of an event the client is describing, asking questions about the participants, their moods, attitudes, and relationships, and when, where, and how the incident started, progressed, and ended in a step-by-step progression.

- The goal of the therapeutic communication process is to guide the client to identify a client-centered goal and to solve his or her own problems. The steps of the therapeutic communication session are introduction and making a verbal contract with the client, assessing the client's problem, constructing a client-centered goal, getting the story, and guiding the client to solve problems.

- The Interpersonal Process Analysis is a way to record the therapeutic communication between nurse and client. Components are goal, developmental factors, interaction between nurse and client, interpretation, and self-evaluation. Interaction consists of nurse–client communication, interpretation (technique rationale), thoughts, feelings, and needs.

- The nurse may be the major caregiver and resource person for increasingly high-risk clients treated in the home and for the client's family, and nurses will become more responsible for primary prevention in wellness and health maintenance. Therapeutic communication techniques and skills are essential to successful management of clients in the community.

REFERENCES

American Nurses Association. (1985). *Code of ethics with interpretive statements.* Kansas City, MO: American Nurses Association.

Andrews, M., & Boyle J. (1999). *Transcultural concepts on nursing care*, 3rd ed. Philadelphia: Lippincott Williams & Wilkins.

Arnold, E., & Boggs, K.. (1995). *Interpersonal relationships: professional communication skills for nurses*, 2nd ed. Philadelphia: W. B. Saunders.

Balzer-Riley, J. W. (1996). *Communications in nursing: communicating assertively and responsibly in nursing: a guidebook*, 3rd ed. Philadelphia: Mosby.

Bandler, R., &. Grinder, J. (1982). *Reframing: neurolinguistic programming and the transformation of meaning.* Moab, UT: Real People Press.

Boyd, M. A., & Nihart, M. A. (1998). *Psychiatric nursing: contemporary practice.* Philadelphia: Lippincott-Raven.

Campbell, J. (1980). The relationship of nursing and self-awareness. *Advances in Nursing Science, 2*, 15.

Cormier, L. S., Cormier, W. H., & Weisser, R. J. (1997). *Interviewing and helping skills for health professionals.* Boston: Jones & Bartlett.

Deering, C. G. (1999). To speak or not to speak? Self-disclosure with patients. *American Journal of Nursing, 99*(1), 34–39.

deVito, J. (1991). *Human communication: the basic course*, 7th ed. New York: Longman.

Geissler, E. (1998). *Pocket guide to cultural assessment*, 2nd ed. Philadelphia: Mosby.

Hall, E. (1963). Proxemics: the study of man's spatial relationships. In J. Gladstone (Ed.). *Man's image in medicine and anthropology* (pp. 109–120). Philadelphia: Mosby.

Hancock, C. (1998). How to decide about self-disclosure. *Nursing 98*(3), 12–13.

Knapp, M., & Hall, J. (1992). *Nonverbal behavior in human interaction*, 3rd ed. New York: Holt, Rinehart & Winston.

Knapp, M. L. (1980). *Essentials of nonverbal communication*, New York: Holt, Rinehart & Winston.

Kreps, G. L., & Kunimoto, E. N. (1994). *Effective communication in multicultural health care settings.* Thousand Oaks, CA: Sage Publications.

Luft, J. (1970). *Group processes: an introduction in group dynamics.* Palo Alto, CA: National Press Books.

McGhee P. (1998). Rx: Laughter. *RN, 7*(3), 50–53.

Morley, W. E., et al. (1967). Crisis: paradigms of intervention. *Journal of Psychiatric Nursing, 5*, 537–538.

Northouse, L. L., & Northouse, P. G. (1998). *Health communication: strategies for health professionals*, 3rd ed. Stamford, CT: Appleton & Lange.

Peplau, H. (1952). *Interpersonal relations in nursing.* New York: G. P. Putnam.

Satir, V. (1967). *Conjoint family therapy: a guide to theory and technique*, revised ed. Palo Alto, CA: Science and Behavior Books, Inc.

Schrank, J. (1998). *Reading people: the unwritten language of the body* [videotape]. Geneva, IL: Stage Fright Productions.

Tarasoff v. Regents of the University of California. 17 Cal. 3d 425; 131 Cal.Reptr. 14 (1976).

van Servellen, G. (1997). *Communication skills for the health care professional: concepts and techniques.* Gaithersburg, MD: Aspen.

Weaver, R. L. (1996). *Understanding interpersonal communication.* New York: Harper-Collins College Publishers.

Wilson, H. S., & Kneisl, C. R. (1996). *Psychiatric nursing,* 5th ed. Philadelphia: Addison-Wesley Nursing.

ADDITIONAL READINGS

Gallois, C., & Callan, V. (1997). *Communication and culture: a guide for practice.* Chichester, England: John Wiley & Sons, Ltd.

Haddad, A. (1998). Ethics in action. *RN,* July, 21.

Hall, E. T. (1976). *Beyond culture.* New York: Anchor Press/Doubleday.

Kahn, S., & Saulo, M. (1994). *Healing yourself: a nurse's guide to self-care and renewal.* Albany, NY: Delmar Publishers, Inc.

Lukas, S. (1993). *Where to start and what to ask: an assessment handbook.* New York: W. W. Norton & Co.

Sundeen, S. J., Stuart, G. W., Rankin, E. A., & Cohen, S. A. (1994). *Nurse–client interaction: implementing the nursing process,* 5th ed. Philadelphia: Mosby.

➤ MULTIPLE-CHOICE QUESTIONS

Select the best answer for each of the following questions.

1. "Good afternoon, Mr. Hollick. My name is John Toth and I am a student nurse from Ocean College Nursing Department. I will be your nurse today from 3 to 10:30 p.m." This statement is made for the purpose of:

    A. Giving recognition and providing self

    B. Offering both first and last name so the client can choose a comfortable way to address the nurse

    C. Setting the limits of the relationship

    D. All of the above

2. Client: "I had an accident."
   Nurse: "Tell me about your accident." This exemplifies which of the following therapeutic communication techniques?

    A. Making observations

    B. Offering self

    C. General lead

    D. Assessing relationship

3. "Earlier today you said you were concerned that your son was still upset with you. When I stopped by your room about an hour ago, you and your son seemed relaxed and smiling as you spoke to one another. How did things go between the two of you?" This is an example of which therapeutic communication technique?

    A. Consensual validation

    B. Encouraging comparison

    C. Accepting

    D. General lead

4. "Why do you always complain about the night nurse? She is a nice woman and a fine nurse, and has five kids to support. You're wrong when you say she is noisy and uncaring." Select the nontherapeutic technique that is not demonstrated in this nurse's response to a client.

    A. Requesting an explanation

    B. Defending

    C. Disagreeing

    D. Advising

5. "How does Jerry make you upset?" is an nontherapeutic communication technique because it:

    A. Gives a literal response

    B. Indicates the existence of an external source of the emotion

    C. Interprets what the client is saying

    D. Is just another stereotyped comment

6. The client says, "The doctor says I have to have my toes amputated. I think the doctor is nuts." Which of the following is an example of a volatile verbiage response from the nurse?

    A. "So you're saying the doctor does not know what she is doing?"

    B. "Tell me more about what the doctor said about amputating your toes."

    C. "This must be difficult for you to hear."

    D. "Don't worry; the surgery is simple and you will be home soon."

7. Client: "I was so upset about my sister ignoring my pain when I broke my leg."
   Nurse: "When are you going to your next diabetes education program?" This is a nontherapeutic response because the nurse has:

    A. Used testing to evaluate the client's insight

    B. Changed the topic

    C. An egocentric focus

    D. Advised the client what to do

8. When the client says, "I met Joe at the dance last week," what is the best way for the nurse to ask the client to describe her relationship with Joe?

    A. "Joe who?"

    B. "Tell me about Joe."

    C. "Tell me about you and Joe."

    D. "Joe, you mean that blond guy with the dark blue eyes?"

9. Which of the following is a concrete message?

    A. "Help me put this pile of books on Marsha's desk."

    B. "Get this out of here."

    C. "When is she coming home?"

    D. "They said it is too early to get in."

➤ SHORT-ANSWER QUESTIONS

Define the following:

1. Culture

2. Proxemics

3. Incongruent message

4. Spirituality

5. Validity or consistent

6. Nonverbal communication

7. Cliché

8. Metaphor

9. Spoken words

10. Johari window

11. Therapeutic use of self

12. Underlying needs

In the following client responses, underline the cues (words, phrases, or issues) that should be followed up with therapeutic communication interventions. Then write therapeutic response.

1. "I feel good."

2. "I can't take it anymore."

3. "I have two children, one from my wife and one from my girlfriend."

4. "We were standing on the corner."

5. "My son is never going to understand the way his wife is ruining them."

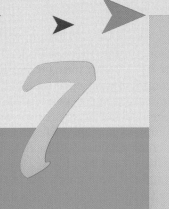

Client's Response to Illness

Nursing philosophies often describe the individual as a biopsychosocial being, possessing unique characteristics and responding to others and the world in various and diverse ways. This view of the individual as unique requires nurses to assess each person and his or her responses to plan and provide meaningful nursing care. This uniqueness of response may partially explain why some people become ill while others do not. It is difficult to understand why two people both raised in a stressful environment, such as one with neglect or abuse, seem to turn out differently: one becomes reasonably successful and maintains a satisfying marriage and family, while the other feels isolated, depressed, and lonely, is divorced, and abuses alcohol. Although we do not know exactly what makes the difference, studies have begun to show that there are certain personal, interpersonal, and cultural factors that influence a person's response.

Culture is all of the socially learned behaviors, values, beliefs, customs, and ways of thinking of a population that guide its members' view of themselves and the world. This view of others and the world affects all aspects of the person's being, including health, illness, and treatment. **Cultural diversity** refers to the vast array of differences that exist among populations.

This chapter examines some of the personal, interpersonal, and cultural factors that create this unique individual response to both illness and treatment. In determining how a person copes with illness, we cannot single out one or two of these factors but must consider each person as a combination of all these overlapping and interacting factors.

INDIVIDUAL FACTORS

Age, Growth, Development

A person's age seems to affect how he or she copes with illness. For instance, the age of onset of schizophrenia is a strong predictor of the prognosis of the disease (Buchanan & Carpenter, 2000). Persons with a younger age of onset have poorer outcomes, such as more negative signs (apathy, social isolation, lack of volition) and less effective coping skills than persons with a later age of onset. Younger clients have not had experiences of successful independent living or the opportunity to work and be self-sufficient, and have a less well-developed sense of personal identity than older clients.

A client's age can also influence how he or she expresses illness. A young child with attention deficit hyperactivity disorder may lack the understanding and ability to describe his or her feelings, so the nurse must be aware of the child's level of language and work to understand the experience as the child describes it.

Erik Erikson described psychosocial development across the life span in terms of developmental tasks to be accomplished in each phase (Table 7-1). Each stage of development is dependent on successful completion of the previous stage. In each stage, the person must complete a critical life task that is essential to well-being and mental health. Failure to complete the critical task results in a negative outcome for that stage of development and impedes completion of future tasks. For example, the infant stage (birth to 18 months) is the stage of trust versus mistrust, when babies must learn to develop basic trust—trust that their parents or caretakers will take care of them, feed them, change their diapers, love them, and keep them safe. If trust is not developed in this stage, the person may be unable to love and trust others later in life, because the ability to trust others is essential in establishing good relationships.

People may get "stuck" at any stage of development. A person who has not completed the developmental task of autonomy may exhibit lack of autonomy or initiative and become overly dependent on others. Failure to develop identity can result in role confusion, or lack of a clear idea of who one is as a per-

Table 7-1

ERIKSON'S STAGES OF PSYCHOSOCIAL DEVELOPMENT

Stage	Task
Trust vs. mistrust (infant)	Viewing the world as safe and reliable
	Viewing relationships as nurturing, stable, dependable
Autonomy vs. shame and doubt (toddler)	Achieving a sense of control and free will
Initiative vs. guilt (preschool)	Beginning development of a conscience
	Learning to manage conflict and anxiety
Industry vs. inferiority (school age)	Emerging confidence in own abilities
	Taking pleasure in accomplishments
Identity vs. role diffusion (adolescence)	Formulating a sense of self and belonging
Intimacy vs. isolation (young adult)	Forming adult, loving relationships and meaningful attachment to others
Generativity vs. stagnation (middle adult)	Being creative and productive
	Establishing the next generation
Ego integrity vs. despair (maturity)	Accepting responsibility for one's self and life

son. Negotiating these developmental tasks affects how the person will respond to stress and illness. Lack of success may result in feelings of inferiority, doubt, lack of confidence, and isolation, and these can affect how a person responds to illness.

Genetics and Biologic Factors

Heredity and biologic factors are not under our control and are a result of our biologic makeup. We cannot change these factors. Research in genetics has identified genetic links to several disorders. For example, some people are born with a gene associated with one type of Alzheimer's disease. Although specific genetic links have not been identified in several mental disorders, research has shown that these disorders tend to appear more frequently among families (e.g., bipolar affective disorder, major depression, alcoholism). Genetic makeup has a tremendous influence on our response to illness and perhaps even our response to treatment. Hence, family history and background is an essential part of the nursing assessment.

Physical Health and Health Practices

Physical health can also influence how a person responds to psychosocial stress or illness. The healthier a person is, the better he or she can cope with stress or illness. Poor nutritional status, lack of sleep, or a chronic physical illness may impair a person's ability to cope. Unlike genetic factors, many of these factors can be altered by how a person lives and takes care of himself or herself. For this reason, nurses must assess the client's physical health even when he or she is seeking help for mental health problems.

Personal health practices, such as exercise, can have an impact on the client's response to illness. Auchus et al. (1995) studied exercise patterns of psychiatric inpatients and found that walking was a common form of exercise. Those who walked one to five times a week reported an improved emotional state, but during the 2 weeks before their hospital admission, they had reduced or stopped walking altogether. This study suggests that walking had a positive influence on these clients' health and that cessation of walking was an indicator that their health was declining.

Response to Drugs

Biologic differences can affect a client's response to treatment, specifically to psychotropic drugs. Ethnic groups differ in the metabolism and efficacy of psychoactive compounds (Mohr, 1998). Some ethnic groups metabolize drugs more slowly (meaning the serum level of the drug is higher), and this increases

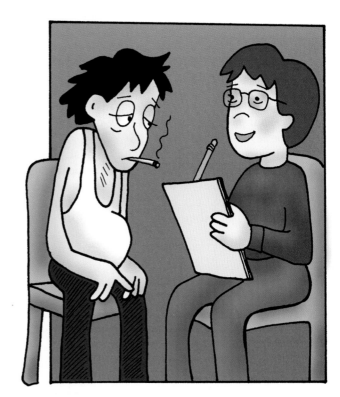

Assess client's physical health

the frequency and severity of side effects. Clients who metabolize drugs more slowly generally need lower doses of a drug to produce the desired effect. Mohr (1998) reported that in general, nonwhites treated with Western dosing protocols will have higher serum levels per dose and suffer more side effects. Although many non-Western countries report successful treatment with lower dosages of psychotropic drugs, Western dosage protocols continue to drive prescribing practices in the United States (Mohr, 1998). When evaluating the efficacy of psychotropic medications, the nurse must be alert to the presence of side effects and serum drug levels in clients from different ethnic backgrounds.

Self-Efficacy

Self-efficacy is a belief that personal abilities and efforts affect the events in our lives (Bandura, 1997). A person who believes that his or her actions will make a difference is more likely to take action. People with high self-efficacy set personal goals, are self-motivated, cope effectively with stress, and attract support from others when it is needed. Persons with low self-efficacy have low aspirations, experience much self-doubt, and may be plagued by anxiety and depression. Bandura (1997) suggests that rather than focusing on solving specific problems, treatment should focus on developing a client's skills to take control of his or her life (developing self-efficacy) so that he or she can make life changes. The four main ways to accomplish this are:

- Experience of success or mastery in overcoming obstacles
- Social modeling (observing successful people instills the idea that one can also succeed)
- Social persuasion (persuading people to believe in themselves)
- Reducing stress, building physical strength, and learning how to interpret physical sensations in a positive way (e.g., viewing fatigue as a sign that one has accomplished something rather than as a lack of stamina).

Hardiness

Hardiness is a person's ability to resist illness when under stress. First described by Kobasa (1979), hardiness is viewed as having three components:

- Commitment: active involvement in life's activities
- Control: ability to make appropriate decisions in life activities
- Challenge: ability to perceive change as beneficial rather than just a stressful event.

Hardiness has been found to have a moderating or buffering effect on persons experiencing stress. Kobasa (1979) found that male executives who had high stress but low illness occurrence scored higher on the hardiness scale than executives with high stress and high illness occurrence. The study suggested that people with low hardiness were more harmed by stressful life events. Other studies have found that hardiness seems to have a moderating effect on the occurrence of burnout among nurses (Boyle et al., 1991; Keane et al., 1985; Topf, 1989).

Hardiness has also been studied in relation to chronic illness. Pollack (1986) studied people with diabetes mellitus and found that those scoring higher on hardiness exhibited better physiologic adaptation than those with low hardiness scores, although hardiness was not related to adaptation to hypertension and arthritis. Lambert (1990) found that for women with rheumatoid arthritis, hardiness was a significant predictor of psychological well-being, along with social support.

Although hardiness has been described as a trait, some researchers believe they can increase health-related hardiness through education. People who believed their lives were affected by stress participated in a study designed to improve their abilities to manage stress. They were referred by local health providers, therapists, and physicians or obtained information about the study through newspaper ads or literature at the local mental health center. The Wellness Program focused on identifying and managing feelings, developing coping strategies, taking time for oneself, and improving communication. After the psychoeducation groups, people were found to have increased control and commitment (hardiness components) and a significant reduction in symptoms such as obsessive-compulsive behaviors, hostility, withdrawal/isolation, and level of distress (Webster & Austin, 1999).

Some believe that the concept of hardiness is vague and indistinct and may not be helpful to everyone. Some research on hardiness suggests it is not the same for men and women (Benishek & Lopez, 1997) and that hardiness is more prevalent as a stress moderator in men. Low (1999) suggested that hardiness may be useful only to those who value individualism, such as some people in Western cultures; however, for people and cultures who value relationships over individual achievement, hardiness may not be beneficial.

Resilience and Resourcefulness

Two closely related concepts, resilience and resourcefulness, help people to cope with stress and minimize the effects of illness. **Resilience** is defined as having healthy responses to stressful circumstances or risky situations (Hill, 1998). This concept helps us understand why one person reacts to a slightly stressful event with severe anxiety symptoms, while another person may not experience distress even when confronted by a major disruption or stressful event (Dyer & McGuinness, 1996). Studies on resiliency first focused on factors that resulted in positive outcomes for children who were at risk because their parents had alcohol or mental health problems (Rutter, 1987). Factors that enhanced outcomes were children's abilities to develop self-esteem and self-efficacy through relationships with others, the ability to have new experiences, and assistance with life transitions as they matured.

Studies have shown that families that use their strengths show improved resiliency and more positive outcomes than families who are viewed as victims of multiple problems, such as poverty, unemployment, and low socioeconomic status. Hill (1998) identified family protective mechanisms that improved the resiliency of the children, such as instilling positive family values, promoting positive communication and social interactions, maintaining flexible family roles, exercising control over children, and providing academic support to children. Other protective factors in the family have been shown to improve the resiliency of adolescents, including caring and supportive relationships with adult caregivers; high expectations of the children for good citizenship, academic achievement, and spiritual involvement; and encouragement of involvement in caring for siblings, household chores, part-time work, and carefully selected, safe activities outside the home (Calvert, 1997).

Resourcefulness involves using problem-solving abilities and believing that one can cope with adverse or novel situations. It is acquired through interactions with others and is demonstrated in one's ability to manage daily activities (Zauszniewski, 1995a,b). Resourcefulness may help prevent depressed feelings (Warheit, 1979). Studies indicate that clients with depression may be able to use resourcefulness as a means of coping with stressful circumstances and the accompanying feelings of depression (Zauszniewski, 1995a,b). Examples of resourcefulness include performing health-seeking behaviors, learning self-care, monitoring one's thoughts and feelings about stressful situations, and taking action to deal with stressful circumstances.

Spirituality

Spirituality involves the essence of a person's being and his or her beliefs about the meaning of life and the purpose for living. It may include belief in God or a higher power, the practice of religion, cultural beliefs and practices, and a relationship with the environment. Although many clients with mental disorders have disturbing religious delusions, for many in the general population, religion and spirituality are a source of comfort and help in times of stress or trauma. Studies have shown that spirituality is a gen-

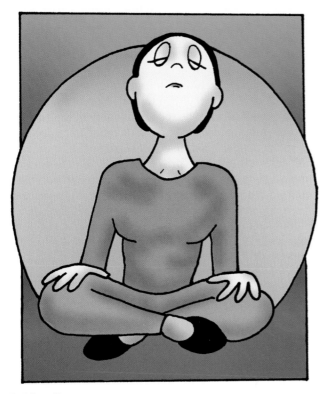

Spirituality

uine help to many mentally challenged adults, serving as a primary coping device and a source of meaning and coherence in their lives, or helping to provide a social network (Sullivan, 1993).

Religion and activities such as church attendance, praying, and the social support associated with religion have been shown to be very important for many people and are associated with better health and a sense of well-being (Stolley & Koenig, 1997). These activities have also been found to help people cope with poor health. Adams and Partee (1998) identified hope as a critical factor in psychiatric rehabilitation as well as physical rehabilitation.

Some studies have shown that religion and spirituality can be helpful to families who have a family member with mental illness: religion was found to play an important role in providing support to caregivers and was a major source of solace (Stolley & Koenig, 1997). In a study of factors that enhanced the dying process for elderly people, Siefken (1993) reported that having a physician who focused on the person's inner aspects and who respected the person's spirituality and religious beliefs was of major importance. Nelson (1989) found that religious orientation was helpful as a coping mechanism and a source of social support for elderly persons who were depressed.

Because spiritual or religious beliefs and practices help many clients to cope with stress and illness, the nurse must be particularly sensitive to and accepting of clients' spiritual beliefs and practices. Incorporating those practices into the care of clients can help them cope with illness and find meaning and purpose in the situation, and can offer a strong source of support.

INTERPERSONAL FACTORS
Sense of Belonging

A **sense of belonging** is the feeling of connectedness or involvement in a social system or environment of which a person feels an integral part (Hagerty & Patusky, 1995). Abraham Maslow described a sense of belonging as a basic human psychosocial need. A sense of belonging involves both feelings of value and fit. Value refers to the person's feeling valued, needed, and accepted. Fit refers to the person's characteristics meshing or fitting in with the system or environment (Hagerty & Patusky, 1995). This means that when a person feels that he or she is a part of a system or group, within that support system the person feels valued and worthwhile. These social systems can include family, friends, coworkers, club or social groups, and even health care providers.

A person's sense of belonging is closely related to his or her social and psychological functioning. A sense of belonging was found to promote health, whereas

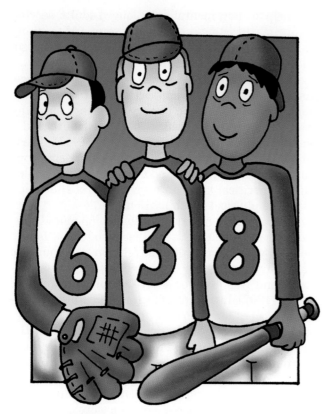

Sense of belonging

a lack of belonging impaired health (Hagerty et al., 1996). An increased sense of belonging was also associated with lower levels of anxiety (Hagerty & Patusky, 1995). Persons with a sense of belonging are less alienated and isolated, have a sense of purpose, believe they are needed by others, and feel productive socially. Hence, the nurse should focus on interventions that help increase a client's sense of belonging.

Social Networks and Social Support

Social networks are groups of people whom one knows and with whom one feels connected. Studies have found that having a social network can help reduce stress and diminish illness (Bisconti & Bergeman, 1999) and can have a strong positive influence on the person's ability to cope and adapt (Buchanan, 1995).

Social support is emotional sustenance that comes from friends, family members, and even health care providers who help a person when a problem arises. It is different from social contact, which does not always provide emotional support. Social contact can be the friendly talk that goes on at parties.

Persons who are supported emotionally and functionally have been found to be healthier than those who are not supported (Buchanan, 1995). Meaningful social relationships with family or friends were found

to improve the health and well-being outcomes for older adults (Bisconti & Bergeman, 1999). These researchers also found that an essential element of these improved outcomes was that the family or friends responded with support when it was requested. In other words, the person must be able to count on these friends or family to help or support him or her, such as going to visit or talking on the phone. Thus, the primary components of satisfactory support are the person's ability and willingness to request support when needed and the ability and willingness of the support system to respond.

Family members and friends should be encouraged to maintain contact with clients in institutional care. Social support has been found to be beneficial for older adults with chronic mental illness in an institutional setting. Beeler et al. (1999) found that 75% of people living in the institution had family contact; this is contrary to the stereotypical notion that persons with mental illness in institutions lose family ties. Siblings and mothers accounted for the majority of contacts. Residents with family contact were happier and felt connected to their families even though they lived in an institution.

Knisely and Northouse (1994) also found that among adult psychiatric inpatients, social support and help-seeking behaviors were highly correlated: in other words, having a social network and being able to ask for and receive support when needed are vital steps in the recovery process. Clients with social support were more likely to seek help and participate in their treatment and felt more satisfied with their hospital stay.

Buchanan (1995) focused on the specific elements required for a support system to be effective for the client. In a study of social support in adults with schizophrenia, Buchanan found that two key components were necessary: the client's perception of the support system, and the responsiveness of the support system (mobilization). The client must perceive that the social support system bolsters his or her confidence and self-esteem and provides such stress-related interpersonal help as offering assistance in solving a problem. The client must also perceive that the actions of the support system are consistent with the client's desires and expectations—in other words, the support provided is what the client wants, not what the supporter thinks would be good for the client. Also, the support system must be able to provide direct help or material aid (e.g., providing transportation, making a follow-up appointment). Buchanan explained that some people have the capacity to seek help when needed, while a lack of well-being may cause others to withdraw from potential providers of support. The nurse can help the client find support people who will be available and helpful and can teach the client to request support when needed.

Family Support

Family as a source of social support can be a key factor in the recovery of clients with psychiatric illnesses. Although family members are not always a positive resource in mental health, they are most often an important part of recovery (Kumfo, 1995). Health care professionals cannot totally replace family members. The nurse must encourage family members to continue to support the client even while in the hospital and should identify family strengths, such as love and caring, as a resource for the client.

CULTURAL FACTORS

According to the U.S. Census Bureau, in 2000, 33% of U.S. residents are members of ethnically diverse cultures, and by 2050, the nonwhite population will more than triple. This changing composition of society has implications for health care professionals, who are predominantly white and unfamiliar with different cultural beliefs and practices (Bechtel et al., 1998). **Culturally competent** nursing care means being sensitive to issues related to culture, race, gender, sexual orientation, social class, economic situation, and other factors (Lipson et al., 1996).

Nurses and other health care providers must learn about other cultures and become skilled at providing care to people with different cultural backgrounds than their own. Finding out about another's cultural beliefs and practices and understanding their meaning is essential to providing holistic care that is meaningful to the client (Table 7-2).

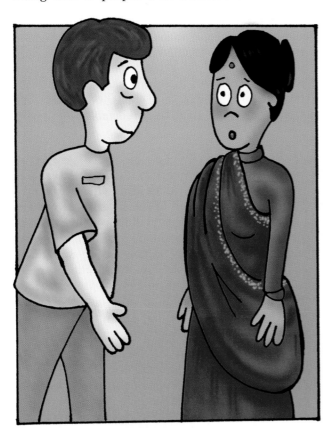

Initial meeting: Various cultures

grounds than their own. Finding out about another's cultural beliefs and practices and understanding their meaning is essential to providing holistic care that is meaningful to the client (Table 7-2).

Beliefs About Causes of Illness

Culture has the most influence on a person's health beliefs and practices (Campinha-Bacote, 1994). Culture has been shown to influence one's concept of disease and illness. There are two prevalent types of beliefs about what causes illness in non-Western cultures: personalistic and naturalistic. Personalistic beliefs attribute the cause of illness to the active, purposeful intervention of an outside agent, spirit, or supernatural force or deity. The naturalistic view is rooted in a belief that natural conditions or forces, such as cold, heat, wind, or dampness, are responsible for the illness (Campinha-Bacote, 1994). A sick person with these beliefs would not see the relationship between his or her behavior or health practices and the illness. Thus, he or she would try to counteract the negative forces or spirits using traditional cultural remedies rather than taking medication or changing his or her health practices.

Factors in Cultural Assessment

Bechtel et al. (1998) recommend a model for assessing clients using six cultural phenomena: communication, physical distance or space, social organization, time orientation, environmental control, and biologic variations (Box 7-1 and Table 7-3).

COMMUNICATION

Verbal communication can be difficult when the client and nurse do not speak the same language. The nurse should be aware that nonverbal communication has different meanings in various cultures. For example, touch is welcomed and considered supportive in some cultures but is offensive to other cultures. Some Asian women avoid shaking hands with each other or men. Some Native American tribes believe that vigorous handshaking is aggressive, whereas people from Spain and France consider a firm handshake a sign of strength and good character (Bechtel et al., 1998).

Direct eye contact is considered rude to Native Americans and Asians, and they often avoid looking strangers in the eye when talking to them. People from Middle Eastern cultures can maintain very intense eye contact, which may appear to be glaring to those from different cultures. These differences are important to note, because inferences about a person's behavior are often made based on the frequency or duration of eye contact.

Table 7-2

CULTURAL BELIEFS ABOUT HEALTH AND ILLNESS

	Illness Beliefs: Causes of Mental Illness	Concept of Health
African Americans	Lack of spiritual balance	Feelings of well-being, able to fulfill role expectations, free of pain or excess stress
American Indians	Loss of harmony with natural world, breaking of taboos, ghosts	Holistic and wellness-oriented
Arab Americans	Wrath of God, sudden fears, pretending to be ill to manipulate family	Gift of God manifested by eating well, meeting social obligations, good mood, no stressors or pain
Cambodians	Khmer Rouge brutalities	Health as equilibrium, individually maintained but influenced by family and community
Chinese	Lack of harmony of emotions, evil spirits	Health maintained by balance of *yin* and *yang*, body, mind, and spirit
Filipinos	Disruption of harmonious function of individual and spirit world	Maintaining balance; good health involves good food, strength, and no pain
Japanese Americans	Loss of mental self-control caused by evil spirits, punishment for behavior or not living good life	Balance and harmony between oneself, society, and universe
Mexican Americans	Humoral, God, spirituality, and interpersonal relationships all can contribute	Feeling well and being able to maintain role function
Russians	Stress and moving into new environment	Regular bowel movements and absence of symptoms
South Asians	Spells cast by enemy, falling prey to evil spirit	Balance of digestive fire, bodily humors, and waste products; senses functioning normally; body, mind, and spirit in harmony
Vietnamese	Disruption of harmony in individual; ancestral spirit haunting	Harmony and balance within oneself

Chapter 6 provides a detailed discussion of communication techniques.

PHYSICAL DISTANCE OR SPACE

Various cultures have different perspectives on what is considered a comfortable physical distance from another while communicating. In the United States and many Western cultures, 2 to 3 feet is a comfortable distance. Latin Americans and people from the Middle East tend to stand closer to each other and health care providers than people in Western cultures (Bechtel et al., 1998). People from Asian and Native American cultures are usually more comfortable with distances greater than 2 or 3 feet. The nurse should be conscious of these cultural differences in space and should allow enough room for clients to be comfortable.

SOCIAL ORGANIZATION

Social organization refers to family structure and organization, religious values and beliefs, ethnicity, and culture, all of which affect a person's role and therefore his or her health and illness behavior (Bechtel et al., 1998). The role of family in making health care decisions is strongly valued among many Chinese, Mexican, Vietnamese, and Puerto Rican Americans. Decisions may be delayed until appropriate family members can be consulted. Autonomy in health care decisions is an unfamiliar and undesirable concept because the collective is considered greater than the individual.

TIME ORIENTATION

Time orientation, or how time is viewed as precise or approximate, can be different for some cultures. Western and some European countries focus on the urgency

Box 7-1

➤ IMPORTANT FACTORS IN CULTURAL ASSESSMENT

Communication
Physical distance or space
Social organization
Time orientation
Environmental control
Biologic variations

Bechtel, G., Giger, J. N., & Davidhizar, R. (1998). Case managing patients from other cultures. Journal of Care Management, *4(5), 87–91.*

Table 7-3

CULTURAL ASSESSMENT FACTORS OF VARIOUS CULTURES AFFECTING RESPONSE TO ILLNESS

Culture	Communication	Space	Social Organization	Time Orientation
African Americans	**Nonverbal:** affectionate, hugging, touching, eye contact **Tone:** may be loud and animated	Respect privacy, respectful approach, handshake appropriate	Family: nuclear, extended, matriarchal, may include close friends	Flexible, nonlinear; life issues may take priority over keeping appointments
American Indians/Native Americans	**Nonverbal:** respect communicated by avoiding eye contact **Tone:** quiet, reserved,	Light-touch handshake	Family: vary; may be matrilineal clan or patrilineal	Flexible, nonlinear; flow with natural cycles rather than scheduled, rigid appointments
Arab Americans	**Nonverbal:** expressive, warm, other-oriented, shy and modest **Tone:** flowery, loud voice means message is important	Prefer closeness in space and with same sex	Family: nuclear and extended, often in same household	More past and future than present
Cambodians	**Nonverbal:** silence welcomed rather than chatter, eye contact acceptable but "polite" women lower their eyes. **Tone:** quiet	Small personal space with each other	Family-oriented, usually three generations in one house	Flexible attitude, tardiness for appointments expected. Emphasis on past (remembering ancestors) but also on present as actions will determine future
Chinese	**Nonverbal:** eye contact and touching among family and friends, eye contact avoided with authority figures **Tone:** expressive and may appear loud	Keep respectful distance	Extended families common, wife expected to be part of husband's family	Being on time not valued
Filipinos	**Nonverbal:** shy and affectionate, little direct eye contact with authority figures **Tone:** soft-spoken, tone changes with emotion	Handshakes not usually practiced, personal space is constricted	Family-oriented, nuclear and extended, may have several generations in one household	Both past and present orientations; tardy for social events but on time for business events like appointments
Japanese Americans	**Nonverbal:** quiet and polite, reserved and formal, little eye contact with authority figures **Tone:** soft, conflict avoided	Touching uncommon, small bow, handshake with younger generation	Family-oriented, self subordinate to family unit; family structure hierarchical, interdependence	Promptness important, often early for appointments

(continued)

Table 7-3

(*Continued*)

Culture	Communication	Space	Social Organization	Time Orientation
Mexican Americans	**Nonverbal:** direct eye contact avoided with authority figures **Tone:** respectful and polite	Touch by strangers not appreciated, handshake polite and welcomed	Mostly nuclear families with extended family and godparents; family comes first	Present-oriented, time viewed as relative to situation
Russians	**Nonverbal:** direct eye contact, nodding means approval **Tone:** sometimes loud even in pleasant conversations	Space close for family and friends and more distant until familiarity is established	Extended family with strong family bonds and great respect for elders	On time or early
South Asians	**Nonverbal:** direct eye contact considered rude; modesty, humility, shyness emphasized **Tone:** soft, may boss younger persons	Personal space constricted; handshake okay with men but not common among women	Extended family common, daughter expected to move in with husband's family	Not extremely time-conscious in social situations, but on time for appointments
Vietnamese	**Nonverbal:** gentle touch may be okay in conversation, no eye contact with authority **Tone:** soft-spoken	Personal space more distant than in European Americans	Highly family-oriented, may be nuclear or extended	Fashionably late at social functions, but understand the importance of being on time for appointments

of time, and punctuality and precise schedules are important and valued. In other cultures, clients may not perceive the importance of adhering to specific follow-up appointments or procedures or time-related treatment regimens. Health care providers can become resentful and angry when these clients miss appointments or fail to follow specific treatment regimens, such as taking medications at prescribed times. The nurse should not label such a client as noncompliant when his or her behavior may be due to a different cultural orientation to the meaning of time. When possible, the nurse should be sensitive to the client's time orientation, as with follow-up appointments. When timing is essential, as with some medications, the nurse can explain the importance of more precise timing.

ENVIRONMENTAL CONTROL

Environmental control refers to a client's ability to control the surroundings or direct factors in the environment (Bechtel et al., 1998). People who be-

lieve they have control of their health are more likely to seek care, to change their behavior, and to follow treatment recommendations. Those who believe that illness is a result of nature or natural causes (personalistic or naturalistic view) are less likely to seek traditional health care because they do not believe it can help them.

BIOLOGIC VARIATIONS

Biologic variations exist between people from different cultural backgrounds, and research is just beginning to help us understand these variations (Bechtel et al., 1998). For example, we now know that people of some ethnic/cultural origins respond differently to psychotropic drugs (discussed earlier). Biologic variations based on physical makeup are said to arise from one's race, whereas other cultural variations arise from ethnicity. For example, sickle-cell anemia is found almost exclusively in African Americans, and Tay-Sachs disease is most prevalent in the Jewish community (Bechtel et al., 1998).

Socioeconomic Status and Social Class

Socioeconomic status refers to one's income, education, and occupation (Lipson et al., 1996). It has a strong influence on a person's health, including whether the person has insurance and adequate access to health care or can afford prescribed treatment. People who live in poverty are also at risk for threats to health such as inadequate housing, lead paint, gang-related violence, drug trafficking, or substandard schools.

Social class has less influence in the United States, where there are loose barriers among the social classes and more mobility: people can gain access to better schools, housing, health care, and lifestyle as they increase their income (Lipson et al., 1996). In many other countries, however, social class is a powerful influence on social relationships and can determine how people relate to one another, even in a health care setting. For example, the caste system still exists in India, and people in the lowest caste may feel unworthy or undeserving of the same level of health care as persons in higher castes. The nurse must determine whether social class is a factor in how clients relate to health care providers and the health care system.

Cultural Patterns and Differences

Knowledge of expected cultural patterns provides a starting place for the nurse to begin to relate to persons with different ethnic backgrounds than his or her own (Andrews & Boyle, 1999). Being aware of the usual differences can help the nurse know what to ask or how to assess preferences and health practices. However, there is a wide range of variations among people from any culture: not everyone fits the general pattern. Individual assessment of each person and family is necessary to provide culturally competent care that meets the client's needs. The following information about various ethnic groups should be a starting place for the nurse in terms of learning about greetings, acceptable communication patterns and tone of voice, and beliefs about mental illness, healing, spirituality, and medical treatment.

AFRICAN AMERICANS

Several terms are used to refer to African Americans, such as Afro-American, black, or person of color; therefore, it is best to ask what the client prefers.

During illness, families are often a support system for the sick person, although the client maintains his or her independence, such as making his or her own health care decisions. Families often feel comfortable demonstrating public affection, such as hugging and touching each other. Conversation among family and friends may be animated and loud. Greeting a stranger usually includes a handshake, and direct eye contact indicates interest and respect. Silence may indicate a lack of trust of the caregiver or the situation (Locks & Boateng, 1996).

The church is an important and valued support system for many African Americans, and they may receive frequent hospital visits from ministers or congregation members. Prayer is an important part of healing. For some in the black community, the cause of mental illness may be viewed as a spiritual imbalance (Locks & Boateng, 1996) or as punishment for sin (Andrews & Boyle, 1999). Folk remedies may be used in conjunction with Western medicine (Locks & Boateng, 1996).

AMERICAN INDIANS OR NATIVE AMERICANS

Older adults usually prefer the term American Indian, whereas younger adults prefer Native American. Many Native Americans refer to themselves by a tribal name, such as Winnebago or Navajo. A light-touch handshake is a respectful greeting, with minimal direct eye contact. Communication is slow and may be punctuated by many long pauses. It is important not to rush the speaker or interrupt with questions. This is a culture accustomed to communicating by telling stories, so communicating is a long, detailed process. Family members are reluctant to provide information about the client if he or she can do so, believing it violates the client's privacy to talk about him or her. Orientation to time is flexible and does not coincide with rigidly scheduled appointments.

Mental illness is a culturally specific concept, and beliefs about causation may include ghosts, breaking taboos, or loss of harmony with the environment (Kramer, 1996). Clients are often quiet and stoic, making few if any requests. Experiences that involve seeing visions or hearing voices may have spiritual meaning and may not be viewed as illness. Native Americans with traditional religious beliefs may be reluctant to discuss their beliefs and practices with strangers. If the client wears a medicine bag, it should not be removed if possible. The medicine bag or other ritual healing objects should not be casually discussed or touched by others. Other Native Americans belong to Christian denominations, but they may incorporate healing practices or use a spiritual healer along with Western medicine.

ARAB AMERICANS

The preferred term of address may be by region, such as Arab Americans or Middle Eastern Americans, or by country of origin, such as Egyptian or Palestinian. Greetings include a smile, direct eye contact, and a social comment about family or the client. Using a loud voice indicates the importance of the topic, as does repeating the message. To appear respectful, those of Middle Eastern background commonly express agreement in front of a stranger, but it does not necessarily reflect their true feelings. Families make collective decisions, with the father, eldest son, uncle, or husband as the family spokesperson. Most appointments, viewed as official, will be kept, although human concerns are more valued than adhering to a schedule (Meleis, 1996).

Mental illness is believed to result from sudden fears, attempts to manipulate family, wrath of God, or God's will, all focused on the individual. Loss of country, family, or friends may also cause mental illness. Mental health care is sought only as a last resort after all family and community resources are exhausted. When sick, these clients expect to be taken care of by family or health care professionals. The client's energy is reserved for healing, so complete rest and abdication from all responsibilities are practiced during illness. Mental illness is viewed more negatively than physical illness and is believed to be something the person can control. Although early immigrants were Christians, more recent immigrants are Muslims. Prayer is very important to Muslims: strict Muslims pray five times a day, washing before every prayer and praying in silence.

Western medicine is the primary treatment sought, but some may use home remedies and amulets (charms or objects used for their protective powers) (Meleis, 1996).

CAMBODIANS

The preferred term for people from Cambodia is Khmer (pronounced Kami), or Sino-Khmer (if they are Chinese-Cambodians). Those who have assimilated into Western culture use a handshake for greeting, whereas others may slightly bow, bringing the palms together with the fingers pointed upward, and make no contact with the person they are greeting. Asians often speak softly, so it is important to listen carefully rather than asking them to speak louder. Politeness is highly valued. Eye contact is acceptable, but women may lower their eyes to be polite. Silences are common and appropriate; meaningless chatter should be avoided. It is considered impolite to disagree, so clients may say yes when not really agreeing or intending to comply. It is inappropriate to touch

someone's head without permission because some believe the soul is in the head. Family members are usually included in making decisions. Orientation to time can be flexible (Kulig, 1996).

Most Khmer immigrated to the United States after 1970 and believe that mental illness is caused by the Khmer Rouge war and associated brutalities. When ill, they assume a passive role, expecting others to care for them. Western medicine and traditional healing practices are used simultaneously. Buddhism is the primary religion, although some have converted to Christianity. An *accha* (holy person) may perform many elaborate ceremonies in the person's home but will not do so in the hospital. Healers may visit the client in the hospital but are unlikely to disclose that they are healers, much less what their practices are. Some still have a naturalistic view of illness and may be reluctant to have blood drawn, believing they will lose body heat needed for harmony and balance (Kulig, 1996).

CHINESE

The Chinese are often shy in unfamiliar environments, so socializing or friendly greetings are helpful. Direct eye contact with authority figures is avoided to show respect, and keeping a respectful distance is recommended (Chin, 1996). Asking questions can be a sign of disrespect; silence is a sign of respect. Chinese is an expressive language, so loudness is not necessarily a sign of agitation or anger. Time urgency is not highly valued by traditional Chinese societies. Extended families are common, with the eldest male member of the household making decisions and serving as the spokesperson for the family.

Mental illness is thought to result from a lack of harmony of emotions, or evil spirits. Health practices may vary according to the length of time immigrants have lived in the United States. Immigrants from 40 to 60 years ago are strong believers in Chinese folk medicine, whereas immigrants from the last 20 years combine folk and Western medicine. First- and second-generation Chinese Americans are mostly oriented to Western medicine (Chin, 1996). However, many Chinese use herbalists and acupuncture either before or in conjunction with Western medicine. Rarely, a spiritual healer will be sought to rid psychiatric clients of evil spirits. Many Chinese are Buddhists, but Catholic and Protestant religions are also common.

FILIPINOS

Smiles rather than handshakes are a common form of greeting. Facial expressions are animated and may be used to convey emotion rather than words. Direct eye contact is considered impolite, so there is little direct eye contact with authority figures such as nurses and physicians. Typically, Filipinos are soft-spoken and avoid expressing disagreement (Cantos & Rivera, 1996); however, their tone of voice may get louder to emphasize what is being said, or as a sign of anxiety or fear. Medical appointments are seen as business, and clients are likely to be punctual.

Causes of mental illness are both religious and mystical. Mental illness is thought to result from a disruption of the harmonious function of the whole person and the spiritual world. These causes can include contact with a stronger life force, ghosts, or souls of the dead; disharmony among wind, vapors, diet, and shifted body organs; or physical and emotional strain, sexual frustration, and unrequited love. Most Filipinos are Catholic and when very ill may want to see a priest and a physician. Prayer is important to the client and family, and they often want to receive the religious sacraments while sick. Filipinos often seek both Western medical treatment and the help of healers who help remove evil spirits. The ill client assumes a passive role, and decisions are made by the eldest male in the household after conferring with family members (Cantos & Rivera, 1996).

JAPANESE AMERICANS

Japanese Americans identify themselves by the generation in which they were born. Issei, the first generation of Japanese Americans in the United States, have a strong sense of Japanese identity. Nisei, second-generation Japanese Americans born and educated in the United States, appear westernized but have strong roots in Japanese culture. Sansei (third generation) and Yonsei (fourth generation) are assimilated into Western culture and are less connected to Japanese culture (Shiba & Oka, 1996).

Greetings tend to be formal, such as a smile or small bow for older generations and a handshake for younger generations. There is little touching and eye contact is minimal, especially with authority figures. Facial expressions are controlled, and conflict or disagreement is avoided. Elders may nod frequently, but this does not necessarily indicate understanding or agreement. Self-disclosure is unlikely unless trust has been established, and then only if the information is directly requested. Questions should be phrased to elicit more than just a yes or no answer. Promptness is important, so clients are often early for appointments.

Mental illness brings shame and social stigma to the family, so clients are reluctant to seek help. Evil spirits are thought to cause loss of mental self-control as a punishment for bad behavior or failure to live a good life. Persons are expected to use will power to regain their lost self-control and are often perceived as not trying hard enough. Western psychological therapies based on self-disclosure, sharing feelings, and discussing one's family experiences are very difficult for many Japanese Americans. These clients may be seen as unwilling or uncooperative.

Buddhism, Shinto, and Christianity are the most common religions among Japanese Americans, and religious practices vary with the religion. Prayer and offerings are common in Buddhist and Shinto religions and are usually done in conjunction with Western medicine (Shiba & Oka, 1996).

MEXICAN AMERICANS

There is wide diversity among Mexican Americans in terms of health practices and beliefs, depending on the client's education, socioeconomic status, generation, time spent in the United States, and affinity to traditional culture. It is best for the nurse to ask the client how he or she would like to be identified (e.g., Mexican American, Latino, Hispanic). A handshake is considered a polite greeting, but other touch by strangers is not appreciated, although touching and embracing warmly are common among family and friends. Direct eye contact with authority figures may be avoided to convey respect. Polite social interaction before asking health-related questions is preferred to help establish rapport. Generally, one or two questions will produce a wealth of information, so listening is important. Silence is often a sign of disagreement and may be used in place of words. Orientation to time is flexible; the client may be 15 or 20 minutes late for an appointment but will not consider that as being late (de Paula et al., 1996).

There is no clear separation of mental and physical illness. Many have a naturalistic or personalistic view of illness and believe disease is based on the imbalance of the person and the environment, including emotional, spiritual, social, and physical factors. Mexican Americans may seek medical care for severe symptoms while still using folk medicine to deal with spiritual or psychic influences. Eighty percent to 90% of Mexican Americans are Catholic and observe the rites and sacraments of this religion (de Paula et al., 1996).

RUSSIANS

A formal greeting or a handshake with direct eye contact is acceptable. Touching or embracing with kissing on the cheeks is reserved for close friends and family. Tone of voice can be loud even in pleasant conversations. Most clients are on time or early for appointments (Evanikoff, 1996).

The cause of mental illness is seen as stress and moving into a new environment. Some Russian Christians believe illness is God's will or a test of faith. Sick people often put themselves on bed rest. Many Russians do not like to take any medications and will try home remedies first. Some older Russians believe that excessive drug use can be harmful and that many medicines can be more damaging than natural remedies. Primary religious affiliations are Eastern Orthodox, with a minority being Jewish or Protestant (Evanikoff, 1996).

SOUTH ASIANS

South Asians living in America include people from India, Pakistan, Bangladesh, Sri Lanka, Nepal, Fiji, and East Africa. Preferred terms of identification may be related to geography, such as South Asians, East Indians, Asian Indians, or Indo-Americans, or by religious affiliation, such as Sikhs, Hindus, or Muslims. Greetings are expressed orally as well as in gestures. Hindus and Sikhs press their palms together while saying *namaste* (Hindus) or *sasariyakal* (Sikhs). Muslims take the palm of the right hand to their forehead and bow slightly while saying *AsSalamOAlaikuum*. Shaking hands is common among men but not women. Touching is not common among South Asians; rather, feelings are expressed through eyes and facial expression. Direct eye contact, especially with elders, may be considered rude or disrespectful. Silence usually indicates acceptance, approval, or tolerance. Most South Asians have a soft tone of voice, and loudness is considered disrespectful. Although not time-conscious about social activities, most South Asians are punctual for scheduled appointments for health care (Rajwani, 1996).

Mental illness is believed to result from spells cast by an enemy or possession by evil spirits. Those who believe in Ayurvedic philosophy may think a person is susceptible to mental problems related to an imbalance in body humors. Sick people usually assume a passive role and want to rest and be relieved of daily responsibilities. Hindus worship many gods and goddesses and believe in a social caste system. Hindus believe that reciting charms and performing rituals will eliminate diseases, enemies, sins, and demons. Many believe that yoga will eliminate certain mental illnesses. Muslims believe in one God and pray five times daily after washing their hands. Reciting verses from the holy Koran is believed to eliminate diseases and ease suffering. Sikhs also believe in one god and the equality of all people. Spiritual healing practices and prayer are common, but South Asians living in the United States readily seek health care from Western physicians as well (Rajwani, 1996).

VIETNAMESE

Vietnamese greet with a smile and bow. A health care provider should not shake a woman's hand unless she offers her hand first. Touch in communication is more limited among older, more traditional people. The head may be considered sacred and the feet profane, so the order of touching is important. Direct eye contact is avoided with those in authority and elders as a sign of respect. Personal space is more distant than it is for European Americans. Typically, the Vietnamese are soft-spoken and raising the voice is disrespectful, as is a finger-pointing gesture. Open expression of emotions or conflict may be considered bad taste. Punctuality for appointments is usual (Farrales, 1996).

Mental illness is caused by individual disharmony or by an ancestral spirit coming back to haunt the person because of past bad behavior. When sick, clients assume a passive role and expect to have everything their way.

The two primary religions are Catholicism and Buddhism. Catholics recite the rosary and say prayers and may wish to see a priest daily. Buddhists pray silently to themselves.

Vietnamese people believe in both Western medicine and folk medicine. Some believe that traditional healers can exorcise evil spirits. Other health practices include coin rubbing, pinching the skin, acupuncture, and herbal medicine (Farrales, 1996).

NURSE'S ROLE IN WORKING WITH CLIENTS OF VARIOUS CULTURES

To provide culturally competent care, the nurse must find out as much as possible about a client's cultural values, beliefs, and health practices. Often the client is the best source of that information, so the nurse must ask the client what is important to him or her—for instance, "How would you like to be cared for?" or "What do expect (or want) me to do for you?" (Andrews & Boyle, 1999).

At the initial meeting, the nurse may rely on what he or she knows about a client's particular cultural group, such as preferences for greeting, eye contact, physical distance, and so forth. Based on the client's behavior, the nurse can alter that approach as needed. For example, if a client from a culture that does not usually shake hands offers the nurse his or her hand, the nurse should return the handshake. There is a wide variation among members of the same cultural group, and the nurse must remain alert for these individual differences.

A client's health practices and religious beliefs are other important areas to assess. The nurse can ask, "Are there any dietary preferences or restrictions that you follow?" and "How can I assist you in practicing your religious or spiritual beliefs?" The nurse can also gain an understanding of the client's health and illness beliefs by asking, "How do you think this health problem came about?" and "What kinds of remedies have you tried at home?"

An open and objective approach to the client is essential. Clients will be more likely to share personal and cultural information if the nurse is genuinely interested in knowing and does not appear skeptical or judgmental.

The nurse should ask these same questions even to clients from his or her own cultural background. Again, people in a cultural group vary widely, so the nurse should not assume that he or she knows what a client believes or practices just because the nurse shares the same culture.

SELF-AWARENESS ISSUES

The nurse must be aware of the factors that influence a client's response to illness, including the individual, interpersonal, and cultural factors discussed above. Assessment of these factors can help guide the planning and implementation of nursing care. Biologic and hereditary factors cannot be changed. Others, such as interpersonal factors, can be changed, but only with difficulty. For instance, helping a client develop a social support system requires more than simply giving him or her a list of community contacts. The client needs to feel that these resources are valuable to him or her, must perceive them as helpful, responsive, and supportive, and must be willing to use them.

Nurses with limited experience in working with various ethnic groups may feel anxious when encountering someone from a different cultural background and worry about saying "the wrong thing" or doing something offensive or disrespectful to the client or family. Nurses may have stereotypical concepts about some ethnic groups and be unaware of them until they encounter a client from that group. It is a constant challenge to remain aware of one's feelings and to handle them effectively.

Helpful Hints to Remember

- Approach the client with a genuine, caring attitude.
- Ask the client at the beginning of the interview how he or she prefers to be addressed, and ways the nurse can promote spiritual, religious, and health practices.
- Recognize any negative feelings or stereotypes, and discuss them with a colleague so that myths and misconceptions can be dispelled.
- Remember that a client's response to illness is complex and is influenced by a wide variety of factors.

➤ KEY POINTS

- Each client is unique, with different biologic, psychological, and social factors that influence his or her response to illness.
- Individual factors that influence a client's response to illness include age, growth, and development; biologic and genetic factors; hardiness, resilience, and resourcefulness; and self-efficacy and spirituality.
- Biologic makeup includes the person's heredity and physical health.
- Younger clients may have difficulty expressing their thoughts and feelings and thus often have poorer outcomes when experiencing stress or illness at an early age.

INTERNET RESOURCES

Resource	Internet Address
Native American Cultural Society	http://www.negia.net/~linda/NACS.html
National Multicultural Institute	http://www.nmci.org/
Electronic Resources on Diversity	http://scuish.scu.eduSCU/Programs/Diversity/esources.html
ITI's Multicultural Network	http://www.fcg.net/iti/iti_cultnet.html

Critical Thinking

Questions

1. What is the cultural and ethnic background of your family? How does that influence your beliefs about mental illness?
2. How would you describe yourself in terms of the individual characteristics that affect one's response to illness, such as growth and development, biologic factors, self-efficacy, hardiness, resilience and resourcefulness, and spirituality?
3. Which of the categories of factors that influence the client's response to illness—individual, interpersonal, and cultural—do you think is most influential? Why?

• People who have difficulty negotiating the tasks of psychosocial development have less effective skills to cope with illness.
• There are cultural/ethnic differences in how people respond to certain psychotropic drugs; this can affect dosage and side effects. Nurses need to be aware of these cultural differences when treating clients. Clients from non-Western countries generally require lower doses of psychotropic drugs to produce desired effects.
• Self-efficacy is a belief that one's abilities and efforts can have an effect on the events in their lives. A person's sense of self-efficacy is an important factor in coping with stress and illness.
• Hardiness is a person's ability to resist illness when under stress.
• Resilience is a person's ability to respond in healthy manner to stressful circumstances or risky situations.
• Resourcefulness is demonstrated in one's ability to manage daily activities and is a personal characteristic acquired through interactions with others.
• Spirituality involves the inner core of a person's being and his or her beliefs about the meaning of life and the purpose for living. It may include belief in God or a higher power, the practice of religion, cultural beliefs and practices, and a relationship with the environment.
• Interpersonal factors that influence the client's response to illness include a sense of belonging, or personal involvement in a system or environment, and social networks, which provide social support or emotional sustenance.
• The increasing social and cultural diversity in the United States and Canada makes it essential for nurses to be knowledgeable about the health and cultural practices of various ethnic or racial groups. To provide competent nursing care, nurses must be sensitive to and knowledgeable about factors that influence the care of clients, including issues related to culture, race, gender, sexual orientation, and social and economic situation.
• Culture has the most influence on a person's health beliefs and behaviors.
• A model for assessing clients from various ethnic backgrounds includes six cultural phenomena: communication techniques and style, physical distance and space, social organization, time orientation, environmental control, and biologic variations.
• Socioeconomic status has a strong influence on a person's health. It may determine whether the person has insurance, adequate access to health care, or the ability to afford prescribed treatment.
• Knowledge of various cultural patterns and differences helps the nurse begin to relate to persons of different ethnic backgrounds.
• Nurses who are unsure of a person's social or cultural preferences need to ask the client directly during the initial encounter about preferred terms of address and ways the nurse can help support the client's spiritual, religious, or health practices.

REFERENCES

Adams, S. M., & Partee, D. J. (1998). Hope: The critical factor in recovery. *Journal of Psychosocial Nursing, 36*(4), 29–32.

Andrews, M. M., & Boyle, J. S. (1999). *Transcultural concepts in nursing care* (3rd ed.). Philadelphia: Lippincott, Williams & Wilkins.

Auchus, M. P., Wood, K., & Kaslow, N. (1995). Exercise patterns of psychiatric patients admitted to a short-term inpatient unit. *Psychosocial Rehabilitation Journal, 18*(3), 137–145.

Bandura, A. (1997). Insights: self-efficacy. *Harvard Mental Health Letter, 13*(9), 4–6.

Bechtel, G., Giger, J. N., & Davidhizar, R. (1998). Case managing patients from other cultures. *Journal of Care Management, 4*(5), 87–91.

Beeler, J., Rosenthal, A., & Cohler, B. (1999). Patterns of family caregiving and support to older psychiatric patients in long-term care. *Psychiatric Services, 50*(9), 1222–1224.

Benishek, L. A., & Lopez, F. G. (1997). Critical evaluation of hardiness theory: gender differences, perception of life events, and neuroticism. *Work & Stress, 11*(3), 33–45.

Bisconti, T. L., & Bergeman, C. S. (1999). Perceived social control as a mediator of the relationships among social support, psychological well-being, and perceived health. *Gerontologist, 39*(1), 94–103.

Boyle, A., Grap, M. J., Younger, J., & Thornby, D. (1991). Personality hardiness, ways of coping, social support, and burnout in critical care nurses. *Journal of Advanced Nursing, 16*(7), 850–857.

Buchanan, B. W. & Carpenter, W. T. (2000). *Schizophrenia: Introduction and overview.* In B. J. Sadock & V. A. Sadock (Eds.). Comprehensive Textbook of Psychiatry, Vol. 1 (7th ed, 1096–1110). Philadelphia: Lippincott Williams & Wilkins.

Buchanan, J. (1995). Social support and schizophrenia: a review of the literature. *Archives of Psychiatric Nursing, 9*(2), 68–76.

Calvert, W. J. (1997). Protective factors within the family, and their role in fostering resiliency in African American adolescents. *Journal of Cultural Diversity, 4*(4), 110–117.

Campinha-Bacote, J. (1994). Cultural competence in psychiatric mental health nursing: a conceptual model. *Nursing Clinics of North America, 29*(1), 1–8.

Cantos, A., & Rivera, E. (1996). In J. G. Lipson, S. L. Dibble, & P. A. Minarik (Eds.). *Culture & nursing care: a pocket guide* (pp. 115–125). San Francisco: UCSF Nursing Press.

Chin, P. (1996). Chinese Americans. In J. G. Lipson, S. L. Dibble, & P. A. Minarik (Eds.). *Culture & nursing care: a pocket guide* (pp. 74–81). San Francisco: UCSF Nursing Press.

De Paula, T., Lagana, K., & Gonzalez-Ramirez, L. (1996). Mexican Americans. In J. G. Lipson, S. L. Dibble, & P. A. Minarik (Eds.). *Culture & nursing care: a pocket guide* (pp. 203–221). San Francisco: UCSF Nursing Press.

Dyer, J. G., & McGuinness, T. M. (1996). Resilience: analysis of the concept. *Archives of Psychiatric Nursing, 10*(5), 276–282.

Evanikoff, L. J. (1996). Russians. In J. G. Lipson, S. L. Dibble., & P. A. Minarik (Eds.). *Culture & nursing care: a pocket guide* (pp. 239–249). San Francisco: UCSF Nursing Press.

Farrales, S. (1996). Vietnamese. In J. G. Lipson, S. L. Dibble, & P. A. Minarik (Eds.). *Culture & nursing care: a pocket guide* (pp. 280–290). San Francisco: UCSF Nursing Press.

Hagerty, B. M., & Patusky, K. (1995). Developing a sense of belonging measure. *Journal of Nursing Research, 44*(1), 9–13.

Hagerty, B. M., Williams, R. A., Coyne, J. C., & Early, M. R. (1996). Sense of belonging and indicators of social and psychological functioning. *Archives of Psychiatric Nursing, 10*(4), 235–244.

Hill, R. B. (1998). Enhancing the resilience of African American families. *Journal of Human Behavior in the Social Environment, 1*(2/3), 49–61.

Keane, A., Ducette, J., & Adler, D. C. (1985). Stress in ICU and non-ICU nurses. *Nursing Research, 34*(4), 231–236.

Knisely, J. E., & Northouse, L. (1994). The relationship between social support, help-seeking behavior, and psychological distress in psychiatric clients. *Archives of Psychiatric Nursing, 8*(6), 357–365.

Kobasa, S. C. (1979). Stressful life events, personality, and health: An inquiry into hardiness. *Journal of Personality & Social Psychology, 37*(1), 1–11.

Kramer, J. (1996). American Indians. In J. G. Lipson, S. L. Dibble, & P. A. Minrik (Eds.). *Culture & nursing care: a pocket guide* (pp. 11–22). San Francisco: UCSF Nursing Press.

Kulig, J. C. (1996). Cambodians (Khmer). In J. G. Lipson, S. L. Dibble, & P. A. Minarik (Eds.). *Culture & nursing care: a pocket guide* (pp. 55–63). San Francisco: UCSF Nursing Press.

Kumfo, J. (1995). The family as a mental health resource. *Mental Health Nursing, 15*(5), 16–18.

Lambert, V. A., Lambert, C. E., Klipple, G. L., & Mewshaw, E. A. (1990). Relationships among hardiness, social support, severity of illness, and psychological well-being in women with rheumatoid arthritis. *Health Care for Women International, 35*(2), 159–173.

Lipson, J. G., Dibble, S. L., & Minarik, P. A. (Eds.). (1996). *Culture & nursing care: a pocket guide.* San Francisco: USCF Nursing Press.

Locks, S., & Boateng, L. (1996). Black/African Americans. In J. G. Lipson, S. L. Dibble, & P. A. Minarik (Eds.). *Culture & nursing care: a pocket guide* (pp. 37–43). San Francisco: UCSF Nursing Press.

Low, J. (1999). The concept of hardiness: persistent problems, persistent appeal. *Holistic Nursing Practice, 13*(3), 20–24.

Meleis, A. I. (1996). Arab Americans. In J. G. Lipson, S. L. Dibble, & P. A. Minarik (eds.). *Culture & nursing care: a pocket guide* (pp. 23–36). San Francisco: UCSF Nursing Press.

Mohr, W. K. (1998). Cross-ethnic variations in the care of psychiatric patients: a review of contributing factors and practice considerations. *Journal of Psychosocial Nursing, 36*(5), 16–21.

Nelson, P. B. (1989). Ethnic differences in intrinsic/extrinsic religious orientation and depression in the elderly. *Archives of Psychiatric Nursing, 3*(4), 199–204.

Pollock, S. E. (1986). Human responses to chronic illness: Physiological and psychosocial adaptation. *Nursing Research, 35*(2), 90–95.

Rajwani, R. (1996). South Asians. In G. Lipson, S. L. Dibble, & P. A. Minarik (Eds.). *Culture & nursing care: a pocket guide* (pp. 264–279). San Francisco: UCSF Nursing Press.

Rutter, M. (1987). Psychosocial resilience and protective mechanisms. *American Journal of Orthopsychiatry, 57*(3), 316–331.

Shiba, G., & Oka, R. (1996). Japanese Americans. In J. G. Lipson, S. L. Dibble., & P. A. Minarik (Eds.). *Culture & nursing care: a pocket guide* (pp. 180–190). San Francisco: UCSF Nursing Press.

Siefken, S. (1993). The Hispanic perspective on death and dying: a combination of respect, empathy, and spirituality. *Pride Institute Journal of Long-Term Home Health Care, 12*(2), 26–28.

Stolley, J. M., & Koenig, H. (1997). Religion/spirituality and health among elderly African Americans and Hispanics. *Journal of Psychosocial Nursing, 35*(11), 32–46.

Sullivan, W. P. (1993). "It helps me to be a whole person": the role of spirituality among the mentally challenged. *Psychosocial Rehabilitation Journal, 16*(3), 125–134.

Topf, M. (1989). Personality hardiness, occupational stress, and burnout in critical care nurses. *Research in Nursing & Health, 12*(3), 179–186.

Warheit, G. J. (1979). Life events, coping, stress, and depressive symptomatology. *American Journal of Psychiatry, 136*(4B), 502–507.

Webster, C., & Austin, W. (1999). Health-related hardiness and the effect of a psycho-educational group on client's symptoms. *Journal of Psychiatric and Mental Health Nursing, 6*(3), 241–247.

Zauszniewski, J. A. (1995a). Learned resourcefulness: a conceptual analysis. *Issues in Mental Health Nursing, 16*(1), 13–31.

Zauszniewski, J. A. (1995b). Theoretical and empirical considerations of resourcefulness. *Image, 27*(3), 177–180.

ADDITIONAL READINGS

Baker, F. M. (1994). Psychiatric treatment of older African Americans. *Hospital and Community Psychiatry, 45*(1), 32–37.

Borge, L., Martinsen, E. W., Ruud, T., Watne, O., & Friis, S. (1999). Quality of life, loneliness, and social contact among long-term psychiatric patients. *Psychiatric Services, 50*(1), 81–84.

Bowsher, J. E., & Keep, D. (1995). Toward an understanding of three control constructs: personal control, self-efficacy, and hardiness. *Issues in Mental Health Nursing, 16*(1), 33–50.

Callahan, P., Young-Cureton, G., Zalar, M., & Wahl, S. (1997). Relationship between tolerance/intolerance of ambiguity and perceived environmental uncertainty in hospitals. *Journal of Psychosocial Nursing, 35*(11), 39–44.

Finley, L. Y. (1998). The cultural context: families coping with severe mental illness. *Psychiatric Rehabilitation Journal, 21*(3), 230–40.

Jordan, J. B. (1997). Mental health considerations with the Yupik Eskimo. *Alaska Medicine, 39*(3), 67–70.

Kennedy, M. G. (1999). Cultural competence and psychiatric-mental health nursing. *Journal of Transcultural Nursing, 10*(1), 11.

Low, J. (1996). The concept of hardiness: a brief but critical commentary. *Journal of Advanced Nursing, 24,* 588–590.

Meadows, M. (1997). Mental health and medicine: cultural considerations in treating Asians. *Minority Nurse Newsletter, 4*(4), 1–2.

Millet, P. E., Sullivan, B. F., Schwebel, A. I., & Myers, L. J. (1996). Black Americans' and white Americans' views of the etiology and treatment of mental health problems. *Community Mental Health Journal, 2*(3), 235–241.

Nelson, G., Hall, G. B., & Walsh-Bowers, R. (1998). The relationship between housing characteristics, emotional well-being, and the personal empowerment of psychiatric consumers/survivors. *Community Mental Health Journal, 34*(1), 57–69.

Nicholas, P. K., & Leuner, J. D. (1999). Hardiness, social support, and health status: are there differences in older African American and Anglo-American adults? *Holistic Nursing Practice, 13*(3), 53–61.

Sims, E. M., Pernell-Arnold, A., Graham, R., et al. (1998). Principles of multicultural psychiatric rehabilitation services. *Psychiatric Rehabilitation Journal, 21*(3), 219–223.

Solomon, P., & Draine, J. (1995). Adaptive coping among family members of persons with serious mental illness. *Psychiatric Services, 46*(11), 1156–1160.

Tuck, I. (1997). The cultural context of mental health nursing. *Issues in Mental Health Nursing, 18*(3), 269–281.

Weaver, H. N., & White, B. J. (1997). The Native American family: roots of resiliency. *Journal of Family Social Work, 2*(1), 67–79.

Chapter Review

➤ MULTIPLE-CHOICE QUESTIONS

Select the best answer for each of the following questions.

1. Which of the following is important for nurses to remember when administering psychotropic drugs to nonwhites?

   A. Lower doses may be used to produce desired effects.

   B. Fewer side effects occur with nonwhite clients.

   C. Response to the drug will be similar to that in whites.

   D. No generalization can be made.

2. Which of the following states the naturalistic view of what causes illness?

   A. Illness is a natural part of life and therefore unavoidable.

   B. Illness is caused by cold, heat, wind, and dampness.

   C. Only natural agents will be effective in treating illness.

   D. Outside agents, such as evil spirits, upset the body's natural balance.

3. Which of the following is most influential in determining health beliefs and practices?

   A. Cultural factors

   B. Individual factors

   C. Interpersonal factors

   D. All of the above are equally influential

4. Which of the following groups considers a firm handshake a sign of strength?

   A. White European Americans

   B. Filipinos

   C. Mexican Americans

   D. Native Americans

5. Which of the following groups consider direct eye contact a lack of respect?

   A. African Americans

   B. Arab Americans

   C. Russians

   D. Vietnamese

➤ TRUE-FALSE QUESTIONS

Identify each of the following statements as T (true) or F (false). Correct any false statements.

_____ 1. Self-efficacy refers to the ability to stand up for one's own rights.

_____

_____ 2. Three components of hardiness are commitment, challenge, and control.

_____

_____ 3. Hardiness has no effect on physical illness, just on psychological well-being.

_____

_____ 4. Spirituality and religious practices help older African Americans cope with physical illness.

_____

_____ 5. Social support refers to the number of social contacts a person has in the community.

_____

_____ 6. An increased sense of belonging can decrease anxiety.

_____

_____ 7. Social support from health care providers is more effective than support from family members.

_____

_____ 8. People are born with either high or low resiliency, and it cannot be changed.

_____

*Identify the developmental task that corresponds to
the following age groups, according to Erik Erikson.*

_____ Infant   _____ Young adult

_____ School age   _____ Maturity

_____ Adolescence

➤ SHORT-ANSWER QUESTIONS

1. Briefly explain culturally competent nursing care.

2. What is the result of achieving or failing to achieve a psychosocial
   developmental task, according to Erik Erikson?

3. What is the essential difference between hardiness and resilience?

Assessment

Learning Objectives

After reading this chapter, the student should be able to:

1. Identify the categories used to assess the client's mental status.
2. Formulate questions to obtain information in each category.
3. Describe the client's functioning in terms of self-concept, roles, and relationships.
4. Recognize key physiologic functions that are often impaired in persons with mental disorders.
5. Obtain and organize psychosocial assessment data to use as a basis for planning nursing care.
6. Examine one's own feelings and discomfort in discussing suicide, homicide, or self-harm behaviors with a client.

Key Terms

abstract thinking

affect

automatism

blunted affect

circumstantial thinking

concrete thinking

delusion

duty to warn

flat affect

flight of ideas

hallucinations

ideas of reference

insight

judgment

labile mood

loose associations

mood

neologisms

psychomotor retardation

self-concept

tangential thinking

thought blocking

thought broadcasting

thought content

thought insertion

thought process

waxy flexibility

word salad

Assessment is the first step of the nursing process and involves the collection, organization, and analysis of information (American Nurses Association, 1994). In psychiatric-mental health nursing, this process is often referred to as a psychosocial assessment, which includes a mental status examination. The purpose of the psychosocial assessment is to construct a picture of the client's current emotional state, mental capacity, and behavioral function. This assessment serves as the basis for developing a plan of care to meet the needs of the client. It is also a clinical baseline used to evaluate the effectiveness of treatment and interventions, or a measure of the client's progress (American Nurses Association, 1994).

FACTORS INFLUENCING ASSESSMENT

Client Participation/Feedback

A thorough and complete psychosocial assessment requires active client participation. If the client is unable or unwilling to participate, some areas of the assessment will be incomplete or vague. For example, the client who is extremely depressed may not have the energy to answer questions or complete the assessment. Clients exhibiting psychotic thought processes or impaired cognition may have an insufficient attention span or may be unable to comprehend the questions being asked. The nurse may need to have several contacts to complete the assessment or gather further information as the client's condition permits.

Client's Health Status

The psychosocial assessment can also be affected by the client's health status. If the client is in pain or fatigued or anxious, the nurse may have difficulty eliciting the client's full participation in the assessment. The information obtained may reflect the client's pain or anxiety, not an accurate assessment of the client's situation. The nurse needs to recognize these situations and deal with them before continuing the full assessment. The client may need to rest, receive medications to alleviate pain, or be calmed before the assessment can continue.

Client's Previous Experience/ Misconceptions About Health Care

The client's perception of his or her circumstances can elicit emotions that interfere with obtaining an accurate psychosocial assessment. If the client is reluctant to seek treatment or has had previous unsatisfactory experiences with the health care system, he or she may have difficulty answering questions directly. The client may minimize or maximize symptoms or problems or may refuse to provide information in some areas. The nurse must address the client's feelings and perceptions to establish a trusting, working relationship before proceeding with the assessment.

Client's Ability to Understand

The nurse must also determine the client's ability to hear, read, and understand the language being used in the assessment. If the client's primary language is different from that of the nurse, the client may misunderstand or misinterpret what is being asked, resulting in inaccurate information. A client with impaired hearing may also fail to understand what the nurse is asking. It is important that the information obtained in the assessment reflects the client's health status; it should not be a result of poor communication.

Nurse's Attitude and Approach

The psychosocial assessment can be influenced by the nurse's attitude and approach. If the client perceives the nurse's questions to be short and curt, or the client feels rushed or pressured to complete the assessment, he or she may provide only superficial information or omit discussing problems in some areas altogether. The client may also refrain from providing information of a sensitive nature if the nurse is perceived as unaccepting, defensive, or judgmental. For example, a client may be reluctant to relate instances of child abuse or domestic violence if the nurse seems uncomfortable or unaccepting. The nurse must be aware of his or her own feelings and responses and be able to approach the assessment in a matter-of-fact manner.

HOW TO CONDUCT THE INTERVIEW

Environment

The psychosocial assessment should be conducted in an environment that is comfortable, private, and safe for both the client and the nurse. An environment that is fairly quiet, with few distractions, allows the client to give his or her full attention to the interview. Conducting the interview in a place such as a conference room assures the client that no one will overhear what is being discussed. However, the nurse should not choose an isolated location for the interview, particularly if the client is unknown to the nurse or if any threatening behavior exists. The safety of the client and nurse must be ensured, even if that means another person is present during the assessment.

Input From Family and Friends

If the client has been accompanied by family, friends, or caregivers, the nurse should obtain their perceptions of the client's behavior and emotional state (McBride & Walden-McBride, 1995). How this is done depends on the situation. Sometimes the client does not give permission for the nurse to interview family members outside the presence of the client. The nurse should then be aware that friends or family may not feel comfortable talking about the client in his or her presence and may provide limited information. Likewise, the client may not feel comfortable participating in the assessment without the presence of family or friends. This, too, may limit the amount or type of information the nurse obtains. It is desirable to conduct at least part of the assessment without the presence of others, especially if abuse or intimidation is suspected. The nurse should make every effort to assess the client in privacy if it is suspected that abuse exists.

How to Phrase Questions

The nurse may use open-ended questions to begin the assessment. This allows the client to begin where he or she feels comfortable and also gives the nurse an idea about the client's perception of his or her situation. Examples of open-ended questions are:
- What brings you here today?
- Tell me what has been happening to you.
- How can we be of help to you?

If the client cannot organize his or her thoughts or has difficulty answering open-ended questions, the nurse may need to use more direct questions to obtain information. Questions need to be clear, simple, and focused on one specific behavior or symptom; they should not cause the client to remember several things at once. Questions regarding several different behaviors or symptoms—"How are your eating and sleeping habits, and have you been taking any over-the-counter medications that affect your eating and sleeping?"—can be confusing to the client.

The following are examples of focused or closed-ended questions:
- How many hours did you sleep last night?
- Have you been thinking about suicide?
- How much alcohol have you been drinking?
- How well have you been sleeping?
- How many meals a day do you eat?
- What over-the-counter medications are you taking?

The nurse should use a nonjudgmental tone and language, particularly when asking about sensitive information, such as drug or alcohol use, sexual behavior, abuse or violence, and child-rearing practices.

Using nonjudgmental language and a matter-of-fact tone avoids giving the client verbal cues to become defensive or not tell the truth. For example, when asking a client about his or her parenting role, the nurse should ask, "What types of discipline do you use?" rather than, "How often do you physically punish your child?" The first question is more likely to elicit honest and accurate information; the second question gives the impression that physical discipline is wrong, and it may cause the client to respond dishonestly.

CONTENT OF THE ASSESSMENT

The information gathered in a psychosocial assessment can be organized in many different ways. Most assessment tools or conceptual frameworks contain similar categories, with some variety in arrangement or order. The nurse should use some kind of organizing framework so that the client can be assessed in a thorough and systematic way that lends itself to analysis and serves as a basis for the client's care. The framework for psychosocial assessment discussed here and used throughout this textbook contains the following components:
- History
- General appearance and motor behavior
- Mood and affect
- Thought process and content
- Sensorium and intellectual processes
- Judgment and insight
- Self-concept
- Roles and relationships
- Physiologic and self-care concerns.

Box 8-1 lists the factors that should be included in each of these areas of the psychosocial assessment.

History

Background assessments include the client's history, age and developmental stage, cultural and spiritual beliefs, and beliefs about health and illness. The history of the client, as well as the client's family history, may provide some insight into the client's current situation—for example, has the client experienced similar difficulties in the past? Has the client been admitted to the hospital, and if so, what was that experience like? A family history that is positive for alcoholism, bipolar disorder, or suicide is significant because it places the client at higher risk for these problems.

The client's chronologic age and developmental stage are important factors in the psychosocial assessment. The nurse evaluates the client's age and developmental level for congruence with expected norms. For example, a client may be struggling with personal identity and attempting to achieve independence from his or her parents. If the client is 17 years

Box 8-1

➤ PSYCHOSOCIAL ASSESSMENT COMPONENTS

History
    Age
    Developmental stage
    Cultural considerations
    Spiritual beliefs
    Previous history
General assessment and motor behavior
    Hygiene and grooming
    Appropriate dress
    Posture
    Eye contact
    Unusual movements or mannerisms
    Speech
Mood and affect
    Expressed emotions
    Facial expression
    Self-harm or suicide urges
Thought process and content
    Content (what client is thinking)
    Process (how client is thinking)
    Clarity of ideas
Sensorium and intellectual processes
    Orientation
    Confusion

Memory
    Abnormal sensory experiences or misperceptions
    Concentration
    Abstract thinking abilities
Judgment and insight
    Judgment (interpretation of environment)
    Decision-making ability
    Insight (understanding one's own part in current situation)
Self-concept
    Personal view of self
    Description of physical self
    Personal qualities or attributes
Roles and relationships
    Current roles
    Satisfaction with roles
    Success at roles
    Significant relationships
    Support systems
Physiologic and self-care considerations
    Eating habits
    Sleep patterns
    Health problems
    Compliance with prescribed medications
    Ability to perform activities of daily living

old, these struggles may be normal and anticipated, because these are two of the primary developmental tasks for the adolescent. However, if the client is 35 years old and still struggling with these issues of self-identity and independence, the nurse will need to explore these issues. The client's age and developmental level may also be incongruent with expected norms if the client has a developmental delay or mental retardation.

The nurse must be sensitive to the client's cultural and spiritual beliefs to avoid making inaccurate assumptions about his or her psychosocial functioning (Schultz & Videbeck, 1998). Many cultures have beliefs and values about a person's role in society or acceptable social or personal behavior that may differ from those of the nurse. In Western cultures, it is generally expected that as a person reaches adulthood, he or she becomes financially independent, leaves home, and makes his or her own life decisions. In contrast, in some Eastern cultures, three generations may live in one household, and major life decisions are made by the elders of the family. Another example is the assessment of eye contact. In Western cultures, good eye contact is considered a positive characteristic, indicating self-esteem and paying attention. For people from other countries, such as Japan, it is a sign of disrespect.

The nurse must not stereotype clients. Just because a person's physical characteristics are consistent with a particular race, the person may not have the attitudes, beliefs, and behaviors traditionally attributed to that group. For example, many people of Asian ancestry have beliefs and values that are more consistent with Western beliefs and values than those typically associated with people from Asian countries. To avoid making inaccurate assumptions, the nurse must ask clients about the beliefs or health practices that are important to them, or how they view themselves in the context of society or relationships. (See the section on cultural considerations in Chap. 7).

The client's beliefs about health and illness must also be considered when the nurse is assessing the client's psychosocial functioning. Some people may view emotional or mental problems as family concerns, to be handled only among family members. Seeking outside or professional help may be viewed as a sign of individual weakness. Others may believe that their problems can be solved only with the right medication and will not accept other forms of therapy. Another common problem is the misconception that one should take medication only when feeling sick. Many mental disorders, like some medical conditions, may require clients to take medications on a long-term basis, perhaps even for a lifetime. Just like diabetic persons must take insulin and persons with high blood pressure need antihypertensive medications, persons with recurrent depression may need to take antidepressants on a long-term basis.

General Appearance and Motor Behavior

The nurse assesses the client's overall appearance, including dress, hygiene, and grooming. Is the client appropriately dressed for his or her age and the weather? Is the client unkempt or disheveled? Does the client appear to be his or her stated age? The nurse also observes the client's posture, eye contact, facial expression, and any unusual tics or tremors. Observations and examples of behaviors should be documented to avoid personal judgment or misinterpretation. Specific terms used in making assessments of general appearance and motor behavior include:

- **Automatisms**: repeated, purposeless behaviors often indicative of anxiety, such as drumming fingers, twisting locks of hair, or tapping the foot
- **Psychomotor retardation**: overall slowed movements
- **Waxy flexibility**: maintenance of posture or position over time, even when it is awkward or uncomfortable.

The nurse assesses the client's speech for quantity, quality, and any abnormalities. Does the client talk nonstop? Does the client perseverate (seem to be stuck on one topic, unable to move to another idea)? Are responses a minimal "yes" or "no" without elaboration? Is the content of the client's speech relevant to the question being asked? Is the rate of speech fast or slow? Is the tone audible or loud? Does the client speak in a rhyming manner? Does the client use **neologisms** (invented words that have meaning only for the client)? The nurse notes any speech difficulties, such as stuttering or lisping.

Mood and Affect

Mood refers to the client's pervasive and enduring emotional state. **Affect** is the outward expression of the client's emotional state. The client may make statements about feelings, such as, "I'm depressed" or "I'm elated," or the nurse may infer the client's mood from data such as posture, gestures, tone of voice, and facial expression. The nurse also assesses for consistency between the client's mood, affect, and situation. For instance, the client may have an angry facial expression but deny feeling angry or upset in any way. Or the client may be talking about the recent loss of a family member while laughing and smiling. Such inconsistencies need to be noted.

Common terms used in assessing mood and affect include:

- **Blunted affect**: showing little expression; facial expression slow to respond
- **Flat affect**: absence of facial expression
- **Labile mood**: unpredictable and rapid mood swings from depressed and crying to euphoria with no apparent stimuli.

It sometimes helps to have the client estimate the intensity of his or her mood. This can be accomplished by asking the client to rate his or her mood on a scale of 1 to 10. For example, if the client reports being depressed, the nurse might ask, "On a scale of 1 to 10, with 1 being least depressed and 10 being most depressed, where would you place yourself right now?"

ASSESSMENT OF SUICIDE OR HARM TOWARD OTHERS

For the depressed or hopeless client, the nurse must determine whether the client has suicidal ideation or a lethal plan. This is accomplished by asking the client directly, "Do you have thoughts of suicide?" or "What thoughts of suicide have you had?" Box 8-2 lists assessment questions the nurse should ask any client who has suicidal ideas.

Likewise, if the client is angry or hostile or making threatening remarks about a family member, spouse, or any other person, the nurse must ask whether the client has thoughts or plans about hurting that person. This is accomplished by asking the client directly:

- What thoughts have you had about hurting [person's name]?
- What is your plan?
- What do you want to do to [person's name]?

When a client makes specific threats or has a plan to harm another person, health care providers are legally obligated to warn the person who is the

---

Box 8-2

> ## SUICIDE ASSESSMENT QUESTIONS

Ideation: "Are you thinking about killing yourself?"

Plan: "Do you have a plan to kill yourself?"

Method: "How do you plan to kill yourself?"

Access: "How would you carry out this plan? Do you have access to the means to carry out the plan?"

Where: "Where would you kill yourself?"

When: "When do you plan to kill yourself?"

Timing: "What day or time of day do you plan to kill yourself?"

target of the threats or plan. The legal term for this is **duty to warn**. This is one situation when the client's confidentiality is breached to protect the person being threatened.

Thought Process and Content

Thought process refers to how the client thinks. It is inferred from the client's speech and speech patterns. **Thought content** is what the client actually says. The nurse assesses whether the client's verbalizations make sense—whether ideas are related and flow logically from one to the next. The nurse must also determine whether the client seems preoccupied, as if talking to or paying attention to someone or something else. When the nurse encounters clients with marked difficulties in thought process and content, it may be helpful to try asking focused questions requiring short answers. Common terms used in assessing thought processes and content include the following (DSM-IV, 1994):

- **Circumstantial thinking**: client eventually answers the question being asked, but only after an excessive amount of unnecessary detail is given
- **Delusion**: a fixed, false belief, not based in reality
- **Flight of ideas**: excessive amount and rate of speech composed of fragmented or unrelated ideas
- **Ideas of reference**: client's inaccurate interpretation that general events are personally directed to the client, such as hearing a speech on the news and believing the message had personal meaning for the client
- **Loose associations**: disorganized thinking that jumps from one idea to another, with little or no evident relation between the thoughts
- **Tangential thinking**: client wanders off the topic and never provides the information requested
- **Thought blocking**: client stops abruptly in the middle of a sentence or train of thought, sometimes unable to continue the idea
- **Thought broadcasting**: delusional belief that others can hear or know what the client is thinking
- **Thought insertion**: delusional belief that others are putting ideas or thoughts into the client's head—that is, the ideas are not those of the client
- **Word salad**: flow of unconnected words that convey no meaning to the listener.

Sensorium and Intellectual Processes

ORIENTATION

Orientation refers to the client's recognition of person, place, and time—knowing who and where one is and the correct day, date, and year. This is often documented as "oriented ×3." Occasionally a fourth sphere, situation, is added (whether the client accurately perceives his or her current circumstances). Absence of correct information about person, place, and time is referred to as disorientation, or "oriented ×1" (person only) or "oriented ×2" (person and place). The order of person, place, and time is significant. When a person is disoriented, he or she first loses track of time, then place, and lastly person. Orientation returns in the reverse order: first, the person knows who he or she is, then realizes place, and finally time.

Disorientation is not synonymous with confusion. A confused person cannot make sense of his or her surroundings or figure things out, even though he or she may be fully oriented.

MEMORY

Memory, both recent and remote, is assessed. Memory is assessed directly by asking questions whose answers the nurse can verify. For example, if the nurse asks, "Do you have any memory problems?" the client may inaccurately respond "no," and the nurse cannot verify that. Similarly, if the nurse asks, "What did you do yesterday?" the nurse may be unable to verify the accuracy of that answer. Hence, questions to assess memory generally include ones such as:

- What is the name of the current president?
- Who was the president before that?
- In what county do you live?
- What is the capital of this state?
- What is your social security number?

ABILITY TO CONCENTRATE

The ability to concentrate is assessed by asking the client to perform certain tasks, such as:

- Spell the word "world" backwards.
- Begin with the number 100, subtract seven, subtract seven again, and so on. This is called "serial sevens."
- Repeat the days of the week backward.
- Ask the client to perform a three-part task, giving the instructions at one time, such as, "Take a piece of paper in your right hand, fold it in half, and put it on the floor."

ABILITY TO THINK ABSTRACTLY AND INTELLECTUAL ABILITIES

When assessing intellectual functioning, the nurse must bear in mind the client's level of formal education. Lack of formal education could hinder performance in many of the tasks in this section.

The nurse assesses the client's ability to use **abstract thinking**, or make associations or interpretations about a situation or comment. This can usually be assessed by asking the client to interpret a common proverb, such as "a stitch in time saves nine." If the client can explain the proverb correctly, his or her abstract thinking abilities are intact. However, if the client provides a literal translation of the proverb and cannot interpret the meaning, abstract thinking abilities are lacking. When the client continually gives literal translations, this is evidence of **concrete thinking**. For instance:

- *Proverb*: A stitch in time saves nine.
  Abstract meaning: If you take the time to fix something now, you'll avoid bigger problems in the future.
  Literal translation: Don't forget to sew up holes in your clothes (concrete thinking).
- *Proverb*: People who live in glass houses shouldn't throw stones.
  Abstract meaning: Don't criticize others for things you may also be guilty of doing.
  Literal translation: If you throw a stone at a glass house, it will break (concrete thinking).

The nurse may also assess the client's intellectual functioning by asking him or her to identify the similarities between pairs of objects—for example, "What is similar about an apple and an orange?" or "What do the newspaper and the television have in common?"

Sensory-Perceptual Alterations

Some clients experience **hallucinations** (false sensory perceptions, or perceptual experiences that do not really exist). Hallucinations can involve the five senses and bodily sensations. Auditory hallucinations (hearing voices) are the most common and visual hallucinations (seeing things that don't really exist) are the second most common. Initially clients perceive hallucinations as real experiences, but at a later point in the illness they may recognize them as hallucinations.

Judgment and Insight

Judgment refers to the ability to interpret one's environment and situation correctly and to adapt one's behavior and decisions accordingly (Chow & Cummings, 2000). Problems with judgment may be evidenced as the client describes recent behavior and activities that reflect a lack of reasonable care for self or others. For example, the client may spend large sums of money on frivolous items when he or she cannot afford basic necessities, such as food or clothing. Risky behaviors such as picking up strangers in bars or unprotected sexual activity may also indicate poor judgment. Judgment can also be assessed by asking the client hypothetical questions, such as, "If you found a stamped, addressed envelope on the ground, what would you do?"

Insight is the ability to understand the true nature of one's situation and accept some personal responsibility for that situation. Insight is often inferred from the client's ability to describe realistically the strengths and weaknesses of their behavior. An example of poor insight would be a client who places all blame on others for his own behavior, saying, "It's my wife's fault that I drink and get into fights, because she nags me all the time." This client is not accepting responsibility for his drinking and fighting. Another example of poor insight would be the client who expects all problems to be solved with little or no personal effort, saying, "The problem is my medication. As soon as the doctor gets the medication right, I'll be just fine."

Self-Concept

Self-concept is the way one views oneself in terms of personal worth and dignity. To assess a client's self-concept, the nurse can ask the client to describe himself or herself and what characteristics he or she likes and what he or she would change. The client's description of self in terms of physical characteristics gives the nurse information about the client's body image, which is also part of self-concept.

Also included in an assessment of self-concept is the emotions the client frequently experiences, such as sadness or anger, and whether the client is comfortable with those emotions. The client's coping strategies need to be assessed. This can be accomplished by asking, "What do you do when you have a problem? How do you solve it? What usually works to deal with anger or disappointment?"

Roles and Relationships

People function in their community through a variety of roles, such as mother, wife, son, daughter, teacher, secretary, or volunteer. The nurse assesses the roles the client occupies, satisfaction with the roles, and whether the client believes he or she is fulfilling the roles adequately (Roy & Andrews, 1991). The number and type of roles may vary, but they usually include family, occupation, and hobbies or activities. Family roles include son or daughter, sibling, parent, child, and spouse or partner. Occupation roles can be related to a career or school, or both. The ability to fulfill a role or the lack of a desired role is often central to the client's psychosocial functioning. Changes in roles may also be part of the client's difficulty.

Relationships with other people are important to one's social and emotional health. Relationships vary in terms of significance, level of intimacy or closeness, and intensity. The inability to sustain satisfying relationships can result from mental health problems or can contribute to the worsening of some problems. The nurse needs to assess the relationships in the client's life, the client's satisfaction with those relationships, or any loss of relationships. Common questions include:

- Do you feel close to your family?
- Do you have or want a relationship with a significant other?
- Are your relationships meeting your needs for companionship or intimacy?
- Can you meet your sexual needs in a satisfactory manner?
- Have you been involved in any relationships that were abusive?

If the client's family relationships seem to be a significant source of stress, or if the client is closely involved with his or her family, a more in-depth assessment of this area may be useful. Box 8-3 is the McMaster Family Assessment Device, an example of such an in-depth family assessment.

Physiologic and Self-Care Considerations

When doing a psychosocial assessment, the nurse must include physiologic functioning. Although a full physical health assessment may not be indicated, some areas of physiologic function are often affected adversely by emotional problems. Eating and sleeping patterns can be greatly affected by emotional problems: under stress, people may eat excessively or not at all, and may sleep up to 20 hours a day or be unable to sleep more than 2 or 3 hours a night. Clients with bipolar affective disorder may not eat or sleep for days. Clients with major depression may not be able to get out of bed. Therefore, the nurse must assess the client's usual patterns of eating and sleeping and then determine how those patterns have changed (Chow & Cummings, 2000).

The nurse should also ask the client whether he or she has any major or chronic health problems and whether he or she takes prescribed medications as ordered and follows dietary recommendations. The client's use of alcohol and over-the-counter or illicit drugs should also be explored. These questions need to be asked in a nonjudgmental manner; the client should be reassured that truthful information is needed to determine his or her plan of care.

Noncompliance with prescribed medications is an important area. If the client has stopped taking medication or is taking medication other than as prescribed, the nurse must help the client feel comfortable enough to reveal this information. The nurse should also explore the barriers to compliance. Is the client choosing noncompliance because of undesirable side effects? Has the medication failed to produce the desired results? Does the client have difficulty obtaining the medication? Is the medication too expensive for the client?

DATA ANALYSIS

After completing the psychosocial assessment, the nurse must analyze all the data that have been collected. Data analysis involves thinking about the overall assessment rather than focusing on isolated bits of information. The nurse looks for patterns or themes in the data that lead to conclusions about the client's strengths and needs and a particular nursing diagnosis. No one statement or behavior is adequate to reach such a conclusion. The nurse must also consider the congruence of all information provided by the client, family, or caregivers and his or her own observations. It is not uncommon for the client's perception of his or her behavior and situation to differ from that of others. Assessments in a variety of areas are needed to support nursing diagnoses such as Low Self-Esteem or Ineffective Individual Coping.

Traditionally, data analysis leads to the formulation of nursing diagnoses as a basis for the client's plan of care. Nursing diagnoses have been an integral part of the nursing process for many years. However, with the sweeping changes occurring in health care, the nurse must also be able to articulate the client's needs in ways that are clear to health team members in other disciplines, as well as families and caregivers. For example, a multidisciplinary treatment plan or critical pathway may be the vehicle for planning care in some agencies. A plan of care that is useful to the client's family for home care may be needed. The nurse must describe and document goals and interventions that can be understood by many others, not just professional nurses. The descriptions must be free of jargon or terms that are not clear to the client, family, or other providers of care.

Psychological Tests

Psychological tests are another source of data for the nurse to use in planning care for the client. Two basic types of tests are intelligence tests and personality

Box 8-3

➤ **McMaster Family Assessment Device**

Instructions: Following are a number of statements about families. Please read each statement carefully, and decide how well it describes your own family. You should answer according to how you see your family. For each statement there are four (4) possible responses:

Strongly Agree (SA)	Check SA if you feel that the statement describes your family very accurately.
Agree (A)	Check A if you feel that the statement describes your family for the most part.
Disagree (D)	Check D if you feel that the statement does not describe your family for the most part.
Strongly Disagree (SD)	Check SD if your feel that the statement does not describe your family at all.

Try not to spend too much time thinking about each statement, but respond as quickly and honestly as you can. If you have trouble with one, answer with your first reaction. Please be sure to answer every statement and mark all your answers in the space provided next to each statement.

STATEMENTS	SA	A	D	SD
1. Planning family activities is difficult because we misunderstand each other.	—	—	—	—
2. We resolve most everyday problems around the house.	—	—	—	—
3. When someone is upset the others know why.	—	—	—	—
4. When you ask someone to do something, you have to check that they did it.	—	—	—	—
5. If someone is in trouble, the others become too involved.	—	—	—	—
6. In times of crisis we can turn to each other for support.	—	—	—	—
7. We don't know what to do when an emergency comes up.	—	—	—	—
8. We sometimes run out of things that we need.	—	—	—	—
9. We are reluctant to show our affection to each other.	—	—	—	—
10. We make sure members meet their family responsibilities.	—	—	—	—
11. We cannot talk to each other about the sadness we feel.	—	—	—	—
12. We usually act on our decisions regarding problems.	—	—	—	—
13. You only get the interest of others when something is important to them.	—	—	—	—
14. You can't tell how a person is feeling from what they are saying.	—	—	—	—
15. Family tasks don't get spread around enough.	—	—	—	—
16. Individuals are accepted for what they are.	—	—	—	—
17. You can easily get away with breaking the rules.	—	—	—	—
18. People come right out and say things instead of hinting at them.	—	—	—	—
19. Some of us just don't respond emotionally.	—	—	—	—
20. We know what to do in an emergency.	—	—	—	—
21. We avoid discussing our fears and concerns.	—	—	—	—
22. It is difficult to talk to each other about tender feelings.	—	—	—	—
23. We have trouble meeting our bills.	—	—	—	—
24. After our family tries to solve a problem, we usually discuss whether it worked or not.	—	—	—	—
25. We are too self-centered.	—	—	—	—
26. We can express our feelings to each other.	—	—	—	—
27. We have no clear expectations about toilet habits.	—	—	—	—
28. We do not show our love for each other.	—	—	—	—
29. We talk to people directly rather than through go-betweens.	—	—	—	—
30. Each of us has particular duties and responsibilities.	—	—	—	—
31. There are lots of bad feelings in the family.	—	—	—	—
32. We have rules about hitting people.	—	—	—	—
33. We get involved with each other only when something interests us.	—	—	—	—

Continued

Box 8-3

➤ MCMASTER FAMILY ASSESSMENT DEVICE—cont'd

STATEMENTS	SA	A	D	SD
34. There's little time to explore personal interests.	—	—	—	—
35. We often don't say what we mean.	—	—	—	—
36. We feel accepted for what we are.	—	—	—	—
37. We show interest in each other when we can get something out of it personally.	—	—	—	—
38. We resolve most emotional upsets that come up.	—	—	—	—
39. Tenderness takes second place to other things in our family.	—	—	—	—
40. We discuss who is to do household jobs.	—	—	—	—
41. Making decisions is a problem for our family.	—	—	—	—
42. Our family shows interest in each other only when they can get something out of it.	—	—	—	—
43. We are frank with each other.	—	—	—	—
44. We don't hold to any rules or standards.	—	—	—	—
45. If people are asked to do something, they need reminding.	—	—	—	—
46. We are able to make decisions about how to solve problems.	—	—	—	—
47. If the rules are broken, we don't know what to expect.	—	—	—	—
48. Anything goes in our family.	—	—	—	—
49. We express tenderness	—	—	—	—
50. We confront problems involving feelings.	—	—	—	—
51. We don't get along well together.	—	—	—	—
52. We don't talk to each other when we are angry.	—	—	—	—
53. We are generally dissatisfied with the family duties assigned to us.	—	—	—	—
54. Even though we mean well, we intrude too much into each other's lives.	—	—	—	—
55. There are rules about dangerous situations.	—	—	—	—
56. We confide in each other.	—	—	—	—
57. We cry openly.	—	—	—	—
58. We don't have reasonable transport.	—	—	—	—
59. When we don't like what someone has done, we tell them.	—	—	—	—
60. We try to think of different ways to solve problems.	—	—	—	—

From Schutle, N. S., & Malouff, J. M. (1995). Sourcebook of adult assessment strategies. *New York: Plenum Press. Brown University/ Butler Hospital Family Research Program. © 1982.*

tests. Intelligence tests are designed to evaluate the client's cognitive abilities and intellectual functioning. Personality tests reflect the client's personality in areas such as self-concept, impulse control, reality testing, and major defenses (Adams & Culbertson, 2000). Personality tests may be objective (constructed of true-false or multiple-choice questions). Table 8-1 describes selected objective personality tests. The client's answers are compared with standard answers or criteria, and a score or scores are obtained.

Other personality tests, called projective tests, are unstructured and are usually conducted by the interview method. The stimuli for these tests, such as pictures or Rorschach's ink blots, are standard, but clients may respond with answers that are very different. The client's responses are analyzed, and a narrative result of the testing is given by the evaluator. Table 8-2 lists commonly used projective personality tests.

Both intelligence tests and personality tests are frequently criticized as being culturally biased. It is important to consider the client's culture and environment when evaluating the importance of scores or projections from any of these tests. They can provide useful information about the client in some circumstances but may not be suitable for all clients.

Table 8-1

OBJECTIVE MEASURES OF PERSONALITY

Test	Description
Minnesota Multiphasic Personality Inventory (MMPI)	566 multiple-choice items; provides scores on 10 clinical scales such as hypochondriasis, depression, hysteria, paranoia; 4 special scales such as anxiety and alcoholism; 3 validity scales to evaluate the truth and accuracy of responses
MMPI-2	Revised version of MMPI with 567 multiple-choice items; provides scores on same areas as MMPI
Milton Clinical Multiaxial Inventory (MCMI) and MCMI-II (revised version)	175 true-false items; provides scores on various personality traits and personality disorders
Psychological Screening Inventory (PSI)	103 true-false items; used to screen for the need for psychological help
Beck Depression Inventory (BDI)	21 items rated on scale of 0–3 to indicate level of depression
Tennessee Self-Concept Scale (TSCS)	100 true-false items; provides information on 14 scales related to self-concept

Adams, R. L., & Culbertson, J. L. (2000). Personality assessment: Adults and children. In B. J. Sadock & V. A. Sadock (Eds.). *Comprehensive textbook of psychiatry*, Vol. 1 (7th ed.), 702–722. Philadelphia: Lippincott Williams & Wilkins.

Psychiatric Diagnoses

Medical diagnoses of psychiatric illness are found in the *Diagnostic and Statistical Manual of Mental Disorders*, fourth edition (DSM-IV-TR). This taxonomy is universally used by psychiatrists and some therapists in the diagnosis of psychiatric illnesses. The DSM-IV-TR classifies mental disorders into categories. Each disorder is described, and diagnostic criteria are provided to distinguish one from another (Schultz & Videbeck, 1998). Although the DSM-IV-TR is not a substitute for a thorough psychosocial nursing assessment, the descriptions of disorders and related behaviors can be a valuable resource for the nurse to use as a guide. The DSM-IV-TR uses a multiaxial system to provide the format for a complete psychiatric diagnosis:

- Axis I: clinical disorders, other conditions that may be a focus of clinical attention
- Axis II: personality disorders, mental retardation
- Axis III: general medical conditions
- Axis IV: psychosocial and environmental problems

Table 8-2

PROJECTIVE MEASURES OF PERSONALITY

Test	Description
Rorschach test	10 stimulus cards of ink blots; client describes perceptions of ink blots; narrative interpretation discusses areas such as coping styles, interpersonal attitudes, characteristics of ideation
Thematic Apperception Test (TAT)	20 stimulus cards with pictures; client tells a story about the picture; narrative interpretation discusses themes about mood state, conflict, quality of interpersonal relationships
Sentence completion test	Client completes a sentence from beginnings such as, "I often wish," "Most people," "When I was young."

Adams, R. L., & Culbertson, J. L. (2000). Personality assessment: Adults and children. In B. J. Sadock & V. A. Sadock (Eds.). *Comprehensive textbook of psychiatry*, Vol. 1 (7th ed.), 702–722. Philadelphia: Lippincott Williams & Wilkins.

- Axis V: global assessment of functioning (GAF).

The psychosocial and environmental problems categorized on axis IV include educational, occupational, housing, financial, and legal problems, as well as difficulties with the social environment, relationships, and access to health care.

The GAF is used to make a judgment about the client's overall level of functioning (Box 8-4). The GAF score given to the client may describe his or her current level of functioning, as well as the highest level of functioning in the past year or 6 months. This information is useful in setting appropriate goals for the client's care.

SELF-AWARENESS ISSUES

Self-awareness is crucial when a nurse is trying to obtain accurate and complete information from the client during the assessment process. The nurse must be aware of any feelings, biases, and values that could interfere with the psychosocial assessment of a client with different beliefs, values, and behaviors. The nurse cannot let personal feelings and beliefs influence the treatment of a client. Self-awareness does not mean the nurse's beliefs are wrong or must change, but it does help the nurse to be open and accepting of others' beliefs and behaviors, even when the nurse does not agree with them.

Two areas that may be uncomfortable or difficult for the nurse to assess are sexuality and self-harm

Box 8-4

➤ GLOBAL ASSESSMENT OF FUNCTIONING (GAF) SCALE

Consider psychological, social, and occupational functioning on a hypothetical continuum of mental health—illness. Do not include impairment in functioning due to physical (or environmental) limitations. (**Note:** Use intermediate codes when appropriate, e.g., 45, 68, 72.)

Code

100 | 91	**Superior functioning in a wide range of activities, life's problems never seem to get out of hand, is sought out by others because of his or her many positive qualities. No symptoms.**
90 | 81	**Absent or minimal symptoms** (e.g., mild anxiety before an exam), **good functioning in all areas, interested and involved in a wide range of activities, socially effective, generally satisfied with life, no more than everyday problems or concerns** (e.g., an occasional argument with family members).
80 | 71	**If symptoms are present, they are transient and expectable reactions to psychosocial stressors** (e.g., difficulty concentrating after family argument); **no more than slight impairment in social, occupational, or school functioning** (e.g., temporarily falling behind in schoolwork).
70 | 61	**Some mild symptoms** (e.g., depressed mood and mild insomnia) **OR some difficulty in social, occupational, or school functioning** (e.g., occasional truancy, or theft within the household), **but generally functioning pretty well, has some meaningful interpersonal relationships.**
60 | 51	**Moderate symptoms** (e.g., flat affect and circumstantial speech, occasional panic attacks) **OR moderate difficulty in social, occupational, or school functioning** (e.g., few friends, conflicts with peers or coworkers).
50 | 41	**Serious symptoms** (e.g., suicidal ideation, severe obsessional rituals, frequent shoplifting) **OR any serious impairment in social, occupational, or school functioning** (e.g., no friends, unable to keep a job).
40 | 31	**Some impairment in reality testing or communication** (e.g., speech is at times illogical, obscure, or irrelevant) **OR major impairment in several areas, such as work or school, family relations, judgment, thinking, or mood** (e.g., depressed man avoids friends, neglects family, and is unable to work; child frequently beats up younger children, is defiant at home, and is failing at school).
30 | 21	**Behavior is considerably influenced by delusions or hallucinations OR serious impairment in communication or judgment** (e.g., sometimes incoherent, acts grossly inappropriately, suicidal preoccupation) **OR inability to function in almost all areas** (e.g., stays in bed all day; no job, home, or friends).
20 | 11	**Some danger of hurting self or others** (e.g., suicide attempts without clear expectation of death; frequently violent; manic excitement) **OR occasionally fails to maintain minimal personal hygiene** (e.g., smears feces) **OR gross impairment in communication** (e.g., largely incoherent or mute).
10 | 1	**Persistent danger of severely hurting self or others** (e.g., recurrent violence) **OR persistent inability to maintain minimal personal hygiene OR serious suicidal act with clear expectation of death.**
0	Inadequate information.

The rating of overall psychological functioning on a scale of 0–100 was operationalized by Luborsky in the Health-Sickness Rating Scale (Luborsky L: "Clinicians' Judgments of Mental Health." Archives of General Psychiatry 7:407–417, 1962). Spitzer and colleagues developed a revision of the Health-Sickness Rating Scale called the Global Assessment Scale (GAS) (Endicott J, Spitzer RL, Fleiss JL, Cohen J: "The Global Assessment Scale: A Procedure for Measuring Overall Severity of Psychiatric Disturbance." Archives of General Psychiatry 33:766–771, 1976). A modified version of the GAS was included in DSM-III-R as the Global Assessment of Functioning (GAF) Scale.

behaviors. The beginning nurse may feel uncomfortable asking questions about a client's intimate relationships and behavior and any self-harm behaviors or suicide, as if such questions are prying into personal matters. However, it is important to ask these questions to obtain a thorough and complete assessment. The nurse needs to remember that it may be uncomfortable for the client to discuss these topics as well.

The nurse may hold beliefs that differ from the client's, but he or she must not make judgments about the client's practices. For example, the nurse may believe abortion is a sin, but the client might have had several elective abortions. Or the nurse may believe that adultery is wrong, but during the course of an assessment he or she may discover that a client has had several extramarital affairs.

Being able to listen to the client nonjudgmentally and to support the discussion of personal topics takes practice and usually gets easier with experience. Talking to more experienced colleagues about such discomfort and methods of alleviating it often helps. It may also be helpful for the nurse to preface uncomfortable questions by saying to the client, "I need to ask you some personal questions. Remember, this is information that will help the staff provide better care for you."

The nurse must assess the client for suicidal thoughts. Some beginning nurses feel uncomfortable discussing suicide or feel that asking about suicide might suggest it to a client who had not previously thought about it. This is not the case. It has been shown that the safest way to assess a client with suspected mental disorders is to ask him or her clearly and directly about suicidal ideas. It is the nurse's professional responsibility to keep the client's safety needs first and foremost, and this includes overcoming any personal discomfort in talking about suicide (Schultz & Videbeck, 1998).

Helpful Hints When Doing a Psychosocial Assessment

- The nurse is trying to gain all the information needed to help the client. Judgments are not part of the assessment process.
- Being open, clear, and direct when asking about personal or uncomfortable topics will help alleviate the client's anxiety or hesitancy about discussing the topic.
- Examining one's own beliefs and gaining self-awareness is a growth-producing experience for the nurse.
- If the nurse's beliefs differ strongly from those of the client, the nurse should vent his or her feelings to colleagues or discuss the differences with them. The nurse's own beliefs must not

Critical Thinking

Questions

1. The nurse is preparing to do a psychosocial assessment for a client who is seeking help because she has been physically abusive to her children. What feelings might the nurse experience? How does the nurse view this client?
2. The nurse has discovered through the assessment process that the client drinks a quart of vodka every 2 days. The client states this is not a problem. How does the nurse proceed? What could the nurse say to this client?
3. The nurse is assessing a client who is illiterate. How will the nurse assess the intellectual functioning of this client? What other areas of a psychosocial assessment might be impaired by the client's inability to read or write?

be allowed to interfere with the nurse–client relationship and the assessment process.

➤ KEY POINTS

- The purpose of the psychosocial assessment is to construct a picture of the client's current emotional state, mental capacity, and behavioral function. This baseline clinical picture serves as the basis for developing a plan of care to meet the needs of the client.
- The components of a thorough psychosocial assessment include the client's history, general appearance and motor behavior, mood and affect, thought process and content, sensorium and intellectual process, judgment and insight, self-concept, roles and relationships, and physiologic and self-care considerations.
- Several important factors can influence the psychosocial assessment: the client's ability to participate and give feedback, physical health status, emotional well-being and perception of the situation, and ability to communicate, and the nurse's attitude and approach.
- The psychosocial assessment can be greatly influenced by the nurse's attitude and approach. The nurse must conduct the assessment in a professional, nonjudgmental, and matter-of-fact manner, not allowing his or her personal feelings to influence the interview.
- The nurse must be sensitive to the client's cultural and spiritual beliefs to avoid making inaccurate assumptions about the client's psychosocial functioning. Many cultures have values and beliefs about a person's role

in society or acceptable social or personal behavior that may differ from the beliefs and values of the nurse.

- Self-awareness on the nurse's part is crucial to obtain an accurate, objective, and thorough psychosocial assessment.
- Areas that are often difficult for nurses to assess include sexuality and self-harm behaviors and suicidality. Discussion with colleagues and experience with clients can help the nurse deal with uncomfortable feelings.
- The client's safety is a priority; therefore, asking clients clearly and directly about suicidal ideation is essential.
- Accurate analysis of assessment data involves considering the entire assessment and identifying patterns of behavior as well as congruence among components and sources of information.

REFERENCES

Adams, R. L., & Culbertson, J. L. (2000). Personality assessment: Adults and children. In B. J. Sadock & V. A. Sadock (Eds.). *Comprehensive textbook of psychiatry, Vol. 1* (7th ed., pp. 702–722). Philadelphia: Lippincott Williams & Wilkins.

American Nurses Association. (1994). *Statement on psychiatric-mental health nursing practice and standards of psychiatric and mental health nursing practice.* Washington, DC: American Nurses Publishing.

American Psychiatric Association. (2000). *Diagnostic and statistical manual of mental disorders, fourth edition, text revision.* Washington, DC: American Psychiatric Association.

Chow, T. W., & Cummings, J. L. (2000). Neuropsychiatry: Clinical assessment and approach to diagnosis. In B. J. Sadock & V. A. Sadock (Eds.). *Comprehensive textbook of psychiatry, Vol. 1* (7th ed., pp. 221–253). Philadelphia: Lippincott Williams & Wilkins.

McBride, L., & Walden-McBride, D. (1995). Balancing the heart of patient care. *Home Healthcare Nurse, 13*(4), 46–49.

Roy, S. C., & Andrews, H. (1991). *The adaptation model: A definitive statement* (2d ed.). Norwalk, CT: Appleton & Lange.

Schultz, J. M., & Videbeck, S. (1998) *Lippincott's manual of psychiatric nursing care plans* (5th ed.). Philadelphia: Lippincott-Raven.

Schutle, N. S. & Malouff, J. M. (1995). *Sourcebook of adult assessment strategies.* New York: Plenum Press.

Chapter Review

➤ **MULTIPLE-CHOICE QUESTIONS**

Select the best answer for each of the following questions.

1. Which of the following is an example of an open-ended question?
   A. Who is the current president of the United States?
   B. What concerns you most about your health?
   C. What is your address?
   D. Have you lost any weight recently?

2. Which of the following is an example of a closed-ended question?
   A. How have you been feeling lately?
   B. How is your relationship with your wife?
   C. Have you had any health problems recently?
   D. Where are you employed?

3. Which of the following is not included in the assessment of sensorium and intellectual processes?
   A. Concentration
   B. Memory
   C. Judgment
   D. Orientation.

4. Assessment data about the client's speech patterns are categorized in which of the following areas?
   A. History
   B. General appearance and motor behavior
   C. Sensorium and intellectual processes
   D. Self-concept.

5. When the nurse is assessing whether the client's ideas are logical and make sense, the nurse is examining which of the following?
   A. Thought content
   B. Thought process
   C. Memory
   D. Sensorium.

➤ **TRUE-FALSE QUESTIONS**

Identify each of the following statements are T (true) or F (false). Correct any false statements.

_____ 1. The client with circumstantial thinking never really answers the question being asked.

_____ 2. A client's belief that a news broadcast has special meaning for him is an example of ideas of reference.

_____ 3. A delusion is defined as a fixed, false belief.

_____ 4. The client who believes everyone is out to get him is hallucinating.

_____ 5. The client who looks sad and complains of being depressed is said to have a labile mood.

_____ 6. A neologism is a word that is made up and has meaning for the client only.

_____ 7. The Thematic Apperception Test (TAT) is an example of a projective personality test.

_____ 8. Objective personality tests are those that are free of cultural bias.

➤ FILL-IN-THE-BLANK QUESTIONS

Identify each of the following terms being described.

_____ 1. Repeated, purposeless behaviors, often indicating anxiety

_____ 2. The belief that others can read one's thoughts

_____ 3. Generally slowed body movements

_____ 4. Flow of unconnected words that have no meaning

➤ SHORT-ANSWER QUESTIONS

Identify a question the nurse might ask to assess each of the following.

1. Abstract thinking ability

2. Insight

3. Self-concept

4. Judgment

5. Mood

6. Orientation

The nurse at a mental health clinic is meeting a new client for the first time and plans to do a psychosocial assessment. When the client arrives, the nurse finds a young woman who looks somewhat apprehensive and is crying and twisting facial tissues in her hands. She can tell the nurse her name and age but begins crying before she can provide any other information. The nurse knows it is essential to obtain information from this young woman, but it is clear she will have trouble answering all the interview questions at this time.

1. What should the nurse do with the crying client?

2. Identify five questions that the nurse would choose to ask this client initially. Give a rationale for the chosen questions.

3. What, if any, assumptions might the nurse make about this client and her situation?

4. If the client decided to leave the clinic before the assessment formally began, what would the nurse need to do?

Unit 3

Current Social and Emotional Concerns

Grief and Loss

Key Terms

acculturation

adaptive denial

anticipatory grieving

attachment behaviors

attentive presence

avoiders

complicated grieving

dysfunctional grieving

grief

grieving

homeostasis

mourning

phase of numbing

phase of yearning and searching

phase of disorganization and despair

phase of reorganization

psychogenic

psychospiritual

sensitizers

somatic

spirituality

Clinical Vignette: Grief

"If I had known what the grief process was like, I would never have married, or I would have prayed every day of my married life that I would be the first to die," reflects Margaret, 9 years after the death of her husband.

She recalls her initial thought, denying and acknowledging reality simultaneously, when James was diagnosed with multiple myeloma in October 1987: "It's a mistake . . . but I know it isn't."

For 2 ½ years, Margaret and James diligently followed his regimen of treatment while taking time for work and play, making the most of their life together in the moment. "We were not melodramatic people. We told ourselves, 'This is what's happening; we'll deal with it.'"

For Margaret, it was a shock to realize that some friends who had been so readily present for social gatherings were no longer available. She waited alone in the wee hours of the night when James had emergency surgery. Again, she was shocked when she told a priest who came into the room, "My husband is having surgery," and his reply was "Oh, sorry to bother you; I'm looking for the paper."

Margaret began to undergo a shift in her thinking: "You begin to evaluate your perceptions of others. I asked myself, 'Who is there for me?' Friends, *are* they *really?* It can be painful to find out they really aren't. It frees you later, though. You can let them go."

When James died, Margaret remained "level-headed and composed" until one day shortly after the funeral when she suddenly became aware of her exhaustion. While shopping, she found herself in protest of the emotional pain and wanting to shout, "Doesn't anybody know that I have just lost my husband?"

Surprised with how overwhelmed she felt, one of her hardest moments was putting her sister on the plane and going home to "an empty house." It was at this time that she began to feel the initial shock of her loss. Her body felt like it was "wired with electricity." She felt as though she was "just going through the motions," doing routine chores like grocery shopping and putting gas in the car, all the while feeling numb.

Crying spells lasted 6 months. She became "tired of mourning" and would ask herself, "When is this going to be relieved?" She also felt anger. "I was upset with James, wondering why he didn't go for his complete physical. Maybe James' death may not have happened so soon."

After a few months and well into her journey with grief, Margaret knew she needed to "do something constructive." She did. She attended support groups, traveled, and became involved with church activities.

Her faith in God was a plus. Exercising this faith, she trusted that eventually her emotions would catch up with the intellectual understanding of all that had transpired in James' dying. She developed an "inner knowing that God is all-seeing, all-knowing." This belief gave her spiritual strength and empowered her as she grieved.

Nearly a decade after James' death, Margaret views the painful journey of grief as a profound and poignant "search for meaning in life. If he had not gone, I would not have come to where I am in life. I am content, confident, and happy with how authentic life is."

Even so, a sense of James' presence remains with her as she pictures the way he was before he became ill. She states, "This is good for me."

Experiences of loss and grief are essential and normal in the life of a human. Letting go, relinquishing, and moving on happen as one travels between stages of normal growth and development. Saying "goodbye" to places, people, dreams, and familiar objects, such as a favorite blanket or toy, a first-grade teacher, or the teenage hope of becoming a famous rock star, are all examples of necessary loss that comes with growth. The loss allows one to change and move toward development and fulfillment of one's innate human potential. Loss may be planned, expected, or sudden, and the grieving that follows is rarely comfortable or pleasant. Although uncomfortable, loss is sometimes beneficial; other times it is devastating and debilitating.

Grief refers to the subjective emotions and affect that are a normal response to the experience of loss (Varcarolis, 1998). **Grieving** refers to the process by which the grief is experienced. **Mourning**, the outward sign of grief, is a way of integrating loss and grief into the life of the bereaved (Marrone, 1997; Webb, 1993). Grieving involves not only the content (*what* a person thinks, says, and feels) but also the process (*how* a person thinks, says, and feels). Thus, we will be examining what a person who has suffered loss experiences in terms of what he or she thinks, feels, and does.

All people grieve when they experience life's changes and losses, and often the process is one of the most difficult and challenging of human existence. To meet the challenge that grief brings to a client, the nurse must have a basic understanding of the journey involved in grieving for a loss. The grief process should be familiar terrain to the nurse who is interacting with clients responding to a myriad of losses along the continuum of health and illness.

Although all losses relevant to human need are cause for grieving, probably the most devastating loss is that of a loved one—a child, parent, spouse, or significant other. The discussions that follow deal

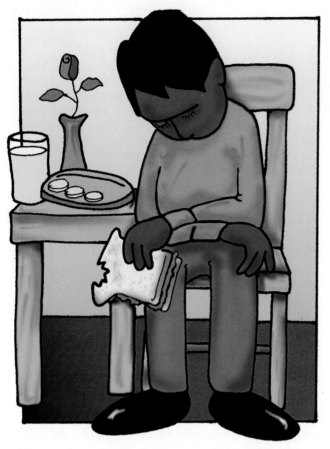

Grief

primarily with the grieving that occurs in response to the loss of a loved one.

Grief can and perhaps should be the focus of treatment at times. Although it is not a mood disorder, grief sometimes appears so to the inexperienced eye. It can be more difficult to assess grief in a person who has a coexisting psychiatric disability such as depression or schizophrenia because the flat affect, depressed mood, or cognitive disorganization that accompanies many mental disorders can camouflage the client's grieving behaviors. Nurses must be particularly alert to clients with psychiatric disorders who are also grieving. These clients can experience grief and a sense of loss not only when they lose an important relationship through death but also when they experience changes in treatment settings, routine, environment, or even staff.

This chapter focuses on the human experience of loss and the process by which a person moves through it—we will view it as a journey of grieving. The process of grieving is discussed in terms of the stages through which a person integrates a loss into his or her life. To support and care for the grieving client, the nurse needs to understand these phases and cultural responses to loss. The nursing process section outlines the nurse's role in the grieving

process and gives guidelines for offering support and teaching necessary coping skills to the client who is grieving. The importance of self-awareness and competency as a facilitator is outlined as well.

TYPES OF LOSSES

A useful way to examine types of losses is by using Maslow's hierarchy of human needs. According to Maslow (1954), human actions are motivated by a hierarchy of needs, beginning with physiologic needs (food, air, water, and sleep), then safety needs (a safe place to live and work), then needs of security and belonging. When those needs are met, the person is motivated by the need for self-esteem that leads to feelings of adequacy and confidence. The last and final need is self-actualization, an attempt to realize one's full innate potential. When these human needs are not met or are taken away for some reason, the person experiences a loss. Some examples of the losses relevant to specific human needs identified in Maslow's hierarchy are:

- Physiologic losses: Loss of adequate air exchange, loss of adequate functioning of the pancreas, loss of a limb, and other somatic related symptoms or conditions represent physiologic losses.
- Safety losses: Loss of a safe environment, such as in domestic and public violence, may be the starting point of a long journey of grief—for instance, posttraumatic stress syndrome. A breach of confidentiality in the professional relationship can be perceived as a loss of psychological safety secondary to broken trust between client and provider.
- Loss of security and a sense of belonging: Loss occurs when relationships change through birth, marriage, divorce, illness, and death. When the meaning of a relationship changes, roles may be lost within families or groups. The loss of a loved one affects the need to love and be loved.
- Loss of self-esteem: Self-esteem needs are threatened or perceived as losses whenever there is a change in how a person is valued at work and in relationships. One's sense of self-worth may be challenged and experienced as a loss when perceptions of oneself change. A loss of role function, and thus self-perception and worth as it is tied to a particular role, may come with the death of a loved one.
- Loss related to self-actualization: Personal goals and individual potential may be threatened or lost when some external or internal

crisis blocks or inhibits the strivings toward fulfillment (Parkes, 1998). A change in goals or direction will bring an inevitable grief period as one gives up a creative thought to make room for new ideas and direction. Examples of losses related to self-actualization include having to give up plans to go to graduate school, losing the hope of marriage and family, or losing one's sight or hearing while pursuing the goal of becoming an artist or composer.

THEORETICAL UNDERSTANDING OF THE GRIEF PROCESS

Regardless of the kind of loss, nurses must be ready to recognize the characteristics of the grieving process for all clients. By understanding the phenomena that clients experience as they deal with the discomfort of loss, the nurse may promote the expression and release of emotional as well as physical pain, thus supporting the grieving process. Supporting the process means ministering to psychological as well as physical needs.

The therapeutic relationship and communication skills such as active listening are paramount when assisting the grieving client. Recognizing the verbal and nonverbal communication content of the various stages of grieving can help the nurse select interventions that will meet the patient's psychological and physical needs.

Kubler-Ross's Stages of Grieving

Elisabeth Kubler-Ross's work helped set the stage for understanding how loss affects human life. As she attended to her clients with terminal illnesses, a process of dying became apparent. Through observations of and work with dying clients and their families, she developed a model for understanding what people experience as they grieve or mourn for a loss of life. She described the stages of denial, anger, bargaining, depression, and acceptance (Kubler-Ross, 1969):

- Denial is shock and disbelief regarding the loss.
- Anger may be expressed toward God, a relative, friends, or health care providers.
- Bargaining occurs when the person bargains for more time in an effort to prolong the inevitable loss.
- Depression results when awareness of the loss becomes acute.
- Acceptance occurs when the person shows evidence of coming to terms with death.

This model became a prototype for care providers as they looked for ways to understand and assist their clients in the grieving process.

Bowlby's Theory of Attachment Behaviors

John Bowlby, a British psychoanalyst, developed a theory of attachment that proposed that humans instinctively attain and retain affectional bonds with significant others by attachment behaviors. These **attachment behaviors** are crucial to the development of a sense of security and survival. Behaviors used to attain or retain a sense of attachment can include following, clinging, calling out, or crying. Bowlby saw these attachment behaviors as being modified and adapted as a child matures into adulthood in an effort to maintain affectional bonds. Patterns of attachment behavior begun early in life endure throughout the life cycle. The most intense emotions are experienced when forming a bond, such as falling in love; maintaining a bond, such as loving someone; disrupting the bond, when loss occurs; and renewing attachment (Bowlby, 1980).

An attachment that is maintained is a source of security, and the renewing of an attachment is a source of joy. However, when a bond is threatened or broken, there is a response of anxiety, protest, and anger. Actual loss leads to sorrow. These emotions reflect affectional bonds, according to Bowlby. In loss, attachment behaviors are strongly aroused or activated—thus, the clinical picture of increased anxiety, sorrow, anger, looking for the lost person or object, calling out, crying, and protesting in an attempt to restore the affectional bond that was lost.

Phases of the Grieving Process

Bowlby's understanding of grieving will be the predominant framework for this chapter. He described the process of grieving for a loss as having four phases:

1. Numbness and denial of the loss
2. Emotional yearning for the lost loved one and protesting the permanence of the loss
3. Cognitive disorganization and emotional despair, finding it difficult to function in the everyday world
4. Reorganizing and reintegrating the sense of self so to pull life back together.

Another theorist, John Harvey (1998), described similar phases of grieving as:

1. Shock, outcry, and denial
2. Intrusion of thoughts, distractions, and obsessive reviewing of the loss

3. Confiding in others as a way to emote and cognitively restructure an account of the loss.

Rodebaugh et al. (1999) view the process of grief as a journey through four stages:

1. Reeling: clients experience shock, disbelief, or denial
2. Feelings: clients express anguish, guilt, profound sadness, anger, lack of concentration, sleep disturbances, appetite changes, fatigue, and general physical discomfort
3. Dealing: clients begin to adapt to the loss by engaging in support groups, grief therapy, reading, and spiritual guidance
4. Healing: clients integrate the loss as part of life, and acute anguish lessens. Healing does not imply that the loss is forgotten or accepted.

Theorists believe that a dynamic interaction exists throughout the myriad of expressions in grieving. Nurses must listen and observe for fluidity (emotions flowing together or easily changing from one to another) as a person goes through the phases of the process.

Table 9-1 compares theories of grieving.

Nurses should not expect a client to follow predictable steps in the grieving process. Indeed, such an expectation may put added pressure or stress on the client when he or she most needs acceptance, reflection, and support from care providers to ease the journey of grieving (Weisman, 1974). Later in the chapter, we will discuss interventions that can help the grieving process.

Tasks of the Grieving Process

Tasks inherent to grieving are described by Rando (1984) as:

- Undoing psychosocial bonds to the loved one and eventually creating new ties
- Adding new roles, skills, and behaviors and revising old ones into a "new identity and sense of self"
- Pursuing a healthy lifestyle that includes people and activities
- Integrating the loss into life. This does not mean that a final end to the grieving is achieved but, rather, that "accommodation" is made as the reality of the loss is integrated into life.

The clinical vignette gives an example of integrating loss into life: Margaret viewed James' death and the painful journey of grief as a profound and poignant "search for meaning in life." The sense of his presence remains with her as she pursues her life without him, and she often pictures him before he

Table 9-1

THEORETICAL UNDERSTANDING OF THE GRIEVING PROCESS

Theorist/Clinician	Phase I	Phase II	Phase III	Phase IV
Kubler-Ross (1969)	Stage I: denial	Stage II: anger Stage III: depression	Stage IV: bargaining	Stage V: acceptance
Bowlby (1980)	Numbness; denial	Emotional yearning for the loved one; protesting permanence of the loss	Cognitive disorganization; emotional despair; difficulty functioning	Cognitive reorganization; reintegrating sense of self
Harvey (1998)	Shock; outcry; denial	Intrusion of thoughts, distractions; obsessive reviewing of the loss	Confiding in others to emote and to cognitively restructure account of loss	
Rodebaugh et al. (1999)	Reeling: shock, disbelief, or denial	Feeling: anguish, guilt, sadness, anger, lack of concentration, sleep disturbances, appetite changes, fatigue, general discomfort	Dealing: adapting to the loss	Healing: integration of loss; acute anguish dissipated; loss may or may not be forgotten or accepted

became ill. Viewing the journey in a more positive light, she believes his death in some way has encouraged her to become more independent and to engage in other opportunities.

DIMENSIONS OF GRIEVING

The nurse must observe and listen to what the grieving client says and does as cues to what he or she is thinking and feeling. The content of grieving is what the grieving person thinks, speaks, feels, acts out, and physiologically experiences during the process. It might also be referred to as human response and correlates with what Schneider (1984) proposed as a holistic model of grieving with cognition, emotion, spirit, behavior, and physiology as five dimensions of the process.

Cognitive Responses to Grief

The pain in grieving is in some respects a result of the disturbance in a person's beliefs (Parkes, 1998). Basic assumptions and beliefs about life's meaning and purpose are disrupted, if not shattered. Grieving often causes one to change beliefs about oneself and the world, such as one's perception of the world's benevolence, the meaning of life as it relates to justice, and a sense of destiny or life path (Janoff-Bulman, 1989). Other changes in thinking and attitude include reviewing and ranking one's values, becoming wiser, shedding illusions about one's immortality, viewing the world more realistically, and re-evaluating religious or spiritual beliefs (Schwartzberg & Halgin, 1991).

QUESTIONING AND TRYING TO MAKE SENSE OF THE LOSS

The grieving person needs to make sense of the loss (Schwartzberg & Halgin, 1991). He or she will undergo self-examination and question accepted ways of thinking. Old assumptions about life are challenged. For example, when a loved one is lost prematurely, the grieving person often questions the belief that "life is fair" or that "one has control over one's life or destiny." He or she searches for answers to why this trauma has happened. The goal of the search is to make sense of the loss and to give meaning and purpose to the loss. The nurse might hear the following questions:

- "Why did this have to happen? He took such good care of himself!"
- "Why didn't she go in earlier for a thorough exam. If they found the cancer sooner, she might not have died!"
- "He was such a good person! Why did this happen to him?"

Questioning may help the person accept the reality of why someone died. For example, perhaps death does relate to the person's health practices—maybe the person did not take good care of himself and have regular check-ups. Or it may include coming to the realization that loss and death are a reality of life, that we must all face death one day. Others may discover explanations and meaning and even gain comfort from a religious or spiritual perspective, such as believing that the dead person is with God and is at peace.

ATTEMPTING TO KEEP THE LOST ONE PRESENT

Believing in an afterlife and believing that the lost one becomes a personal guide are cognitive responses that serve to keep the lost one present. Carrying on an internal dialogue with the loved one while doing an activity such as a household chore is an example: "John, I wonder what you would do in this situation. I wish you were here to show me. Let's see, I think you would probably . . ." This method of keeping the lost one present helps to soften the impact of the loss as the person continues to assimilate the reality of it.

Emotional Responses to Grief

Feelings of anger, sadness, and anxiety are the predominant emotional experiences of loss. Anger and resentment may be directed toward the dead person and his or her health practices, at family members, and at health care providers or institutions. Common reactions the nurse might hear are:

- "He should have stopped smoking years ago."
- "If you had taken her to the doctor earlier, this might not have happened."
- "It took you too long to diagnose his illness."

Guilt over things not done or said in the lost relationship is another painful emotion. Feelings of hatred and revenge can be expected when death has been due to extreme circumstances such as suicide, murder, or war (Henderson, 1994).

Emotional responses are evident in all the phases of Bowlby's grief process. During the **phase of numbing**, a common first response to news of a loss is a feeling of being stunned, as though unable to perceive the reality of the loss. Emotions vacillate in frequency and intensity. Contrasting emotions are common, such as one moment experiencing an impulsive outburst of anger toward the deceased, oneself, or others, and then feeling an unexpected elation at the sense of union with the deceased (Bowlby, 1980) At one moment, one may be functioning automatically in a state of calm; the next, one suddenly becomes overwhelmed with panic. In the clinical vignette, Margaret feels " a numbness" going through the routine functions of her life immediately after her husband's death and then one day finds herself in the department store overwhelmed with frustration and wanting to shout, "Doesn't anyone realize I've just lost my husband?"

In the second phase, **yearning and searching**, reality begins to set in and the grieving one exhibits anger, profound sorrow, and crying. The client often reverts back to the attachment behaviors of a child—for example, a child who loses his mother in a store or park. Irritability, bitterness, and hostility may be expressed and targeted toward clergy, medical providers, relatives, comforters, and even the dead person. The hopeless yet intense desire to restore the bond with the lost person compels the bereaved to search for and recover him or her. Sounds, sights, and smells associated with the lost person are interpreted as signs of the deceased's presence and intermittently comfort the client and ignite hope for a reunion. For example, the ring of the telephone at a time in the day when the deceased may have phoned on a routine basis will trigger the excited expectation of hearing his or her voice, or the scent of the deceased's perfume will spur her late husband to scan the room for her smiling face. As hopes for the lost one's return diminish, sadness and loneliness become constant.

In the vignette, Margaret became angry with her husband for not going in for his physical examination sooner and angry with friends who seemed to disappear after her husband became critically ill. This emotional tumult may last several months and seems necessary for the person to begin to acknowledge the true permanence of the loss.

During the **phase of disorganization and despair**, the bereaved person begins to understand the permanence. Patterns of thinking, feeling, and acting that have been attached to life with the deceased need to change. As all hope of recovering the lost one is relinquished, the person inevitably experiences moments of depression, apathy, or despair. Night is a time of acute loneliness during this phase.

In the final **phase of reorganization**, the bereaved person begins to re-establish a sense of personal identity, direction, and purpose for living; a sense of independence and confidence is felt (Bowlby, 1980). Experimenting with and accomplishing newly defined roles and functions, the bereaved becomes personally empowered. This emotional and affective experience is closely associated with the inherent cognitive recognition that life without the loved one is a reality and therefore needs to be different. In this reorganization phase, the deceased is still missed, but thinking of him or her no longer evokes painful feelings. In the vignette, hearing Spanish music, which was associated with James' love and her sense of being loved, was unbearable for Margaret for many months. Spanish music now inspires warm memories of their love for one another and is comforting to her.

Spiritual Responses to Grief

Thus far, we have been discussing how a person responds to loss through the human dimensions of cognition and emotion. Closely associated with cognitive and emotional dimensions are the deeply embedded personal values that give us meaning and purpose in life. These values and the belief systems that sustain them are central components of **spirituality** and the spiritual response to grief. At times of loss, it is in the spiritual dimension of human experience that a person may be most comforted, challenged, or devastated. The grieving one may become disillusioned and angry with God or other religious figures such as the priest, who in Margaret's situation seemed more concerned about getting a paper than being aware of her loneliness in the surgical waiting room. The anguish of abandonment, loss of hope, or loss of meaning is cause for deep spiritual suffering.

Ministering to the spiritual needs of those grieving, then, is an essential aspect of nursing care. The client's emotional and spiritual responses become intertwined as he or she grapples with pain. With an astute awareness of the client's suffering, the nurse can promote a sense of well-being. Providing opportunities for the client to share his or her suffering assists in the **psychospiritual** (involving both psychological and spiritual aspects of experience) transformation that often evolves in grieving. Finding explanations and meaning through religious or spiritual beliefs, the client may begin to identify positive and perhaps joyful aspects of the journey. The loss can also be experienced as significant in the client's own growth and development. In the vignette, although Margaret was "disillusioned" with aspects of her religious support system, she eventually found much comfort, hope, and strength in her spiritual beliefs. She began to see that her husband's death gave her life new direction and empowered her to act in new ways. She states, "If he hadn't gone, I wouldn't be the person I am today. I'm very content and peaceful about who I am and what I am doing." She became a volunteer and comforted others with terminal illness.

Behavioral Responses to Grief

Behavioral responses are often the easiest to observe (Fig. 9-1). Recognizing behaviors common to grieving, the nurse can provide supportive guidance for the client's exploration of emotionally and cognitively rough terrain. To promote the process, the nurse must provide a context of acceptance in which the client's behavior is explored. For example, observing the grieving one as functioning "automatically" or routinely without much thought can indicate that the person is in the numbness phase of grieving—the re-

▶ DIMENSIONS (RESPONSES) AND SYMPTOMS OF THE GRIEVING CLIENT

Cognitive responses
- Disruption of assumptions and beliefs
- Questioning and trying to make sense of the loss
- Attempting to keep the lost one present
- Believing in an afterlife and as though the lost one is a guide

Emotional responses
- Anger, sadness, anxiety
- Resentment
- Guilt
- Feeling numb
- Vacillating emotions
- Profound sorrow, loneliness
- Intense desire to restore bond with lost one or object
- Depression, apathy, despair during phase of disorganization and despair
- Sense of independence and confidence as phase of reorganization evolves

Spiritual responses
- Disillusioned and angry with God
- Anguish of abandonment or perceived abandonment
- Hopelessness; meaninglessness

Behavioral responses
- Functioning "automatically"
- Tearful sobbing; uncontrollable crying
- Great restlessness; searching behaviors
- Irritability and hostility
- Seeking and avoiding places and activities shared with lost one
- Keeping valuables of lost one while wanting to discard them
- Possibly abusing drugs or alcohol
- Possible suicidal or homicidal gestures or attempts
- Seeking activity and personal reflection during phase of reorganization

Physiologic responses
- Headaches, insomnia
- Impaired appetite, weight loss
- Lack of energy
- Palpitations, indigestion
- Changes in immune and endocrine system

ality of the loss has not set in. Tearful sobbing, uncontrollable crying, great restlessness, and searching behaviors are evidence of yearning and searching for the lost figure. The person may actually call out for the deceased and visually scan the room looking for the lost one. Irritability and hostility toward others reveal feelings of anger and frustration in the process. Seeking out as well as avoiding places or activities once shared with the deceased, and keeping valuables belonging to or shared with the deceased while wanting to discard belongings illustrate fluctuating emotions and perceptions of hope for a reconnection with the dead person.

During the phase of disorganization, the cognitive act of redefining the bereaved person's self-identity, although difficult, is essential in moving through the grief. Although superficial at first, efforts made in social or work activities are behavioral means to support the person's cognitive and emotional shifts. Drug or al-

cohol abuse indicates a maladaptive behavioral response to the emotional and spiritual despair. Suicide and homicide attempts may be extreme responses if the bereaved person cannot move through the grieving process.

In the reorganization phase, the bereaved person participates in activities and reflection that is personally meaningful and satisfying. Margaret became involved in creative outlets and personal growth, stating, "I'm happy with who I am and what I do. My life is more authentic."

Physiologic Responses to Grief

Physiologic symptoms and problems associated with grief responses are often a source of anxiety and concern for the grieving person as well as friends or caregivers. Clients may complain of insomnia, headaches, impaired appetite, weight loss, lack of energy,

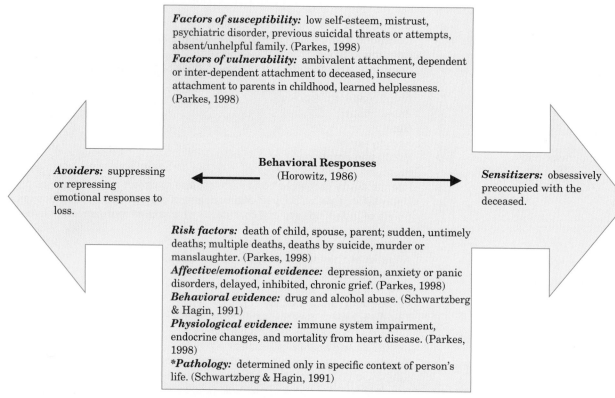

Factors of susceptibility: low self-esteem, mistrust, psychiatric disorder, previous suicidal threats or attempts, absent/unhelpful family. (Parkes, 1998)
Factors of vulnerability: ambivalent attachment, dependent or inter-dependent attachment to deceased, insecure attachment to parents in childhood, learned helplessness. (Parkes, 1998)

Behavioral Responses
(Horowitz, 1986)

Avoiders: suppressing or repressing emotional responses to loss.

Sensitizers: obsessively preoccupied with the deceased.

Risk factors: death of child, spouse, parent; sudden, untimely deaths; multiple deaths, deaths by suicide, murder or manslaughter. (Parkes, 1998)
Affective/emotional evidence: depression, anxiety or panic disorders, delayed, inhibited, chronic grief. (Parkes, 1998)
Behavioral evidence: drug and alcohol abuse. (Schwartzberg & Hagin, 1991)
Physiological evidence: immune system impairment, endocrine changes, and mortality from heart disease. (Parkes, 1998)
*Pathology: determined only in specific context of person's life. (Schwartzberg & Hagin, 1991)

Figure 9-1. Overview of complicated grief. Adapted from work of Parkes, 1998; Schwartzberg & Halgin, 1990; Horowitz, 1986.

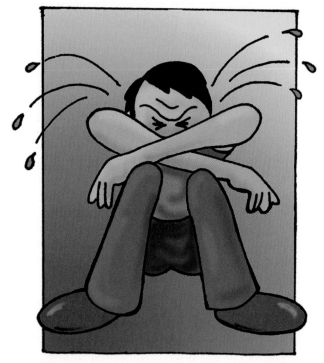

Sobbing

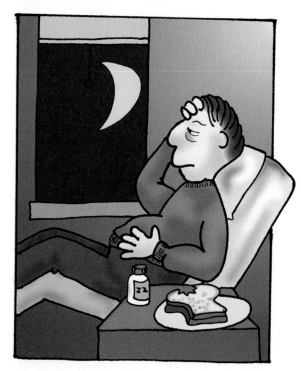

Physiologic symptoms

palpitations and indigestion, and changes in the immune and endocrine system. Some believe that these **psychogenic** (originating in mental or emotional turmoil) or **somatic symptoms** (pertaining to the body) after major loss reflect a loss of security.

CULTURAL CONSIDERATIONS
Universal Reactions to Loss

Although all cultures grieve for lost loved ones, the rituals and habits surrounding death vary from culture to culture. Each culture defines the process of grieving and integration of loss into life in ways consistent with their beliefs about life, death, and an afterlife. Certain aspects of the experience may be considered more important, others less so (Shapiro, 1996).

Universal reactions include the initial reaction of shock and social disorientation, trying to continue a relationship with the deceased, feeling angry with those responsible for the death, and a time for mourning. However, a specific culture may define acceptable ways of exhibiting shock and sadness, acceptable forms of anger, or how long the mourning should last (Bowlby, 1980). Cultural awareness of rituals for mourning can help the nurse understand an individual client or family's behavior.

Culture-Specific Rituals

Because cultural bereavement rituals have their roots in several of the world's major religions, such as Buddhism, Christianity, Hinduism, Islam, and Judaism, the client's religious or spiritual beliefs and practices regarding death will guide him or her in the manner of mourning. In the United States, a variety of mourning rituals and practices exist. We will summarize a few of the major ones.

AFRICAN AMERICANS

Most of the ancestors of today's African Americans came to the United States as slaves and lived under the influence of European American and Christian religious practices. However, African Americans have maintained unique patterns of worship. In Catholic and Episcopalian services, hymns may be sung, poetry read, and a eulogy spoken; less formal Baptist and Holiness traditions involve singing, speaking in tongues, and body movements. Typically, the deceased is viewed in church before burial takes place in a cemetery. Mourning may also be expressed through public prayers, wearing black clothing, and decreasing social activities. The mourning period may last a few weeks to several years. For persons from the Middle East and an increasing number of African Americans

who are Muslim, cremation is not permitted, and the deceased is wrapped with special cloths before burial.

HAITIAN AMERICANS

Some Haitian Americans practice *vodun* (voodoo), also called "root medicine." Derived from Roman Catholic rituals and saints and cultures of the Republic of West Africa and the Sudan, *vodun* is the practice of calling on a group of spirits with whom one periodically makes peace during specific events in life. The death of a loved one may be one of those times. This practice can be found in Alabama, Louisiana, the Carolinas, and Virginia and in some New York City communities.

CHINESE AMERICANS

As the largest Asian population in the United States, the Chinese have strict norms for announcing death, preparing the body, arranging the funeral and burial, and mourning after burial. The burning of incense and reading of scripture are ways of assisting the spirit of the deceased in the afterlife journey. For a year after death, bowls of food may be placed on a table for the spirit.

JAPANESE AMERICANS

For Japanese Americans who are Buddhist, death is viewed as a life passage. The deceased is bathed with warm water by close family members and after purification rites is dressed in a white kimono. For 2 days, family and friends may visit, bearing gifts or offering money for the deceased while prayers are said and incense is burned.

FILIPINO AMERICANS

Most Filipino Americans are Catholic. The wearing of black clothing or armbands is customary, depending on how close a person was to the deceased. Wreaths are placed on the casket and a broad black cloth may be draped on the home of the deceased. It is common for announcements to be placed in local newspapers asking for prayers and blessings on the soul of the deceased.

VIETNAMESE AMERICANS

Vietnamese Americans are predominately Buddhist. The deceased is bathed and dressed in black clothes. A few grains of rice may be put in the mouth and money is placed with the deceased so that he or she can buy a drink as the spirit moves on in the afterlife.

Viewing of the body before burial may be done at home. When friends enter, music is played as a way to warn the deceased of the arrival.

HISPANIC AMERICANS

Hispanic or Latino Americans have their origins in Spain, Mexico, Cuba, Puerto Rico, and the Dominican Republic. Because those countries were colonized by the Spanish several centuries ago, they are predominately Roman Catholic. Hispanics pray for the soul of the deceased during a novena (9-day devotion) and a rosary (devotional prayer). *Luto* (mourning) is manifested by the wearing of black or black and white, and by a subdued manner. Respect for the deceased may include not watching TV, going to the movies, listening to the radio, or attending dances or other social events for a period of time. Friends and relatives bring flowers and crosses to decorate the grave.

Americans from Guatemala may include a marimba band in the funeral procession and services. Lighting of candles and blessing the dead one during a wake in the home are common practices.

NATIVE AMERICANS

Ancient beliefs and practices influence the more than 500 Native American Indian tribes in the United States, even though most are now Christians. The medicine man or priestly healer of a tribe is an essential spiritual guide for the friends and family of the deceased as he assists them in regaining their spiritual equilibrium after the loss of a loved one. Ceremonies of baptism for the spirit of the deceased seem to help ward off depression that may be experienced. Perceptions about the meaning of death and its impact on family and friends are as varied as the number of tribal communities.

Viewing death as a state of unconditional love where the spirit of the deceased remains present is comforting for the Cherokee and encourages movement toward life's purpose of being happy and living in harmony with nature and others. The Navajo believe in and fear ghosts; death signifies the end of all that is good, and touching the body of the deceased is avoided. The Dakotah believe in a happy afterlife called the land of the spirits; they believe that proper mourning is essential not only for the soul of deceased but also to protect members of the community. To designate the end of mourning, a ceremony is held at the burial grounds where the grave is covered with a blanket or cloth for making clothes and later given to a tribe member. A dinner is served where songs are sung, speeches are made, and money is given away.

ORTHODOX JEWISH AMERICANS

A custom of Orthodox Jews is that a relative stays with a dying person so that the soul will not leave the body while the person is alone. To leave the body alone after death is a sign of disrespect. The eyes of the deceased should be closed while the body is covered and untouched until family, a rabbi, or a Jewish undertaker can begin rites. Although organ donation is permitted, autopsy is not; burial must occur within 24 hours unless delayed by the Sabbath.

Nurse's Role

The diverse cultural environment of the United States offers the sensitive nurse much opportunity to individualize care when relating to grieving clients. In extended families, varying expressions and responses to loss can exist, depending on the degree of **acculturation** (altering cultural values or behaviors as a way to adapt to another culture). Rather than assuming that he or she understands a particular culture's appropriate grieving behaviors, the nurse must encourage clients to discover and use what is effective and meaningful for them. For example, the nurse could ask an Hispanic or Latino practicing Catholic if he or she would like to pray for the deceased. If an Orthodox Jew has just died, the nurse could offer to stay with the body while relatives are notified.

COMPLICATED GRIEVING

The descriptions of grieving discussed in this chapter so far are considered normal responses to the loss of a loved one. Some believe that **complicated grieving** is a response that lies outside the norm and occurs when a person may be void of emotion, grieve for prolonged periods of time, and have expressions of grief that seem out of proportion.

Although it is important to recognize that complications may arise in the arduous journey of grief, and although many descriptions demonstrate a pattern to grieving, the process remains a unique and dynamic experience. Immense variety exists in terms of the cultural determinants in communicating the experience and in terms of individual differences in emotional reactions, depth of pain, and the amount of time needed to acknowledge and grasp the personal meaning or assimilate the loss. Box 9-1 discusses styles of grieving.

For some people, the impact of grief is particularly devastating because their personality or emotional state or situation makes them susceptible to complications during the process. Sometimes mental illness can develop (Parkes, 1998).

➤ STYLES OF GRIEVING

When determining whether a person may be experiencing a complicated grieving process, the nurse should consider viewing the person's behavior as a unique style of grieving. Silver and Wortman (1980) have suggested three styles of grieving:

- The bereaved vacillates from high to low distress over time.
- The bereaved shows no distress either as an immediate response to loss or subsequently.
- The bereaved remains in a high state of distress for a period beyond what others would consider appropriate.

Characteristics of Susceptibility

Characteristics of people vulnerable to complicated grief include those with (Parkes, 1998):

- Low self-esteem
- Low trust in others
- A previous psychiatric disorder
- Previous suicide threats or attempts
- Absent or unhelpful family members
- An ambivalent, dependent, or interdependent attachment to the deceased person. In an ambivalent attachment, one or both of the partners are unclear about how they love or do not love each other. In a dependent attachment, one partner is reliant on the other to provide for his or her needs. With an interdependent attachment, both partners are givers and takers in the relationship; the needs of both are mutually met.
- An insecure attachment to parents in childhood, especially where the child has learned fear and helplessness. For example, the person may have been intimidated through abuse and not given opportunities to make choices as a child and could not depend on the parent to meet the needs of safety and security.

A person's perception is another factor in the experience of vulnerability: one's perception, or how one thinks or feels about a situation, is not always the reality. After the death of a loved one, a person may believe that he or she really is incapable of going on in life and is at a great disadvantage in surviving. Therefore, he or she may become increasingly sad and depressed, not eating or sleeping and perhaps entertaining thoughts of suicide.

Risk Factors Leading to Vulnerability

Parkes (1998) identified experiences that increase the risk for complicated grieving for the vulnerable persons mentioned above. These experiences are related to trauma or individual perceptions of vulnerability. These risk factors for complicated grieving include:

- Death of a spouse or child
- Death of a parent (particularly in early childhood or adolescence)
- Sudden, unexpected, and untimely death
- Multiple deaths
- Death by suicide or murder.

Complicated Grieving as a Unique and Varied Experience

Human behavioral responses to complicated grief illustrate the process on a continuum. At one end are persons who hold back, suppressing or repressing emotional response to loss (often called **avoiders**). At the other end are those who are obsessively preoccupied with the deceased and express emotions with great intensity and duration (often called **sensitizers**) (Horowitz, 1986). Sensitizers often have loved the dead person in an ambivalent way (never quite sure of the degree to which they were committed to the person) or believe that they cannot survive without the dead person (Parkes, 1998).

The person with complicated grieving can also experience physiologic and emotional reactions. Physical reactions can include impairment of the immune system, increased adrenocortical activity, increased levels of serum prolactin and growth hormone, psychosomatic disorders, and an increased mortality rate from heart disease. Characteristic emotional responses include depression, anxiety or panic disorders, delayed or inhibited grief, and chronic grief (Parkes, 1998).

Because the grieving process is unique to each person, the nurse must assess the degree of impairment with regard to each client's life and experiences—for example, examining current coping responses compared with previous experiences, and assessing whether the client is involved in maladaptive behaviors such as drug and alcohol abuse as a means of dealing with the painful experience (Schwartzberg & Halgin, 1991).

SELF-AWARENESS ISSUES

Clients who are grieving need more than someone who is equipped with skills and basic knowledge; they need the support of someone they can trust with their emotions and thoughts. For nurses to be seen as trustworthy, they need to be willing to examine their personal attitudes about loss and the grieving process. Taking a self-awareness inventory means periodic reflection on such questions as:

- What are the losses in my life, and how do they affect my life?
- Am I currently grieving for a significant loss? How does my loss affect my ability to be present to my client?
- Who is there for me as I am grieving?
- How am I coping with my loss?
- Is the pain of my personal grief spilling over as I listen and watch for cues of the client's grieving?
- Am I making assumptions about the client's experience based on my own process?
- Can I keep appropriate nurse–client boundaries as I attend to the client's needs?
- Do I have the strength to be present and to guide the client on his or her journey?
- What does my supervisor or a trusted colleague observe about my current ability to support a client on his or journey through grief?

Ongoing self-examination is an effective method of keeping the therapeutic relationship goal-directed and acutely attentive to the client's needs.

APPLICATION OF THE NURSING PROCESS

Because the strong emotional attachment created in a significant relationship is not easily released, loss through death of a loved one is a major crisis that has a momentous impact on a person's life. Aquilera and Messick (1982) developed a broad approach to assessment and intervention in their work on crisis intervention. The state of disequilibrium produced by the crisis (or loss) causes great consternation and extreme discomfort, compelling the person to return to **homeostasis**, a state of equilibrium or balance. The factors that influence the grieving person's return to homeostasis are adequate perception of the situation, adequate situational support, and adequate coping. These factors help the person regain a sense of balance and return to his or her previous level of functioning, or even to use the crisis as opportunity to grow. Because any loss may be perceived as a personal crisis, it seems appropriate that the nurse apply understanding of crisis theory to the nursing process.

For the nurse to support and guide clients on this difficult journey of grieving, he or she must observe and listen for the cues from the client. These include cognitive, emotional, spiritual, behavioral, and physiological cues. Although the nurse must be familiar with the phases or tasks to be accomplished and the dimensions of human response to loss, the nurse must realize that each client has a unique experience. Skillful communication is the key to performing assessment and providing interventions.

The nurse should be a trustworthy guide for the client. The nurse must examine his or her personal attitudes, maintain an attentive presence, and provide a psychologically safe environment for the client's deeply intimate sharing. Maintaining attentive presence can be accomplished by using open body language such as standing or sitting with arms down and facing the client and maintaining moderate eye contact, especially as the client speaks. Creating a psychologically safe environment includes assuring the client of confidentiality, refraining from giving specific advice, and allowing the client freedom to share thoughts and feelings without fear of judgment.

Assessment

Assessment includes observing and hearing the content of a client's grieving: what is thought, spoken, felt, and indicated through behavior. Sometimes, in dealing with a grieving client, interventions actually take place during assessment. Some of the conversations that are part of assessment actually become interventions as the client comes to a better understanding of what he or she is thinking and feeling.

Three major areas need to be explored in assessment:

- Adequate perception regarding the loss
- Adequate support while grieving for the loss

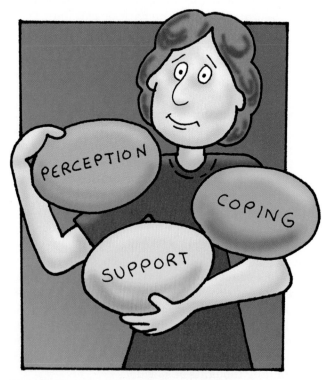

Three major areas to explore to facilitate grieving client.

- Adequate coping behaviors during the process.

ASSESSMENT REGARDING PERCEPTION OF THE LOSS

Assessment should begin with exploring the client's perception of the loss: what does the loss mean to the client? This question may have different answers and should be considered as a valuable intervention in grieving. Other questions that assess perception or meaning as well as encourage the client's movement on the grieving journey include:

- What does the client think and feel about the loss?
- How is the loss going to have an impact on the client's life?
- What information needs to be clarified or shared with the client?

Assessing the client's "need to know" in plain and simple language can invite the client to verbalize perceptions that may need clarification. This is especially true for the person who is anticipating a loss, such as in a life-ending illness. The nurse should use open-ended questions and help clarify misperceptions the client may have.

The doctor has just informed Ms. Morrison that the lump on her breast is cancerous and that she is scheduled for a mastectomy in 2 days. The nurse visits the client after rounds and finds her quietly watching TV.

Nurse: *"How are you?"* (offering presence; giving a broad opening)

Client: *"Oh, I'm fine. Really, I am."*

Nurse: *"The doctor was just here. Tell me, what is your understanding of what he said?"* (open-ended questions asking for description of perception)

Client: *"Well, I think he said that I will have to have surgery on my breast."*

Nurse: *"How was that news for you?"* (open-ended question asking what it means for the client)

Exploring what the person believes about the process of grieving is another important assessment. Does the client have preconceived ideas about the time allotted for grieving or about the way in which it should happen? The nurse can help the client realize that grieving is a very personal and unique experience: each person grieves in his or her own way.

The nurse finds Ms. Morrison hitting her pillow and crying. This is her second postoperative day. She has eaten little food and has refused visitors since the surgery.

Nurse: *"Ms. Morrison, I see that you are upset. Tell me, what is happening right now?"* (sharing observation; encouraging description)

Client: *"Oh, I'm so disgusted with myself. I'm sorry you had to see me act this way. I should be snapping out of this and getting on with my life."*

Nurse: *"You're pretty upset with yourself, thinking you should be feeling different than you are."* (using reflection)

Client: *"Yes, exactly. Don't you think so?"*

Nurse: *"You have had to deal with quite a shock these past few days. Sounds to me like you are expecting quite a bit of yourself, beyond what would be expected. What do you think?"* (using reflection; sharing perceptions; seeking validation)

Client: *"I don't know, maybe. How long is this going to go on? I'm a wreck emotionally."*

Nurse: *"You are grieving, and there is no fixed timetable for what you are having to deal with. Everyone has a unique time and way of doing this work."* (informing; validating her experience)

ASSESSMENT REGARDING ADEQUATE SUPPORT

Purposeful assessment of the client's support system is a way to provide the grieving client with an awareness of those around who can meet the client's emotional and spiritual needs of security and love. The nurse can help the client to identify his or her support system and to reach out and accept what they have to offer.

Nurse: *"Who is a person in your life who should or would really want to know what you've just heard from the doctor?"* (seeking information about situational support for the client)

Client: *"Oh, I'm really alone. I'm not married and don't have any relatives in town."*

Nurse: *"There's no one who would care about this news?"* (voicing doubt)

Client: *"Oh, maybe a friend I talk with on the phone now and then."*

ASSESSMENT REGARDING ADEQUATE COPING BEHAVIORS

The client's behavior is likely to give the nurse the easiest and most concrete information about his or her coping skills. The nurse must be careful to observe the client's behavior at various junctures on the grieving journey, never assuming that a client is at a particular phase. The nurse must use effective communication skills to assess how the client's behavior is a reflection of coping as well as what he or she is feeling and thinking.

The nurse has heard in report that Ms. Morrison received the news of her upcoming mastectomy. She entered Ms. Morrison's room and saw her crying, with a full tray of food untouched.

Nurse: *"You must be quite upset about the news you received from the doctor today."* (an observation made assuming the client was crying as an expected behavior of loss and grief)

Client: *"I'm not having surgery. You have me mistaken for someone else."* (using denial as coping)

The nurse must also consider several other questions when assessing the client's adequacy of coping. How has the person dealt with loss previously? How is the person currently impaired? How does the current experience compare with what has gone before? What does the client perceive as a problem, and is it related to unrealistic ideas about what he or she should be feeling or doing? (Schwartzberg & Halgin, 1991).

The interaction that exists among the dimensions of human response is fluid and dynamic. What a person is thinking about during grieving affects his or her feelings, and what is felt influences how he or she behaves. The critical factors of perception, support, and coping are interrelated as well and provide a framework for assessing and assisting the client.

Data Analysis and Planning

The nursing diagnosis for the person experiencing loss must be based on the subjective and objective assessment data collected by the nurse. In this chapter, we have discussed assessment data in terms of the dimensions of grieving and have applied components of crisis theory in the gathering and clustering of data. We have also emphasized the importance of understanding cultural influences in grieving and mourning, as well as recognizing that the process is a fluid one for clients.

Lynda Carpenito (1995), in *Nursing Diagnoses: Application to Clinical Practice,* describes three nursing diagnoses for the process of grieving. Statements of etiology for the diagnoses may be based on the types of losses as described earlier in this chapter:

- **Grieving,** related to actual or perceived loss, such as a physiologic loss (e.g., loss of a limb), is defined as a normal process in the human experience of loss and can be applied, in this chapter, to Margaret in the vignette.
- **Grieving, Anticipatory**, related to actual or perceived loss is defined as a response to a loss that is expected or anticipated. This diagnosis would apply to the example of Ms. Morrison, whose loss of one of her breasts may affect her presurgery body image.
- **Grieving, Dysfunctional,** related to (a specific factor) is defined as a complicated process of experiencing loss. Complicated grieving was discussed earlier in the chapter.

Outcome Identification

Examples of outcomes for the three nursing diagnoses are:

- Grieving: The client will identify the impact of his or her loss, seek adequate support, and apply effective coping strategies while expressing and assimilating the experience of loss in his or her life.
- Grieving, Anticipatory: The client will identify the meaning of the expected loss in his or her life, seek adequate support while expressing grief, and develop a plan for coping with the loss as it becomes a reality in his or her life.
- Grieving, Dysfunctional: The client will identify the meaning of his or her loss, recognize its deleterious effects on his or her life, and seek or accept professional assistance as a means to promote the grieving process.

Interventions

The nurse's guidance helps the client examine and make changes in any one of the dimensions. Changes imply movement as the client trudges up the trail, sometimes one painful step at a time and over what seems like old terrain as each switchback is conquered on the journey.

INTERVENTIONS REGARDING THE PERCEPTION OF LOSS

Cognitive responses in grieving are significantly connected with the intense emotional turmoil that occurs in grieving. For example, in the vignette, Margaret's disillusionment with those not available after her husband's death added great pain to her loss. She had counted on them to be there for her as she dealt with James' death. A cognitive shift occurred when she realized they would not be there for her, meaning she was alone and they no longer cared. She felt abandoned. She then had two immediate losses: James' death and realizing that people she had counted on were not available to her.

Exploring the client's perception and meaning of his or her loss is a first step that can help alleviate the pain of what some would call the initial emotional overload in grieving. Using the example of Margaret, it might be useful to ask what it means to her that she experiences being alone, and to explore the possibility of others being supportive of her. Further exploration could focus on her perception that those who had abandoned her no longer cared. Perhaps, in her thinking, she would discover that her need to be cared for could be met by others. She may begin to think that it was fear or discomfort about death that kept former friends away. In fact, it was in just this way that she could accept the caring of some friends and release the importance of those who would not or could not be there for her. In this situation, exploring perceptions and the meaning of the loss helped the bereaved to make cognitive shifts that had a valuable impact on her emotional experience.

When a death or loss occurs, especially if it happens suddenly and without warning, the cognitive defense mechanism of denial acts as a cushion in softening the impact. Typical verbal responses are, "I can't believe this has happened. It can't be true. There's been a mistake."

Adaptive denial, where the client gradually adjusts to the reality of the loss, can help the client to make cognitive shifts that require letting go of previous (before the loss) perceptions while creating new ways of thinking about himself or herself, others, and the world. For example, Margaret had to face the reality that although she believed that a priest, because he was a priest, would care about her being alone in the surgery waiting room, he was actually only concerned about getting a paper. Only gradually did she relinquish this assumption about priests. Effective communication skills can be useful in helping the client in adaptive denial toward acceptance.

The nurse has heard in report that Ms. Morrison received the news of her upcoming mastectomy. She entered Ms. Morrison's room and saw her crying, with a full tray of food untouched.

Nurse: *"You must be quite upset about the news you received from your doctor about your surgery."* (reflection, assuming the client was crying as an expected response of grief. Focusing on the surgery is an indirect approach regarding the subject of cancer.)

Client: *"I'm not having surgery. You have me mistaken for someone else."* (denial)

Nurse: *"I saw you crying and wonder what is upsetting you. I'm interested in how you are feeling."* (focusing on behavior and sharing observation while indicating concern and accepting the client's denial)

Client: *"I'm just not hungry. I don't have an appetite and I'm not clear what the doctor said."* (focusing on physiologic response; nonresponsive to nurse's encouragement to talk about feelings; acknowledging doctor's visit but unsure of what he said—beginning to adjust cognitively to reality of condition)

Nurse: *"I wonder if your not wanting to eat may be related to what you are feeling. Are there times when you don't have an appetite and you feel upset about something?"* (suggesting a connection between physiologic response and feelings; promoting adaptive denial)

Client: *"Well, as a matter of fact, yes. But I can't think what I would be upset about."* (acknowledging a connection between behavior and feeling; continuing to deny reality)

Nurse: *"You said you were unclear about what the doctor said. I wonder if things didn't seem clear because it may have upset you to hear what he had to say. Then, tonight you don't have an appetite."* (using client's experience while making connection between doctor's news and client's physiologic response and behavior)

Client: *"What did he say, do you know?"* (Requesting information demonstrates a readiness to hear it again while continuing to adjust to reality.)

In this example, the nurse gently but persistently guides the client toward acknowledging the reality of her impending loss.

INTERVENTIONS REGARDING ADEQUATE SUPPORT

The nurse can help the client to reach out and accept what others want to give in support of his or her grieving process.

Nurse: *"Who is a person in your life would really want to know what you've just heard from the doctor?"* (seeking information about situational support for the client)

Client: *"Oh, I'm really alone. I'm not married."*

Nurse: *"There's no one who would care about this news?"* (voicing doubt)

Client: *"Oh, maybe a friend I talk with on the phone now and then."*

Nurse: *"Why don't I get the phone book for you and you can call her right now?"* (continuing to offer presence, an immediate source of support, and suggesting a plan of action providing further support)

Resources for the Grieving Client. Many Internet resources are available to the nurse who wants to help a client find information, support groups, and activities related to the grieving process. Bereavement and Hospice Support Netline is one source that has numerous Internet links throughout the United States to a variety of organizations providing support and education. If a client does not have Internet access, most public libraries can help locate groups and activities that would serve his or her needs. Depending on the state where a person lives, specific groups exist for those who have lost an infant or suffered a miscarriage, lost a child, lost a spouse, or lost a loved one to suicide, murder, a motor vehicle accident, or cancer.

INTERVENTIONS REGARDING ADEQUATE COPING BEHAVIORS

When attempting to focus Ms. Morrison on the reality of her surgery, the nurse was helping Ms. Morrison make the shift from an unconscious mechanism of

> ▶ INTERVENTIONS FOR THE CLIENT
> WHO IS GRIEVING

Explore client's perception and meaning of his or her loss.

Allow adaptive denial.

Encourage or assist client to reach out for and accept support.

Encourage client to examine patterns of coping in past and present situation of loss.

Encourage client to review personal strengths and personal power.

Encourage client to care for himself or herself.

Offer client food without pressure to eat.

Use effective communication:
- Offer presence and give broad openings
- Use open-ended questions
- Encourage description
- Share observations
- Use reflection
- Seek validation of perceptions
- Provide information
- Voice doubt
- Use focusing
- Attempt to translate into feelings or verbalize the implied

Establish rapport and maintain interpersonal skills such as:
- Attentive presence
- Respect for client's unique grieving process
- Respect for client's personal beliefs
- Being trustworthy: honest, dependable, consistent
- Periodic self-inventory of attitudes and issues related to loss

denial to conscious coping with reality. The nurse used communication skills to encourage Ms. Morrison to look at her experience and behavior as possible ways in which she might be coping with the news of loss. Margaret and James' logical approach to life allowed them to cope by continuing to have fun together while attending to medical regimens as they faced the reality of his impending death.

Intervention involves giving the client the opportunity to compare and contrast ways that he or she has coped with significant loss in the past, helping him or her to review strengths and renew a sense of personal power. Remembering and practicing old behaviors in a new situation may lead to experimentation with new methods and self-discovery. Having an historical perspective eases the person's journey by allowing shifts in thinking about himself or herself, the loss, and perhaps the meaning of the loss in his or her life. Margaret's religious practices of

prayer and spiritual reading helped her discover new depths of meaning and purpose in her life.

Encouraging the client to care for himself or herself is another intervention that helps the client cope. The nurse can offer food without pressuring the client to eat. Being careful to eat, sleep well, exercise, and take time for comforting activities are ways the client can nourish himself or herself. Just as the tired hiker needs to stop, rest, and replenish himself or herself, so must the bereaved person take a break from the exhausting process of grieving. Going back to a routine of work or focusing on other members of the family may provide that respite. Volunteer activities— volunteering at a hospice or botanical garden, taking part in church activities, or speaking to bereavement education groups, for example—can affirm the client's talents and abilities and can renew feelings of self-worth.

Communication and interpersonal skills are tools of the effective nurse, just like his or her stethoscope, scissors, and gloves. The client trusts that the nurse will have what it takes to assist him or her in this difficult journey. In addition to previously mentioned skills, these tools include:

- Use simple, nonjudgmental statements to acknowledge loss: "I want you to know I'm thinking of you."
- Refer to a loved one or object of loss by name (if acceptable in the client's culture)
- Words are not always necessary; a light touch on the elbow, shoulder, or hand or just being there will indicate caring.

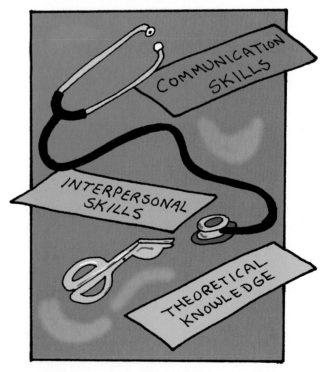

Nurses' tools

INTERNET RESOURCES

Resource	Internet Address
▶ Grief, bereavement, resource and change	www.therapeuticresources.com/2854text.htm
▶ Sites devoted to grief and bereavement	www.growthhouse.org
▶ Books on grief, bereavement, and life after death	www.azsids.org/family/bookstore/griefbooks.html
▶ Practical grief resources	www.isis.csuhayward.edu/ALSS/soc/NAN/dd/ddgrief.htm
▶ Bereavement and hospice support	http://www.ubalt.edu/bereavement/
▶ What Can I Say? What Can I Do?	http://members.aol.com/Jeri10/Death.html
▶ Poems about the loss of a child	http://www.thelaboroflove.com/prose/loss.html
▶ Grief and healing	http://www.webhealing.com/cgi-bin/main.pl

- Respect the client's unique process of grieving.
- Respect the client's personal beliefs.
- Be worthy of the client's trust: honest, dependable, and consistent.

A welcoming smile and eye contact from the client during intimate conversations indicate the nurse's trustworthiness.

Evaluation

Evaluation of progress depends on the goals established for the client. A review of the tasks and phases of grieving (discussed earlier in the chapter) can be useful in making a statement about the client's status at any given moment. We could say that while Margaret, in the vignette, still misses James, she is in the reorganization phase of grieving. She has a sense of independence and confidence and has accomplished several tasks of grieving—creating new ties, developing a new sense of self, pursuing new activities, and integrating the loss of James into her life.

➤ KEY POINTS

- Grief refers to the subjective emotions and affect that are a normal response to the experience of loss.

- Grieving is the process through which a person travels as he or she experiences grief.
- Types of losses can be identified as unfulfilled or unmet human needs. Maslow's hierarchy of human needs is a useful model for understanding loss as it relates to unfulfilled human needs: physiologic, safety, security and sense of belonging, self-esteem, and self-actualization losses.
- The arduous journey of grieving is one of life's most difficult challenges. The challenge to integrate a loss requires all that the person can give of mind, body, and spirit.
- Because the nurse constantly interfaces with clients at various points on the health–illness continuum, he or she must understand loss and the process of grieving.
- Attachment behaviors are activated or aroused when loss of a significant other occurs. Attachment behaviors range from quiet glances toward the significant other or following, clinging to, searching for, and calling out for the other, to wails of protest when the significant other or object is lost.
- The process of grieving has been described in terms of phases that are dynamically interrelated: numbness and denial; yearning and protesting; cognitive disorganization and

(text continues on page 207)

SAMPLE CARE PLAN GRIEF

Nursing Diagnosis

➤ **Dysfunctional Grieving** (9.2.1.1)
A state in which an individual's response to a loss (actual, perceived, or anticipated) is prolonged, distorted, exaggerated, or delayed and which may impair the individual's functioning.

ASSESSMENT DATA

- Questioning and trying to make sense of the loss
- Experiencing disillusionment
- Feeling numb
- Feelings of sorrow, loneliness
- Tearful, sobbing
- Vacillating emotions, including anger
- Hopelessness
- Helplessness, powerlessness
- Great restlessness; searching for the deceased
- Headaches
- Insomnia
- Lack of energy
- Functioning "automatically"
- Keeping valuables of loved one while wanting to discard them

EXPECTED OUTCOMES

The client will:
- Identify the loss and its meaning for self (adequate perception)
- Express feelings, verbally and non-verbally
- Establish and maintain adequate nutrition, hydration, and elimination (adequate coping)
- Establish and maintain an adequate balance of rest, sleep, and activity (adequate coping)
- Establish or maintain an adequate support system
- Verbalize knowledge of the grief process
- Demonstrate initial integration of loss into his or her life (adequate coping)
- Verbalize realistic future plans integrating loss (adequate perception)

IMPLEMENTATION

Nursing Interventions

After establishing rapport with the client, bring up the loss in a supportive manner; if the client refuses to discuss it, withdraw and state your intention to return. ("I can understand that you may not want to talk with me about this now. I will come to talk with you again at 11:00, maybe we can talk about it then.") Return at the stated time, then continue to be as supportive as possible rather than confronting the client.

Rationale

Your presence demonstrates interest and caring. Telling the client you will return conveys your support. The client may need emotional support to face and express uncomfortable or painful feelings. Confronting the client or pushing him or her to express feelings may increase anxiety and lead to further denial or avoidance.

continued on page 205

continued from page 204

Talk with the client in realistic terms concerning his or her loss; discuss concrete changes that have occurred in his or her life as a result of the loss and changes that the client must now begin to make.

Discussing the loss on this level may help to make it more real for the client.

Encourage the expression of feelings in ways with which the client is comfortable—for example, talking, writing, drawing, crying, and so forth. Convey your acceptance of these feelings and means of expression. Offer the client verbal support for attempts to express feelings.

Expression of feelings can help the client to identify, accept, and work through his or her feelings, even if these are painful or otherwise uncomfortable for the client.

Encourage the client to recall experiences, talk about what was involved in his or her relationship with the lost person or object, and so forth. Discuss with the client the changes in his or her feelings toward self, others, and the lost person or object as a result of the loss and grief process.

Discussing the lost object or person can help the client identify and express the loss, what the loss means to him or her, and his or her emotional response.

Encourage appropriate (that is, safe) expression of all feelings that the client has toward the lost person or object and convey acceptance. Assure the client that even "negative" feelings like anger and resentment are normal and healthy in grieving.

Feelings are not inherently bad or good. Giving the client support for expressing feelings may help the client accept uncomfortable feelings.

Convey to the client that although feelings may be uncomfortable, they are natural and necessary to this process, that he or she can withstand having these feelings, and that the feelings will not harm him or her.

The client may fear the intensity of his or her feelings.

Discourage rumination if the client is ruminating on his or her guilt or worthlessness. After listening to the client's feelings, tell the client you will talk about other aspects of grief and feelings.

The client needs to identify and express the feelings that underlie the rumination and to proceed through the grief process.

Referral to the facility chaplain, clergy, or other spiritual resource person may be indicated.

The client may be more comfortable discussing spiritual issues with an advisor who shares his or her belief system.

Provide opportunities for the release of tension, anger, guilt, and so forth through physical activities. Promote regular exercise as a healthy means of dealing with stress and tension.

Physical activity provides a way to relieve tension in a healthy, nondestructive manner.

continued on page 206

continued from page 205

Limit times and frequency of therapeutic interactions with the client. Encourage independent, spontaneous expression of feelings (writing, initiating interactions with other clients or with other staff members, getting involved in a physical activity). Plan staff-initiated interactions at times that allow the client to fulfill responsibilities (activities, unit duties) and maintain personal care (sleeping, eating, hygiene).

The client needs to develop independent skills of communicating feelings and to integrate the loss into his or her daily life, while meeting his or her own basic needs.

Encourage the client to talk with others, individually and in small groups (larger as tolerated), about the loss in terms of his or her own and others' feelings and about experiences and changes resulting from the loss.

The client needs to develop independent skills of communicating feelings and expressing grief to others.

Promote sharing, communicating, ventilating feelings, and support among clients. Use larger groups (such as open report) for a general discussion of loss and grief (with or without focusing on this client's loss). However, help the client also realize that there are limits to sharing grief in a social context.

Sharing grief and experiences with others can help the client identify and express feelings and feel normal in grieving. Dwelling on grief in social interactions, however, can result in other people's discomfort with their own feelings and may lead to the client being avoided by friends and significant others.

Point out to the client that a major aspect of loss is a real physical stress. Encourage good nutrition, hydration, and elimination, as well as adequate rest and daily physical exercise (such as walking, running, swimming, or cycling), in the hospital and after discharge.

The client may be unaware of the physical stress of the loss of may lack interest in the activities of daily living. Physical exercise can relieve tension or pent-up feelings in a healthy, nondestructive manner.

Teach the client (and his or her family or significant others) about the grief process.

The client and family or significant others may have little or no knowledge of grief or the process involved in recovery

Point out to the client that time spent grieving can be a nurturing time, a time of learning and growth from which to gather the strength to go forward.

The grief process allows the client to adjust to a change in his or her life and to begin to move toward opportunities in the future.

Adapted from Schultz, J. M. & Videbeck, S. D. (1998). *Lippincott's manual of psychiatric nursing care plans,* (5th ed.). Philadelphia: Lippincott Williams & Wilkins.

Critical Thinking

Questions

1. Although grieving is explained in terms of a process of stages, the client experiences a myriad of emotions and thoughts. What phenomena of the grieving process give the nurse concrete information about the client's progress? Of these phenomena, which is the easiest to observe? How must the nurse investigate the meaning of this phenomenon?

2. What issues of loss does the critical care nurse deal with every day? What are the nurse's most valuable tools for dealing with these losses? How might the nurse in this setting use understanding of critical factors for integration of loss?

3. A client in the psychiatric setting has recently lost his mother. How will the nurse differentiate between the client's psychiatric illness and a normal response to grief? How will the nurse determine the risk of complicated grief for this client?

4. How might the nurse maintain his or her professional responsibility toward the therapeutic relationship with those who are grieving for a loss? What components of trustworthiness must the nurse cultivate in relation to the client who is grieving?

5. Think about a time in the past 5 years when you have experienced a loss. Using Maslow's hierarchy of needs, identify what human needs were jeopardized, unfulfilled, or lost in your experience. After reviewing the dimensions of grieving, describe your predominant responses to the loss. Using Bowlby's description of the grief process, explain your grieving process. What perceptual changes did you make as a result of your process? Who were the most supportive people in your life during the process? List a few of the most effective things people said or did that helped you integrate the loss into your life. What new coping behaviors did you develop because of this loss? What did you gain from this experience that will make a difference in your professional practice as a nurse? You may want to take time to share your reflections with a classmate or record them as a way to honor your personal growth and development.

- emotional despair; and reorganization and reintegration.
- Dimensions of human response include cognitive, emotional, spiritual, behavioral, and physiologic responses. They may be experienced in more than one phase of the grieving process.
- When experiencing the loss of a loved one, many basic assumptions and beliefs about life's meaning and purpose are disrupted. The grieving persons searches for answers, and often perceptions of the world, others, and oneself change.
- Emotional responses to loss can range from sadness to hate or revenge. They may be directed toward the lost object or person, significant others, health care providers, and oneself.
- It is in the spiritual dimension that the greatest strength or greatest devastation may be experienced while grieving. Attending to the spiritual response of the bereaved is an essential aspect of promoting the grieving process.
- Behaviors can indicate thoughts or feelings that are too painful for direct expression and may provide important information about the person's progress. The nurse must not assume what a behavior means; rather, he or she should gently explore its meaning in the context of acceptance.
- Complicated grieving is a response that lies outside the norm. The person may be void of emotion, grieve for a prolonged period, or express feelings that seem out of proportion. Because there are so many variables in the grieving process, what may appear to be complicated grieving may be only the person's unique style of grieving.
- Low self-esteem, distrust of others, a psychiatric disorder, previous suicide threats or attempts, and absent or unhelpful family members increase the risk of complicated grieving.
- Situations considered to be risk factors for complicated grief in those already vulnerable include death of a spouse or child; a sudden, unexpected death; and murder.
- During assessment, the nurse observes and listens for cues in what the person thinks and feels and how he or she behaves, then uses this relevant data to guide the client in the grieving process.
- Crisis theory can be used to help the nurse working with a grieving client. Adequate perception, adequate support, and adequate coping are critical factors.

- Effective communication skills are the key to successful assessment and interventions.
- Interventions focused on the perception of loss include exploration of the meaning of the loss and allowing adaptive denial, the process of gradually adjusting to the reality of a loss.
- Being there to help the client while assisting him or her to seek other sources of support is an essential intervention.
- Encouraging the client to care for himself or herself promotes adequate coping.
- To earn the client's trust, the nurse must examine his or her own attitudes about loss and periodically take a self-awareness inventory.

REFERENCES

Aquilera, D. C., & Messick, J. M. (1982). *Crisis intervention: theory and methodology.* St. Louis: C. V. Mosby.

Bowlby, J. (1980). *Attachment and loss, Vol. 3: Loss, sadness, and depression.* New York: Basic Books.

Carpenito, L. J. (1995). *Nursing diagnoses: application to clinical practice.* Philadelphia: J. B. Lippincott.

Harvey, J. H., & Miller, E. D. (1998). Toward a psychology of loss. *Psychological Science, 9*(6), 429. *http://web6.infotrac.galegroup.com/itw/in*

Henderson, A. S. (1994). Coping with bereavement. *World Health, 47*(3), 25. http://web6.infotrac.galegroup.co/itw/in

Horowitz, M. (1986). *Stress response syndromes.* Northvale, NJ: Aronson.

Janoff-Bulman, R. (1989). Assumptive worlds and the stress of traumatic events: application of the schema construct. *Social Cognition, 7,* 113–136.

Kubler-Ross, E. (1969). *On death and dying.* New York: Macmillan.

Marrone, R. (1997). *Death, mourning & caring.* California State University: Brooks/Cole.

Maslow, A. H. (1954). *Motivation and personality.* New York: Harper.

Parkes, C. M. (1998). Coping with loss: Bereavement in adult life. *British Medical Journal, 316*(7134), 856–859.

Rando, T. A. (1984). *Grief, dying and death: clinical interventions for caregivers.* Champaign, IL: Research Press.

Rodebaugh, L. S., Schwindt, R. G., & Valentine, F. M. (1999). How to handle grief with wisdom. *Nursing, 29,* 52.

Schneider, J. (1984). Stress, loss and grief. In S. Schonebaum & B. Friedman (Eds.). *Death, mourning & caring* (p. 110). California State University: Brooks/Cole.

Schultz, J. M. & Videbeck, S. D. (1998). *Lippincott's manual of psychiatric nursing care plans,* (5th ed.). Philadelphia: Lippincott Williams & Wilkins.

Schwartzberg, S. S., & Halgin, R. P. (1991). Treating grieving clients: the importance of cognitive change. *Professional Psychology: Research and Practice, 22*(3), 240–246.

Shapiro, E. R. (1996). *Grief as a family process: a developmental approach to clinical practice.* New York: Guilford Press.

Silver, R. K., & Wortman, C. B. (1980). Coping with undesirable life events. In J. Garber & M. E. P. Seligman (Eds.). *Human helplessness: theory and applications* (pp. 220–231). New York: Academic Press.

Varcarolis, E. M. (1998). *Foundations of psychiatric mental health nursing.* Philadelphia: W. B. Saunders.

Webb, N. B. (1993). Helping bereaved children: a handbook for practitioners. In S. Schonebaum & B. Friedman (Eds.). *Death, mourning & caring* (p. 108). California State University: Brooks/Cole.

Weisman, A. D. (1974). The realization of death. In S. Schonebaum & B. Friedman (Eds.). *Death, mourning & caring.* California State University: Brooks/Cole.

ADDITIONAL READINGS

Aldrige, D. (1993). Is there evidence for spiritual healing? *Advances, 9*(4), 421.

Customs of bereavement: a guide for providing cross-cultural assistance. Washington, D.C.: American Association of Retired Persons, 1990.

Geissler, E. M. (1998). *Pocket guide to cultural assessment.* St. Louis: Mosby.

Humphrey, G. M., & Zimpfer, D. G. (1996). *Counseling for grief and bereavement.* Thousand Oaks, CA: Sage Publications Ltd.

Rando, T. A. (1993). *Treatment of complicated mourning.* Champaign, IL: Research Press.

Chapter Review

➤ **MULTIPLE-CHOICE QUESTIONS**

Select the best answer for each of the following questions.

1. Which of the following identify phases of the grieving process according to Bowlby?

   A. Denial, anger, depression, bargaining, acceptance

   B. Shock, outcry, and denial; intrusion of thought, distractions, and obsessive reviewing of the loss; confiding in others to emote and cognitively restructure an account of the loss

   C. Numbness and denial of the loss, emotional yearning for the loved one and protesting permanence of the loss, cognitive disorganization and emotional despair, reorganizing and reintegrating a sense of self

   D. Reeling, feeling, dealing, healing.

2. Which of the following give cues to the nurse that a client may be grieving for a loss?

   A. Sad affect, anger, anxiety, and sudden changes in mood

   B. Thoughts, feelings, behavior, and physiologic complaints

   C. Hallucinations, panic level of anxiety, sense of impending doom

   D. Complaints of abdominal pain, diarrhea, and loss of appetite.

3. Situations that are considered risk factors for complicated grief are:

   A. Inadequate support and old age

   B. Childbirth, marriage, and divorce

   C. Death of a spouse or child, death by suicide, sudden and unexpected death

   D. Inadequate perception of the grieving crisis.

4. Physiologic responses of complicated grieving include:

   A. Tearfulness when recalling significant memories of the lost one

   B. Impaired appetite, weight loss, lack of energy, palpitations

   C. Depression, panic disorders, chronic grief

   D. Impaired immune system, increased serum prolactin level, increased mortality rate from heart disease.

5. Critical factors for successful integration of loss during the grieving process are:

   A. The client's adequate perception, adequate support, and adequate coping

   B. The nurse's trustworthiness and healthy attitudes about grief

   C. Accurate assessment and intervention by the nurse or helping person

   D. The client's predictable and steady movement from one stage of the process to the next.

➤ TRUE-FALSE QUESTIONS

Identify each of the following statements as T (true) or F (false). Correct any false statements.

_____ 1. Grief is an abnormal response to loss.

_____

_____ 2. A person who is grieving does so in a strictly predictable manner.

_____

_____ 3. Anger and depression are cognitive expressions of grieving.

_____

_____ 4. When assessing a client's adequacy in coping, the nurse collects data about the person's behavior.

_____

➤ FILL-IN-THE-BLANK QUESTIONS

Identify the dimension of grieving for each of the following client expressions or behaviors.

_____ "I have this insatiable yearning to be with him."

_____ Irritability and hostility toward others

_____ "I thought a priest would certainly be able to see my need to be supported at this time. Why didn't he ask how I was feeling when I told him my husband was having surgery?"

_____ "Why has God done this to me?"

_____ "I've lost my appetite, and I just can't seem to get to sleep at night when I go to bed."

➤ SHORT-ANSWER QUESTIONS

1. Give an example of each of the following:

   Styles of grieving

Critical factor of adequate support

Emotional response during phase of numbing in the grieving process

2. For each of the following client statements, write a response the nurse might make and the rationale for the nurse's response:

"This is unbearable. I can't believe she's gone."

"No one will want to hire me at this age."

"There's nowhere for me to turn."

"Get out of here! Leave me alone! I don't need your help."

Anger, Hostility, and Aggression

Anger is a normal human emotion that is a strong, uncomfortable, emotional response to a provocation that is either real or perceived by the person (Thomas, 1998). Anger results when a person is frustrated, hurt, or afraid. Handled appropriately and expressed assertively, it can be a positive force that helps the person resolve conflicts, solve problems, and make decisions. Anger energizes the body physically for self-defense, when needed, by activating the "fight-or-flight" response mechanisms of the sympathetic nervous system. When expressed inappropriately or suppressed, anger can cause physical or emotional problems or interfere with relationships.

Hostility is an emotion expressed by verbal abuse, lack of cooperation, violation of rules or norms, or threatening behavior, also called verbal aggression (Schultz & Videbeck, 1998). Hostility may be expressed by a person who feels threatened or powerless. Hostile behavior is intended to intimidate or cause emotional harm to another, and it can lead to physical aggression. **Physical aggression** is behavior that attacks or injures another person or involves destruction of property. Aggressive behavior is meant to harm or punish another person or to force someone into compliance. Some psychiatric clients display hostile or physically aggressive behavior that represents a challenge to nurses and other staff members.

Violence and abuse are discussed in Chapter 11, and self-directed aggression such as suicidal behavior is presented in Chapter 14. The focus of this chapter is the nurse's role in recognizing and managing hostile and aggressive behavior directed toward others in psychiatric settings.

ONSET AND CLINICAL COURSE
Anger

Although anger is a normal human emotion, it is often perceived as a negative feeling. Many are not comfortable expressing anger directly. However, anger is a normal and healthy reaction that can occur in response to situations or circumstances that are unfair or unjust, when someone's rights are not respected, or when one's expectations are not met. If the person can express his or her anger assertively, problem solving or conflict resolution can occur.

Anger becomes a negative concept when the person denies or suppresses angry feelings, or when he or she expresses them inappropriately. Denying or suppressing (i.e., holding in) feelings of anger may occur if the person is uncomfortable expressing anger. This can lead to physical problems such as migraine headaches, ulcers, or coronary artery disease, or emotional problems such as depression and low self-esteem.

Anger that is expressed inappropriately can lead to hostility and aggression. The nurse can help clients express anger appropriately by serving as a model and by role-playing assertive communication techniques. Assertive communication uses "I" statements that express feelings and are specific to the situation—for example, "I feel angry when you interrupt me," "I am angry that you changed the work schedule without talking to me." Statements such as these allow appropriate expression of anger and can lead to a productive problem-solving discussion and reduction of anger.

Some people try to vent their angry feelings by engaging in aggressive but safe activities, such as hitting a punching bag or yelling. Such activities, called *catharsis*, are supposed to provide a release for anger. However, Bushman and Stack (1999) found that catharsis could increase rather than alleviate angry feelings. Therefore, cathartic activities may be contraindicated for angry clients. Activities that are not aggressive, such as walking or talking with another person, are more likely to be effective in decreasing anger.

Phillips (1998) found that men who experience angry outbursts have twice the risk of stroke as men who control their tempers. Angry, aggressive outbursts of temper such as yelling or throwing things should be replaced by effective methods of anger expression, such as using assertive communication. Controlling one's temper or managing anger effec-

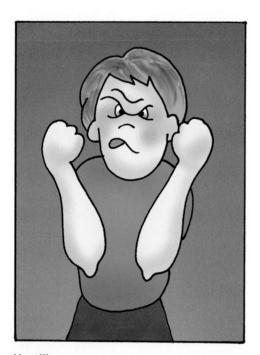

Hostility

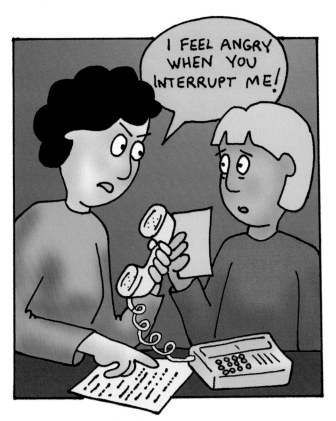

I FEEL ANGRY WHEN YOU INTERRUPT ME!

Assertive communication

tively should not be confused with suppressing angry feelings, which can lead to the problems described earlier.

Hostility and Aggression

Hostile and aggressive behavior can occur suddenly without much warning. However, there often are stages or phases that can be identified in aggressive incidents: a triggering phase, an escalation phase, a crisis phase, a recovery phase, and a postcrisis phase. These phases and their signs, symptoms, and behaviors are discussed later in the chapter.

As the client's behavior escalates toward the crisis phase, he or she loses the ability to perceive events accurately, solve problems, express feelings appropriately, or control his or her behavior, which may lead to physically aggressive behavior. Therefore, intervention at the triggering or escalation phase is key in preventing physically aggressive behavior (see below).

RELATED DISORDERS

When persons with mental illness commit aggressive acts, there is a great deal of media attention. This gives the general public the mistaken idea that most persons with mental illness are aggressive and should be feared. In reality, psychiatric clients are much more likely to hurt themselves than someone else.

Although most psychiatric clients are not aggressive (Shepherd & Lavender, 1999), clients with a variety of psychiatric diagnoses can exhibit angry, hostile, and aggressive behavior. Clients with paranoid delusions may believe others are out to get them and will retaliate with hostility or aggression in the belief that they are protecting themselves. Some clients have auditory hallucinations commanding them to hurt others. Aggressive behavior also can be seen in clients with dementia, delirium, head injuries, intoxication with alcohol or other drugs, and antisocial and borderline personality disorders.

Fava and Rosenbaum (1999) reported that about 40% of clients with major depression have anger attacks. These sudden, intense spells of anger typically occur in situations where the depressed person feels emotionally trapped. Anger attacks involve verbal expressions of anger or rage but no physical aggression. Clients described these anger attacks as uncharacteristic behavior that was inappropriate for the situation and was followed by remorse. The anger attacks seen in some depressed clients may be related to irritable mood, overreaction to minor annoyances, and decreased coping abilities (Fava & Rosenbaum, 1999).

Intermittent explosive disorder is a rare psychiatric diagnosis characterized by discrete episodes of aggressive impulses that result in serious assaults or destruction of property. The aggressive behavior displayed is grossly out of proportion to any provocation or precipitating factor. This diagnosis is made only if there are no other comorbid psychiatric disorders, as discussed above. The person describes a period of tension or arousal that is relieved after the aggressive outburst. Afterward, the person is remorseful and embarrassed by the aggressive behavior, and there is no sign of aggressiveness between the episodes (Burt & Katzman, 2000). Intermittent explosive disorder is seen between late adolescence and the third decade of life (DSM-IV-TR, 2000). Burt and Katzman noted that clients with intermittent explosive disorder typically are large men with dependent personality features who respond to feelings of uselessness or ineffectiveness with violent outbursts.

Acting out is an immature defense mechanism in which the person deals with emotional conflicts or stressors by actions rather than by reflection or feelings. The person engages in acting-out behavior, such as verbal or physical aggression, to feel temporarily less helpless or powerless. Children and adolescents often "act out" when they cannot verbally handle intense feelings or deal with emotional conflict. To understand acting-out behaviors, it is important to consider the situation and the person's ability to deal with feelings and emotions.

ETIOLOGY

Neurobiologic Theories

The role of neurotransmitters in the study of aggression has been examined in animals and humans, but no single cause has been found. Findings reveal that serotonin plays a major inhibitory role in aggressive behavior; therefore, low serotonin levels may cause an increase in aggressive behavior. This may be related to the anger attacks seen in some depressed clients. In addition, increased activity of dopamine and norepinephrine in the brain is associated with an increase in impulsively violent behavior (Kavoussi et al., 1997). Further, structural damage to the limbic system and the frontal and temporal lobes of the brain may alter the person's ability to modulate aggression, leading to aggressive behavior.

Psychosocial Theories

Infants and toddlers express themselves loudly and intensely; this is normal for these stages of growth and development. Temper tantrums are a common response from a toddler whose wishes are not granted. As the child matures, he or she is expected to develop impulse control (the ability to delay gratification) and socially appropriate behavior. Failure to develop these qualities can result in a person who is impulsive, easily frustrated, and prone to aggressive behavior.

CULTURAL CONSIDERATIONS

The nurse must be aware of cultural norms to provide culturally competent care, and the expression of anger is strongly influenced by what is culturally acceptable. In the United States, women were traditionally not permitted to express anger openly and directly, because that would not be "feminine" and would challenge male authority. That cultural norm has slowly changed in the past 25 years. In some cultures, such as the Asian or Native American community, expressing anger may be seen as rude or disrespectful and is avoided at all costs. In these cultures, trying to help a client express anger verbally to an authority figure would be unacceptable.

Two culture-bound syndromes involve aggressive behavior. *Bouffée delirante,* a condition observed in West Africa and Haiti, is characterized by a sudden outburst of agitated and aggressive behavior, marked confusion, and psychomotor excitement. These episodes may include visual and auditory hallucinations and paranoid ideation, resembling brief psychotic episodes (Mezzich et al., 2000). *Amok* is a dissociative episode characterized by a period of brooding followed by an outburst of violent, aggressive, or homicidal behavior directed at other people and objects. This behavior is precipitated by a perceived slight or insult and is seen only in men. Originally reported from Malaysia, similar behavior patterns are seen in Laos, the Philippines, Papua New Guinea, Polynesia (*cafard*), Puerto Rico (*mal de pelea*), and among the Navajo (*iich'aa*) (Mezzich et al., 2000).

TREATMENT

The treatment of aggressive clients often is aimed at treating the underlying or comorbid psychiatric diagnosis, such as schizophrenia or bipolar disorder. Successful treatment of comorbid disorders results in successful treatment of aggressive behavior. Lithium has been effective in treating aggressive clients with bipolar disorder, conduct disorders (in children), and mental retardation. Carbamazepine (Tegretol) and valproate (Depakote) are used to treat aggression associated with dementia, psychosis, and personality disorders. Atypical antipsychotic agents such as clozapine (Clozaril), risperidone (Risperdal), and olanzapine (Zyprexa) have been effective in treating aggressive clients with dementia, brain injury, mental retardation, and personality disorders. Benzodiazepines can reduce irritability and agitation in elderly clients with dementia, but they can result in the loss of social inhibition for other aggressive clients, thereby increasing rather than reducing their aggression (Fava, 1997).

For aggressive psychotic clients, the cocktail or chaser approach may be used to produce rapid sedation. The cocktail method involves giving two medications, usually haloperidol (Haldol) and lorazepam (Ativan), in successive doses until the client is sedated. The first dose is given at the time of the aggressive behavior, a second dose is given 30 minutes to 1 hour after the behavior, and a third dose is given 1 to 2 hours after the behavior. The chaser approach involves giving only lorazepam at the specified time intervals, followed by an antipsychotic medication after the client is sedated with the lorazepam (Hughes, 1999) (Table 10-1). Both of these methods require careful assessment for the development of extrapyramidal side effects, which can be quickly treated with benztropine (Cogentin). Chapter 2 provides a full discussion of these medications and side effects.

Although not a treatment per se, the short-term use of seclusion or restraint may be required during the crisis phase of the aggression cycle to protect the client and others from injury. Many legal and ethical safeguards govern the use of seclusion and restraint.

Table 10-1

RAPID TRANQUILIZATION OF THE ACUTELY AGGRESSIVE PSYCHOTIC CLIENT

	At the Time of the Behavior	30 Minutes to 1 Hour After the Behavior	1 to 2 Hours After the Behavior
Cocktail	Lorazepam 1–2 mg PO or IM Haloperidol 5–10 mg PO or IM	Lorazepam 1–2 mg PO or IM; total dose of 2–4 mg Haloperidol 5–10 mg PO or IM; total dose of 10–20 mg	Lorazepam 1–2 mg PO or IM; total dose of 3–6 mg Haloperidol 5–10 mg PO or IM; total dose of 15–30 mg
Chaser*	Lorazepam 1–2 mg PO or IM	Lorazepam 1–2 mg PO or IM; total dose of 2–4 mg	Lorazepam 1–2 mg PO or IM; total dose of 3–6 mg

*Redosing is for clients who have not achieved sedation from the previous dose of medication. When the client becomes sedated, then antipsychotic medication is offered. (Hughes, D. H. [1999]. Acute psychopharmacological management of the aggressive psychotic patient. *Psychiatric Services, 50*[9], 1135–1137.) © 1999, American Psychiatric Association. Reprinted with permission.

LEGAL AND ETHICAL CONSIDERATIONS

Psychiatric clients have legal rights, just like clients in other settings. The legal and ethical issues discussed in this section are particularly pertinent to the topic of hostile and aggressive clients, but they apply to all clients in any mental health setting.

Involuntary Hospitalization

Most clients are admitted to an inpatient setting on a voluntary basis. This means they are willing to seek treatment and agree to be hospitalized. However, some clients do not wish to be hospitalized and treated. Their wishes are respected unless they are a danger to themselves or others (i.e., they are threatening or have attempted suicide or represent a danger to others). Clients who are hospitalized against their will under these conditions are committed to the hospital for psychiatric care until they are no longer a danger to themselves or anyone else. Each state has laws that govern the civil commitment process, but they are similar. A person can be detained in a psychiatric facility for 48 to 72 hours on an emergency basis until a hearing can be conducted to determine whether the client should be committed to a facility for treatment for a specified period of time. Many states have similar laws governing the commitment of clients with substance abuse problems who represent a danger to themselves or others when under the influence of the substance. Civil commitment or involuntary hospitalization curtails the client's right to freedom, or to leave the hospital when he or she wishes. All other client rights remain intact.

Release From the Hospital

Clients who are admitted voluntarily to the hospital have the right to leave, provided they do not represent a danger to themselves or others. Clients can sign a written request for discharge and be released from the hospital against medical advice if they are not dangerous. If a voluntary client who is dangerous to himself or herself or others signs a request for discharge, the psychiatrist may file for a civil commitment to detain the client against his or her will until a hearing can take place to decide the matter.

While in the hospital, the committed client may take medications and improve fairly rapidly, making him or her eligible for discharge when he or she no longer represents a danger. Some clients stop taking their medications after discharge and once again become threatening, aggressive, or dangerous. Mental health clinicians have increasingly been held legally liable for the criminal actions of such clients, raising the debate about extended civil commitment for dangerous clients. A study by Weinberger et al. (1998) showed that the court accepted fewer than 50% of mental health professionals' petitions for extended civil commitment of dangerous psychiatric clients. The court's concern is that psychiatric clients have civil rights and should not be unreasonably detained against their will in a hospital when they are no longer dangerous. Communities counter by claiming they deserve to be protected from dangerous persons who have a history of not taking their medications and thus may become a threat to the community.

Rights of Clients

Mental health clients retain all of the civil rights afforded to all persons, except the right to leave the hospital in the case of involuntary commitment. Clients have the right to refuse treatment, to send and receive sealed mail, and to have or refuse visitors (Box 10-1). Any restrictions (e.g., mail, visitors, clothing) must be made by a court or a physician's order for a verifiable, documented reason. Examples include:

Box 10-1

➤ A PATIENT'S BILL OF RIGHTS

1. The patient has the right to considerate and respectful care.
2. The patient has the right and is encouraged to obtain from physicians and other direct caregivers relevant, current, and understandable information concerning diagnosis, treatment, and prognosis.
3. The patient has the right to make decisions about the plan of care prior to and during the course of treatment and to refuse a recommended treatment or plan of care to the extent permitted by law and hospital policy and to be informed of medical consequences of this action. In case of such refusal, the patient is entitled to other appropriate care and services that the hospital provides, or transfer to another hospital. The hospital should notify patients of any policy that might affect patient choice within the institution.
4. The patient has the right to have an advance directive (such as a living will, health care proxy, or durable power of attorney for health care) concerning treatment, with the expectation that the hospital will honor the intent of that directive to the extent permitted by law and hospital policy.
5. The patient has the right to every consideration of privacy. Case discussion, consultation, examination, and treatment should be conducted so as to protect each patient's privacy.
6. The patient has the right to expect that all communications and records pertaining to his or her care will be treated as confidential by the hospital, except in cases such as suspected abuse and public health hazards, when reporting is permitted or required by law. The patient has the right to expect that the hospital will emphasize the confidentiality of this information when it releases it to any other parties entitled to review information in these records.
7. The patient has the right to review the records pertaining to his or her medical care and to have the information explained or interpreted as necessary, except when restricted by law.
8. The patient has the right to expect that, within its capacities and policies, a hospital will make a reasonable response to the request of a patient for appropriate and medically indicated care and services.
9. The patient has the right to ask and be informed of the existence of business relationships among the hospital, educational institutions, other health care providers, or payers that may influence the patient's treatment and care.
10. The patient has the right to consent or decline to participate in proposed research studies or human experimentation affecting care and treatment or requiring direct patient involvement, and to have those studies fully explained prior to consent. A patient who declines to participate in research or experimentation is entitled to the most effective care that the hospital can otherwise provide.
11. The patient has the right to expect reasonable continuity of care when appropriate and to be informed by physicians and other caregivers of available and realistic patient care options when hospital care is no longer appropriate.
12. The patient has the right to be informed of hospital policies and practices that relate to patient care, treatment, and responsibilities. The patient has the right to be informed of available resources for resolving disputes, grievances, and conflicts, such as ethics committees, patient representatives, or other mechanisms available in the institution. The patient has the right to be informed of the hospital's charges for services and available payment methods.

American Hospital Association. (1992). A patient's bill of rights. *Chicago: AHA. Reprinted with permission of the AHA, © 1992.*

• A suicidal client may not be permitted to keep a belt, shoelaces, or scissors, because these items may be used for self-harm.
• A client who becomes aggressive after having a particular visitor may have that person restricted from visiting for a period of time.
• A client making threatening phone calls to others outside the hospital may be permitted only supervised phone calls until his or her condition improves.

Conservatorship

The appointment of a conservator or legal guardian is a separate process from civil commitment. Persons who are gravely disabled; are found to be incompetent; cannot provide food, clothing, and shelter for themselves even when resources exist; and cannot act in their own best interests may require appointment of a conservator. In these cases, the court appoints a person to act as a legal guardian. This guardian assumes many responsibilities for the person, such as giving informed consent, writing checks, and entering into contracts. The client with a guardian loses the right to enter into legal contracts or agreements (e.g., marriage or mortgage) that require a signature: this affects many daily activities we take for granted. Because conservators or guardians speak for clients, the nurse must obtain consent or permission from the conservator of the client.

Least Restrictive Environment

Clients have the right to treatment in the **least restrictive environment** that is appropriate to meet their needs. This concept was central to the deinstitutionalization movement discussed in Chapters 1 and 6. This means that a client does not have to be hospitalized if he or she can be treated in an outpatient setting or a group home. It also means that the client must be free of restraint or seclusion unless it is necessary.

Restraint is the direct application of physical force to a person, without his or her permission, to restrict his or her freedom of movement. The physical force may be human, a mechanical device, or a combination. Human restraint is when staff members physically control the client and move him or her to a seclusion room. Mechanical restraints are devices, usually ankle and wrist restraints, that are fastened to the bed frame to curtail the client's physical aggression, such as hitting, kicking, and hair pulling.

Seclusion is the involuntary confinement of a person in a specially constructed, locked room, equipped with a security window or camera for direct visual monitoring of the client (JCAHO, 2000). The room often has a bed bolted to the floor and a mattress for safety. Any sharp or potentially dangerous objects such as pens, glasses, belts, and matches are removed from the client as a safety precaution. Seclusion provides decreased stimulation, protection of others from the client, prevention of property destruction, and privacy for the client. The goal of seclusion is to give the client the opportunity to regain physical and emotional self-control.

Short-term use of restraint or seclusion is permitted only when the client is imminently aggressive and dangerous to himself or herself or others. Box 10-2 lists the standards that govern the use of restraint and seclusion. The use of restraint and seclusion requires a physician's order every 24 hours, assessment by the nurse every 2 to 4 hours, and close supervision of the client. The nurse assesses the client for any injury that may have occurred and provides treatment as needed. Clients are checked at least every 10 to 15 minutes in person and may be continuously monitored on a video camera as well. The client's skin condition, circulation of the hands and feet, and emotional well-being are monitored and documented. The nurse must monitor the client closely for side effects of medications, which may be given in large doses in emergency situations. Offers of food, fluids, and opportunities to use the bathroom are made per facility policies and procedures and documented.

As soon as possible, the client is informed of what behavioral criteria will be used to determine whether the use of restraint or seclusion should be decreased or ended. Criteria may include the ability to verbalize feelings and concerns in a rational manner, absence of verbal threats, decreased muscle tension, and the client's stated ability to be in control. If a client remains in restraints for 1 to 2 hours, two staff members can free one limb at a time for movement and exercise. Frequent contact by the nurse allows ongoing assessment of the client's well-being and self-control, and reassurance that restraint is a restorative, not a punitive, procedure.

 CLINICAL VIGNETTE: SECLUSION

The goal of seclusion is to give the client the opportunity to regain self-control, both emotionally and physically. However, most clients who have been secluded have very different feelings and thoughts about seclusion. Clients reported feeling angry, agitated, bored, frustrated, helpless, and afraid while in seclusion. Seclusion was perceived as a punishment and gave the message that the client was "bad." Many clients were not clear about the reasons for seclusion or the criteria for exiting seclusion. Most believed they were secluded for too long. In general, clients thought that other interventions such as interaction with staff, a place to calm down, or scream when needed, or the presence of a family member could reduce or eliminate the need for seclusion. Clients who had not been secluded described seclusion in more positive terms, such as helpful, caring, fair, and good. Both secluded and nonsecluded clients agreed that clients would be "worse off" without the seclusion room.

Adapted from Martinez, R. J., Grimm, M., & Adamson, M. (1999). From the other side of the door. Journal of Psychosocial Nursing, 37(3), 13–22.

Box 10-2

> ### ➤ RESTRAINT AND SECLUSION STANDARDS FOR BEHAVIORAL HEALTH

- The leaders (medical director, director of patient services) establish and communicate the organization's philosophy on the use of restraint and seclusion to all staff who have direct care responsibility.
- Staffing levels and assignments are set to minimize circumstances that give rise to restraint or seclusion use and to maximize safety when restraint and seclusion are used.
- Staff are trained and competent to minimize the use of restraint and seclusion and in their safe use.
- The initial assessment of each client at the time of admission or intake is used to obtain information about the client that could help minimize the use of restraint or seclusion.
- Nonphysical techniques are the preferred intervention in the management of behavior.
- Restraint or seclusion use is limited to emergencies in which there is an imminent risk of a client physically harming himself or herself, staff, or others, and nonphysical interventions would not be effective.
- A licensed independent practitioner orders the use of restraint or seclusion.
- The client's family is notified promptly of the initiation of restraint or seclusion.
- A licensed independent practitioner sees and evaluates the client in person.
- Written or verbal orders for initial and continuing use of restraint and seclusion are time-limited.
- Clients who are in restraint or seclusion are regularly re-evaluated.
- Clinical leadership is informed of instances in which clients experience extended or multiple episodes of restraint or seclusion.
- Individuals in restraint or seclusion are assessed and assisted.
- Individuals in restraint or seclusion are monitored.
- Restraint and seclusion are discontinued when the individual meets the behavior criteria for their discontinuation.
- The individual and staff participate in a debriefing about the restraint or seclusion episode.
- Medical records document that the use of restraint or seclusion is consistent with organization policy.
- The organization collects data on the use of restraint and seclusion in order to monitor and improve its performance of processes that involve risks or may result in sentinel events.
- Organizational policies and procedures address the prevention of the use of restraint and seclusion, and, when employed, guide their use.

© Joint Commission on Accreditation of Healthcare Organizations. Restraint and seclusion standards for behavioral health. Oakbrook Terrace, IL: Joint Commission on Accreditation of Healthcare Organizations, 2000. Reprinted with permission.

The nurse should also offer support to the client's family. Families may be angry or embarrassed when the client is restrained or secluded. A careful and thorough explanation about the client's behavior and the subsequent use of restraint or seclusion is important. If the client is an adult, however, such a discussion requires a signed release of information. In the case of minor children, a signed consent is not required to inform parents or guardians about the use of restraint or seclusion. Providing the family with information may help avoid legal or ethical difficulties, and it keeps the family involved in the client's treatment.

Duty to Warn Third Parties

One exception to the client's right to confidentiality is the **duty to warn**, based on the California Supreme Court decision in *Tarasoff* vs. *Regents of the University of California* (Box 10-3). As a result of this decision, mental health clinicians have a duty to warn identifi-able third parties of threats made by a person, even if these threats were discussed during therapy sessions that are otherwise protected by privilege. Based on the Tarasoff decision, many states have enacted laws regarding warning a third party of threats or danger. The clinician should ask four questions to determine whether a duty to warn exists (Felthous, 1999):

- Is the client dangerous to others?
- Is the danger due to serious mental illness?
- Is the danger imminent?
- Is the danger targeted at identifiable victims?

For example, if a man were admitted to a psychiatric facility stating he was going to kill his wife, there is a clear duty for his wife to be warned. However, if a paranoid person is admitted saying, "I'm going to get them before they get me" but provides no other information, there is no specific third party to warn. Decisions about the duty to warn third parties are usually made by the psychiatrist or, in outpatient settings, the qualified mental health therapist.

> **Box 10-3**

> ## ➤ TARASOFF VS. REGENTS OF THE UNIVERSITY OF CALIFORNIA (1976)

In 1969, a graduate student at the University of California, Prosenjit Poddar, dated a young woman named Tatiana Tarasoff for a short time. After the brief relationship ended, Poddar sought counseling with a psychologist at the university. He confided to the therapist that he intended to kill his former girlfriend when she returned from Brazil at the end of the summer. The psychologist contacted the university campus police, who detained and questioned Poddar. He was released because he appeared rational, promised to stay away from Tarasoff, and claimed he would not harm her. Two months later, shortly after her return from Brazil, Tatiana Tarasoff was murdered by Poddar on Oct. 27, 1969. Her parents sued the University of California, claiming that the therapist had a duty to warn their daughter of Poddar's threats. The California Supreme Court concluded that the protective privilege ends where the public peril begins.

Mason, T. (1998). Tarasoff *liability. International Journal of Nursing Studies, 35(1/2), 109–114.*

APPLICATION OF THE NURSING PROCESS

Assessment

Assessment and effective intervention with angry or hostile clients can often prevent aggressive episodes. Early assessment, judicious use of medications, and verbal interaction with an angry client can often prevent anger from escalating into physical aggression.

The nurse should be aware of factors that influence aggression in the psychiatric environment (unit milieu). Shepherd and Lavender (1999) found that aggressive behavior was less common on psychiatric units where there was strong psychiatric leadership, staff roles were clear, and events such as staff–client interaction, group interaction, and activities were planned and adequate in number. Conversely, when there was a lack of predictability of meetings or groups and staff–client interactions, clients often felt frustrated and bored, and aggression was more common and intense.

In addition to assessing the unit milieu, the nurse needs to assess individual clients carefully. A history of violent or aggressive behavior is one of the best predictors of future aggression. It is helpful to determine how the client with a history of aggression handles anger and what the client thinks can help him or her control or manage angry feelings in a nonaggressive manner. Clients who are angry and frustrated and believe that no one is listening to them are more prone to behave in a hostile or aggressive manner.

The nurse should assess the client's behavior to determine which phase of the aggression cycle he or she is in so that appropriate interventions can be implemented. The five phases of aggression and their signs, symptoms, and behaviors are presented in Table 10-2. Assessment of clients must take place at a safe distance. The nurse can approach the client while maintaining an adequate distance so the client does not feel trapped or threatened. To ensure staff safety and exhibit teamwork, it may be prudent for two staff members to approach the client.

Data Analysis

Nursing diagnoses commonly used when working with aggressive clients include:
- Risk for Violence: Self-Directed or Directed at Others
- Ineffective Individual Coping

If the client is intoxicated, depressed, or psychotic, additional nursing diagnoses may be indicated.

Outcome Identification

Expected outcomes for aggressive clients may include:
1. The client will not harm or threaten others.
2. The client will refrain from behaviors that are intimidating or frightening to others.
3. The client will describe his or her feelings and concerns without aggression.
4. The client will be compliant with treatment.

Intervention

Hostility or verbally aggressive behavior can be intimidating or frightening, even for the experienced nurse. Clients exhibiting these behaviors are also threatening to other clients, staff, and visitors. In social settings, the most frequent response to hostile people is to get as far away from them as possible. However, in the psychiatric setting, it is most helpful to engage the hostile person in dialogue to prevent the behavior from escalating to physical aggression.

Interventions are most effective and least restrictive when implemented early in the cycle of aggression. This section presents interventions for the man-

Table 10-2

FIVE-PHASE AGGRESSION CYCLE

Phase	Definition	Signs, Symptoms, and Behaviors
Triggering	An event occurs or circumstances in the environment initiate the client's response, which is often anger or hostility.	Restlessness, anxiety, irritability, pacing, muscle tension, rapid breathing, perspiration, loud voice, anger
Escalation	Client's responses represent escalating behaviors that indicate movement toward a loss of control.	Pale or flushed face, yelling, swearing, agitated, threatening, demanding, clenched fists, threatening gestures, hostility, loss of ability to solve the problem or think clearly
Crisis	A period of emotional and physical crisis in which the client loses control	Loss of emotional and physical control, throwing objects, kicking, hitting, spitting, biting, scratching, shrieking, screaming, inability to communicate clearly
Recovery	Client regains physical and emotional control.	Lowering of voice, decreased muscle tension, clearer, more rational communication, physical relaxation
Postcrisis	Client attempts reconciliation with others and returns to the level of functioning before the aggressive incident and its antecedents.	Remorse, apologies, crying, quiet withdrawn behavior

Adapted from Keltner, N. L., Schwecke, L. H., & Bostrom, C. E. (1999). *Psychiatric nursing* (3d ed.). St. Louis: Mosby, Inc.

agement of the milieu, which benefit all clients, and specific interventions for each phase of the aggression cycle.

MANAGING THE ENVIRONMENT (MILIEU THERAPY)

It is important to consider the environment for all clients when trying to reduce or eliminate aggressive behavior. Planned activities or groups such as card games, watching and discussing a movie, or informal discussions give clients the opportunity to talk about events or issues when they are calm. Activities also engage clients in the therapeutic process and minimize boredom. Scheduling one-to-one interactions with clients indicates the nurse's genuine interest in the client and a willingness to listen to the client's concerns, thoughts, and feelings. Knowing what to expect enhances the client's feelings of security.

If clients have a conflict or dispute with one another, the nurse can offer the opportunity for problem solving or conflict resolution. Expressing angry feelings appropriately, using assertive communication statements, and negotiating a solution are important skills clients can practice. These skills will be useful for the client when he or she returns to the community.

If a client is psychotic, hyperactive, or intoxicated, the nurse must consider the safety and security of other clients, who may need protection from the intrusive or threatening demeanor of that client. Talking with other clients about their feelings is helpful,

and close supervision of the client who is potentially aggressive is essential.

MANAGING THE CLIENT

In the *triggering phase,* the nurse should approach the client in a nonthreatening, calm manner. Conveying empathy for the client's anger or frustration is important. The nurse can encourage the client to express his or her angry feelings verbally, suggesting that the client is still in control and can maintain that control. Use of clear, simple, short statements is helpful. The nurse should allow the client time to express himself or herself. The nurse can suggest that the client go to a quiet area, or may get assistance to move other clients to decrease stimulation. Medications (PRN) should be offered, if ordered. As the client's anger subsides, the nurse can help the client to use relaxation techniques and look at ways to solve any problem or conflict that may exist (Maier, 1996). Physical activity, such as walking, also may help the client relax and become calmer.

If these techniques are unsuccessful and the client progresses to the *escalation phase*, the nurse must take control of the situation. The nurse should provide directions to the client in a calm, firm voice. The client should be directed to take a time out for cooling off in a quiet area or his or her room. The nurse should tell the client that aggressive behavior is not acceptable, and the nurse is there to help the client regain control. If the client refused medications during the triggering phase, the nurse should offer them again.

If the client's behavior continues to escalate and he or she is unwilling to accept direction to a quiet area, the nurse should obtain assistance from other staff members. Initially, four to six staff members should remain ready, in sight of the client, but not as close as the primary nurse talking with the client. This technique is sometimes called a "show of force," indicating to the client that the staff will control the situation if the client cannot do so. Sometimes the presence of additional staff convinces the client to accept medication and take the time out necessary to regain control.

When the client becomes physically aggressive (*crisis phase*), the staff must take charge of the situation for the safety of the client, staff, and other clients. Psychiatric facilities offer training and practice in safe techniques for managing behavioral emergencies, and only staff with such training should participate in the restraint of a physically aggressive client. The nurse's decision to use seclusion or restraint should be based on the facility's protocols and standards for restraint and seclusion. The nurse should obtain a physician's order as soon as possible after deciding to use restraint or seclusion.

Four to six trained staff members are needed to restrain an aggressive client safely. Children, adolescents, and female clients can be just as aggressive as adult male clients. The client is informed that his or her behavior is out of control, and that the staff are taking control to provide safety and prevent injury. Four staff members each take a limb, another protects the client's head, and another helps control the client's torso, if needed. The client is transported by gurney or carried to a seclusion room, and restraints are applied to each limb and fastened to the bed frame. If PRN medication has not been taken earlier, the nurse may obtain an order for intramuscular medication in this type of emergency situation. As noted above, the nurse performs close assessment of the client in seclusion or restraint and documents the actions.

As the client regains control (*recovery phase*), he or she is encouraged to talk about the situation or triggers that led to the aggressive behavior. The nurse should help the client relax, perhaps sleep, and return to a calmer state. It is important to help the client explore alternatives to aggressive behavior by asking what the client or staff can do next time to avoid an aggressive episode. The nurse also should assess staff members for any injuries and complete the required documentation, such as incident reports and flow sheets. The staff usually has a debriefing session, discussing the aggressive episode, how it was handled, what worked well or needed improvement, and how the situation could have been defused more effectively. It also is important to encourage other clients to talk about their feelings regarding the incident. However, the aggressive client should not be discussed in detail with other clients.

In the *postcrisis phase*, the client is removed from restraint or seclusion as soon as he or she meets the behavioral criteria. The nurse should not lecture or chastise the client for the aggressive behavior but should discuss the behavior in a calm, rational manner. The client can be given feedback for regaining control, with the expectation that he or she will be able to handle feelings or events in a nonaggressive manner in the future. The client should be reintegrated into the milieu and its activities as soon as he or she can participate.

Evaluation

Care is most effective when the client's anger can be defused in an earlier stage (Morales & Duphorne, 1995), but restraint or seclusion is sometimes needed to handle physically aggressive behavior. The goal is to teach angry, hostile, and potentially aggressive

---

 CLINICAL VIGNETTE: ESCALATION PHASE

John, 35, was admitted to the hospital for schizophrenia. John has a history of aggressive behavior, usually precipitated by voices telling him he will be harmed by staff and must kill them to protect himself. John had not been taking his prescribed medication for 2 weeks before hospitalization. The nurse observes John pacing in the hall, muttering to himself, and avoiding close contact with anyone else.

Suddenly, John begins to yell, "I can't take it. I can't stay here!" His fists are clenched, and he is very agitated.

The nurse approaches John, remaining 6 feet away from him, and says, "John, tell me what is happening." John runs to the end of the hall and will not talk to the nurse. The nurse asks John to take a PRN medication and go to his room. He refuses both. As he begins to pick up objects from a nearby table, the nurse summons other staff to assist.

clients to express their feelings verbally and safely without threats or harm to others or destruction of property.

COMMUNITY-BASED CARE

For many clients with aggressive behavior, effective management of the comorbid psychiatric disorder is the key to controlling aggression. Regular follow-up appointments, compliance with prescribed medication, and participation in community support programs help the client achieve stability. Anger management groups are available to help clients express their feelings and to learn problem-solving and conflict-resolution techniques.

(*text continues on page 227*)

NURSING CARE PLAN

Nursing Diagnosis

➤ **Risk for Violence: Self-Directed or Directed at Others** (9.2.2)
A state in which an individual experiences behaviors that can be physically harmful either to the self or to others

RISK FACTORS

- Actual or potential physical acting out of violence
- Destruction of property
- Homicidal or suicidal ideation
- Physical danger to self or others
- History of assaultive behavior or arrests
- Disordered thoughts
- Agitation or restlessness
- Lack of impulse control
- Delusions, hallucinations, or other psychotic symptoms
- Substance use

EXPECTED OUTCOMES

The client will:
- Not harm others or destroy property
- Decrease acting-out behavior
- Experience decreased restlessness or agitation
- Experience decreased fear, anxiety, or hostility
- Demonstrate the ability to exercise internal control over his or her behavior
- Identify ways to deal with tension and aggressive feelings in a nondestructive manner
- Express feelings of anxiety, fear, anger, or hostility verbally or in a nondestructive manner

IMPLEMENTATION

Nursing Interventions	Rationale
Build a trust relationship with this client as soon as possible, ideally well in advance of aggressive episodes.	Familiarity with and trust in the staff members can decrease the client's fears and facilitate communication.
Be aware of factors that increase the likelihood of violent behavior or that signify a build-up of	A period of building tension often precedes acting out or violent behavior; however, a client who is

continued on page 225

continued from page 224

agitation. Use verbal communication or PRN medication to intervene before the client's behavior reaches a destructive or violent point and physical restraint becomes necessary.

intoxicated or psychotic may become violent without warning. Signs of increasing agitation include increased restlessness; verbal cues ("I'm afraid of losing control"); threats; increased motor activity (pacing, tremors); increased voice volume; decreased frustration tolerance; frowning; clenching fists.

Decrease environmental stimulation by turning stereo or television off or lowering the volume; lowering the lights; asking other clients, visitors, or others to leave the area (or you can go with the client to another room).

If the client is feeling threatened, he or she can perceive any stimulus as a threat. The client cannot deal with excess stimuli when agitated.

If the client tells you (verbally or nonverbally) that he or she is beginning to feel hostile, aggressive, or destructive, try to help the client express these feelings, verbally or physically, in nondestructive ways (remain with the client and listen; use communication techniques; or take the client to the gym or outside with adequate supervision for physical exercise).

The client may need to learn nondestructive ways to express feelings. The client can try out new behaviors with you in a nonthreatening environment and learn to focus on expressing emotions rather than acting out.

Calmly and respectfully assure the client that you (the staff) will provide control if he or she cannot control himself or herself, but do not threaten the client.

The client may fear loss of control and will be reassured that control will be provided. The client may be afraid of what he or she may do if he or she begins to express anger. Show that you are in control without competing with the client and without lowering his or her self-esteem.

Always maintain control of yourself and the situation; remain calm. If you do not feel competent in dealing with a situation, obtain assistance as soon as possible.

Your behavior provides a role model for the client and communicates that you can and will provide control.

Do not use physical restraints or techniques without sufficient reason.

The client has a right to the fewest restrictions possible within the limits of safety and prevention of destructive behavior.

Remain aware of the client's body space or territory; do not trap the client.

Potentially violent people have a body space zone much larger than that of other people (up to four times as large). Allow them more space and stay farther away from them for them to not feel trapped or threatened.

continued on page 226

continued from page 225

Allow the client freedom to move around (within safety limits) unless you are trying to restrain him or her.

Interfering with the client's mobility without the intent of restraint may increase the client's frustration, fears, or perception of threat.

Talk with the client in a low, calm voice. You may need to reorient the client: call the client by name, tell the client your name and where you are, and so forth.

Using a low voice may help calm the client or prevent increasing agitation. The client may be disoriented or unaware of what is happening.

Tell the client what you are going to do and what you are doing. Use simple, clear, direct speech; repeat if necessary. Do not threaten the client, but state limits and expectations.

The client's ability to understand the situation and to process information is impaired. Clear limits let the client know what is expected of him or her.

When a decision has been made to subdue or restrain the client, act quickly and cooperatively with other staff members. Tell the client in a matter-of-fact manner that he or she will be restrained, subdued, or secluded; allow no bargaining after the decision has been made. Reassure the client that he or she will not be hurt and that restraint or seclusion is to ensure safety.

Firm limits must be set and maintained. Bargaining interjects doubt and will undermine the limit.

While subduing or restraining the client, talk with other staff members to ensure coordination of effort (e.g., don't attempt to carry the client until you are sure that everyone is ready).

Direct communication will promote cooperation and safety.

Do not strike the client.

Physical safety of the client is a priority.

Do not help to restrain or subdue the client if you are angry (if enough other staff members are present). Do not restrain or subdue the client as a punishment.

Staff members must maintain self-control at all times and act in the client's best interest. There is no justification for being punitive to a client.

If possible, do not allow other clients to watch the situation of staff subduing or restraining the client. Take them to a different area, and involve them in activities or discussion.

Other clients may be frightened, agitated, or endangered by an aggressive client. They need safety and reassurance at this time.

When placing the client in restraints or seclusion, tell the client what you are doing, the reason for this (to regain control or to protect the client from injuring himself, herself, or others). Use simple, concise language in a nonjudgmental, matter-of-fact manner.

The client's ability to understand what is happening to him or her may be impaired.

continued on page 227

continued from page 226

Tell the client where he or she is and that he or she will be safe. Assure the client that staff members will check on him or her, and if possible tell the client how to summon the staff.	Being placed in seclusion or restraints can be terrifying to a client. Your assurances may help alleviate the client's fears.
Reassess the client's need for continued seclusion or restraint as you observe him or her. Reorient the client or remind him or her of the reason for restraint if necessary. Release the client or decrease restraint as soon as it is safe and therapeutic to do so. Base your decisions and actions on the client's, not the staff's, needs.	The client has a right to the restrictions possible within the limits of safety and prevention of destructive behavior.
Remain aware of the client's feelings (including fear), dignity, and rights.	The client is a worthwhile person regardless of his or her unacceptable behavior.
Carefully observe the client, and promptly complete charting and reports in keeping with hospital or unit policy. Bear in mind possible legal implications.	Accurate recording of information is essential in situations that may later be reviewed in court. Restraint, seclusion, assault, and so forth are situations that may involve legal action.

Adapted from Schultz, J. M. & Videbeck, S. L. (1998). Lippincott's manual of psychiatric nursing care plans *(5th ed.) Philadelphia: Lippincott-Raven.*

SELF-AWARENESS ISSUES

The nurse must be aware of how he or she deals with anger before he or she can help clients to do so. The nurse who is afraid of angry feelings may avoid a client's anger, allowing the client's behavior to escalate. If the nurse makes an angry response, this will escalate the situation because it sets up a power struggle, and the opportunity to "talk down" the client's anger will be lost.

It is important to practice and gain experience in using techniques for restraint and seclusion before

INTERNET RESOURCES

Resource	Internet Address
▶ **Mental Health Patient's Bill of Rights**	http://www.apa.org/pubinfo/rights
▶ **APA: Warning Signs**	http://helping.apa.org/warningsigns/
▶ **LifeSkills Resource Center**	http://www.rpeurifoy.com
▶ **Anger Alternatives**	http://angeralternatives.anthill.com
▶ **Anger Management Institute**	http://www.manageanger.com

attempting the techniques with clients in crisis. There is a risk of staff injury whenever a client is aggressive. Ongoing education and practice of safe techniques are essential to minimize or avoid injury to both staff and clients. The nurse must be calm, nonjudgmental, and nonpunitive when using techniques to control a client's aggressive behavior. Inexperienced nurses can learn from watching experienced nurses deal with clients who are hostile or aggressive.

When verbal techniques fail to defuse a client's anger and the client becomes aggressive, the nurse may feel frustrated or angry, as if he or she failed. However, the client's aggressive behavior does not necessarily reflect the nurse's skills and abilities. Some clients have a limited capacity to control their aggressive behaviors, and the nurse can help them learn alternative ways to handle angry or aggressive impulses.

Helpful Hints for Working With Clients Who are Angry, Hostile, or Aggressive

- Identify how you handle angry feelings; assess your use of assertive communication and your conflict-resolution skills. Increasing your skills in dealing with your angry feelings will help you work more effectively with clients.
- Discuss situations or the care of potentially aggressive clients with experienced nurses.
- Do not take the client's anger or aggressive behavior personally, or as a measure of your effectiveness as a nurse.

Critical Thinking

Questions

1. Some psychiatric clients make headlines when they commit crimes against others that involve serious injury or death. With treatment and medication, these clients are rational and represent no threat to others, but they have a history of stopping their medications when released from treatment facilities. Where and how should these clients be treated? What measures can protect their individual rights as well as the public right to safety?
2. If an aggressive client injures another client or a staff person, should criminal charges be filed against the client? Why or why not?

➤ KEY POINTS

- Anger, expressed appropriately, can be a positive force that helps the person solve problems and make decisions.
- Hostile behavior, also called verbal aggression, is intended to intimidate or cause emotional harm to another and can lead to physical aggression. Physical aggression is behavior meant to harm or punish another person, or to force someone into compliance.
- Most psychiatric clients are not aggressive. Clients with schizophrenia, bipolar disorder, dementia, head injury, antisocial or borderline personality disorders, or conduct disorder, or those intoxicated with alcohol or other drugs may be aggressive. Rarely, clients may be diagnosed with intermittent explosive disorder.
- Treatment of aggressive clients often involves treating the comorbid psychiatric disorder with mood stabilizers or antipsychotic medications.
- The Patient's Bill of Rights includes the right to receive and refuse treatment, to be involved in the plan of care, to refuse to participate in research, and to have unrestricted visitors, mail, and phone calls.
- The use of seclusion and restraint falls under the domain of the patient's right to the least restrictive environment. Short-term use is permitted only if the client is imminently aggressive and dangerous to himself or herself and others. The use of restraint and seclusion requires a physician's order every 24 hours, assessment by the nurse every 2 to 4 hours, and documentation of the patient's condition and provision for basic needs. Restraint and seclusion are ended as soon as the client has met the established behavioral criteria.
- Assessment and effective intervention with angry or hostile clients can often prevent aggressive episodes.
- Aggressive behavior is less common and less intense on units where there is strong psychiatric leadership, staff roles are clear, and events such as staff–client interaction, group interaction, and activities are planned and adequate in number.
- The nurse must be familiar with the signs, symptoms, and behaviors associated with the triggering, escalation, crisis, recovery, and postcrisis phases of the aggression cycle.
- In the triggering phase, nursing interventions include speaking in a calm, nonthreatening manner; conveying empathy;

listening; offering PRN medication; and suggesting retreat to a quiet area.

- In the escalation phase, interventions include using a directive approach; taking control of the situation; using a calm, firm voice for giving directions; directing the client to take a time out in a quiet place; offering PRN medication; and making a "show of force" from the presence of other staff.
- In the crisis phase, the client's aggression is dealt with quickly by experienced, trained staff, using the techniques of seclusion or restraint.
- During the recovery phase, clients are helped to relax, regain self-control, and talk about the aggressive event in a rational manner.
- In the postcrisis phase, the client is reintegrated into the milieu.
- Important self-awareness issues include examining how one handles angry feelings and deals with one's own reactions to angry clients.

REFERENCES

American Hospital Association. (1992). *A patient's bill of rights.* Chicago: AHA.

American Psychiatric Association. (2000). *Diagnostic and statistical manual of mental disorders-Text Revision.* (4th ed.). Washington, D.C.: American Psychiatric Association.

Burt, V. K., & Katzman, J. W. (2000). Impulse-control disorders not elsewhere classified. In B. J. Sadock & V. A. Sadock (Eds.). *Comprehensive textbook of psychiatry,* Vol. 2, (7th ed., pp. 1701–1713). Philadelphia: Lippincott Williams & Wilkins.

Bushman, B. J., & Stack, A. D. (1999). Catharsis, aggression, and persuasive influence: self-fulfilling or self-defeating prophecies? *Journal of Personality & Social Psychology, 76*(3), 367–376.

Fava, M. (1997). Psychopharmacologic treatment of pathological aggression. *Psychiatric Clinics of North America, 20*(2), 427–451.

Fava, M., & Rosenbaum, J. F. (1999). Anger attacks in patients with depression. *Journal of Clinical Psychiatry, 60*(15), 21–24.

Felthous, A. R. (1999). The clinician's duty to protect third parties. *Psychiatric Clinics of North America, 22*(1), 49–61.

Hughes, D. H. (1999). Acute psychopharmacological management of the aggressive psychotic patient. *Psychiatric Services, 50*(9), 1135–1137.

Joint Commission on Accreditation of Healthcare Organizations. (2000). *Restraint and seclusion standards for behavioral health,* May 3, 2000. Document available: http://www.jcaho.org/standard/restraint/restraint_stds.html

Kavoussi, R., Armstead, P., & Coccaro, E. (1997). The neurobiology of impulse aggression. *Psychiatric Clinics of North America, 20*(2), 395–403.

Keltner, N. L., Schwecke, L. H., & Bostrom, C. E. (1999). *Psychiatric nursing* (3rd ed.). St. Louis: Mosby, Inc.

Maier, G. J. (1996). Managing threatening behavior: the role of talk up and talk down. *Journal of Psychosocial Nursing & Mental Health Services, 34*(6), 25.

Martinez, R. J., Grimm, M., & Adamson, M. (1999). From the other side of the door: patient views of seclusion. *Journal of Psychosocial Nursing, 37*(3), 13–22.

Mason, T. (1998). *Tarasoff* liability: its impact for working with patients who threaten others. *International Journal of Nursing Studies, 35*(1/2), 109–114.

Mezzich, J. E., Lin, K., & Hughes, C. C. (2000). Acute and transient psychotic disorders and culture-bound syndromes. In B. J. Sadock & V. A. Sadock (Eds.), *Comprehensive textbook of psychiatry,* Vol. 1, (7th ed., pp. 1264–1276). Philadelphia: Lippincott Williams & Wilkins.

Morales, E., & Duphorne, P. L. (1995). Least restrictive measures: alternatives to four-point restraints and seclusion. *Journal of Psychosocial Nursing, 33*(10), 13–16.

Phillips, P. (1998). Study says stay calm and halve the risk of stroke. *Journal of the American Medical Association, 279*(16), 1246–1247.

Schultz, J. M. & Videbeck, S. D. (1998). *Lippincott's manual of psychiatric nursing care plans* (5th ed.). Philadelphia: Lippincott-Raven.

Shepherd, M., & Lavender, T. (1999). Putting aggression into context: an investigation into contextual factors influencing the rate of aggressive incidents in a psychiatric hospital. *Journal of Mental Health, 8*(2), 159–170.

Thomas, S. P. (1998). Assessing and intervening with anger disorders. *Nursing Clinics of North America, 33*(1), 121–133.

Weinberger, L. E., Sreenivasan, S., & Markowitz, E. (1998). Extended civil commitment for dangerous psychiatric patients. *Journal of the American Academy of Psychiatric Law, 26*(1), 75–87.

ADDITIONAL READINGS

Bowers, L. (1999). A critical appraisal of violent incident measures. *Journal of Mental Health, 8*(4), 339–349.

Echternacht, M. R. (1999). Potential for violence toward psychiatric nursing students: risk reduction techniques. *Journal of Psychosocial Nursing, 37*(3), 36–39.

Woods, P., Reed, V., & Robinson, D. (1999). The behavioural status index: therapeutic assessment of risk, insight, communication and social skills. *Journal of Psychiatric and Mental Health Nursing, 6*(2), 79–90.

Wright, S. (1999). Physical restraint in the management of violence and aggression in in-patient settings: a review of issues. *Journal of Mental Health, 8*(5), 459–472.

Chapter Review

➤ **MULTIPLE-CHOICE QUESTIONS**

Select the best answer for each of the following questions.

1. Which of the following is an example of assertive communication?

    A. "I wish you would stop making me angry."

    B. "I feel angry when you walk away when I'm talking."

    C. "You never listen to me when I'm talking."

    D. "You make me angry when you interrupt me."

2. Which of the following statements about anger is true?

    A. Expressing anger openly and directly usually leads to arguments.

    B. Anger is the result of being frustrated, hurt, or afraid.

    C. Suppressing anger is a sign of maturity.

    D. Angry feelings are a negative response to one's situation.

3. Which of the following types of drugs should be used cautiously with potentially aggressive clients?

    A. Antipsychotic medications

    B. Benzodiazepines

    C. Mood stabilizers

    D. Lithium.

4. Which of the following would indicate a duty to warn a third party?

    A. A delusional client states, "I'm going to get them before they get me."

    B. A hostile client says, "I hate all police."

    C. A client says he plans to blow up the federal government.

    D. A client states, "If I can't have my girlfriend back, then no one can have her."

5. A client is pacing in the hallway with clenched fists and a flushed face. He is yelling and swearing. Which phase of the aggression cycle is he in?

    A. Anger

    B. Triggering

    C. Escalation

    D. Crisis.

➤ **TRUE-FALSE QUESTIONS**

Identify each of the following statements as T (True) or F (False). Correct any false statements.

_____ 1. Once a client is involuntarily committed, he or she must remain in the hospital until symptom-free.

_____ 2. Hostile behavior is intended to intimidate others.

_____ 3. Verbally aggressive clients often calm down on their own if staff don't bother them.

_____ 4. Holding a client's arms to prevent him from hitting someone is a form of restraint.

_____ 5. Clients who have a history of aggressive behavior should be secluded to protect others.

_____

_____ 6. A client who is involuntarily committed loses the right to freedom of movement.

_____

_____ 7. Under no circumstances can a client's rights be restricted.

_____

_____ 8. During the postcrisis phase of the aggression cycle, clients may express remorse for their behavior.

_____

➤ FILL-IN-THE-BLANK QUESTIONS

Indicate which phase of the aggression cycle would be appropriate for each of the following interventions.

_____ Talking about the incident

_____ Reintegrating the client into the milieu

_____ Encouraging a description of feelings or events

_____ Directing the client to go to a quiet place for time out

_____ Using physical restraint techniques.

➤ SHORT-ANSWER QUESTIONS

1. Describe the medication administration techniques of cocktail and chaser.

2. Discuss the concept of the least restrictive environment

Abuse and Violence

Violent and abusive behavior has been identified as a national health concern and a priority for intervention in the United States (Tyra, 1996), where the incidence of violence exceeds 2 million occurrences per year (Denham, 1995). Violent behavior permeates our society. The most alarming statistics relate to violence in the home: **abuse**, or the wrongful use and maltreatment of another person. Victims of abuse occur across the life span. They can be a spouse or partner, a child, or an elderly parent. Statistics show that abuse occurs most frequently at the hands of someone known to the victim.

The Centers for Disease Control and Prevention (CDC, 1999), the U.S. Department of Education, the Department of Justice, and the National School Safety Center have been examining homicides and suicides associated with schools. The study examined events occurring on the way to and from school, on school property, and at school-sponsored events and found that 83% of the victims of school homicide or suicide were male and 65% of school-associated violent deaths were students, 11% were teachers or staff, and 23% were community members killed on school property.

The original study was expanded to cover school-associated violent deaths from July 1994 to June 1998. The study results showed 173 incidents, most of which were homicides committed with firearms. The total number of events decreased since the 1992–93 school year, but the number of multiple-victim events during that period increased. This means that fewer events involving one individual have occurred, but multiple-victim events increased from one per year in 1992–95 to five per year from August 1995 through July 1998. One only has to watch the evening news to know that this is the trend.

The CDC has been working with schools to develop curricula that emphasize problem-solving skills, anger management, and social skills development. In addition, parenting programs that promote strong bonding between parents and children and conflict management in the home, as well as mentoring programs for young people, show promise in dealing with school-related violence. A few of the people responsible for such violence have actually been diagnosed with a psychiatric disorder, often conduct disorder, which is discussed in Chapter 18. Often, however, this violence seems to occur when alienation, disregard for others, and little regard for self predominate.

In this chapter we will discuss domestic abuse (child abuse/neglect, spouse abuse, elder abuse) and rape. Because many of the survivors of abuse suffer long-term emotional trauma, we will also discuss two disorders associated with abuse and violence, posttraumatic stress disorder and dissociative disorders. Other long-term problems associated with abuse and trauma include substance abuse (see Chap. 17) and depression (see Chap. 14).

CLINICAL PICTURE OF ABUSE AND VIOLENCE

Victims of trauma or abuse certainly can have physical injuries that need medical attention, but they also experience psychological injuries that can include a broad range of responses. Some may be agitated and visibly upset; others are withdrawn and aloof, appearing numb or oblivious to their surroundings. Many times, domestic violence goes undisclosed for months or even years because victims fear their abusers. Victims often suppress their anger and resentment for years and cannot tell anyone. This is particularly true in situations involving childhood sexual abuse.

These survivors of abuse often suffer in silence and continue to feel guilt and shame. Children in particular come to believe that somehow they are at fault and did something to deserve or provoke the abuse. Adults often feel guilt or shame for not trying to stop the abuse. Abuse survivors feel degraded, humiliated, and dehumanized. Their self-esteem is extremely low, and they view themselves as unlovable. They believe they are unacceptable to others and contaminated or ruined (Humphreys, 1997).

Victims of abuse have problems relating to other people in relationships. They have difficulty trusting others, especially authority figures. When relating to other people, their emotional reactions are likely to be erratic, intense, and perceived as unpredictable. Engaging in intimate relationships may trigger extreme emotional responses, such as panic anxiety, fear, or terror. Even when these victims of abuse desire the closeness of another person, once someone gets close to them, they may feel it is intrusive and threatening. The nurse should be sensitive to the client's need to feel safe, secure, and in control of his or her body. The nurse should take care to maintain the client's personal space and should assess the client's level of anxiety and ask permission before touching him or her for any reason.

CHARACTERISTICS OF VIOLENT FAMILIES

Family violence encompasses the physical, emotional, and sexual abuse of children, child neglect, spouse battering, marital rape, and elder abuse. Abusive and violent behavior that would not be acceptable from strangers is often tolerated for years within a family. In violent families, the family, which is normally a safe haven where members feel loved and protected, may be the most dangerous place for the victim. Research studies have identified some common characteristics of the violent family, regardless of the type of abuse that exists (Box 11-1).

Box 11-1

► CHARACTERISTICS OF VIOLENT FAMILIES

Social isolation
Abuse of power and control
Alcohol and other drug abuse
Intergenerational transmission process

Social Isolation

One characteristic of violent families is social isolation. Members of these families keep to themselves and often do not invite others into the home or tell others what is going on. Often, abused children and women are threatened by the abuser with even greater harm if they reveal the secret. Children may be threatened that their mother, sibling, or pet will be killed if anyone outside the family learns of the abuse. They are frightened into keeping the secret or preventing others from interfering with "private family business."

Power and Control

The abusive family member is almost always in a position of power and control over the victim, whether the victim is a child, spouse, or elderly parent. The abuser not only exerts physical power over the victim, but also economic and social control. The abuser is often the only member of the family who makes decisions, spends money, or is permitted to spend time outside the home with other people. The abuser uses emotional abuse by belittling and blaming the victim and often threatening him or her. Any indication of independence or disobedience by family members, either real or imagined, usually results in an escalation of violence (Singer et al., 1995).

Alcohol and Other Drug Abuse

There is an association between substance abuse, especially alcohol, and family violence. This does not imply a cause-and-effect relationship—alcohol does not cause the person to be abusive; rather, a person who is abusive is also likely to use alcohol or other drugs. Fifty to ninety percent of men who batter their domestic partners have a history of substance abuse as well. Up to 50% of women who have been abused seek refuge in alcohol as well (Commission on Domestic Violence, 1999). However, many researchers believe that alcohol may diminish inhibitions and make violent behavior more intense or frequent (Denham, 1995).

Alcohol is also cited as a factor in acquaintance or date rape. The CDC's Division of Violence Prevention reports that studies identify heavy alcohol or drug use to be associated with sexual assault. In addition, the use of flunitrazepam (Rohypnol) to subdue potential victims of date rape on the rise in the United States, even though the drug is illegal (Smith, Wesson, & Calhoun, 1999).

Intergenerational Transmission Process

Intergenerational transmission process means that patterns of violent behavior are perpetuated from one generation to the next by means of role modeling and social learning (Humphreys, 1997; Tyra, 1996). Intergenerational transmission suggests that family violence is a learned pattern of behavior. For example, children who witness family violence learn from watching their parents that violence is a means of resolving conflict and an integral part of a close relationship. Statistics show that one third of abusive men are likely to have come from violent homes where they witnessed wife-beating or were abused themselves. Women who grew up in violent homes are 50% more likely to expect or accept violence in their own relationships (Singer et al., 1995). However, not all persons exposed to family violence become abusive or violent as adults, so this single factor alone does not explain the perpetuation of violent behavior.

CULTURAL CONSIDERATIONS

The Commission on Domestic Violence (1999) has stated that domestic violence affects families from all ethnic, racial, age, national origin, sexual orientation, religious, and socioeconomic backgrounds. However, a specific population addressed by the commission is immigrant women. Battered immigrant women face legal, social, and economic problems different from those of U.S. citizens, even those from other cultural, racial, or ethnic origins:

- The battered woman may come from a culture that accepts domestic violence.
- She may believe she has less access to legal and social services than do citizens.
- If she is not a citizen, she may be forced to leave the United States if she seeks legal sanctions against her husband or attempts to leave him.
- She is isolated by cultural dynamics that do not permit her to leave her husband; economically, she may be unable to gather the resources to leave, work, or go to school.
- Language barriers may interfere with her ability to call 911, learn about her rights or legal options, or obtain shelter, financial assistance, or food.

SPOUSE OR PARTNER ABUSE

Spouse or partner abuse is the mistreatment or misuse of one person by another in the context of an intimate relationship. The abuse can be emotional or psychological, physical, sexual, or a combination of all types, which is common (Singer et al., 1995). Psychological or emotional abuse includes name-calling, belittling, screaming and yelling, destroying property, and making threats, as well as more subtle forms such as refusing to speak to the victim or pretending she is not there. Physical abuse can range from shoving and pushing to severe battering and choking, involving broken limbs and ribs, internal bleeding, brain damage, and even homicide. Sexual abuse includes physical assaults during sexual relations, such as biting nipples, pulling hair, slapping and hitting, as well as rape (which is discussed later).

Spouse abuse is estimated to occur in 2 to 12 million homes in the United States each year. Eight percent of homicides in the U.S. involve the killing of one spouse by another, and three of every 10 female homicide victims are murdered by their spouse, ex-spouse, boyfriend, or ex-boyfriend (Commission on Domestic Violence, 1999). Ninety to ninety-five percent of domestic violence victims are women, and it has been estimated that one in three women in the United States have been beaten by their spouses at least once (Commission on Domestic Violence, 1999).

Pregnancy seems to escalate violent behavior, with an estimated 15% to 25% of women experiencing violence while pregnant, according to a CDC survey. Battering during pregnancy leads to adverse pregnancy outcomes, such as miscarriage and stillbirth, as well as further physical and psychological problems for the woman (Mattson & Rodriguez, 1999; Scobie & McGuire, 1999).

According to the Commission on Domestic Violence (1999), domestic violence occurs in same-sex relationships with the same statistical frequency as in heterosexual relationships. Although same-sex battering mirrors heterosexual battering in prevalence, its victims receive fewer protections. Seven states define domestic violence in a way that excludes same-sex victims. Twenty-one other states have **sodomy laws** that designate sodomy (anal intercourse) as a crime; thus, same-sex victims must first confess to the crime of sodomy to prove a domestic relationship exists between partners (Commission on Domestic Violence, 1999). The same-sex batterer has an additional weapon to use against the victim: the threat of revealing the partner's homosexuality to friends, family, employers, or the community.

CLINICAL VIGNETTE: SPOUSE ABUSE

Darlene sat in the bathroom, trying to regain her balance and holding a cold washcloth to her face. She looked in the mirror and saw a large red, swollen area around her eye and cheek where her husband, Frank, hit her. They had been married for only 6 months, and this was the second time since they married that he had gotten angry and struck her in the face several times before storming out of the house. Last time he was so sorry the day after it happened and brought her flowers and took her out for dinner to apologize. He said he loved her more than ever and felt terrible about what he had done. He said it was because he had had an argument with his boss over getting a raise and went out drinking after work before coming home. He had promised not to go out drinking anymore and promised it would never happen again. For several weeks after he quit drinking, he was wonderful and it felt like it was before they got married. She remembered thinking that she must try harder to keep him happy because she knew he really did love her.

But during the past 2 weeks, he had been increasingly silent and sullen, complaining about everything. He didn't like the dinners she cooked and said he wanted to go out to dinner, even though money was tight for

them right now and their credit cards were loaded with charges they couldn't pay off. That's when this argument happened and he began drinking. After a few hours of drinking, he yelled at her and said she was the cause of all his money problems. She tried to reason with him, but he hit her and this time he knocked her to the floor and her head hit the table. She was really frightened now, but what should she do? She couldn't move out; she had no money of her own and her job just didn't pay enough to support her right now. Go to her parents? She couldn't tell them about what happened because they never wanted her to marry Frank in the first place. They would probably say, "We told you so and you didn't listen. Now you married him and you'll have to deal with his problems." She was too embarrassed to tell her friends, most of whom were "their" friends and had never seen this violent side of Frank. They probably wouldn't believe her. What should she do? Her face and head were really beginning to hurt now. I'll talk to him tomorrow when he is sober and tell him he must get some help for the drinking problem. When he's sober, he is reasonable and he'll see that this drinking is causing a big problem for our marriage.

Clinical Picture

An abusive husband often believes his wife belongs to him, like property, and he becomes increasingly violent and abusive if she shows any sign of independence, such as getting a job or threatening to leave the marriage. The typical abuser is usually emotionally immature and needy, has strong feelings of inadequacy and low self-esteem, has poor problem-solving and social skills, and is irrationally jealous and possessive. He is even jealous of his wife's attention to their own children, and the abuser often beats his children as well as his wife. By bullying his family and physically punishing them, the abuser often experiences a sense of power and control over family members, a feeling that eludes him in life outside the family. Therefore, the violent behavior is often rewarding to him and boosts his self-esteem.

The trait most commonly found in abused wives who stay with their husbands is dependency. Personal and financial dependency is often cited as a reason women find it extremely difficult to leave an abusive relationship. Regardless of the victim's talents or abilities, she perceives herself as unable to function without her husband. She too often suffers from low self-esteem and defines her success as a person by her ability to remain loyal to her marriage and "make it work." Some women internalize the criticism they receive and mistakenly believe they are to blame. Women also fear their abuser will kill them if they try to leave. This fear seems to be a realistic one given the national statistics showing that women who are murdered by their spouse or boyfriend often were attempting to leave or had left (Hattendorf & Tollerud, 1997).

Cycle of Abuse and Violence

Another reason often given for why women have difficulty leaving an abusive relationship is the **cycle of violence** or abuse (Fig. 11-1). There is a typical pattern of how abuse occurs. Usually, the initial episode of battering or violent behavior is followed by a period when the abuser expresses his regret and apologizes, promising it will never happen again. He professes his love for his wife and may even engage in romantic behavior, buying gifts and flowers. This period of contrition or remorse is sometimes called the honeymoon period. The woman naturally wants to believe her husband and is hopeful that the violence was an isolated incident. After this honeymoon period, the tension-building phase begins; there may be arguments, stony silence, or more complaints from the husband. The tension ends in another violent episode, after which the abuser once again feels regret and remorse and promises to change. This cycle

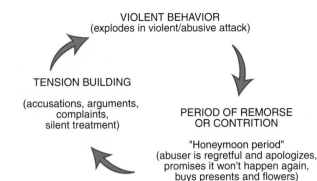

Figure 11-1. Cycle of violence.

repeats itself again and again. Each time the victim keeps hoping that this time the violence is going to stop.

Initially, the honeymoon period may last weeks or even months, allowing the woman to believe that the relationship has improved and her husband's behavior has changed. Over time, the violent episodes become more frequent, the period of remorse disappears altogether, and the level of violence and the severity of injuries become worse. Eventually, the violent behavior occurs routinely, several times a week or even daily.

Treatment and Intervention

Every state in the United States allows police to make arrests in domestic violence cases, and more than half of the states have laws requiring police to make arrests for at least some domestic violence crimes (Commission on Domestic Violence, 1999). Sometimes, after police have been called to the scene, the abuser is allowed to remain at home after talking with police and calming down. If an arrest is made, sometimes he is held only for a few hours or overnight. Often the abuser retaliates when he is released and goes home; hence, women have a legitimate fear of calling the police. Studies have shown that arresting the batterer may reduce violence in the short term but increase violence in the long term (Commission on Domestic Violence, 1999). A woman can obtain a **restraining order** (protection order) from the county where she lives that legally prohibits the abuser from approaching or contacting her. However, a restraining order provides only limited protection. The abuser may decide to violate the order, and the woman may be severely injured or killed before police can intervene. In one study, 60% of women reported acts of abuse after receiving a protection order, and 30% reported acts of severe violence (Commission on Domestic Violence, 1999).

Because most abused women do not seek direct help for the abuse, nurses must be able to help identify abused women in a variety of settings. Nurses may encounter abused women in emergency rooms, clinics, or a pediatrician's office. Some may be seen when seeking treatment for other medical conditions not directly related to the abuse, or when they are pregnant. Identifying abused women who need assistance is a top priority of the Department of Health and Human Services. The generalist nurse is not expected to deal with this complicated problem alone. However, the nurse can make the referrals and contact appropriate health care professionals who are experienced in working with abused women. Above all, the nurse can offer the client caring and support throughout. Table 11-1 summarizes techniques for working with victims of partner violence.

Many hospitals, clinics, and doctor's offices ask all women about safety issues as part of any health history or intake interview. Because this is a delicate and sensitive issue, and many abused women are afraid or embarrassed to admit they are being abused, nurses must be skilled in asking the appropriate questions regarding abuse. Box 11-2 gives an example of questions to ask using the acronym SAFE (**S**tress/**S**afety, **A**fraid/**A**bused, **F**riends/**F**amily, and **E**mergency plan). The first two categories are designed to detect abuse. Questions in the other two categories should be asked if abuse is present. These questions should be asked when the woman is alone and can be paraphrased or edited as needed in any given situation.

Battered women's shelters can provide temporary housing and food for an abused woman and her children when she decides to leave the abusive relationship. However, in many cities shelters are crowded, some have waiting lists, and the relief they provide is

---

Box 11-2

▶ SAFE QUESTIONS

- **S**tress/**S**afety: What stress do you experience in your relationships? Do you feel safe in your relationships? Should I be concerned for your safety?
- **A**fraid/**A**bused: Are there situations in your relationships where you have felt afraid? Has your partner ever threatened or abused you or your children? Have you ever been physically hurt or threatened by your partner? Are you in a relationship like that now? Has your partner ever forced you to engage in sexual intercourse that you did not want? People in relationships/marriages often fight; what happens when you and your partner disagree?
- **F**riends/**F**amily: Are your friends aware that you have been hurt? Do your parents or siblings know about this abuse? Do you think you could tell them, and would they be able to give you support?
- **E**mergency plan: Do you have a safe place to go and the resources you (and your children) need in an emergency? If you are in danger now, would you like help in locating a shelter? Would you like to talk to a social worker/counselor/me to develop an emergency plan?

Ashur, M. L. C. (1993). Asking about domestic violence: SAFE questions. JAMA, 269, (18), p. 2367. © American Medical Association.

---

temporary. The woman leaving an abusive relationship may have no means of financial support and limited job skills or experience, and she often has dependent children. These are difficult barriers to overcome, and public or private assistance is limited.

Table 11-1

DO'S AND DON'TS OF WORKING WITH VICTIMS OF PARTNER ABUSE

Don'ts	Do's
Don't disclose client communications without the client's consent.	Do ensure and maintain the client's confidentiality.
Don't preach, moralize, or imply you doubt the client.	Do listen, affirm, and say "I am sorry you have been hurt."
Don't minimize the impact of violence.	Do express: "I'm concerned for your safety."
Don't express outrage with the perpetrator.	Do tell the victim: "You have a right to be safe and respected."
Don't imply the client is responsible for the abuse.	Do say: "The abuse is not your fault."
Don't recommend couples counseling.	Do recommend a support group or individual counseling.
Don't direct the client to leave the relationship.	Do identify community resources and encourage the client to develop a safety plan.
Don't take charge and do everything for the client.	Offer to help the client contact a shelter, police, or other resources.

Commission on Domestic Violence (1999). Domestic Violence Resources. http://www.abanet.org.domviol/stats/html.

In addition to the many physical injuries that abused women may experience, there are emotional and psychological consequences as well. Individual psychotherapy or counseling, group therapy, or support and self-help groups can help abused women deal with the trauma they have experienced and begin to build new, healthier relationships. Battering also may result in posttraumatic stress disorder, which is discussed later in this chapter.

CHILD ABUSE

Child abuse or maltreatment is generally defined as the intentional injury of a child and can include physical abuse or injuries, neglect or failure to prevent harm, failure to provide adequate physical or emotional care or supervision, abandonment, sexual assault or intrusion, and overt torture or maiming (Biernet, 2000). In the United States, each state defines child maltreatment, identifies specific reporting procedures, and establishes service delivery systems. Although there are similarities between the laws of the 50 states, there is also a great deal of variation. For this reason, accurate data on the type, frequency, and severity of child maltreatment across the country are difficult to obtain.

In 1997, child protective service agencies in 49 states investigated an estimated 2 million reports alleging the maltreatment of 3 million children, with more than half younger than 7 years and 26% younger than 4 years. Every day, on average, more than three children die in the United States as a result of abuse or neglect (Paulk, 1999). More than 3 million children were reported to child protective services for suspected child abuse or neglect (Paulk, 1999). Children are also affected by domestic violence in their homes. One study reported that 27% of domestic violence homicide victims were children, with 56% of those child victims younger than 2 years (Paulk, 1999).

Sexual abuse is most often perpetrated on girls by fathers, stepfathers, uncles, older siblings, and live-in partners of the child's mother. About 75% of reported cases involve father–daughter incest; mother–son incest occurs much less frequently. It is estimated that 15 million women in the United States have been sexually abused as children, and one third of all sexually abused victims were molested before 9 years of age. Accurate statistics on sexual abuse are difficult to obtain because many incidences go unreported due to shame and embarrassment, or women do not acknowledge sexual abuse until they are adults (Singer et al., 1995).

Types of Child Abuse

Physical abuse of children is often the result of unreasonably severe corporal punishment, or unjustifiable punishment, such as hitting an infant for crying or soiling his or her diapers. Intentional deliberate assaults on children include burning, biting, cutting, poking, twisting limbs, or scalding with hot water. The victim often has evidence of old injuries, such as scars, fractures that were not treated, or multiple bruises of various ages, that cannot be adequately explained by the history provided by parents or caregivers (Lego, 1996).

Sexual abuse involves sexual acts performed by an adult on a child younger than 18 years. These acts can include incest, rape, and sodomy, performed by a person or with an object, oral–genital contact, and acts of molestation such as rubbing, fondling, or exposure of the adult's genitals. Sexual abuse may consist of a single incident or multiple episodes over a protracted period of time. A second type of sexual abuse involves exploitation, such as making, promoting, or selling pornography involving minors and coercion of minors to participate in obscene acts.

Neglect is the malicious or ignorant withholding of the physical, emotional, or educational necessities for the child's well-being. Child abuse by neglect is the most prevalent type of maltreatment and includes refusal to seek health care or a delay in

---

 CLINICAL VIGNETTE: CHILD ABUSE

Johnny is a 7-year-old boy who has been sent to the school nurse because of a large bruise on his face. The teacher says Johnny is quiet, shy, and reluctant to join games or activities with others at recess. He stumbled around with no good explanation of what happened to his face when the teacher asked him about it this morning.

The nurse has seen Johnny before for a variety of bruises, injuries, and even a burn on his hands. In the past, Johnny's mother has described him as clumsy, always tripping and falling down. She says he's a "dare-devil," always trying stunts with his bike or Rollerblades or climbing trees and falling or jumping to the ground. She says she has tried everything but can't slow him down.

When the nurse talks to Johnny, he is reluctant to discuss the bruise on his face. He does not make eye contact with the nurse and gives a vague explanation for his bruise: "I guess I ran into something." The nurse suspects that Johnny is being abused by someone in his home.

doing so; abandonment; inadequate supervision; reckless disregard for the child's safety; punitive, exploitive, or abusive emotional treatment; spousal abuse in the child's presence; giving the child permission to be truant; or failing to enroll him or her in school.

Psychological abuse (emotional abuse) includes verbal assaults, such as blaming, screaming, name-calling, and sarcasm; constant family discord, characterized by fighting, yelling, and chaos; and emotional deprivation or withholding of affection, nurturing, and normal experiences that engender feelings of acceptance, love, security, and self-worth. Emotional abuse often accompanies other types of abuse, such as physical or sexual abuse. Exposure to parental alcoholism, drug use, or prostitution, and the neglect that results, can also be included in this category.

Clinical Picture

Parents who abuse their children often have minimal parenting knowledge and skills. They may not understand or know what their children need, or they may be angry or frustrated because they are emotionally or financially unequipped to meet those needs. Although lack of education and poverty are some of the factors that contribute to child abuse and neglect, they by no means explain the entire phenomenon. There are many incidences of abuse and violence in families who seem to have everything—the parents are well-educated and have successful careers, and the family is financially stable.

Parents who abuse their children are often emotionally immature and needy, incapable of meeting their own needs, much less those of a child. As in spousal abuse, children who are abused are often viewed as the property of the abuser, belonging to the abusing parent. Children are not valued as people

with rights and feelings. In some instances, the parent feels the need to have children to replace his or her own faulty and disappointing childhood; the parent wants to feel the love between child and parent that he or she missed as a child. These unrealistic expectations of having a child who will give the parent love and fulfill all the parent's needs are often shattered by the reality of the tremendous emotional, physical, and financial demands of raising children. When the parent's unrealistic expectations are not met, he or she often reverts to using the same methods his or her parents used.

This tendency for adults to raise their children in the same way they were raised perpetuates the cycle of family violence. Adults who have been victims of abuse as children often become abusers of their own children (Biernet, 2000).

Assessment

As with all types of family violence, detection and accurate identification are the first steps. Box 11-3 lists signs that might lead the nurse to suspect neglect or abuse. Burns or scald injuries are present in 10% of abused children. The burns may have an identifiable shape, such as cigarette burns, or may have a "stocking and glove" distribution, indicating scalding injuries. The parent of an infant with a severe skull fracture may report that he or she "rolled off the couch," even though the child is too young to do so or the injury is much too severe for a fall of 20 inches (Ladebauche, 1997).

Children who have been sexually abused may have urinary tract infections; bruised, red, or swollen genitalia; tears of the rectum or vagina; and bruising. The emotional response of children who are abused may vary widely. Often these children talk or behave in ways that indicate more advanced knowledge of sexual issues than would be expected for their age.

Box 11-3

> **WARNING SIGNS OF ABUSED/NEGLECTED CHILDREN**

- Serious injury such as fractures, burns, and lacerations with no reported history of trauma
- Delay in seeking treatment for a significant injury
- Child or parent gives a history inconsistent with severity of injury, such as a baby with *contre-coup* injuries to the brain (shaken baby syndrome) that the parents claim was caused when the infant rolled off the sofa
- Inconsistencies or changes in the child's history during the evaluation by either the child or the adult
- Unusual injuries for a child's age and level of development, such as a fractured femur on a 2-month-old or a dislocated shoulder in a 2-year-old
- High incidence of urinary tract infections; bruised, red, or swollen genitalia, tears or bruising of rectum or vagina
- Evidence of old injuries not reported, such as scars, fractures not treated, multiple bruises that cannot be adequately explained by the parent/caregiver

Other times, victims are frightened and anxious and may either cling to an adult or reject adult attention entirely.

The key is to recognize when the child's behavior is outside what is normally expected for the child's age and stage of development. Seemingly unexplained behavior, from refusal to eat to aggressive behavior with peers, may indicate abuse. The nurse does not have to decide with certainty that abuse has occurred. Nurses are responsible for reporting suspected child abuse with accurate and thorough documentation of assessment data. All 50 states have laws requiring nurses to reported suspected abuse, often called mandatory reporting laws. The nurse, alone or in consultation with other health team members, such as the physician or social worker, may report suspected abuse to appropriate local governmental authorities. In some states, that authority is Child Protective Services, Children and Family Services, or the Department of Health. The number to call can be located in the local telephone book. The reporting person may remain anonymous if desired.

Persons who work in such agencies have special education in the investigation of abuse. Questions must be asked in ways that do not further traumatize the child or impede any legal actions that may result. The generalist nurse should not pursue investigation with the child: it may do more harm than good.

Treatment and Intervention

The first part of treatment for child abuse or neglect is to ensure the child's safety and well-being (Biernet, 2000). This may involve removing the child from the home, which can also be traumatic. A thorough psychiatric evaluation is also indicated, given the high risk for psychological problems. Developing a trust relationship with a therapist is crucial to helping the child deal with the trauma of abuse. Therapy may be indicated over a significant period of time, depending on the severity and duration of abuse and the child's response.

Long-term treatment for the child usually involves professionals from a variety of disciplines, such as psychiatry, social work, psychology, and other therapists. The very young child may communicate best through play therapy, where he or she draws or acts out situations with puppets or dolls rather than talking about what has happened or his or her feelings. Social service agencies are involved in determining whether it is possible to return the child to the parental home if parents can show benefit from treatment. Family therapy may be indicated if it is feasible to reunite the family. Parents may require psychiatric or substance abuse treatment. If the child is not likely to return home, foster care services may be indicated on either a short- or long-term basis.

ELDER ABUSE

Elder abuse is the maltreatment of older adults by family members or caretakers. It may include physical and sexual abuse, psychological abuse, neglect, self-neglect, financial exploitation, and denial of adequate medical treatment. It has been estimated that a half-million elders are abused or neglected in domestic settings, and that as many as five unreported incidents of abuse or neglect occur for each one that is reported. Nearly 60% of the perpetrators are spouses, 20% are adult children, and 20% are other persons, such as siblings, grandchildren, and boarders (Lego, 1996).

CLINICAL VIGNETTE: ELDER ABUSE

Margaret is an elderly woman who has moved in with her son, daughter-in-law, and two grandchildren after the death of her husband. She lives in a finished basement apartment with her own bath. Friction with her daughter-in-law begins to develop when Margaret tries to help out around the house. She comments on the poor manners and outlandish clothes of her teen-aged grandchildren. She adds spices to food her daughter-in-law is cooking on the stove. She comments on how late the children stay out, their friends, and how hard her son works. All of this is annoying but harmless.

Margaret's daughter-in-law gets very impatient, telling her husband, "I'm the one who has to deal with your mother all day long." One day, after another criticism from Margaret, the daughter-in-law slaps her. She then tells Margaret to go downstairs to her room and stay out of sight if she wants to have a place to live. A friend of Margaret's calls on the phone and the daughter-in-law lies and tells her Margaret is sleeping.

Margaret spends more time alone in her room, becomes more isolated and depressed, and is eating and sleeping poorly. She is afraid she will be placed in a nursing home if she doesn't get along with her daughter-in-law. Her son seems too busy to notice what is happening, and Margaret is afraid to tell him for fear he won't believe her or will take his wife's side. Her friends don't seem to call much anymore, and she has no one to talk to about how miserable she is. She just stays to herself most of the day.

Most victims of elder abuse are 75 years or older, and 60% to 65% are women. Abuse is more likely when the elder has multiple, chronic mental and physical health problems, and when the elder is dependent on others for food, medical care, and various activities of daily living.

Persons who abuse elders are almost always in a caretaking position, or the elder is dependent on them in some way. Most cases of elder abuse occur when one older spouse is taking care of another. This type of spousal abuse usually occurs over many years after a disability renders the abused spouse unable to care for himself or herself. When the abuser is an adult child, it is twice as likely to be a son than a daughter. Abuse of elders may also be aggravated by a psychiatric disorder or substance abuse of the caretaker (Goldstein, 2000).

Elders are often reluctant to report abuse, even when they can do so, because it usually involves family members whom the elder wishes to protect. Victims also often fear losing their support and being moved to an institution.

There are no national estimates of abuse of elders living in institutions. Under a 1978 federal mandate, ombudsmen are allowed to visit nursing homes to check on the care of the elderly. These ombudsmen still report that elder abuse is common in institutions (Goldstein, 2000).

Clinical Picture

The victim may have bruises or fractures, may lack needed eyeglasses or hearing aids, may be denied food, fluids or medications, or may be restrained in a bed or chair. The abuser may use the victim's financial resources for his or her own pleasure, while the elder cannot afford food or medications. Medical care itself may be withheld from an elder with acute or chronic illness. Self-neglect involves the elder's failure to provide for himself or herself.

Assessment

Careful assessment of elderly persons and their caregiving relationships is essential in detecting elder abuse. It is often difficult to determine whether the elder's condition results from deterioration associated with a chronic illness or from abuse. There are several potential indicators of abuse that require further assessment and careful evaluation (Box 11-4). However, these indicators by themselves do not necessarily signify abuse or neglect.

Abuse should be suspected if there are injuries that have been hidden or untreated or injuries that are incompatible with the explanation provided. These injuries can include cuts, lacerations, puncture wounds, bruises or welts, or burns. Burns can be cigarette burns, acid or caustic burns, or friction burns of the wrists or ankles caused from being restrained by ropes, clothing, or chains. Signs of physical neglect include a pervasive smell of urine or feces, dirt, rashes, sores, or lice, or inadequate clothing. Dehydration or malnourishment that is not a result of a specific illness is also a strong indicator of abuse.

Possible indicators of emotional or psychological abuse may include an elder who is hesitant to talk openly to the nurse or is fearful, withdrawn, depressed, and helpless. The elder may also exhibit anger or agitation for no apparent reason. He or she may deny that any problems exist, even when the facts indicate otherwise.

Possible indicators of self-neglect include inability to manage money (hoarding or squandering while failing to pay bills), inability to perform activities of daily living (personal care, shopping, food preparation, and cleaning), and changes in intellectual function (confusion, disorientation, inappropriate responses, and memory loss and isolation). Other indicators of self-neglect include signs of malnutrition or dehydration, rashes or sores on the body, an odor of urine or feces, or failure to keep needed medical appointments. For self-neglect to be diagnosed, the elder must be evaluated as unable to manage day-to-day life and take care of himself or herself. Self-neglect cannot be established based solely on family members' beliefs that the elder cannot manage his or her finances. For example, an older adult cannot be considered to have self-neglect just because he or she gives away large sums of money to a group or charity or invests in some venture of which family members disapprove.

Warnings of financial exploitation or abuse may include numerous unpaid bills (when the client has enough money to pay them), unusual activity in bank accounts, checks signed by someone other than the elder, or recent changes in a will or power of attorney when the elder cannot make such decisions. The elder may lack amenities that he or she can afford, such as clothing, personal products, or a television. The elder may report losing valuable possessions and report that he or she has no contact with friends or relatives.

The nurse may also detect possible indicators of abuse from the caregiver. The caregiver may complain about how difficult it is to care for the elder or complain about incontinence, difficulties in feeding, or excessive costs of medication. The caregiver may display anger or indifference toward the elder and try to keep the nurse from talking with the elder alone. Elder abuse is more likely to occur when the caregiver has a history of family violence or alcohol or drug problems.

Some states have mandatory reporting laws for elder abuse, and others have only voluntary report-

Box 11-4

➤ POSSIBLE INDICATORS OF ELDER ABUSE

PHYSICAL ABUSE INDICATORS

- Frequent, unexplained injuries, accompanied by a habit of seeking medical assistance from a variety of locations
- Reluctance to seek medical treatment for injuries, or denial of their existence
- Disorientation or grogginess, indicating misuse of medications
- Fear or edginess in the presence of family member of caregiver

PSYCHOLOGICAL OR EMOTIONAL ABUSE INDICATORS

- Helplessness
- Hesitance to talk openly
- Anger or agitation
- Withdrawal or depression

FINANCIAL ABUSE INDICATORS

- Unusual or inappropriate activity in bank accounts
- Signatures on checks that are different from the elder's
- Recent changes in will or power of attorney when elder is not capable of making those decisions
- Missing valuable belongings that are not just misplaced
- Lack of television, clothes, or personal items that could be afforded easily
- Unusual concern by the caregiver over the expense of the elder's treatment when it is not the caregiver's money being spent

NEGLECT INDICATORS

- Dirt, fecal or urine smell, or other health hazards in the elder's living environment
- Rashes, sores, or lice on the elder
- Elder has an untreated medical condition or is malnourished or dehydrated not related to a known illness
- Inadequate clothing

INDICATORS OF SELF-NEGLECT

- Inability to manage personal finances, such as hoarding, squandering, or giving away money while not paying bills
- Inability to manage activities of daily living, such as personal care, shopping, housework
- Wandering, refusing needed medical attention, isolation, substance use
- Failure to keep needed medical appointments
- Confusion, memory loss, unresponsiveness
- Lack of toilet facilities, living quarters infested with animals or vermin

WARNING INDICATORS FROM CAREGIVER

- Elder is not given opportunity to speak for self, to have visitors, or to see anyone without the presence of the caregiver
- Attitudes of indifference or anger toward the elder
- Blaming the elder for his or her illness or limitations
- Defensiveness
- Conflicting accounts of elder's abilities, problems, and so forth
- Previous history of abuse or problems with alcohol or drugs

Adapted from the California Registry, Elder Abuse Prevention (1999). http://www.calregistry.com/resources/eldabpag.html

ing laws. Nurses should be familiar with the laws or statutes for reporting abuse in their own state. Many cases still go unreported. The local agency on aging can provide procedures for reporting abuse in accordance with state laws. To find the local agency, call the national information center at 1-800-677-1116.

Treatment and Intervention

Elder abuse may develop gradually over time as the burden of caregiving exceeds the caretaker's physical or emotional resources. Relieving the caregiver's stress and providing additional resources may help correct the abusive situation and leave the caregiving relationship intact. In other cases, the neglect or abuse is intentional and designed to provide personal gain to the caregiver, such as access to the victim's financial resources. In these situations, removal of the elder or caregiver is necessary.

RAPE

Rape is a crime of violence and humiliation of the victim expressed through sexual means. Rape is the perpetration of an act of sexual intercourse with a female, against her will and without her consent, whether her will is overcome by force or fear of force or by drugs or intoxicants. It is also considered rape if the woman is incapable of exercising rational judgment because of mental deficiency, or when she is below the age of consent (which varies among states from 14 to 18 years of age) (Singer et al., 1995). The crime of rape requires only slight penetration of the outer vulva; full erection and ejaculation are not necessary. Forced acts of fellatio and anal penetration, although they frequently accompany rape, are legally considered sodomy. The woman who is raped may also be physically beaten and injured.

Rape can occur between strangers, acquaintances, married persons, and persons of the same sex, although seven states define domestic violence in a way that excludes same-sex victims (Commission on Domestic Violence, 1999). About half of rapes are committed by strangers and the other half by men known to the victims. **Date rape (acquaintance rape)** is rape committed by someone known to the victim or someone she is dating. It may occur on a first date, on a ride home from a party, or when the two people have known each other for a period of time. Date rape is more

prevalent near college and university campuses. The CDC Division of Violence Prevention (1999) reports that with increased consumption of alcohol by either the victim or perpetrator, the rate of serious injuries associated with dating violence increases.

Rape is a highly underreported crime: it is estimated that only 1 rape is reported for every 4 to 10 rapes that occur. The underreporting is attributed to the victim's feelings of shame and guilt, the fear of further injury, and the belief that she has no recourse in the legal system. Victims of rape can be of any age: reported cases have ranged from 15 months to 82 years of age. The highest incidence is in girls and women ages 16 to 24 years. Girls younger than 18 were the victims in 61% of the rapes reported (American Medical Association, 1999).

Rape most commonly occurs in a women's neighborhood, often inside or near her home. Most rapes are premeditated. Seven percent are perpetrated by close relatives of the victim and 10% involve more than one attacker. Rape results in pregnancy about 10 of the time (Singer et al., 1995).

Male rape is a significantly underreported crime. It can occur between gay partners or strangers but is most prevalent in institutions such as prisons or maximum-security hospitals. It is estimated that 2% to 5% of male inmates are sexually assaulted, but the figure may be much higher. This type of rape is particularly violent, and the dynamics of power and control are the same as for heterosexual rape.

Dynamics of Rape

Most men who commit rapes are 25 to 44 years old. In terms of race, 51% are white and tend to rape white victims, and 47% are African American and

---

CLINICAL VIGNETTE: RAPE

Cynthia is a 22-year-old college student who spent Saturday afternoon with a group of friends at the football game. Afterwards, they were going to attend a few parties held to celebrate the victory. Alcohol was served freely at these parties. At one of the parties, Cynthia got separated from her friends but started talking to Ron, whom she recognized from her English Lit course. They spent the rest of the evening together, talking, dancing, and drinking. She had had more drinks then she was used to, as Ron kept bringing her more drinks every time her glass was empty. At the end of the night, Ron asked if she wanted him to drive her home. Her friends were staying longer at the party.

When Ron and Cynthia arrived at her apartment, none of her roommates had gotten back yet, so she asked Ron to come in. She was feeling a little tipsy and

they began kissing and she could feel Ron really getting excited. He began to try to remove her skirt, but she said, "No" and tried to move away from him. She remembered him saying, "What's the matter with you? Are you a prude or what?" She told him she had had a good time but didn't want to go further. He responded, "Come on, you've been trying to turn me on all night. You want this as much as I do." He forced himself on top of her and held his arm over her neck and raped her.

When her roommates return in about 1 hour, Cynthia is huddled in the corner of her room and seems stunned and is crying uncontrollably. She feels sick and confused. Did she do something to cause this whole thing? She kept asking herself whether she might not have gotten into that situation had she not been a little tipsy. She was so confused.

tend to rape African American victims; the remaining 2% come from all other races. Alcohol is involved in 34% of all rapes. Rape often occurs as an accompaniment to another crime. Almost three fourths of arrested rapists have prior criminal histories, including other rapes, assault, robbery, and homicide (Singer et al., 1995).

Recent research has categorized male rapists into four categories: sexual sadists who are aroused by the pain of their victims; exploitive predators who impulsively use their victims as objects for gratification; inadequate men who believe that no woman would voluntarily have sexual relations with them and are obsessed with fantasies about sex; and men for whom rape is a displaced expression of anger and rage (Singer et al., 1995). Feminist theory proposes that women have historically served as objects for aggression, dating back to the time when women (and children) were legally the property of men. In 1982, for the first time, a married man was convicted of raping his wife, signaling the end to the notion that sexual intercourse could not be denied in the context of marriage.

Women who are raped are frequently in a life-threatening situation, so their primary motivation is to stay alive. At times, attempts to resist or fight off the attacker can be successful, but in other situations, fighting and yelling results in more severe physical injuries or even death. There is a higher degree of submission when the attacker has a weapon, such as a gun or knife. In addition to forcible penetration, the more violent rapist may urinate or defecate on the woman or insert foreign objects into her vagina and rectum.

The physical and psychological trauma suffered by rape victims is severe. Medical problems resulting from rape can include acute injury, risk of sexually transmitted diseases, risk of pregnancy, and lingering medical complaints. A cross-sectional study of medical patients found that women who had been raped rated themselves as significantly less healthy, visited a physician twice as often, and incurred medical costs more than twice as high as women who had not experienced any criminal victimization (American Medical Association, 1999). The level of violence experienced during the assault was found to be a powerful predictor of future use of medical services. Many victims of rape experience fear, helplessness, shock and disbelief, guilt, humiliation, and embarrassment. They may also avoid the place or circumstances of the rape, avoid previously pleasurable activities, and experience depression, sexual dysfunction, insomnia, and impaired memory (American Medical Association, 1999).

Until recent years, the rights of rape victims were often ignored. For example, when rape victims reported a rape to authorities, they were often faced with doubt and embarrassing questions by male officers. The rights of the victims were not protected in court, either—for example, a woman's past sexual behavior was admissible in court, although the past criminal record of her accused attacker was not. Laws to correct these problems have been enacted on a state-by-state basis since the mid-1980s.

Although the treatment of rape victims and the prosecution of rapists have improved in the past two decades, many people still believe that somehow a woman provokes rape by her behavior and that the woman is partially responsible for this crime. Box 11-5 summarizes common myths and misunderstandings about rape.

Treatment and Intervention

The victim of rape fares best when she receives immediate support and can ventilate her fear and rage to family members, nurses, physicians, and law enforcement officials who believe her (Singer et al., 1995). Education about rape and the needs of victims is an ongoing need for health care professionals, law enforcement officers, and the general public.

Box 11-6 lists warning signs of relationship violence. These signs, used at the State University of New York at Buffalo to educate students about date rape, can alert women to the characteristics of men who are likely to commit dating violence, such as negativity about women, acting tough, heavy drinking, jealousy, belittling comments, and anger and intimidation.

Rape treatment centers (emergency services that coordinate psychiatric, gynecologic, and physical trauma services in one location and work with law enforcement agencies) are most helpful to the victim. In the emergency setting, the nurse is an essential part

---

Box 11-5

> ### COMMON MYTHS ABOUT RAPE

- When a woman submits to rape, she really wants it to happen.
- Women who dress in a provocative manner are asking for trouble.
- Some women like rough sex, but later call it rape.
- Once a man is aroused by a woman, he cannot stop his actions.
- Walking alone at night is an invitation for rape.
- Rape cannot happen between persons who are married.
- Rape is exciting for some women.

Adapted from University of Buffalo Counseling Center (1999). http://ub-counseling.buffalo.edu/Relationships/Violence/warnings.html.

Box 11-6

> WARNING SIGNS OF RELATIONSHIP VIOLENCE

- Emotionally abuses you (insults, belittling comments, acting sulky or angry when you initiate an idea or activity)
- Tells you with whom you may be friends or how you should dress, or tries to control other elements of your life
- Talks negatively about women in general
- Gets jealous when there is no reason
- Drinks heavily, uses drugs, or tries to get you drunk
- Acts in an intimidating way by invading your personal space, such as standing too close or touching you when you don't want him to
- Is unable to handle sexual or emotional frustration without becoming angry
- Does not view you as an equal: sees himself as smarter or socially superior
- Guards his masculinity by acting tough
- Is angry or threatening to the point that you have changed your life or yourself so you won't anger him.

Adapted from the State University of New York at Buffalo Counseling Center (1999).

of the team in providing emotional support to the victim. The nurse should allow the woman to proceed at her own pace, not rush her through any interview or examination procedures. To preserve possible evidence, the physical examination should occur before the woman has showered, brushed her teeth, douched, changed her clothes, or had anything to drink. This may not be possible, because the woman may have done some of these things before seeking care. If there is no report of oral sex, then rinsing the mouth or drinking fluids can be permitted immediately.

To assess the woman's physical status, the nurse asks the victim to describe what happened. If the woman cannot do so, the nurse may ask questions as needed in a gentle and caring manner. Rape kits and rape protocols are available in most emergency room settings and provide the equipment and instructions needed for the collection of physical evidence. The physician is primarily responsible for this step of the examination.

It is important to give as much control back to the victim as is possible. This is done by allowing her to make decisions, when possible, about whom to call, what to do next, what she would like done, and so forth. It is the woman's decision about whether to file charges and testify against the perpetrator. Consent forms must be signed before any photographs or hair and nail samples can be taken for future evidence.

Prophylactic treatment for sexually transmitted diseases, such as chlamydia or gonorrhea, is offered. It is cost-effective to do so, and many victims of rape will not return to get definitive test results for these diseases. HIV testing is strongly encouraged in high-risk areas such as New York, California, New Jersey, and Florida, but it is not required for low-risk areas (Ledray & Arndt, 1994). Women are also encouraged to engage in safe-sex practices until the results of

HIV testing are available. Prophylaxis with ethinyl estradiol and norgestrel (Ovral) can be offered to prevent pregnancy. Some women may elect to wait to initiate intervention until they have a positive pregnancy test or miss a menstrual period.

Rape crisis centers, women's advocacy groups, and other local resources often provide a counselor or volunteer to be with the victim from the emergency room through longer-term follow-up. This person provides emotional support to the woman, serves as an advocate for her throughout the process, and can be totally available to the victim. This type of complete and unconditional support is often crucial to recovery.

Therapy is usually supportive in approach and focuses on restoring the victim's sense of control over her life; relieving the feelings of helplessness, dependency, and obsession with the assault that frequently follow rape; regaining trust; improving daily functioning; finding adequate social support; and dealing with feelings of guilt, shame, and anger. Group therapy with other women who have been raped is a particularly effective form of treatment. Some women will attend both individual and group therapy.

It often takes a year or more for victims of rape to regain previous levels of functioning. In some cases, victims of rape have long-term consequences such as posttraumatic stress disorder, which is discussed below.

PSYCHIATRIC DISORDERS RELATED TO ABUSE AND VIOLENCE

Posttraumatic Stress Disorder

Posttraumatic stress disorder (PTSD) is a disturbing pattern of behavior demonstrated by someone who has experienced a traumatic event—for example, a natural disaster, combat, or an assault. The person with PTSD was exposed to an event that posed a threat of death or serious injury and responded with intense fear, helplessness, or terror. He or she persistently re-experiences the trauma through memories, dreams, flashbacks, or reactions to external cues about the event and avoids stimuli associated with the trauma. The victim feels a numbing of general responsiveness and shows persistent signs of increased arousal, such as insomnia, hypervigilance, irritability, or angry outbursts. In PTSD, the symptoms occur 3 months or more after the trauma. PTSD is distinguished from **acute stress disorder**, which is the DSM-IV-TR diagnosis given when the symptoms appear within the first month after the trauma and do not persist longer than 4 weeks.

PTSD can occur at any age, including childhood. It is estimated that up to 60% of persons at risk, such as combat veterans and victims of violence and natural disasters, develop PTSD. Complete recovery occurs within 3 months for about 50% of people. The severity and duration of the trauma and the proximity of the person to the trauma are the most important factors affecting the likelihood of developing PTSD (DSM-IV-TR, 2000).

Dissociative Disorders

Dissociation is a subconscious defense mechanism that helps a person protect his or her emotional self from recognizing the full impact of some horrific or traumatic event by allowing the mind to forget or remove itself from the painful situation or memory. Dissociation can occur both during and after the event. As with any other protective or coping mechanism, dissociating becomes easier with repeated use.

Dissociative disorders have the essential feature of a disruption in the usually integrated functions of consciousness, memory, identity, or perception of the environment. This often interferes with the person's ability to function in daily life, with relationships, and with the person's ability to cope with the realities of the abusive or traumatic event. This disturbance varies greatly in intensity in different people, and the onset may be sudden or gradual, transient or chronic. Dissociative symptoms are seen in clients with PTSD. The DSM-IV-TR describes different types of dissociative disorders:

- *Dissociative amnesia*: The client cannot remember important personal information, usually of a traumatic or stressful nature.
- *Dissociative fugue*: The client has episodes of suddenly leaving the home or place of work without any explanation, traveling to another city, and being unable to remember his or her past or identity. He or she may assume a new identity.
- *Dissociative identity disorder* (formerly multiple personality disorder): The client displays two or more distinct identities or personality states that recurrently take control of his or her behavior. This is accompanied by the inability to recall important personal information.
- *Depersonalization disorder*: The client has a persistent or recurrent feeling of being detached from his or her mental processes or body. This is accompanied by intact reality testing—that is, the client is not psychotic or out of touch with reality.

Dissociative disorders are relatively rare in the general population but are much more prevalent among persons with histories of childhood physical and sexual abuse. Some believe the recent increase in the diagnosis of dissociative disorders in the United States is due to a greater awareness of this disorder by mental health professionals (DSM-IV-TR, 2000).

Much media attention has been focused on the theory of **repressed memories** in victims of abuse. Many professionals believe that memories of childhood abuse can be deeply buried in the subconscious mind or repressed because they are too painful for the victim to acknowledge, and victims can be helped to recover or remember such painful memories. If a person comes to a mental health professional experiencing serious problems in relationships, symptoms of PTSD, or flashbacks involving abuse, the mental health professional may help the person remember or recover those memories of abuse (Hall, 1996). Some believe that mental health professionals may be overzealous in helping the client "remember" abuse that really did not happen (Moyers, 1996). This so-called false memory syndrome has created problems in families where groundless accusations of abuse were made. However, it is feared that people who were abused in childhood will be more reluctant to talk about their abuse history because, once again, no one will believe them (Hall, 1996).

Treatment and Interventions

Survivors of trauma and abuse who have PTSD or dissociative disorders are often involved in group or individual therapy in the community to address the long-term effects of their experiences. The nurse is most likely to encounter these clients in a hospital setting when there are concerns for their safety or the safety of others, or when acute symptoms have become intense and require stabilization.

SELF-AWARENESS ISSUES

Nurses sometimes are reluctant to ask women about abuse (Henderson, 1994), partly because they may believe some of the common myths about abuse. They may believe that the woman will be offended by questions about abuse, or may fear that incorrect interventions will worsen the situation. Nurses may even believe that a woman who stays in an abusive relationship might deserve or enjoy the abuse, or that abuse is a private matter between husband and wife (Henderson, 1994). Some nurses may believe that abuse is a societal or legal problem, not a health care problem.

It can be difficult to listen to stories of family violence or rape; the nurse may feel horror or revulsion. Because clients often watch for the nurse's reaction, it is important to contain these feelings and focus on the client's needs. The nurse must be prepared to listen to the client's story, no matter how disturbing, and support and validate the client's feelings with comments such as, "That must have been terrifying" or "Sounds like you were afraid for your life." The nurse must convey acceptance and regard for the client as a person with worth and dignity, regardless of the circumstances. These clients often have low self-esteem and guilt feelings. They must learn to accept and face what has occurred. If the client believes that the nurse can accept him or her after hearing what has happened, this may help him or her accept himself or herself. Although this acceptance is often painful, it is essential to healing. The nurse must remember that he or she cannot fix or change things; the nurse's role is to listen and convey acceptance and support for the client.

Nurses with a personal history of abuse or trauma must seek professional assistance to deal with these issues before working with survivors of trauma or abuse. Such nurses can be very effective and supportive of other survivors, but only after engaging in therapeutic word and accepting and understanding their own trauma.

Helpful Hints for Working With Clients Who Have Been Abused or Traumatized

- These clients have many strengths they may not realize. The nurse can help them move from being victims to being survivors.
- Nurses should ask all women about abuse. Some will be offended and angry, but it is more important not to miss the opportunity of helping the woman who replies, "Yes. Can you help me?"
- The nurse should have the client focus on the here and now rather than dwelling on the horrific things that happened in the past.
- Usually a nurse works best with either the survivors of abuse, or the abusers themselves. Most find it too difficult emotionally to work with both groups.

APPLICATION OF THE NURSING PROCESS
Assessment
BACKGROUND

The client has a history of experiencing trauma or abuse. It may be abuse as a child, or abuse in a current or recent relationship. It is generally not necessary or desirable for the client to detail specific events of the abuse or trauma; rather, in-depth discussion of the actual abuse is usually undertaken during individual psychotherapy sessions.

GENERAL APPEARANCE AND MOTOR BEHAVIOR

The client often appears hyperalert and reacts to even small environmental noises with a startle response. He or she may be very uncomfortable if the nurse is too close physically and may require greater distance or personal space than most people (Applegate, 1997). The client may appear anxious or agitated and may have difficulty sitting still, often needing to pace or move around the room. Sometimes the client may sit very still, seeming to curl up with arms around knees.

MOOD AND AFFECT

A wide range of emotions is possible, from passivity to anger. The client may look frightened or scared, or agitated and hostile, depending on what he or she is experiencing at the time. When the client experiences a flashback, he or she appears terrified and may cry or scream or attempt to hide or run away. When the client is dissociating, he or she may speak in a different tone of voice or appear numb, with a vacant stare. The client may report intense feelings of rage or anger or may report feeling dead inside, unable to identify any feelings or emotions.

THOUGHT PROCESS AND CONTENT

Clients who have been abused or traumatized report reliving the trauma, often through nightmares or flashbacks. Intrusive, persistent thoughts about the trauma interfere with the client's ability to think about other things or to focus on daily living. Some clients report hallucinations or buzzing voices in their head. Self-destructive thoughts and impulses as well as intermittent suicidal ideation are also common. Some clients report fantasies in which they take revenge on their abuser.

SENSORIUM AND INTELLECTUAL PROCESSES

The client is oriented to reality, except when experiencing a flashback or dissociative episode. During those experiences, the client may not respond to the nurse or may be unable to communicate at all. Clients who have been abused or traumatized may have memory gaps, periods of time for which they have no clear memories. These periods of time may be short or extensive and are usually related to the time of the abuse or trauma. The client's ability to concentrate or pay attention is often impaired by intrusive thoughts or ideas of self-harm.

JUDGMENT AND INSIGHT

The client's insight is often related to the length of time he or she has had problems with dissociation or PTSD. Early in treatment, the client may have little idea about the relationship of past trauma to his or her current symptoms and problems. Other clients may be quite knowledgeable in this area if they have progressed further in treatment. The client's ability to make decisions or solve problems may be impaired.

SELF-CONCEPT

Usually clients have low self-esteem. They may believe they are bad people, somehow deserving or provoking the abuse that occurred. Many clients think they are unworthy or damaged by their abusive experiences to the point that they will never be worthwhile or valued people. Clients may think they are going crazy and are out of control, with no hope of regaining control. Clients may see themselves as helpless, hopeless, and worthless.

ROLES AND RELATIONSHIPS

Clients generally report a great deal of difficulty with all types of relationships. Problems with authority figures often lead to problems at work, such as being able to take directions from another or having one's performance monitored by another person. Close relationships are difficult or impossible because the client's ability to trust others is severely compromised. Often the client has quit work or been fired, and he or she may be estranged from family members. The intrusive thoughts and flashbacks or dissociative episodes interfere with the client's ability to socialize with family or friends, and the client's avoidant behavior may keep him or her from participating in social or family events.

PHYSIOLOGIC CONSIDERATIONS

Most clients report difficulty sleeping due to nightmares or anxiety from anticipating nightmares. Overeating or lack of appetite is also common. Frequently, clients use alcohol or other drugs to attempt to sleep or blot out intrusive thoughts or memories.

Data Analysis

Nursing diagnoses commonly used when working with clients who dissociate or have PTSD related to trauma or abuse include the following:

- Risk for Self-Abuse or Self-Mutilation
- Ineffective Individual Coping
- Post-Trauma Response
- Self-Esteem Disturbance.

Outcome Identification

Treatment outcomes for clients who have survived trauma or abuse may include:
1. The client will be physically safe.
2. The client will distinguish between ideas of self-harm and taking action on those ideas.
3. The client will demonstrate healthy, effective ways of dealing with stress.
4. The client will express emotions in a non-destructive manner.
5. The client will establish a social support system in the community.

Intervention

PROMOTING THE CLIENT'S SAFETY

The client's safety is a priority. The nurse must assess on an ongoing basis the client's potential for self-harm or suicide, and take action accordingly. The nurse and treatment team must provide safety measures when the client cannot do so (see Chaps. 10 and 14). To increase the client's sense of personal control, it is important for him or her to manage his or her safety needs as soon as possible. The nurse can talk with the client about the difference between having self-harm thoughts and taking action on those thoughts: having the thoughts does not mean the thoughts must be acted on. Gradually, the nurse can help the client find ways to tolerate the thoughts until they diminish in intensity.

The nurse can help the client learn to go to a safe place when having destructive thoughts and impulses so that he or she can calm down and wait until they pass. Initially, this may mean just sitting with the nurse or around other people. Later, the client can find a safe place at home, often a closet or small room, that he or she feels is safe and soothing (Benham, 1995). The client may want to keep a blanket or pillows there for comfort and pictures or a tape recording to serve as reminders of the present.

HELPING THE CLIENT COPE WITH STRESS AND EMOTIONS

Grounding techniques are helpful to use with the client who is dissociating or experiencing a flashback (Benham, 1995). Grounding techniques remind the client that he or she is in the present, as an adult, and is safe. It is also important to validate what the client is feeling during these experiences: "I know this is frightening, but you are safe now." In addition, the nurse can increase contact with reality and diminish the dissociative experience by helping the client focus on what he or she is currently experiencing through their senses:
- "What are you feeling?"
- "Are you hearing something?"

> ## SUMMARY OF NURSING INTERVENTIONS
>
> **PROMOTE CLIENT'S SAFETY**
> - Discuss self-harm thoughts.
> - Help client develop plan for going to safe place when having destructive thoughts or impulses.
>
> **HELP CLIENT COPE WITH STRESS AND EMOTIONS**
> - Use grounding techniques to help client who is dissociating or experiencing flashbacks.
> - Validate client's feelings of fear, but try to increase contact with reality.
> - During dissociative experience or flashback, help client change body position, but do not grab or force client to stand up or move.
> - Use supportive touch if client responds well to it.
> - Teach deep breathing and relaxation techniques.
> - Use distraction techniques such as physical exercise, listening to music, talking with others, or engaging in a hobby or other enjoyable activity.
> - Help make a list of activities and keep materials on hand to engage client when feelings are intense.
>
> **HELP PROMOTE CLIENT'S SELF-ESTEEM**
> - Refer to client as "survivor" rather than "victim."
> - Establish social support system in community.
> - Make a list of people and activities in the community to contact when help is needed.

Nursing Care Plan   FOR A CLIENT WHO IS BEING ABUSED

Nursing Diagnosis

➤ **Ineffective Individual Coping** (5.1.1.1)
Impairment of adaptive behaviors and problem-solving abilities of a person in meeting life's demands and roles

ASSESSMENT DATA

- Verbalization of inability to cope
- Inability to solve problems
- Difficulty in interpersonal relationships
- Lack of trust
- Self-destructive behavior
- Denial of abuse
- Guilt
- Fear
- Anxious, withdrawn, or depressive behavior
- Manipulative behavior
- Social isolation

EXPECTED OUTCOMES

The client will:
- Express feelings of helplessness, fear, anger, guilt, anxiety, and so forth
- Demonstrate decreased withdrawn, depressive, or anxious behaviors
- Demonstrate a decrease in stress-related symptoms
- Identify support systems outside the hospital

IMPLEMENTATION

Nursing Interventions	Rationale
Spend time with the client, and encourage the client to express his or her feelings through talking, writing, crying, and so forth. Be accepting of the client's feelings, including guilt, anger, fear, and caring for the abuser.	Abusive situations engender a variety of feelings that the client needs to express, including grief for the loss of an ideal or healthy relationship, trust, health, hope, plans, financial security, and home. In addition, victims of abuse often feel that they deserved abuse, or it would not have happened. Finally, abuse in a relationship does not preclude feelings of caring.
When interacting with the client, point out and give support for decision making, seeking assistance, expressions of strengths, problem solving, and successes. Recognize the client's efforts in interactions, activities, and his or her treatment plan.	The client may not see his or her strengths or work as valuable and may have suffered abuse when displaying strengths in the past. Positive support may help reinforce the client's efforts and promote the client's growth and self-esteem.
Give the client choices as much as possible. Structure some activities at the client's present level of accomplishment to provide successful experiences.	Offering choices to the client conveys that the client has the right to make choices and is capable of making them. Achievement at any level is an opportunity for the client to receive positive feedback.

continued on page 251

continued from page 250

Use role-playing and group therapy to explore and reinforce effective behaviors.

The client can try out new or unfamiliar behaviors in a nonthreatening, supportive environment.

Teach the client problem-solving and coping skills. Support his or her efforts at decision making; do not make decisions for the client or give advice.

The client needs to learn effective skills and to make his or her own decisions. When the client makes a decision, he or she can enjoy the achievement of a successful decision or learn that he or she can survive a mistake and identify alternatives.

Encourage the client to pursue educational, vocational, or professional avenues as desired. Refer the client to a vocational rehabilitation or educational counselor, a social worker, or other mental health professionals as appropriate.

Development of the client's strengths and abilities can increase self-confidence and enable the client to see and work toward self-sufficiency and independence from the abusive relationship.

Encourage the client to interact with other clients and staff members and to develop relationships with others outside the hospital. Assist the client, or facilitate interactions as necessary.

Clients in abusive relationships often are socially isolated and lack social skills or confidence.

Refer the client to appropriate resources and professionals to obtain child care, economic assistance, and other social services.

Abusive behavior often occurs when economic or other stressors are present or increased.

Help the client identify and contact support systems, crisis centers, shelters, and other community resources. Provide written information to the client (e.g., telephone numbers of these resources), especially if he or she chooses to return to an abusive situation.

Clients in abusive relationships often are isolated and unaware of support or resources available. Contacting people or groups before discharge can be effective in ensuring continued contact.

Adapted from Schultz, J. M. & Videbeck, S. L. (1998). Lippincott's manual of psychiatric nursing care plans (5th ed.). Philadelphia: Lippincott-Raven.

- "What are you touching?"
- "Can you see me and the room we're in?"
- "Do you feel your feet on the floor?"
- "Do you feel your arm on the chair?"
- "Do you feel the watch on your wrist?"

For the client who is experiencing dissociative symptoms, the nurse can use grounding techniques to focus the client on the present. For example, the nurse approaches the client and speaks in a calm, reassuring tone. First, the nurse should call the client by name and then introduce himself or herself, by name and by role. If the area is dark, turn on the lights. The nurse can reorient the client by saying: *"Janet, I'm here with you. My name is Sheila. I'm the nurse working with you today. Today is Tuesday, Feb. 3, 2000. You're here in the hospital. This is your room at the hospital. Can you open your eyes and look at me? Janet, my name is Sheila."* This reorienting information is repeated as needed. Asking the client to look around the room will encourage him or her to move his or her eyes and avoid being locked in a daze or flashback (Benham, 1995).

As soon as possible, the nurse encourages the client to change positions. Often during a flashback the client is curled up in a defensive posture. Getting the client to stand and walk around helps dispel the dissociative or flashback experience. At this time, the client can focus on his or her feet moving on the floor or the swinging movements of the arms. The nurse must not grab the client or attempt to force him or her to stand up or move. The client experiencing a flashback may respond to such attempts in an aggressive or defensive way, even striking out at the nurse. Ideally, the nurse asks the client how he or she responds to touch when dissociating or experiencing a flashback before one occurs; then the nurse will know whether using touch is beneficial for that client. Also, the nurse may ask the client to touch the nurse's arm. If the client does so, then supportive touch is beneficial for this client.

Many clients have difficulty identifying their emotions or gauging the intensity of emotions. They may also report that extreme emotions appear out of nowhere with no warning. The nurse can help clients get in touch with their feelings by using a log or journal. Initially, clients may use a "feelings list" so they can select the feeling that most closely matches what they are experiencing. Clients are encouraged to write down their feelings throughout the day at specified intervals—for example, every 30 minutes (Benham, 1995). Once clients have identified their feelings, then they can gauge the intensity of those feelings—for example, rating the feeling on a scale of 1 to 10. Using this process, clients have a greater awareness of their feelings and the different intensities of those feelings; this is an important step toward managing and expressing those feelings.

After identifying feelings and their intensities, clients can begin to find triggers, or feelings that precede the flashbacks or dissociative episodes. Clients can then begin to use grounding techniques to diminish or avoid these episodes. They can use deep breathing and relaxation, focus on sensory information or stimuli in the environment, or engage in positive distractions until the feelings subside. Such distractions may include physical exercise, listening to music, talking to others, or engaging in a hobby or activity (Clark, 1997). Clients must find which of these distractions work for them, and then write them down and keep the list and the necessary materials for the activity close at hand. When clients begin to experience intense feelings, they can look at the list and pick up a book, listen to a tape, or draw a picture, for instance.

HELPING TO PROMOTE
THE CLIENT'S SELF-ESTEEM

Often it is useful to view the client as a **survivor** of trauma or abuse rather than a victim. For these clients, who believe they are worthless and have no power over the situation, it helps to refocus their view of themselves from being a victim to being a survivor. Defining themselves as survivors allows them to see themselves as being strong enough to survive their ordeal. It is a more empowering image than seeing oneself as a victim.

ESTABLISHING SOCIAL SUPPORT

The client needs to find support people or activities in the community. The nurse can help the client prepare a list of support people. Problem-solving skills are difficult for these clients when under stress, so having a prepared list eliminates confusion or stress. This list should include a local crisis hotline to call when the client experiences self-harm thoughts or urges, and friends or family to call when feeling lonely or depressed. The client can also identify local activities or groups that provide a diversion and a chance to get out of the house. The client needs to establish community supports to reduce dependency on health care professionals.

Local support groups can be located by calling the county mental health services or the Department of Health and Human Services. A variety of support groups, both on-line and in person, can be found on the Internet.

Evaluation

Long-term treatment outcomes for clients who have survived trauma or abuse may take years to achieve. These clients usually make gradual progress in being able to keep themselves safe, learning to manage stress and emotions, and being able to function in their daily lives. But although clients learn to manage their feelings and responses, the effects of trauma and abuse can be far-reaching and can last a lifetime.

Critical Thinking

Questions

1. Is spanking a child an acceptable form of discipline, or is it abusive? What determines the appropriateness of discipline? Who should make these decisions, and why?
2. How can the nurse continue to have a positive relationship with the client who returns to an abusive relationship? What should the nurse say to the client who has decided to return to an abusive relationship?
3. A client has just told the nurse that in the past he has lost his temper and has beaten his child. How should the nurse respond? What factors would affect the nurse's response?

INTERNET RESOURCES*

Resource	Internet Address
▶ Community support groups	http://www.clinicaltrials.com
▶ National Center on Elder Abuse	http://www.gwjapan.com/NCEA
▶ National Center on Child Abuse	http://www.acf.dhhs.gov/programs/cb
▶ Centers for Disease Control	http://cdc.gov
▶ American Medical Association	http://ww.ama.org
▶ Agency on Aging	http://aoa.dhhs.gov
▶ Commission on Domestic Violence	www.abanet.org/domviol
▶ Trauma Anonymous (PTSD support group)	www.bein.com/trauma/index.html

*All of the Websites have multiple links to other sites on the topic.

➤ KEY POINTS

- Violence and abusive behavior have been identified as national health concerns by the U.S. Department of Health and Human Services.
- Women and children are the most likely victims of abuse and violence.
- Characteristics of violent families include an intergenerational transmission process, social isolation, power and control, and the use of alcohol and other drugs.
- Spousal abuse can be emotional, physical, sexual, or a combination of all three.
- Women have difficulty leaving abusive relationships due to financial and emotional dependence on the abuser and the risk of suffering increased violence or death.
- Nurses can uncover abuse in a variety of settings by asking women about their safety in relationships. Many hospitals and clinics now ask women about safety issues as an integral part of the intake interview or health history.
- Rape is a crime of violence and humiliation of the victim through sexual means. Half of reported cases are perpetrated by someone the victim knows.
- Child abuse includes neglect and physical, emotional, and sexual abuse. It affects 3 million children in the United States.

- Elder abuse may include physical and sexual abuse, psychological abuse, neglect, exploitation, and medical abuse.
- Survivors of abuse and trauma often experience guilt and shame, low self-esteem, substance abuse, depression, posttraumatic stress disorder, and dissociative disorders.
- Posttraumatic stress disorder occurs as a response to a traumatic event. It can include flashbacks, nightmares, insomnia, mistrust of others, avoidance behaviors, and intense psychological distress.
- Dissociation is a defense mechanism that protects the emotional self from the full reality of abusive or traumatic events, both during and after those events.
- Dissociative disorders have the essential feature of a disruption in the usually integrated functions of consciousness, memory, identity, or perception of the environment. There are four types: dissociative amnesia, dissociative fugue, dissociative identity disorder, and depersonalization disorder.
- Important self-awareness issues for the nurse include managing his or her own feelings and reactions about the abuse that has occurred, being willing to ask about the existence of abuse, and recognizing and dealing

with any abuse issues the nurse may have personally.

- Survivors of trauma and abuse may be admitted to the hospital for safety concerns or stabilization of intense symptoms, such as flashbacks or dissociative episodes.
- The nurse can help the client minimize dissociative episodes or flashbacks through grounding techniques and reality orientation.
- Important nursing interventions for survivors of abuse and trauma include helping to keep the client safe, helping the client learn to manage stress and emotions, and helping the client build a network of support in the community.

REFERENCES

American Medical Association. (1999). *http://www.ama-assn.org/*

American Psychiatric Association. (2000). *DSM-IV-TR: Diagnostic and statistical manual of mental disorders-text revision* (4th ed.). Washington, DC: American Psychiatric Association.

Applegate, M. (1997). Multiphasic short-term therapy for dissociative identity disorder. *Journal of the American Psychiatric Nurses Association, 3*(1), 1–9.

Ashur, M. L. C. (1993). Asking about domestic violence: SAFE questions. *JAMA, 269*(18), 2367.

Benham, E. (1995). Coping strategies: A psychoeducational approach to post-traumatic symptomatology. *Journal of Psychosocial Nursing, 33*(6), 30–35.

Biernet, W. (2000). Child maltreatment. In B. J. Sadock & V. A. Sadock (Eds.). *Comprehensive textbook of psychiatry,* Vol. 2 (7th ed.), pp. 2878–2889.

Centers for Disease Control. (1999). *http://www.cdc.gov/cdc.html*

Clark, C. C. (1997). Posttraumatic stress disorder: How to support healing. *American Journal of Nursing, 97*(8), 27–32.

Commission on Domestic Violence (1999). Statistics on domestic violence. *http://www.abanet.org.domviol/stats/html*

Denham, S. (1995). Confronting the monster of family violence. *Nursing Forum, 30*(3), 12–19.

Goldstein, M. Z. (2000). Edler abuse, neglect, and exploitation. In B. J. Sadock & V. A. Sadock (Eds.). *Comprehensive textbook of psychiatry,* Vol. 2 (7th ed., pp. 3179–3184). Philadelphia: Lippincott Williams & Wilkins.

Hall, J. M. (1996). Delayed recall of childhood sexual abuse: Psychiatric nursing's responsibilities to clients. *Archives of Psychiatric Nursing, 10*(6), 342–346.

Hattendorf, J., & Tollerud, T. R. (1997). Domestic violence: Counseling strategies that minimize the impact of secondary victimization. *Perspectives in Psychiatric Care, 33*(1), 14–23.

Henderson, A. D. (1994). Enhancing nurses' effectiveness with abused women. *Journal of Psychosocial Nursing, 32*(3), 11–15.

Humphreys, J. (1997). Nursing care of children of battered women. *Pediatric Nursing, 23*(2), 122–128.

Ladebauche, P. (1997). Childhood trauma: When to suspect abuse. *RN, 60*(9), 38–43.

Ledray, L. E., & Arndt, S. (1994). Examining the sexual assault victim: A new model for nursing care. *Journal of Psychosocial Nursing, 32*(2), 7.

Lego, S. (1996). Repressed memory and false memory. *Archives of Psychiatric Nursing, 10*(2), 110–115.

Mattson, S., & Rodriguez, E. (1999). Battering in pregnant Latinos. *Issues in Mental Health Nursing, 20*(4), 405–422.

Moyers, F. (1996). Oklahoma City bombing: Exacerbation of symptoms in veterans with PTSD. *Archives of Psychiatric Nursing, 10*(1), 55–59.

Paulk, D. (1999). Recognizing child abuse, child abusers, and individuals who are likely to abuse. *Physician's Assistant, 23*(5), 38–42.

Schultz, J. M. & Videbeck, S. D. (1998). *Lippincott's manual of psychiatric nursing care plans* (5th ed.). Philadelphia: Lippincott-Raven.

Scobie, J., & McGuire, M. (1999). Professional issues: The silent enemy: Domestic violence during pregnancy. *British Journal of Midwifery, 7*(4), 259–262.

Singer, M. I., Anglin, T. M., Song, L., & Lunghofer, L. (1995). Adolescents' exposure to violence and associated symptoms of psychological trauma. *JAMA, 273*(6), 477–482.

Smith, D. E., Wesson, D. R., & Calhoun, S. R. (1999). Rohypnol information fact sheet. San Francisco: Haight Ashbury Free Clinics, Inc. *http://www.lec.org/DrugSearch/Documents/Rohypnol.html*

The State University of New York–University of Buffalo, Counseling Center. (1999). http://ub-counseling.buffalo.edu/Relationships/Violence/warnings.html

Tyra, P. A. (1996). Helping elderly women survive rape using a crisis framework. *Journal of Psychosocial Nursing, 34*(12), 20–25.

ADDITIONAL READINGS

Bekemeier, B. (1995). Public health nurses and the prevention of and intervention in family violence. *Public Health Nursing, 12*(4), 222–227.

Fry-Bowers, E. K. (1997). Community violence: Its impact on the development of children and implications for nursing practice. *Pediatric Nursing, 23*(2), 117–121.

U.S. Department of Health and Human Services. (2000). *Healthy People 2010.* Washington, DC: DHHS.

Chapter Review

➤ **MULTIPLE-CHOICE QUESTIONS**

Select the best answer for each of the following questions.

1. Which of the following is the best action for the nurse to take when assessing a child who might be abused?

   A. Confront the parents with the facts, and ask them what happened.

   B. Consult with a professional member of the health team about making a report.

   C. Ask the child which of his parents caused this injury.

   D. Say or do nothing; the nurse has only suspicions, not evidence.

2. Which of the following interventions would be most helpful for a dissociative client having difficulty expressing feelings?

   A. Distraction

   B. Reality orientation

   C. Journaling

   D. Grounding techniques.

3. Which of the following is true about touching a client who is experiencing a flashback?

   A. The nurse should stand in front of the client before touching.

   B. The nurse should never touch a client who is having a flashback.

   C. The nurse should touch the client only after receiving permission to do so.

   D. The nurse should touch the client to increase feelings of security.

4. Which of the following is true about domestic violence between same-sex partners?

   A. Such violence is less common than in heterosexual partners.

   B. The frequency and intensity of violence are greater than in heterosexual partners.

   C. Rates of violence are about the same as heterosexual partners.

   D. None of the above.

5. The nurse working with a client during a flashback says, "I know you're scared, but you're in a safe place. Do you see the bed in your room? Do you feel the chair you're sitting on?" The nurse is using which of the following techniques?

   A. Distraction

   B. Reality orientation

   C. Relaxation

   D. Grounding

➤ **TRUE-FALSE QUESTIONS**

Identify each of the following statements as T (true) or F (false). Correct any false statements.

_____ 1. Adults who were abused as children often become abusers of their own children.

_____ 2. The type of elder abuse called self-neglect means the elder's caregiver ignores the elder's needs.

_____ 3. The most common type of child abuse is physical battering.

_____ 4. When a woman in an abusive relationship becomes pregnant, the battering usually increases in intensity.

_____ 5. Nurses have a mandatory legal responsibility to report elder abuse only when abuse has actually occurred.

_____ 6. People who develop PTSD after trauma usually had poor coping skills before the trauma.

_____ 7. A woman who has been raped may chose to testify against the perpetrator or not.

_____ 8. Many adults who were abused as children do not desire close relationships as adults.

➤ FILL-IN-THE-BLANK QUESTIONS

Identify the type of abuse being described in the following situations.

_____ A parent does not see a doctor or give medicine to a 3-month-old with a fever of 103°F.

_____ An elderly woman's utilities are cut off for nonpayment of bills, yet she has three uncashed Social Security checks in her possession.

_____ An adult daughter tells her elderly mother, "I'll send you to a nursing home if you don't give me your Social Security check!"

_____ A parent repeatedly tells a child, "You're stupid. You'll never amount to anything!"

➤ SHORT ANSWER QUESTIONS

Explain each of the following concepts, and give an example to illustrate the concept.

Cycle of violence or abuse

Blaming the victim of abuse or rape

Survivor's guilt

Intergenerational transmission process in violent families.

Nursing Practice for Psychiatric Disorders

Anxiety and Stress-Related Illness

Learning Objectives

After reading this chapter, the student should be able to:

1. Distinguish between normal anxiety and the anxiety experienced in anxiety disorders.

2. Differentiate between anxiety, fear, and stress.

3. Explain positive and negative results of anxiety.

4. Describe the levels of anxiety, with behavioral changes related to each level.

5. Discuss the use of defense mechanisms by people with anxiety disorders.

6. Describe the current etiologic theories regarding the major anxiety disorders.

7. Apply the nursing process to the care of clients with anxiety and stress-related disorders.

8. Provide teaching to clients, families, caregivers, and members of the community to increase understanding of anxiety and stress-related disorders.

Key Terms

agoraphobia

anxiety

anxiety disorders

anxiolytic

assertiveness

assertiveness training

compulsion

defense mechanisms

derealization

fear

flooding

mild anxiety

moderate anxiety

obsession

panic attack

panic disorder

phobia

phobic partners

positive reframing

primary gain

secondary gain

severe anxiety

stress

systematic desensitization

Anxiety disorders are a group of conditions that share a key feature of excessive anxiety, with ensuing behavioral, emotional, and physiologic responses. Individuals suffering from an anxiety disorder can demonstrate unusual behaviors such as panic without reason, unwarranted fear of objects or life conditions, uncontrollable repetitive actions, re-experiencing of traumatic events, or unexplainable or overwhelming worry. Many people, on rare occasion, have demonstrated one of these unusual behaviors as a normal response to anxiety. The difference between these singular anxiety responses and having an anxiety disorder is that the anxiety responses are severe enough to interfere in an individual's work, family life, and social spheres.

Many people experiencing anxiety disorders fear they are "going crazy" because of their unusual behaviors or are having a heart attack because of physiologic responses such as palpitations, sweating, and difficulty breathing. They perceive that they have no control over these unusual responses and would desperately like them to stop. People with anxiety disorders are not psychotic—in fact, they function within the boundaries of reality and are well aware that these bizarre episodes they experience are abnormal. In contrast, psychotic people, such as schizophrenics, do not realize their unusual behaviors are different from the norm.

Anxiety is a vague feeling of dread that is unwarranted by the situation. When anxious, a person feels uneasy or apprehensive or may have a sense of impending doom while having no idea why these threatening emotions have occurred. There is no identifiable object as the stimulus for anxiety (Comer, 1992). Anxiety is an internal warning device that issues an alarm to a person.

Fear is virtually indistinguishable from anxiety, because the person experiences the same range of emotional, physiologic, and behavioral response patterns in both. The only difference is that fear arises in response to a specific, identifiable threatening object. Fear is the knowledge that a threat exists; anxiety is the emotion generated by the fear. The threat that stimulates fear can be real or perceived, such as the real fear experienced when confronted by an assailant carrying a gun or the perceived sense of fear when being called in to "see the supervisor."

Anxiety has both healthy and harmful facets, depending on the degree of anxiety, the amount of time anxiety has been present, and how well the person copes with anxiety. Anxiety can be viewed on a continuum from mild, moderate, and severe to panic. Each level causes both physiologic and emotional changes in the person.

Mild anxiety is a sensation that something is different and warrants special attention. Sensory stimulation increases and helps the person to focus attention to learn, solve problems, think, act, feel, and protect himself or herself. For example, mild anxiety helps students to focus on the new information being addressed in class or clinical.

Moderate anxiety is the disturbing feeling that something is definitely different; the person becomes nervous or agitated. For example, a woman visits her mother for the first time in several months and has a sensation that something is very different. The mother comments she has lost a great deal of weight without trying.

Severe anxiety is experienced when the person is sure that something is different and a threat exists; he or she demonstrates fear and distress responses. When a person reaches the highest level of anxiety, full-blown panic, all rational thinking stops and the person experiences the fight, flight, or freeze response—that is, the need to leave quickly, stay and fight, or become frozen and unable to do anything.

The harmful or negative side of anxiety is excessive worry about real or potential problems. This saps energy, creates fear, and inhibits the person from performing adequately in interpersonal, occupational, and social situations. Anxiety disorders are diagnosed when anxiety no longer functions as a signal of danger but becomes chronic and permeates major portions of the person's life, resulting in maladaptive behaviors and emotional disability. For example, generalized anxiety disorder is diagnosed when a person spends much of the day worrying about anything or everything with no real reason, feels restless, tired, and tense, and has had difficulty concentrating for at least the past 6 months. The focus of this chapter is on anxiety disorders that result in extreme and debilitating anxiety that interferes in an individual's daily life.

CATEGORIES OF ANXIETY DISORDERS

Anxiety disorders have many manifestations, but anxiety is the key feature of each disorder (DSM-IV-TR, 2000):

- Panic disorder with or without agoraphobia
- Phobic disorders: social or specific
- Agoraphobia without panic disorder
- Obsessive-compulsive disorder (OCD)
- Posttraumatic stress disorder
- Acute stress disorder
- Generalized anxiety disorder
- Anxiety disorder due to a medical condition
- Substance-induced anxiety disorder.

Panic disorder, phobic disorder, and OCD are the most common and will be the focus of this chapter. Posttraumatic stress disorder is addressed in Chapter 11.

INCIDENCE

Anxiety disorders are the most common emotional disorders in the United States. At least 17% of adults in the United States demonstrate one or more anxiety disorders in any one year. Anxiety disorders are more prevalent in women, persons younger than 45, persons who are divorced or separated, and those of lower socioeconomic status, except for OCD, where there is no gender difference. Eight percent of the population has an anxiety disorder that creates significant interruption in interpersonal, occupational, and social functioning.

Between 5% and 25% of the people in the United States have phobias (specific more often than social), making it the most common anxiety disorder (Kaplan & Sadock, 1995). OCD affects more than 5 million people, and panic disorder affects 1.5% to 3% of the population (Kaplan et al., 1994).

ONSET AND CLINICAL COURSE

The onset and clinical course of anxiety disorders are extremely variable. The onset can be acute or insidious. It can occur without a precipitating event, or it can be traced to an acute stressful event or even to chronic stressors, such as health, work, nutrition, medication, or family problems. Anxiety disorders are manifested by high levels of anxiety that are demonstrated in unusual behaviors, such as worry, panic, obsessive-compulsive thoughts and acts, or fear of objects or events that is disproportionate to the reality of the situation.

PHYSIOLOGIC AND PSYCHOLOGICAL RESPONSES TO ANXIETY

Autonomic nervous system responses to fear and anxiety generate the involuntary activities of the body that are involved in self-preservation. Sympathetic nerve fibers "charge up" the vital signs at any hint of danger to prepare the body's defenses. The adrenal glands release adrenalin (epinephrine), which causes the body to take in more oxygen, dilate the pupils, and increase the arterial pressure and heart rate while constricting the peripheral vessels and shunting blood from the gastrointestinal and reproductive systems and increasing glycogenolysis to free glucose for fuel for the heart, muscles, and central nervous system. When the danger has passed, parasympathetic nerve fibers reverse this process and return the

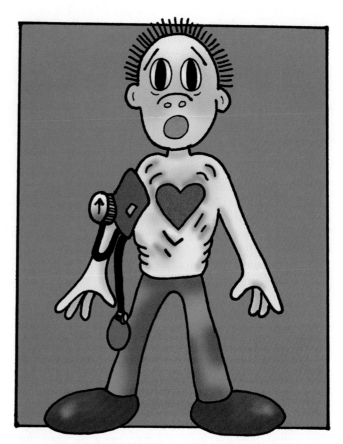

Physiologic response

body to normal operating conditions until the next sign of threat reactivates the sympathetic responses.

Anxiety causes uncomfortable cognitive, psychomotor, and physiologic responses, such as difficulty with logical thought, increasingly agitated motor activity, and increased vital signs. To reduce these uncomfortable feelings, the person tries to reduce the level of discomfort by implementing new adaptive behavior or defense mechanisms. Adaptive behaviors can be positive and can help the person adapt and learn—for example, using imagery techniques to refocus attention on a pleasant scene, sequential relaxation of the body from head to toe, and slow, steady breathing to reduce muscle tension and vital signs. Negative responses to anxiety can result in maladaptive behaviors such as tension headaches, pain syndromes, and stress-related responses that reduce the efficiency of the immune system.

Anxiety can be communicated from one person to another through the use of words, such as hearing someone yell "fire" in a crowded room or listening to the agitated voice of a mother who cannot find her child in a crowded mall. Anxiety can be conveyed nonverbally through empathy, the sense of walking in another person's shoes for a moment in time (Sullivan, 1952). Examples of nonverbal empathetic communication are when the family of a surgical patient can tell from the physician's body language that their loved one has died, when the nurse reads a plea for help in a patient's eyes, or when a person feels the thickened atmosphere of a room where two people have been arguing and are now not speaking to one another.

When adults become anxious, they use defense mechanisms to reduce their anxiety. **Defense mechanisms** are cognitive distortions used by a person to maintain the sense of being in control of a situation, to lessen discomfort, and to deal with the stressful situation. This process involves self-deception, restricted awareness of the situation, or less emotional commitment. Most defense mechanisms arise from the unconscious; thus, the person is unaware of using them. When a patient cannot describe the accident he just had, his mind is using the defense mechanism of repression (unconsciously forgetting the frightening event). A recovering substance abuser who used to beat her children when she was under the influence tries to undo her previously un-acceptable behavior by working with abused children after completing a drug rehabilitation program.

Some people overuse defense mechanisms, and this stops them from learning a variety of appropriate methods to resolve anxiety-producing situations. The dependence on one or two defense mechanisms can also inhibit emotional growth, lead to poor problem-solving skills, and create difficulty with relationships.

LEVELS OF ANXIETY

There are four levels of anxiety (Peplau, 1952): mild, moderate, severe, and panic (Table 12-1). In each of these stages, the person demonstrates changes in be-

havior, cognitive ability, and emotional responses as he or she attempts to deal with the anxiety.

In the low and moderate levels, the person can process information, learn, and solve problems. In fact, these levels of anxiety motivate learning and behavioral change. Cognitive skills predominate in these levels.

As the person progresses to severe anxiety and panic, more primitive survival skills take over, defensive responses occur, and cognitive skills are significantly decreased. A person in severe anxiety has trouble thinking and reasoning, muscles become tight, vital signs are increased, and he or she paces, shows restlessness, irritability, and anger, or uses other similar emotional-psychomotor means to release tension. In a panic state, the person's emotional-psychomotor realm predominates, with fight, flight, or freeze responses. The adrenalin surge has produced greatly increased vital signs, the pupils have enlarged to let in more light, and the only cognitive process focuses on the person's defense.

CULTURAL CONSIDERATIONS

Each culture has rules governing the appropriate way of expressing and dealing with anxiety, and the culturally competent nurse should be aware of them while being careful not to stereotype clients.

Asian Cultural Response

People from Asian cultures believe it is inappropriate to express anxiety and pain; instead, anxiety is somatized (Box 12-1) into expressions of pain in the body, such as headaches, backaches, and stomach problems. However, one intense anxiety reaction that is expressed is *koro*, the profound fear that a man's penis will retract into his abdomen and he will then die. Accepted forms of treatment include having the person keep a firm hold on his penis until the fear passes, often with the assistance of family members or friends, and clamping the penis to a wooden box. In women, *koro* is the fear that the vulva and nipples will disappear (Spector, 2000).

Asian spiritual beliefs focus on harmony and balance. An extension of this Taoist philosophy is the Asian view of health as a balance between *yin* and *yang* forces. *Yin* is female, dark, empty, sleepy, cold, sedentary, negative, and chronic conditions. It represents the inside and the front of the body, the gallbladder, alimentary canal, bladder, and lymph system. *Yin* represents strength of life—for instance, too much *yin* causes anxiety, worry, and colds. *Yin* represents fluids that cool bodies, substantial matter, and earthy things that are close to the ground (Fontaine, 2000; Spector, 2000). *Yang* is male, bright,

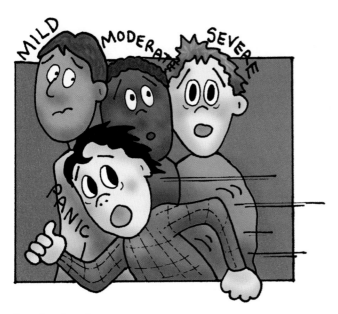

Levels of anxiety

Table 12-1

LEVELS OF ANXIETY RESPONSES

Anxiety Level	Physical Responses	Cognitive Responses	Emotional Responses
Mild (1+)	Mild muscle tension Aware of milieu Relaxed or slight fidgeting Attentive Industrious	Wide perceptual field Secure, confident Low sense of failure Alert, attends to many things Abstracts information Optimal learning level	Automatic behaviors Some impatience Solitary activities Stimulated Secure
Moderate (2+)	Moderate muscle tension Increased vital signs Pupils dilate, sweat starts Some pacing, banging hands Voice changes: tremor, pitch Increased alertness, tension Urinary frequency, headache, sleep changes, backache	Decreased perceptual field Selective inattention Increased focus on stimuli Decreased attention span Problem solving decreased Learning occurs with focusing	Discomfort Irritable Mixed self-confidence Impatient Excited
Severe (3+)	Severe muscle tension Hyperventilation Poor eye contact Increased sweating Speech rapid, high-pitched Random, purposeless actions Clench jaw, gnash teeth Spatial needs increase Pacing, shouting Wringing hands, trembling	Limited perceptual field Fragmented processing Thinking is difficult Poor problem solving Unable to abstract information Attends only to threat Preoccupied with thoughts Egocentric	Frantic Agitation Dread Confusion Inadequacy Withdrawal Denial Wants relief

Panic (4+)	Flight, fight, or freeze
	Extreme muscle tension
	Gross motor agitation
	Dilated pupils
	Increased then decreased
	   vital signs
	Sleepless
	Depleted stress hormones
	   and neurotransmitters
	Facial grimacing, agape
		Tunnel-vision perceptions
		Illogical, distorted thoughts
		Personality disorganized
		Cannot solve problems
		Focused on inner thoughts
		Irrational
		Inaccessible to external stimuli
		Hallucinations, delusions,
		   illusions are possible
			Overwhelmed
			Impotent, helpless
			Out of control
			Rageful, despair
			Anger, terror
			Expects bad outcome
			Aghast, fearful
			Depleted

Adapted from: Beck, A. T. & Emery, C. (1985). *Anxiety disorders and phobias: a cognitive perspective.*
New York: Basic Books; Peplau, H. (1952). *Interpersonal relations in nursing.* New York: GP Putnam's Sons;
Selye, H. (1956). *The stress of life.* New York: McGraw-Hill; Sullivan, H. S. (1954). *The psychiatric interview.*
New York: W. W. Norton.

warm, full, and positive. *Yang* symbolizes aggression and energy, fire and circulation, fever, hypertension, and acute conditions (Fontaine, 2000). It represents the back and the body surface and the heart, liver, lungs, kidney, and spleen. *Yang* foods (bean products, most green vegetables, tubers, pork, water, and white foods) and treatments restore harmony to the body and mind that demonstrate *yin* disharmony. Conversely, *yin* foods and treatments are used to restore harmony in *yang* disorders (Spector, 2000).

Hispanic Cultural Response

The state of balance is a goal of health care in many Hispanic cultures. Each culture assigns hot, cool, or cold values to illnesses, medicines, food, and liquids; for example, Puerto Ricans list bananas, sugar cane, coconuts, and lima beans as cold. Cool items are chicken, fruits, honey, salt cod, milk of magnesia, barley water, and bottled milk. Changes in bowel habits, rashes, ulcers, onions, iron, penicillin, aspirin, and chili peppers are considered hot items. If a person has a cold illness (colds, arthritis, menses), hot treatment and foods are used to restore balance. Conversely, hot illnesses are treated with cold or cool foods and medicines (Andrews & Boyle, 1999). Each Hispanic cultural group or each person may have different views on what is hot and what is cold, so if an Hispanic client refuses to eat, the nurse should ask what food he or she prefers (Spector, 2000).

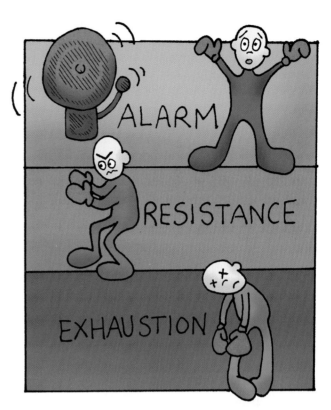

Three reactions or stages of stress

Susto is diagnosed in some Hispanics (Peruvians, Bolivians, Colombians, and Central and South American Indians) when high anxiety, sadness, agitation, weight loss, weakness, and heart rate changes occur. The symptoms are believed to occur because supernatural spirits or bad air from dangerous places and cemeteries invades the body.

ETIOLOGY

Stress is the wear and tear on the body caused by life (Selye, 1956). Anxiety occurs when a person has difficulty dealing with life situations, problems, and goals. Each person handles stress in a different way: one person can thrive in a situation that creates great distress in another. Public speaking is viewed as scary by many people, but for teachers and actors it is an everyday, enjoyable experience. Marriage, children, airplanes, snakes, a new job, a new school, and leaving home are examples of stress-causing events.

Hans Selye (1956, 1974), an endocrinologist, identified the physiologic aspects of stress, which he labeled the general adaptation syndrome. He used laboratory animals to assess biologic system changes, the stages of the body's physical response to pain, heat, toxins, and restraint, and later the mind's emotional response to real or perceived stressors. He determined three stages of reaction to stress.

In the *alarm reaction stage*, stress stimulates the body's physiologic message from the hypothalamus to the glands (such as the adrenal gland to send out adrenalin and norepinephrine for fuel) and organs (for instance, the liver to reconvert glycogen stores to glucose for food) to prepare for potential defense needs. In the *resistance stage*, with continued stress the digestive system reduces function to shunt blood to areas needed for defense, the lungs take in more air, and the heart beats faster and harder so it can circulate this highly oxygenated and highly nourished blood to the muscles to defend the body by fight, flight, or freeze behaviors. If the person adapts to the stress,

the body responses relax and the gland, organ, and systemic responses abate. The *exhaustion stage* occurs when the person has had a negative response to anxiety and stress: body stores are depleted or the emotional components are not resolved, resulting in continual arousal of the physiologic responses and little reserve capacity.

Biologic Theories

Current research focuses on biologic reasons for anxiety as opposed to psychological ones. This research began after it became apparent that benzodiazepine medications, discovered in the 1950s, reduced anxiety. Liberthson et al. (1986) studied a connection between mitral valve prolapse and panic disorder. Some people with episodes of hostility, irritability, asocial behavior, and the sudden sense that things are unreal might be demonstrating an atypical panic disorder. They have electroencephalographic abnormalities of the temporal lobe that generally respond to carbamazepine (an anticonvulsant) or other drugs in this category (Sullivan & Coplan, 2000).

GENETIC THEORIES

Anxiety may have an inherited component, because first-degree relatives of a person with increased anxiety have higher rates of developing anxiety. Panic disorders have an incidence of up to 25% in first-degree relatives, with women having twice the risk of men. Monozygotic twins have a five times greater concordance than dizygotic twins (DSM-IV-TR, 2000). Horwath and Weissman (2000) described a possible "chromosome 13 syndrome." This chromosome is proposed to be involved in the possible genetic linkage of panic disorder, as well as serious headaches, and problems with the kidneys, bladder, or thyroid (mostly hypothyroid) or mitral valve prolapse.

NEUROCHEMICAL THEORIES

Gamma-amino butyric acid (GABA) is the amino acid neurotransmitter believed to be dysfunctional in anxiety disorders. GABA, an inhibitory neurotransmitter, functions as the body's natural antianxiety agent by reducing cell excitability, thus lessening the rate of neuronal firing. It is available in one third of the nerve synapses, especially those in the limbic system and the locus ceruleus, the area where the neurotransmitter norepinephrine, which excites cellular function, is produced. Because GABA reduces anxiety and norepinephrine increases anxiety, it is thought that a problem with the regulation of these neurotransmitters creates anxiety disorders.

The benzodiazepines, a class of anxiolytic drugs (Table 12-2), bind at the same receptor sites as GABA. They help the postsynaptic receptor to be even more receptive to GABA's effects, further reducing the firing rate of cells and decreasing anxiety. Anxiolytics reduce presurgical anxiety and control acute anxiety reactions, but they must be used judiciously because they are addictive. Other neurotransmitters believed to be involved in anxiety dis-

Table 12-2

ANXIOLYTIC DRUGS

Generic Name (Brand Name)	Daily Dose Range	Distribution Rate	Half-Life (hours)	Nursing Implications
chlordiazepoxide (Librium) (Schedule IV)	15–100 mg	Slow	50 – 100	Side effects: drowsiness, lethargy Monitor bilirubin, ALT, AST
clorazepate (Tranxene) (Schedule IV)	15 to 60 mg	Rapid	30 – 200	Side effect: drowsiness Antacids delay absorption.
diazepam (Valium) (Schedule IV)	4–40 mg	Rapid	30 – 100	Side effect: drowsiness Monitor phenytoin and levodopa levels
halazepam (Paxipam) (Schedule IV)	40–80 mg	Intermediate	30 – 200	Side effects: drowsiness, sedation Contraceptives decrease drug effect
clonazepam (Klonopin) (Schedule IV)	1.5–20 mg	Intermediate	18 – 50	Side effects: drowsiness, sedation, ataxia Monitor renal, liver, CBC Overdose: somnolence, sweating, confusion, cramps, coma
lorazepam (Ativan) (Schedule IV)	2–8 mg	Intermediate	10 – 20	Side effects: drowsiness, sedation Cimetidine increases drug effect and side effects Monitor phenytoin and levodopa levels.
alprazolam (Xanax) (Schedule IV)	0.75–1.5 mg	Intermediate	12 – 15	Side effects: drowsiness, sedation Cimetidine & disulfiram increase drug effect and side effects
buspirone (BuSpar)	15–30 mg	Slow onset, rapid distribution	3 – 11	Give with food No dependency

Adapted from McEvoy, R. B. (ed.). (2000). *Facts and comparisons 2000.* St. Louis: Facts and Comparisons, A Wolters Kluwer Company.

orders will be discussed along with each disorder (Sullivan & Coplan, 2000).

Serotonin (5-HT), the indolamine neurotransmitter usually implicated in psychosis and mood disorders, has many subtypes. 5-HT1a plays a role in anxiety, as well as affecting aggression and mood. Serotonin is believed to play a distinct role in OCD, panic disorder, and generalized anxiety disorder. A norepinephrine excess is suspected in panic disorder, generalized anxiety disorder, and posttraumatic stress disorder (Sullivan & Coplan, 2000).

Psychodynamic Theories

INTRAPSYCHIC/PSYCHOANALYTIC

Freud (1936) saw a person's innate anxiety as the stimulus for behavior. He described defense mechanisms as the human's attempt to control awareness of anxiety. For example, if a person has inappropriate thoughts and feelings that raise anxiety, he or she represses them. Repression is the process of filing these inappropriate impulses into the unconscious so they cannot be recalled. Imagine placing a problem into a box, tying the lid on with string, and storing the box in the back of a closet. The knot on this "repression box" can come undone at any point and the problem resurfaces, invading the person's behavior, thoughts, dreams, feelings, and needs. Because all behavior has meaning, anxiety symptoms signal incomplete repression. People with anxiety disorders were believed to overuse one or a specific pattern of several defense mechanisms, stranding them in one of Freud's psychosexual developmental levels.

INTERPERSONAL THEORY

Harry Stack Sullivan (1952) viewed anxiety as being generated from problems in interpersonal relationships. Caregivers can communicate anxiety to an infant or child by inadequate nurturing, agitation in holding or handling the child, and distorted messages. This means of communicating anxiety from one person to another is called empathy. The anxiety empathized by the infant or child can result in dysfunction, such as failure to achieve age-appropriate developmental tasks. In adults, anxiety arises from the person's need to conform to the norms and values of his or her cultural group. The higher the level of anxiety, the lower the ability to communicate and solve problems and the greater chance for anxiety disorders to develop.

Hildegard Peplau (1952) understood that humans existed in interpersonal and physiologic realms; thus, the nurse can better help the client achieve health by attending to both areas. She developed nursing interventions and interpersonal communica-

tion techniques based on Sullivan's interpersonal view of anxiety as empathized and guided the person to use the energy that arose from anxiety to learn and change. Nurses today use Peplau-inspired interpersonal therapeutic communication techniques to develop and nurture the nurse–client relationship and apply the nursing process.

BEHAVIORAL THEORY

Behavioral theorists view anxiety as being learned through one's experiences. Conversely, behaviors can be changed or "unlearned" through new experiences. Behaviorists believe one can modify maladaptive behaviors without gaining insight into the causes of these behaviors. They contend that disturbing behaviors that develop and interfere with a person's life can be extinguished or unlearned by repeated experiences guided by a trained therapist.

PANIC DISORDER

A panic attack is 15- to 30-minute episode of rapid, intense, escalating anxiety in which the person experiences great emotional fear as well as physiologic discomfort. During a panic attack, the person has overwhelmingly intense anxiety and displays four or more of the following symptoms: palpitations, sweating, tremors, shortness of breath, sense of suffocation, chest pain, nausea, abdominal distress, dizziness, paresthesias, chills, or hot flashes.

Panic disorder is diagnosed when the person has recurrent, unexpected panic attacks followed by at least 1 month of persistent concern or worry about having future attacks or worry about their meaning, or a significant behavioral change related to them, when these symptoms are not due to substance abuse or another mental disorder. Slightly more than 75% of people with panic disorder have spontaneous initial attacks with no environmental trigger. The rest have a panic attacks stimulated by a phobic stimulus or are under the influence of a substance that alters the central nervous system and stimulates the same hormonal, organ, and vital sign responses that occur in panic attacks (Keltner et al., 1998).

The prevalence of panic disorder in a given year is 1% to 2%. The lifetime rate is 1.5% to 3.5%. Half of those with panic disorder have accompanying agoraphobia. Panic disorder is more common in people who have not graduated from college and people who are not married. The risk is increased by 18% in depressed persons (Horwath & Weissman, 2000).

Onset and Clinical Course

The onset of panic disorder peaks in late adolescence and in the mid-30s (Keltner et al., 1998). Although

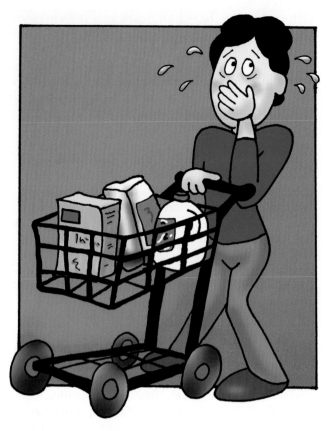

Panic attack

> ▶ SYMPTOMS OF PANIC DISORDER

Recurrent panic attacks are intermittent episodes of the highest level of anxiety or fear, lasting 15 to 30 minutes, with four or more of the following:
- Rapid, pounding heart, or severely increased heart rate
- Sweating
- Quivering, shakiness
- Sense of being unable to breathe
- Choking sensation
- Pain in chest
- Nausea or gastrointestinal distress
- Lightheadedness, dizziness, or faintness
- Sense things are unreal (derealization) or a sense of being disconnected from oneself (depersonalization)
- Worry about going insane or of losing control
- Fear of imminent death
- Tingling or numbness in body
- Hot flashes, chillingly cold
- Worry about the recurrence of a panic attack, staying away from places or people where or with whom panic attacks occurred.

panic is normal in someone experiencing a life-threatening situation, a person with panic disorder experiences these emotional and physiologic responses without this stimulus.

Cultural Considerations

Panic attacks experienced by Latin Americans and Northern Europeans often involve sensations of choking, smothering, numbness, or tingling, as well as fear of dying. Teas of spearmint, chamomile, orange leaves, or sweet basil are used to treat various types of anxiety disorders in some Hispanic groups (Spector, 2000).

Etiology

BIOLOGIC THEORIES

Panic disorder may be genetically inherited. In monozygotic twins, there is a 31% chance that one twin will have panic disorder if the other has it. The rate in first-degree relatives is 15%.

When it was noted that people with anxiety disorders had a greater incidence of anxiety disorder manifestations after vigorous exercise, Pitts and McClure (1967) infused sodium lactate into people with anxiety attacks and found that 13 of 14 had a panic attack after the infusion. Reiman et al. (1989) and Grinspoon (1996) described the use of sodium lactate, carbon dioxide, and caffeine to stimulate panic attacks and found parahippocampal abnormalities. The parahippocampal gyrus (an area of the cerebral cortex associated with the limbic system) showed increased blood flow when persons with panic disorder were challenged with these substances. No effect was seen in the cerebral blood flow of normal persons or those with panic disorders who showed no sensitivity to lactate, suggesting that lactate sensitivity may be associated with only some types of panic disorder. Panic attacks may be initiated when the parahippocampal gyrus is activated by norepinephrine pathways.

The symptoms of a panic attack, such as increased heart rate, are the same as those seen with increased levels of norepinephrine release. Drugs such as yohimbine block the binding receptors of norepinephrine, and anxiety increases. Clonidine, which aids receptor binding of norepinephrine, decreases anxiety symptoms. Serotonin dysfunction is being evaluated, because selective serotonin reuptake inhibitors (SSRIs) have been found to be helpful in the treatment of panic disorder. Adenosine, a purine neurotransmitter that reduces the release of most of the other neurotransmitters, may be implicated in panic disorder. Caffeine, which affects the adenosine receptor, produces anxiety in many people but creates full-scale panic attacks in some people with panic disorder.

Researchers are assessing the role of adenosine receptor agonists in many anxiety disorders (Keltner et al., 1998).

Psychoanalytic

Information that has been repressed into the unconscious can begin to emerge into the conscious mind. This information results in conflict from any of four sources: *superego anxiety*, the guilt felt by the person who has socially and personally inappropriate impulses, and punishment types of conflicts if this information were to become known; *castration anxiety*, related to the fantasy of genital or body mutilation; *separation anxiety*, about the potential loss of significant others; and *id anxiety*, or destruction of the person. The psychoanalytic goal is to face the conflict to assess the true source of anxiety and then intervene (Freud, 1936).

Treatment and Prognosis

Behavioral therapy has been effective in dealing with anxiety disorders, especially when combined with pharmacotherapy (Mavissakalian & Michelson, 1986).

PSYCHOTHERAPY

Several techniques are used by behavioral psychotherapists. **Positive reframing** means turning negative messages into positive messages. The therapist teaches the person to create positive messages to use during panic episodes. For example, instead of thinking, "My heart is pounding. I think I'm going to die!" the client thinks, "I can slow my heart rate. This is just anxiety." These messages can be written down and kept readily accessible, such as in an address book or calendar or on a card in a wallet. **Assertiveness training** helps the person take more control over life situations. Assertiveness training techniques help the person negotiate interpersonal situations and foster self-assurance.

PSYCHOPHARMACOLOGY

Four categories of drugs are used to treat panic disorder: SSRIs, tricyclic antidepressants (TCAs) or heterocyclic antidepressants, benzodiazepine anxiolytics, and monoamine oxidase inhibitor antidepressants (MAOIs).

SSRIs. In general, SSRI antidepressants are the most effective drugs used for treating panic disorders with or without agoraphobia. They are nonaddictive. When given for at least 6 to 18 months and with slow tapering off, the relapse rate is 23%.

SSRIs should not be given concurrently with MAOIs, because this can cause a hypertensive crisis. The MAOI should be discontinued 3 to 5 weeks before starting the SSRI to avoid a hypertensive crisis.

Fluoxetine (Prozac), with a half-life of 4 to 16 days, has been found effective in treating panic disorder in once-weekly doses (Emmanuel et al., in press). Other SSRIs include paroxetine (Paxil), sertraline (Zoloft), and citalopram (Celexa) (Table 12-3).

Anxiolytics. Benzodiazepine anxiolytics are used for a short period (4 weeks or less) and then tapered because of habituation. Anxiolytics, such as alprazolam (Xanax; short-acting) and clonazepam (Klonopin; long-acting, has antiseizure properties), can be used for short-term treatment but must be tapered after a few weeks to a few months because they can cause dependence (see Table 12-3).

Antidepressants. TCAs, an earlier class of antidepressants, are effective in treating panic disorder. They are nonaddictive, and long-term treatment is recommended. TCAs are thought to work by blocking the reuptake of norepinephrine and serotonin. TCAs should not be given concurrently with MAOIs; this can cause a hypertensive crisis. The MAOI should be discontinued 3 to 5 weeks before starting the TCA. There is a lag period of 1 to 3 weeks before TCAs reach serum levels high enough to reduce panic attacks.

MAOIs. The MAOI phenelzine (Nardil) inhibits symptoms of panic disorder (Keltner & Folks, 1997).

APPLICATION OF THE NURSING PROCESS: PANIC DISORDER

Assessment

THOUGHTS, AFFECT, JUDGMENT, AND MOTOR BEHAVIOR

Cognitively, the person feels unreal and detached from the self, fears losing control or going insane, feels like he or she is dying, and has a temporarily disorganized thought process with illogical outcomes. For instance, a young woman has been driving the speed limit of 55 m.p.h. on a toll road starts to have a panic attack. She speeds up to 88 m.p.h. until she sees toll booths and then swerves to a stop at the office building, hysterically trying to get into the locked office because she believes she is dying. Typically during a panic attack, the person attempts to flee from the severe emotions and frightening physiologic responses. Less typically, the person shows the fight or freeze responses distinctive to panic-level anxiety.

Table 12-3

DRUGS USED TO TREAT PANIC DISORDER

Generic Name (Brand Name)	Type	Dose	Nursing Implications
fluoxetine (Prozac)	SSRI	Adult: 20 mg in AM Geriatric: 5–10 mg Max adult dose 80 mg/day	Side effects: headache, nausea/vomiting, dizziness, insomnia, nervousness Monitor for weight loss Increases half-life of diazepam

sertraline (Zoloft)	SSRI	Adult: 50 mg/day
		Geriatric: 25 mg/day
		Give in AM or PM to avoid nighttime insomnia
		Max dose of 200 mg/day
			Side effects: agitation, insomnia, headache, dizziness, somnolence, fatigue
			Monitor
			  Liver function tests
			  Sodium & fluid/geriatric
			  Prothrombin time on warfarin therapy
			Reduces clearance of diazepam and tolbutamide

fluvoxamine (Luvox)	SSRI	Adult: 50 mg hs Geriatric: 25 mg hs	Side effects: headache, insomnia, drowsiness, weight loss, tremor, nervousness, light-headedness, nausea/vomiting, sexual dysfunction, upper respiratory infection, urinary frequency, constipation Monitor liver & renal function
imipramine (Tofranil)	TCA	Adult: 10 mg/day	Side effects: orthostatic hypotension, sedation, confusion, constipation, dry mouth.
nortriptyline (Pamelor)	TCA	Adult: 25 mg tid Geriatric: 10 mg bid or tid	Side effects: sedation, dry mouth, constipation, nausea/vomiting, orthostatic hypotension, seizures, disturbed concentration, confusion
alprazolam (Xanax) (Schedule IV)	Anxiolytic	Adult: 0.25 mg tid; max 24-hour dose 10 mg Geriatric: 0.25 mg bid; max dose 4.5 mg/day Dosage increases made slowly.	Side effects: drowsiness, sedation, depression, lethargy, apathy, fatigue, lightheadedness, anger, hostility, confusion, crying, constipation, drug dependence withdrawal syndrome Tapered gradually No alcohol, hypnotics.
clonazepam (Klonopin) (Schedule IV)	Anxiolytic	Adult: 0.5 bid or tid; max dose 20 mg/day	Side effects: drowsiness, sedation, depression, lethargy, apathy, fatigue, lightheadedness, anger, hostility, confusion, crying, constipation, drug dependence withdrawal syndrome Tapered gradually No alcohol, hypnotics Sedating: give larger doses hs
phenelzine (Nardil)	MAOI	Adult: 45–60 mg; max dose 90 mg/day	Side effects: sedation, weight gain, sexual dysfunction

Adapted from McEvoy, R. B. (Ed.) (2000). *Facts and comparisons 2000.* St. Louis: Facts and Comparisons, A Wolters Kluwer Company.

Judgment is suspended during panic attacks; in an effort to escape, the person can run out of a building and into the street in front of a speeding car before the ability to assess safety has returned.

SELF-CONCEPT

Because of the intense anticipatory fear of having another panic attack, the person begins to alter his or her social, occupational, or family life. The person typically avoids people, places, and events associated with previous panic attacks. For example, the person may no longer ride the bus if he or she once had a panic attack on a bus. Although avoiding these objects does not stop the panic attacks, the person's sense of helplessness is so great that he or she may take even more drastic steps to avoid panic. In some cases, the person becomes homebound or stays in a limited area near home, such as on the block or within town limits. This behavior is known as panic

Box 12-2

> ## HAMILTON RATING SCALE FOR ANXIETY

Instructions: This checklist is to assist the physician or psychiatrist in evaluating each patient as to his degree of anxiety and pathological condition. Please fill in the appropriate rating:

NONE = 0 MILD = 1 MODERATE = 2 SEVERE = 3 SEVERE, GROSSLY DISABLING = 4

Item		Rating	Item		Rating
Anxious mood	Worries, anticipation of the worst, fearful anticipation, irritability	____	Cardiovascular symptoms	Tachycardia, palpitations, pain in chest, throbbing of vessels, fainting feelings, missing beat	____
Tension	Feelings of tension, fatigability, startle response, moved to tears easily, trembling, feelings of restlessness, inability to relax	____	Respiratory symptoms	Pressure or constriction in chest, choking feelings, sighing, dyspnea	____
Fears	Of dark, of strangers, of being left alone, of animals, of traffic, of crowds	____	Gastrointestinal symptoms	Difficulty in swallowing, wind, abdominal pain, burning sensations, abdominal fullness, nausea, vomiting, borborygmi, looseness of bowels, loss of weight, constipation	____
Insomnia	Difficulty in falling asleep, broken sleep, unsatisfying sleep and fatigue on waking, dreams, nightmares, night-terrors	____	Genitourinary symptoms	Frequency of micturition, urgency of micturition, amenorrhea, menorrhagia, development of frigidity, premature ejaculation, loss of libido, impotence	____
Intellectual (cognitive)	Difficulty in concentration, poor memory	____			
Depressed mood	Loss of interest, lack of pleasure in hobbies, depression, early waking, diurnal swing	____	Autonomic symptoms	Dry mouth, flushing, pallor, tendency to sweat, giddiness, tension headache, raising of hair	____
Somatic (muscular)	Pains and aches, twitching, stiffness, myoclonic jerks, grinding of teeth, unsteady voice, increased muscular tone	____	Behavior at interview	Fidgetting, restlessness or pacing, tremor of hands, furrowed brow, strained face, sighing or rapid respiration, facial pallor, swallowing, belching, brisk tendon jerks, dilated pupils, exophthalmos	____
Somatic (sensory)	Tinnitus, blurring of vision, hot and cold flushes, feelings of weakness, picking sensation	____			

ADDITIONAL COMMENTS: _____

Investigator's signature: _____

disorder with **agoraphobia** ("fear of the market-place," or fear of being outside). Some sufferers fear stepping outside the front door, because a panic attack may occur as soon as they are outside. Others can leave the house but feel safe from the anticipatory fear of having a panic attack only within a limited area. Many times these clients come to the attention of health care professionals because they or their family fear that they are having a heart attack.

The behavior patterns of persons with agoraphobia clearly demonstrate the concepts of primary and secondary gain that are associated with many of the anxiety disorders. **Primary gain** is the relief of anxiety achieved by performing the specific anxiety-driven behavior—for example, staying in the house to avoid the anxiety of leaving a safe place. **Secondary gain** is the attention received from others as a result of having these behaviors. For instance, the person with agoraphobia may receive attention and caring concern from family members, who also assume all of the responsibilities of family life outside of the home (work, shopping, and so forth). Essentially, these compassionate significant others become enablers of the agoraphobic person's self-imprisonment.

Data Analysis

The following nursing diagnoses may apply to the client with panic disorder:

- Risk for Injury
- Anxiety
- Fear
- Social Isolation
- Self Esteem Disturbance
- Ineffective Individual Coping
- Powerlessness
- Role Performance, Altered
- Sleep Pattern Disturbance

Outcome Identification

During this phase of treatment, outcomes are related to stabilizing the client's panic response and identifying triggers for panic. This is also a time to evaluate resources and make referrals. Outcomes vary based on the nursing diagnosis chosen. For example, for Sleep Pattern Disturbance, the outcome would be that the client can sleep through the night without awakening. Other examples of outcomes appropriate to panic disorder are as follows:

1. The client will be free of injury to self or others.
2. The client will communicate effectively.
3. The client will demonstrate use of effective coping mechanisms.
4. The client will verbalize knowledge of panic disorder.
5. The client will verbalize a sense of personal control.

Intervention

PROMOTING SAFETY AND COMFORT

The nurse's first concerns is to provide a safe environment and to ensure the client's privacy. If the environment is unsafe or overstimulating, the client

---

▶ SYMPTOMS OF PANIC DISORDER WITH AGORAPHOBIA

Client experiences highest level of anxiety or fear, lasting 15 to 30 minutes with four or more of the symptoms of panic disorder, in addition to the following symptoms:
- Fear of places or situations in which the person believes a panic attack or embarrassing behavior might occur or from which escape is believed impossible
- Avoidance of these places or situations; extreme distress if these situations are unavoidable
- Person is aware response is extreme.

▶ SYMPTOMS OF AGORAPHOBIA WITHOUT PANIC DISORDER

- Intense worry about developing panic-like behaviors when outside the home (or the block or the town where one lives) being with other people in a non-home environment, or traveling
- Avoidance of these situations or tolerance only under great stress and fear. May require accompaniment by another person to attempt these situations.
- Person knows response is extreme.

should move to a safer or quieter place. A quiet place reduces anxiety and provides privacy for the client.

The nurse should remain with the client to help calm him or her down and to assess client behaviors and concerns. After getting the client's attention, the nurse uses a soothing, calm voice and gives brief directions to assure the client that he or she is safe: "John, look around. It's safe, and I'm here with you. Nothing is going to happen. Take a deep breath." Reassurances and a calm demeanor can help reduce the client's fears.

THERAPEUTIC RELATIONSHIP AND THERAPEUTIC COMMUNICATION

Clients with anxiety disorders can collaborate with the nurse in the assessment and planning of their care; thus, the rapport between the nurse and the client is important. Using the therapeutic relationship, the nurse can assess the client's behaviors, needs, situational supports, and milieu to begin planning care. The nurse must establish trust and show unconditional positive regard and genuineness. As the client begins to trust the nurse, together they can begin to plan care.

To establish a therapeutic relationship, the nurse uses the therapeutic communication skills discussed in Chapter 6. Communication should be simple and calm, because the client with severe anxiety cannot pay attention to lengthy messages and may pace to release energy. The nurse should verbally recognize the client's behavior but calmly explain that such behaviors are methods to release anxiety and the energy related to sudden neurotransmitter release. By acknowledging the client's behavior in a calm, nonjudgmental fashion, the nurse expresses unconditional positive regard and genuine interest, helping the client understand that the response is a physiologic one that can be controlled. The nurse should not touch a person with high anxiety: the client may interpret touch by a stranger as a threat and pull away abruptly.

As the client's anxiety diminishes, cognition begins to return. When anxiety has subsided to a manageable level, the nurse uses open-ended communication techniques to discuss the experience:

Nurse: *"It seems your anxiety is subsiding. Is that correct?"* or *"Can you share with me what it was like a few minutes ago?"*

At this point, the client can talk about his or her emotional responses to physiologic processes and behaviors and can try to regain a sense of control.

CLIENT AND FAMILY TEACHING

The nurse can teach the client relaxation techniques to use when he or she is experiencing stress or anxiety. Guided imagery and progressive relaxation are methods to relax taut muscles. Guided imagery involves imagining a safe, enjoyable place to relax. In progressive relaxation, the person progressively tightens, holds, then relaxes muscle groups while letting tension flow out of the body through rhythmic breathing. Thought-stopping is a technique in which the client forcefully orders himself or herself to stop the irrational fears or panicky thoughts, such as believing he or she is dying, cannot breathe, or needs to escape or run. For example, the client may command the heart to stop pounding or command breathing to return to normal. In meditation, another means of thought-stopping, the person ignores distracting thoughts and feelings and uses a repeated word or sound to center his or her thoughts.

Client and family education is of primary importance when working with clients who have anxiety disorders. The client learns ways to manage stress and cope with reactions to stress and stress-provoking situations. With education about the efficacy of combined psychotherapy and medication and the effects of the prescribed medication, the client can become the chief treatment manager of the anxiety disorder. It is important for the nurse to educate the client and family members about the physiology of the anxiety disorder and the merits of using combined psychotherapy and drug management. Such a combined treatment

> ▶ **NURSING INTERVENTIONS FOR CLIENTS WITH PANIC DISORDER**

- Help client focus on breathing slowly and coach to breathe in tandem.
- Help the client maintain regular and balanced eating habits.
- Identify early symptoms and teach the client to use distraction behaviors such as talking to another person, engaging in physical activity (walking, gardening, cleaning), performing repetitive activities (snapping a rubber band against the wrist, counting backwards, reading street signs).
- Help client use preplanned and rehearsed positive self-talk.
- Engage client in exploring how to decrease stressors and anxiety-provoking situations.

approach, along with stress-reduction techniques, can help the client manage these drastic reactions and allow him or her to gain a sense of self-control. The knowledge that one can gain control of one's life again boosts self-esteem and increases compliance with the treatment regimen. The nurse should help the client understand that these therapies and drugs do not "cure" the disorder but are methods to help him or her control and manage it. Client and family teaching regarding medications should include the recommended dosage and the dosage regimen, expected effects, side effects and how to handle them, and substances that have a synergistic or antagonistic effect with the drug.

The nurse should encourage the client to engage in regular exercise, which helps metabolize adrenalin, reduces panic reactions, and increases production of endorphins, which increase feelings of well-being.

Evaluation

Evaluation of the plan of care must be individualized. Ongoing assessment provides data to determine whether the client's outcomes were achieved. The client's perception of the success of treatment also plays a part in evaluation. Even if all outcomes are achieved, the nurse must ask whether the client is comfortable or satisfied with the quality of life.

Evaluation of the treatment of anxiety disorders is based on the following:

- Does the client understand the prescribed medication regimen, and is the client committed to adhere to it?
- Have the client's episodes of anxiety decreased in frequency or intensity?
- Does the client understand various coping methods and when to use them?
- Does the client believe that his or her quality of life is satisfactory?

PHOBIAS

A **phobia** is an illogical, intense, persistent fear of a specific object or a social situation that causes ex-

treme distress and interferes with normal life functioning. Phobias are vastly different from the anxiety and fear stimulated by a real-life situation or threat, such as facing a snarling guard dog or hearing someone trying to get in your apartment door. Phobias are not the natural and realistic responses used in trying to protect one's personal safety. Most phobic objects are usually not threatening to the person's well-being, but the person believes that encountering this object will bring great harm. People with phobias understand that their fear is unusual and irrational and may even joke about how "silly" their behavior is, but they feel powerless to stop it (Burgess, 1997).

People with phobias develop **anticipatory anxiety** even when thinking about the possibility of encountering the dreaded phobic object, and they engage in unusual ritualistic behaviors to attempt to avoid it. For example, a person who has a germ phobia may ritualistically wash his or her hands continuously throughout the day. When these ritualistic behaviors are performed, the person's anxiety is reduced. This feeling of reduced anxiety is the primary gain of performing these ritualistic behaviors. The secondary gain is the attention and assistance the phobic person receives from others.

A specific phobia is an irrational fear of an object (phobic object) or situation, such as an insect or animal, small rooms, water, elevators, or flying. The object or situation causes the person extreme anxiety or produces a panic response when he or she is confronted with it. Other common phobic objects include fear of storms or heights, tunnels, bridges, or even invasive medical procedures. The person takes great trouble to avoid the phobic object; when he or she is faced with the phobic object and unable to escape, he or she experiences symptoms that range from great discomfort to a severe panic attack (DSM-IV-TR, 2000). Often the phobic object is very specific and can be avoided with relative ease. The diagnosis of a phobic disorder is made only when the phobic behavior significantly interferes with the person's life, creating marked distress or difficulty in interpersonal or occupational functioning.

▶ CLIENT AND FAMILY TEACHING: PANIC DISORDER

- Breathing control and relaxation techniques
- Positive coping strategies
- Importance of maintaining prescribed medication regimen and regular follow-up
- Time management techniques such as "to do" lists with realistic estimated time for each activity, crossing off completed items for a sense of accomplishment, and saying "no"
- Counseling and education of family/significant others about biologic causes
- Importance of maintaining contact with community and participation in supportive organizations.

Clinical Vignette: Panic Disorder

Nancy spent as much time in her friend Jennifer's condo as she did in her own home. It was at Jen's place that Nancy had her first panic attack. For no reason at all, she felt the walls closing in on her, no air to breathe, and her heart pounding out of her chest. She needed to get out—Hurry! Run!—so she could live. While a small, still-rational part of her mind assured her there was no reason to run, the need to flee was overwhelming. She ran out of the apartment and down the hall, repeatedly smashing the elevator button with the heel of her hand in hopes of instant response. "What if the elevator doesn't come?" Where were the stairs she so desperately wanted but couldn't find?

The elevator door slid open. Scurrying in the cubicle and not realizing she had been holding her breath, Nancy exhaled with momentary relief. She had the faint perception of someone following her to ask, "What's wrong?" She couldn't answer! She couldn't breathe—again.

Mutely gaping, she held onto the rail on the wall of the elevator. It was the only way to keep herself from falling. "Breathe," she commanded, as she forced herself to inhale. She searched for the right button to push, the one for the ground floor. She couldn't make a mistake, couldn't push the wrong button, couldn't have the elevator take more time, because she might not make it. Heart pounding, no air, run, run!—a mantra she could respond to only in the most primitive ways. With no time for relief when the doors opened, she saw the ground-floor lobby. She ran outside and then bent forward, her hands on her knees. It took 5 minutes for her to realize she was safe and would be OK. Sliding onto a bench, breathing more easily, she sat there long enough for her heart rate to decrease. Exhausted and scared by what had just happened, she wondered, "Is it my heart? Am I going crazy?"

Instead of returning to Jen's, Nancy walked across the street to her own apartment. She couldn't face going into Jen's place until she recovered. She sincerely hoped she would never have this happen to her again; in fact, it might not be a good idea to go to Jen's for a few days or more. As she sat there reasoning out what had happened to her that afternoon and figuring out ways to make sure this horrifying experience never recurred, she realized she might not ever never be able to return to Jen's condo, because this could never happen again.

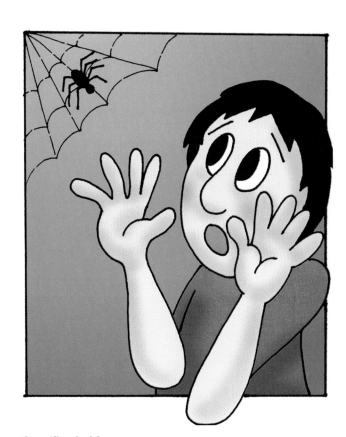

Specific phobias

There are several categories of specific phobias:
- Natural environmental phobias: fear of storms, water, heights, or other natural phenomena
- Blood-injection phobias: fear of seeing one's own or others' blood, traumatic injury, or an invasive medical procedure, such as an injection. There is usually a strong vasovagal response and the person faints. Some people in this category have a phobic response to warning announcements about danger.
- Situational phobias: fear of being in a specific situation, such as a bridge, tunnel, elevator, small room, hospital, or airplane
- Animal phobia: fear of animals or insects, usually a specific one. Often this fear develops in childhood, and it can continue through adulthood in both men and women. Cats and dogs are the most common phobic objects.
- Other types of specific phobias, for example, the fear of getting lost while driving if not able to make all right (and no left) turns to get to one's destination.

In social phobia, a different category of phobia, the person becomes severely anxious to the point of panic or incapacitation when confronted with situations

Box 12-3

> **COMMON PHOBIAS**

Heights	acrophobia	Reptiles	herpetophobia
Open spaces	agoraphobia	Fish	ichthiophobia
Cats	ailurophobia	Germs	microphobia
Pain	algophobia	Mice	muronophobia
Flowers	anthophobia	Dirt	mysophobia
Bees	apiphobia or melissophobia	Numbers	numerophobia
Water	aquaphobia	Night, darkness	nyctophobia
Spiders	arachnophobia	Snakes	ophidiophobia
Lightning	astraphobia	Poverty	peniaphobia
Being alone	autophobia, eremophobia	Ghosts	phasmophobia
Needles	belonophobia	Loud noises	phonophobia
Slime	blennophobia	Light	photophobia
Thunder	brontophobia	Smothering	pnigerophobia
Closed spaces	claustrophobia	Fire	pyrophobia
Feces	coprophobia	Trains	siderodromophobia
Dogs	cynophobia	Buried alive	taphophobia
Mental illness	dementophobia, lyssophobia	Death	thanatophobia
Insects	entomophobia	Hair	trichophobia
Horses	equinophobia	Stage fright	topophobia
Bridge crossing	gephyrophobia	#13	triskaidekaphobia
Sun	heliophobia	Strangers	xenophobia
Blood	hematophobia	Animals	zoophobia

involving people, such as making a speech, attending a social engagement alone, interacting with the opposite sex or with strangers, and making complaints (DSM-IV-TR, 2000). The fear revolves around low self-esteem and concern about others' judgments about one's performance. The person is afraid of being embarrassed, being socially inept, appearing anxious, or doing something embarrassing, such as burping or hiccuping. Other social phobias include fear of eating in public, using public bathrooms, writing in public, or becoming the center of attention. A person may have one or several social phobias; the latter is known as generalized social phobia.

> **SYMPTOMS OF SPECIFIC PHOBIA**

- Irrational fear of an object, such as an animal, the environment (water, storms, heights), an invasive medical procedure, or situation (bridges, tunnels, small rooms, elevators, flying)
- Instant 3+ anxiety to 4+ panic response to feared object
- Client knows response is extreme and excessive to the situation.
- Elaborate avoidance of phobic object
- Behaviors interfere with interpersonal relationships, work performance, or other life activities.

Onset and Clinical Course

Specific phobia occurs more often in women than in men; social phobia occurs equally in the sexes, although it is believed that men seek help more frequently for this phobia. Peak onset times are early childhood and the mid-20s. Specific phobias usually occur in people who are otherwise emotionally normal. In some cases, merely thinking about the dreaded object or handling a plastic model of the object can create a fearful response. The person understands that the phobia is unreasonable but usually feels unable to do anything about it. In some cases the phobias spontaneously remit; in other clients they are lifelong processes, and the person attempts to rationalize the cause. For example, a woman who is terrified of cats may rationalize her fears by saying that as a child, her mother told her to keep the family cat away from the baby, because the cat would smell milk on the baby's breath, would try to lick the milk, and would steal the baby's breath.

Cultural Considerations

Culturally significant taboos must not be interpreted as phobias. For example, some cultures believe in magic or in spirit power. A person from such a culture should not be diagnosed as having a phobia if he or she fears spirits or magic, unless the fear is unusual even in the context of that culture.

> ## ▶ SYMPTOMS OF SOCIAL PHOBIA
>
> - Ongoing and irrational fear of public speaking or other social circumstances (eating, drinking, using public restrooms, writing, meeting new people, speaking to strangers)
> - Fears of humiliating self in front of peers or in situations when client feels others will be appraising his or her behavior or poise
> - Severe to panic response (3+ to 4+) when exposed to feared social situation
> - Client understands fear is extreme and excessive.
> - Behaviors significantly interfere with inter-personal relationships, work performance, or other life activities.

Etiology

BIOLOGIC

Phobias occur more often within families: identical twins have a higher concordance rate of phobias than the general population, and there is a three times higher concordance rate of phobias in first-degree relatives (Andreasen & Black, 1995). Yonkers and Gurguis (1995) hypothesized that women have higher rates of phobias than men because of hormone functions or the activities of neurotransmitters on the central nervous system.

Marks (1966) and McNally (1987) each proposed that certain people have an innate susceptibility to phobic reactions. Oltmanns & Emery (1998) demonstrated a biologic timetable of phobias related to a person's developmental level, such as the startle reflex of the infant, fear of being left by one's mother at age 3, fear of animals at age 5, and fear of social situations in adolescence.

PSYCHODYNAMIC THEORIES

The psychoanalytic view of phobias focuses on a threat of aggression from the same-sex parent because of the child's incestual feelings toward the opposite-sex parent. In this oedipal conflict, the child represses the fear of hostility and displaces it onto another object, which is neutral and easy to avoid. This neutral object, which represents the feared parent, now becomes the phobic stimulus.

Cognitive theorists believe that phobias arise from faulty thinking, such as the person who makes negative statements about himself or herself and holds irrational beliefs. Although the person functions within the boundaries of reality and rational thinking,

the slice of cognition related to the phobia is the irrational portion. The person can often laugh at the phobia, but he or she feels unable to do anything about it.

Social learning theorists believe that phobic people have an external locus of control: "I can't control the environment, so why bother?" Conversely, a person with an internal locus of control believes he or she can control what happens in the future, and when confronted with an unplanned event feels capable of controlling the situation and directing it to a favorable outcome (Johnson & Sarason, 1978).

Learning theorists believe that fears can be learned by modeling: in other words, children are more apt to perform behaviors they have seen enacted, such as fear of cats, germs, or strangers (Bandura, 1973). Observing intense fear reactions is believed to create phobic learning (for example, fear of lightning and thunder, fear of darkness). Specific phobias may be secondary to life experiences and can roughly symbolize that experience: for example, an adult who as a child slipped through thin ice and nearly drowned is now afraid of being in water and never learned to swim. However, phobic people often attempt to rationalize their phobia by attaching it to some reasonable-sounding life event.

Treatment and Prognosis

PSYCHOPHARMACOLOGY

Anxiolytics (see Tables 12-2 and 12-4) can help people with social phobias. Alprazolam (Xanax) is a benzodiazepine useful in the short-term treatment of phobias. The dosage must be increased and decreased gradually; it can be habit-forming. SSRIs have been approved for use in phobias. For example, sertraline (Zoloft) and paroxetine (Paxil) reduce anxiety in social phobic situations. Propranolol hydrochloride (Inderal), a beta blocker, is commonly used to reduce heart rate and lower blood pressure and also diminishes stage fright and fear of public speaking (McEvoy, 2000).

PSYCHOTHERAPY

Behavioral therapy works well in the treatment of phobias. The behavioral therapist initially focuses on teaching what anxiety is, helping the client identify his or her anxiety responses, teaching relaxation techniques, setting goals, discussing methods used to achieve those goals, and helping the client to visualize phobic situations. Therapies that help the client develop self-esteem and self-control are often used, including positive reframing and assertiveness training (explained earlier).

One behavioral therapy often used to treat phobias is **systematic** (serial) **desensitization,** in which

Table 12-4

DRUGS USED FOR PHOBIAS

Type	Generic Name (Brand Name)	Dose Range	Nursing Implications
AGORAPHOBIA			
Anxiolytic	alprazolam (Xanax) (Schedule IV)	Adult: 0.25 mg tid; max 24-hour dose 10 mg Geriatric: 0.25 mg bid; max 24-hour dose 4.5 mg Dosage increases made slowly	Side effects: drowsiness, sedation, depression, lethargy, apathy, fatigue, lightheadedness, anger, hostility, confusion, crying, constipation, drug dependence, withdrawal syndrome. Tapered gradually. No alcohol, hypnotics.
TCA	imipramine (Tofranil)	Adult: 75–100 mg; max dose 300 mg/day	Side effects: orthostatic hypotension, sedation, confusion, constipation, dry mouth
PERFORMANCE ANXIETY			
	propranolol (Inderal)	Adult: 10–80 mg 2 hours before performance	Reduced heart rate, tremor, dry mouth, queasy stomach, and anxiety. Side effects: fatigue, confusion, drowsiness
	sertraline (Zoloft)	Adult: 50 mg/day Geriatric: 25 mg/day Give in AM or PM to avoid nightime insomnia. Increase prn q 2 weeks to max dose of 200 mg	Side effects: agitation, insomnia, headache, dizziness, somnolence, fatigue Liver function tests Sodium & fluid/geriatric PT on warfarin Rx Reduces clearance of diazepam and tolbutamide
	buspirone (BuSpar)	15–45 mg in divided doses max dose 60 mg/day	Side effects: dizziness, headache, drowsiness. ALT/AST. Lag period, can take up to 12 weeks to relieve phobic symptoms. May displace digoxin at binding sites.
	alprazolam (Xanax) (Schedule IV)	Adult: 0.25 mg tid; max 24-hour dose 10 mg Geriatric: 0.25 mg bid; max 24-hour dose 4.5 mg Dosage increases made slowly	Side effects: drowsiness, sedation, depression, lethargy, apathy, fatigue, lightheadedness, anger, hostility, confusion, crying, constipation, drug dependence, withdrawal syndrome. Tapered gradually. No alcohol, hypnotics.
	clonazepam (Klonopin) (Schedule IV)	Adult: 0.5 bid or tid; max 24-hour dose 20 mg	Side effects: drowsiness, sedation, depression, lethargy, apathy, fatigue, lightheadedness, anger, hostility, confusion, crying, constipation, drug dependence, withdrawal syndrome. Tapered gradually. No alcohol, hypnotics. Sedating: give larger doses

Adapted from McEvoy, R. B. (Ed.) (2000). *Facts and comparisons 2000*. St. Louis: Facts and Comparisons, A Wolters Kluwer Company.

the client is progressively exposed to the threatening object, in a safe setting, until his or her anxiety is reduced. During each exposure, the complexity and intensity of exposure gradually increase, but each time the client's anxiety is reduced. The reduced anxiety serves as a positive reinforcement until the anxiety is ultimately eliminated. For example, for the client who fears flying, the therapist would encourage the client to hold a small model airplane while talking about his or her experiences; later, the client would talk about flying while holding a larger model airplane. Later exposures might include walking past an airport, sitting in a parked airplane, and finally taking a short ride in the plane. Each session's challenge is based on the success achieved in previous sessions (Wolpe, 1973).

Flooding is a form of rapid desensitization, performed by a behavioral therapist, in which the person is confronted with the phobic object (either a picture or the actual object) until it no longer produces anxiety. Because the client's worst fear has been realized and the client did not die in the process, there is little reason to fear the situation anymore. The goal is to rid the client of a phobia in one or two sessions. This method is highly anxiety-producing and should be conducted only by a trained psychotherapist under controlled circumstances.

Some people with phobias undertake their own therapy by gradually increasing their experiences with the phobic object—for example, a person with a snake phobia who takes classes in biology, specializing in the study of reptiles, or an adolescent with a phobia of guns who wants to become a police officer.

OBSESSIVE-COMPULSIVE DISORDER

Everyone experiences repetitive behaviors in life—humming the same tune over and over for hours or washing one's hands repeatedly when caring for a sick child. Someone might even nervously decide to mop the clean kitchen floor the night before a big exam while studying for the test. These are all comfort and safety measures that help the person feel in control and less anxious. But obsessive-compulsive behaviors are repeated ritualistic behaviors that are based on unrealistic fears and that interfere with normal life activities.

Obsessions are recurrent thoughts, ideas, visualizations, or impulses that are inappropriate, bothersome, and anxiety-producing and that disturb the person's interpersonal, social, or occupational function. The person knows these thoughts are excessive or unreasonable but believes he or she has no control over them.

Compulsions are the behaviors or rituals continuously carried out to get rid of the obsessive thoughts and reduce anxiety. Some common compulsions include:

- Checking rituals (repeatedly returning to make sure the door is locked or the coffee pot is turned off)
- Counting rituals (each step taken, ceiling tiles, concrete blocks, desks in a classroom)
- Repeated hand-washing until the skin is raw
- Repeating the same words or tunes (perseveration)
- Touching rituals (feeling the texture of each material in a clothing store; touching people, doors, walls, or oneself)
- Symmetry rituals (arranging and rearranging items on a desk, shelf, or furniture into a perfect order; vacuuming the rug pile in one direction)
- Rigid performance rituals (getting dressed in an unvarying pattern)
- Cleanliness (scrubbing the kitchen floor every day)
- Somatic complaints (repetitious announcements of having a specific disease; insisting to the physician that minor pains are cancer)
- Sexual rituals (intrusive sexual thoughts or images accompanied by a need to confess)
- Aggressive impulses (for instance, to throw one's child against a wall).

Obsessive-compulsive behavior is considered a disorder only when the person is consumed by these thoughts, images, and impulses and is compelled to act out the relief behaviors to the point where they interfere with personal, social, and occupational function. Examples of obsessive-compulsive behavior include a man who can no longer work because he spends most of his day aligning and realigning all items in his apartment, or the woman who feels compelled to wash her hands after touching any object or person.

OCD can be manifested through many kinds of behaviors, all of which are repetitive, meaningless, and difficult to conquer. The person understands that these rituals are unusual and unreasonable but feels forced to carry them out to alleviate anxiety. Although a person with OCD may even joke about having these behaviors, it is a source of distress and shame; often sufferers become reclusive and asocial to hide these behaviors.

Onset and Clinical Course

OCD can start in childhood, especially in males. In females, it more commonly begins in the 20s. Overall, there is an equal distribution between the genders. There is a higher incidence in higher socioeconomic and more educated groups (Kaplan & Sadock, 1995). Onset is usually gradual, although there have been acute onsets, with periods of waxing and waning symptoms in this chronic disorder (Barlow, 1993).

Etiology

BIOLOGIC

Many victims of head trauma or infections that affect the central nervous system have later developed OCD. Positron emission tomography scans that assess glucose metabolism in the caudate nuclei and orbital gyri of the basal ganglia of the brain demonstrate differences in persons with and without OCD. These structures affect the brain's command of movement, learned behavior, and patterns of dealing with repetitious stimuli; often after damage to these structures, OCD symptoms develop or subside (Comer, 1992). Positron emission scanning has also been used to demonstrate increased metabolic rates in the prefrontal cortex (Baxter et al., 1987). The neurotransmitter serotonin may play a role in OCD because antidepressants that specifically affect serotonin, such as clomipramine and fluvoxamine, reduce symptoms of this disorder.

There is a greater incidence of OCD in twins, especially identical twins, than in the general population. Also, OCD runs in families where a first-degree relative has OCD, Tourette's syndrome, or trichotillomania (repetitive twisting of hair until it comes out).

PSYCHODYNAMIC

Persons with OCD are thought to use four types of defense mechanisms: regression, isolation, reaction formation, and undoing. The person with OCD is believed to regress and to become fixated in Freud's anal stage. Those who have neat, orderly types of compulsions are said to be anal-retentive; messy or aggressive ones are anal-explosive. For example, the client who does not want to care for an ill parent but realizes this is socially unacceptable regresses to a previous developmental level (anal-retentive) and engages in rituals that are comforting, such as cleaning and orderliness; isolates the event from the emotions and is uncomfortable with the emotions (anxiety); uses reaction formation to keep away the thoughts of not wanting to take care of the parent; and becomes a "super-child," providing excellent care to the parent and keeping the environment spotlessly clean, thereby undoing the original unacceptable impulse to ignore the parent's need.

An interesting parallel relating OCD to regression is the observation that if a person's OCD ritual is interrupted, he or she must start over from the beginning. This is similar to a harried parent who wants to get to the point of a story and interrupts the 4-year-old who is telling the tale, only to discover that the child must start again at the very beginning. In the end, the telling takes twice as long!

Treatment and Prognosis

Like other anxiety disorders, optimal treatment for OCD is a combination of psychotropic drugs and psychotherapy.

PSYCHOPHARMACOLOGY

SSRIs. SSRIs are the most recent drugs approved for treating OCD. Fluvoxamine (Luvox), paroxetine (Paxil), sertraline (Zoloft), and fluoxetine (Prozac) are approved for this use (Table 5). About 70% of persons with OCD have some response to SSRIs; 10% to 15% have full remission. SSRIs are nonaddictive. They cannot be given concurrently with MAOIs, or a hypertensive crisis may occur. The MAOI should be discontinued 3 to 5 weeks before starting the SSRI to avoid a hypertensive crisis. The success of treatment of OCD with SSRIs demonstrates that serotonin plays a role in this disease process.

Antidepressants. The first medication found to reduce the uncontrollable, repetitive behavior of OCD was the TCA clomipramine (Anafranil). This medication is believed to inhibit the reuptake of both norepinephrine and serotonin in the synapses. TCAs are effective in treating OCD probably by blocking the reuptake of norepinephrine and serotonin. They are nonaddictive, and long-term treatment is recommended. MAOIs should be discontinued 3 to 5 weeks before starting a TCA to avoid a hypertensive crisis. There is a 1- to 3-week lag period before symptom abatement begins.

Anxiolytics. The anxiolytics buspirone (BuSpar) and clonazepam (Klonopin) are the only ones effective in relieving OCD.

APPLICATION OF THE NURSING PROCESS: OBSESSIVE-COMPULSIVE DISORDER

Assessment

OCD is usually treated in the community. The nurse must allow adequate time, perhaps several visits, to identify the range of OCD behaviors. For accurate assessment, the nurse needs to gain specific information regarding OCD behaviors to establish a pattern of behavior, including what behaviors or rituals are performed, when and how often they are performed, and the client's response to these relief behaviors.

Nursing assessment should include the following:
* Description of the behaviors
* When the behaviors most often occur
* Specific events or behaviors of other people that increase and decrease the behaviors
* How often during the day the compulsions are demonstrated
* The amount of time required to perform each repetition of the ritual. This information can be used to assess how much time is taken from activities of daily living and will help later to set time limits on rituals.

Table 12-5

DRUGS USED TO TREAT OCD

Generic Name (Brand Name)	Type	Dosage Range	Nursing Implications
fluoxetine (Prozac)	SSRI	Adult: 20 mg in AM Geriatric: 5–10 mg Max adult dose 80 mg/day	Side effects: headache, nausea/ vomiting, dizziness, insomnia, nervousness Monitor for weight loss Increases half-life of diazepam
sertraline (Zoloft)	SSRI	Adult: 50 mg/day Geriatric: 25 mg/day Give in AM or PM to avoid nightime insomnia Increase prn q 2 weeks to max dose of 200 mg	Side effects: agitation, insomnia, headache, dizziness, somnolence, fatigue, constipation Liver function tests Increase fluid and bulk Increase warfarin effect; monitor INR Reduces clearance of diazepam and tolbutamide
fluvoxamine (Luvox)	SSRI	Adult: 50 mg hs Geriatric: 25 mg hs	Side effects: headache, insomnia, drowsiness, weight loss, tremor, nervousness, light-headedness, nausea/vomiting, sexual dysfunction, urinary frequency, constipation Monitor liver & renal function
clomipramine (Anafranil)	TCA	Adult: 75–250 mg/day in divided doses with meals GI SE	Side effects: constipation, dry mouth, sweating, tremors, weight gain
buspirone (BuSpar)	Anxiolytic	Adult: 30 mg tid Geriatric: 10 mg bid or tid	Side effects: dizziness, drowsiness, headache, nausea
clonazepam (Klonopin)	Anxiolytic	Adult: 0.5–1.5 bid or tid; max 24-hour dose: 20 mg	Side effects: drowsiness, sedation, ataxia I & O, LFT, renal function, platelets, CBC, and serum levels of clonazepam. Overdose: sweating, somnolence, confusion, irritability, cramps, reflexes, coma.

Adapted from Wilson, B. A., Shannon, M. T., Stang, C. L. (2000). *Nurses drug guide 2000.* New York: Appleton & Lange; McEvoy, R. B. (Ed.) (2000). *Facts and comparisons 2000.* St. Louis: Facts and Comparisons, A Wolters Kluwer Company.

- The number of repetitions in each set of behaviors. This gives a baseline number that can be used to evaluate when changes occur.
- How the client responds when using these relief behaviors. This documents the physiologic responses and emotional reactions, which gives baseline data for comparison.

DRUG ALERT

Selective serotonin reuptake inhibitors (SSRIs) cannot be given concurrently with monoamine oxidase inhibitors (MAOIs). MAOIs should be discontinued 3 to 5 weeks before starting therapy with SSRIs to avoid a hypertensive crisis.

- The client's actions when something or someone interferes with performance of rituals. This helps determine the degree of rigidity in the need to perform these rituals.

Data Analysis

Depending on the particular obsession and its accompanying compulsions, clients will have varying symptoms. Nursing diagnoses are as varied as the following:
- Anxiety
- Decisional Conflict
- Fatigue
- Loneliness, Risk for
- Perceived Constipation

Box 12-5

➤ Yale-Brown Obsessive-Compulsive Scale

For each item circle the number identifying the response which best characterizes the patient.

1. Time occupied by obsessive thoughts
   How much of your time is occupied by obsessive thoughts?
   How frequently do the obsessive thoughts occur?
   0 None
   1 Mild (less than 1 hr/day) or occasional (intrusion occurring no more than 8 times a day)
   2 Moderate (1–3 hr/day) or frequent (intrusion occurring more than 8 times a day, but most of the hours of the day are free of obsessions)
   3 Severe (greater than 3 and up to 8 hr/day) or very frequent (intrusion occurring more than 8 times a day and occurring during most of the hours of the day)
   4 Extreme (greater than 8 hr/day) or near consistent intrusion (too numerous to count and an hour rarely passes without several obsessions occurring)

2. Interference due to obsessive thoughts
   How much do your obsessive thoughts interfere with your social or work (or role) functioning?
   Is there anything that you don't do because of them?
   0 None
   1 Mild, slight interference with social or occupational activities, but overall performance not impaired
   2 Moderate, definite interference with social or occupational performance but still manageable
   3 Severe, causes substantial impairment in social or occupational performance
   4 Extreme, incapacitating

3. Distress associated with obsessive thoughts
   How much distress do your obsessive thoughts cause you?
   0 None
   1 Mild, infrequent and not too disturbing
   2 Moderate, frequent and disturbing but still manageable
   3 Severe, very frequent and very disturbing
   4 Extreme, near constant and disabling distress

4. Resistance against obsessions
   How much of an effort do you make to resist the obsessive thoughts?
   How often do you try to disregard or turn your attention away from these thoughts as they enter your mind?
   0 Makes an effort to always resist, or symptoms so minimal doesn't need to actively resist
   1 Tries to resist most of the time
   2 Makes some effort to resist

   3 Yields to all obsessions without attempting to control them, but does so with some reluctance
   4 Completely and willingly yields to all obsessions

5. Degree of control over obsessive thoughts
   How much control do you have over your obsessive thoughts?
   How successful are you in stopping or diverting your obsessive thinking?
   0 Complete control
   1 Much control, usually able to stop or divert obsessions with some effort and concentration
   2 Moderate control, sometimes able to stop or divert obsessions
   3 Little control, rarely successful in stopping obsessions
   4 No control, experienced as completely involuntary, rarely able to even momentarily divert thinking

6. Time spent performing compulsive behaviors
   How much time do you spend performing compulsive behaviors?
   How frequently do you perform compulsions?
   0 None
   1 Mild (less than 1 hr/day performing compulsions) or occasional (performance of compulsions occurring no more than 8 times a day)
   2 Moderate (1–3 hr/day performing compulsions) or frequent (performance of compulsions occurring more than 8 times a day, but most of the hours of the day are free of compulsive behaviors)
   3 Severe (greater than 3 and up to 8 hr/day performing compulsions) or very frequent (performance of compulsions occurring more than 8 times a day and occurring during most of the hours of the day)
   4 Extreme (greater than 8 hr/day performing compulsions) or near consistent performance of compulsions (too numerous to count and an hour rarely passes without several compulsions being performed)

7. Interference due to compulsive behaviors
   How much do your compulsive behaviors interfere with your social or work (or role) functioning? Is there anything that you don't do because of the compulsions?
   0 None
   1 Mild, slight interference with social or occupational activities, but overall performance not impaired
   2 Moderate, definite interference with social or occupational performance but still manageable

Continued

Box 12-5

► YALE-BROWN OBSESSIVE-COMPULSIVE SCALE—cont'd

3 Severe, causes substantial impairment in social or occupational performance
4 Extreme, incapacitating

8. Distress associated with compulsive behavior
How would you feel if prevented from performing your compulsions?
How anxious would you become? How anxious do you get while performing compulsions until you are satisfied they are completed?
0 None
1 Mild, only slightly anxious if compulsions prevented or only slightly anxious during performance of compulsions
2 Moderate, reports that anxiety would mount but remain manageable if compulsions prevented or that anxiety increases but remains manageable during performance of compulsions
3 Severe, prominent and very disturbing increase in anxiety if compulsions interrupted or prominent and very disturbing increases in anxiety during performance of compulsions
4 Extreme, incapacitating anxiety from any intervention aimed at modifying activity or

incapacitating anxiety develops during performance of compulsions

9. Resistance against compulsions
How much of an effort do you make to resist the compulsions?
0 Makes an effort to always resist, or symptoms so minimal doesn't need to actively resist
1 Tries to resist most of the time
2 Makes some effort to resist
3 Yields to all compulsions without attempting to control them but does so with some reluctance
4 Completely and willingly yields to all compulsions

10. Degree of control over compulsive behavior
0 Complete control
1 Much control, experiences pressure to perform the behavior but usually able to exercise voluntary control over it
2 Moderate control, strong pressure to perform behavior, can control it only with difficulty
3 Little control, very strong drive to perform behavior, must be carried to completion, can only delay with difficulty
4 No control, drive to perform behavior experienced as completely involuntary

Reprinted with permission from Goodman W. K., Price L. H., Rasmussen S. A., et al. (1989). The Yale-Brown Obsessive-Compulsive Scale, I: Development, use, and reliability. Arch Gen Psychiatry 46:1006.

- Self Esteem, Situational Low
- Skin Integrity, Risk for Impaired.

Outcome Identification

Like the nursing diagnoses, outcomes can be as varied as clients' behaviors. A general outcome is that the client will reduce the time and frequency of ritualistic behaviors. Examples of specific outcomes are:

1. Client will feel a reduced compulsion to clean constantly.
2. Client will show reduced hand-washing and improve skin integrity of hands.
3. Client will drive over bridges.
4. Client will show reduced fear of the animal, person, or situation that previously caused compulsive behavior.

Intervention

Promoting Control and Self-Esteem

The nurse must develop a therapeutic relationship with the client, offering support and compassion and

► SYMPTOMS OF OCD

- Client experiences persistent and recurring thoughts, images, or impulses that are unrealistic and intrusive, disturbing, socially distressing, or morally reprehensible and cause extreme anxiety.
- Obsessions are usually unrelated to any real-life situation and include extreme fear of germs, uncleanliness, infection, need for orderly placement of objects, pornographic fantasies.
- Client is compelled to reduce anxiety by bizarre repetitive and ritualistic behaviors such as counting and recounting, cleaning, hand-washing, praying, checking and rechecking, or precise ordering of objects.
- Compulsive ritualistic behaviors are excessive and interfere with relationships, job, or other functional activities.

> ▶ **NURSING INTERVENTIONS FOR CLIENT WITH OCD**
>
> • Develop a therapeutic relationship.
> • Offer encouragement, support, and compassion.
> • Be clear with the client that you believe he or she can change.
> • Gradually decrease time for the client to carry out ritualistic behaviors.
> • Discuss the function of the rituals in the client's life, without judgment.

believing that the client can change. This encouragement and support from the nurse can boost the client's self-esteem, help him or her overcome feelings of shame and doubt, and instill confidence to bring about slow and gradual behavior changes.

In the early stages of treatment, adequate time (several days to a week) is provided for the client to engage in his or her rituals. After a thorough assessment is completed, the nurse can gradually decrease the amount of time the person has to carry out relief behaviors. Forbidding the client to use relief behaviors results in panic and increases the client's feelings of failure. The nurse should use the therapeutic relationship to discuss the function of rituals in the client's life, being careful not to blame or denigrate either the client or the rituals.

The process of reducing the time spent on these rituals must be gradual so that the person feels some sense of control. For example, if a client takes 20 minutes to wash the chair and table before eating a meal, the nurse should engage the client in some other activity so that he or she has only 19 minutes to complete the ritual. After several days of 19 minutes, when the client seems comfortable with this time limit, the allotted time is reduced to 18 minutes. The client retains some control over ways to carry out the ritual, by speeding it up or deleting one or more repetitions to fit the time limit. This feeling of control decreases the client's helplessness and anxiety, which would be increased if the relief behaviors were prohibited.

To support the client's sense of control in an inpatient setting, the nurse can provide a schedule of daily activities, detailing all events, meals, therapy sessions, rest periods, and visiting hours each day. In a community setting, the nurse and client can create a similar schedule. A person who is focused on scheduled activities has less time for rituals, and the nonritualistic activities are reinforced by providing positive feedback. Ultimately the rituals will be reduced and then extinguished because the person achieves greater acceptance and higher self-worth by engaging in nonritualistic behaviors.

Evaluation

1. Client participated in routine daily activities.
2. Client reduced amount of time spent in ritualistic behaviors.
3. Client used behavioral techniques of imagery, progressive relaxation, thought-stopping, and meditation to reduce anxiety.
4. Client demonstrated safe self-administration of prescribed medication.
5. Client verbalized intent to remain in therapy.
6. Client is resuming family, social, and occupational activities.
7. Family shows decreased participation in client's secondary gains related to OCD behavior and has increased attention during non-OCD activities.

RELATED DISORDERS

Other Anxiety Disorders

Some anxiety disorders are related to the use of medications or other substances, traumatic events, or illnesses. These anxiety disorders also interfere with a person's life, relationships, occupation, and social functioning.

GENERALIZED ANXIETY DISORDER

A person with generalized anxiety disorder worries excessively and feels highly anxious at least half of the time for a period of 6 months or more. Unable to control this focus on worry, the person has three or more of the following symptoms: uneasiness, irritability, muscle tension, fatigue, difficulty thinking, and sleep alterations. Twelve percent of persons who receive treatment for anxiety disorders have generalized anxiety disorder (DSM-IV-TR, 2000).

ANXIETY DISORDER DUE TO A GENERAL MEDICAL CONDITION

Anxiety disorder due to a general medical condition is a diagnostic category in which anxiety disorders such as OCD, generalized anxiety disorder, or panic attacks are directly related to the person's general medical condition. These disorders affect the person's occupational, social, or interpersonal function. Anxiety disorders can be produced by medications, toxins, or substance abuse. Manifested by behaviors related to any of the anxiety disorders, symptoms can appear during use of or withdrawal from the substance. The diagnostic category for these features is substance-induced anxiety disorder (DSM-IV-TR, 2000).

Box 12-6

➤ THERAPEUTIC COMMUNICATION: OCD

A community health nurse walked into the living room to wait until Mrs. Kist finished her conversation with her sister, who was calling from New Mexico. Mrs. Kist had an emergency bowel resection, with a temporary colostomy, and several postoperative complications. This is the nurse's first visit. Mr. Kist is in the living room, and he has arranged and rearranged the magazines on the coffee table four times in 3 minutes.

Nurse (N): "Hi, Mr. Kist. I see you are straightening up the magazines on the coffee table."
Client (C): "Yeah. You caught me."

N: "Caught you?"
C: "Well, my wife complains about my rearranging everything."

N: "Go on."
C: "Sometimes I feel as if I have to sneak this straightening up stuff so she doesn't see me do it and no one else does either."

N: "What's the secrecy about?"
C: "Well, I know this is silly, but I feel as if I have to do this. Yet, I know it drives my wife nuts. Actually, I think I am the one going nuts. I have always been a neat person, but I have been under a lot of stress since my wife has been ill and it seems as if all I do is to make sure all this stuff is precisely arranged."

N: "What does seeing stuff precisely arranged do for you, Mr. Kist?"
C: "Oh, I don't know. I guess I feel as if I have everything under control. (Pauses a few moments) I'm ashamed to admit I have a measuring tape in my pocket, to make sure one item is an equal distance from another."

N: "For how long do you feel better after you have finished your arrangement?"
C: "See, that is just it! The next minute I think I have moved something or it doesn't look right, so I move things around again. I feel so helpless with my wife being sick and needing you nurses and a home health aide to take care of her."

N: "Helpless?"
C: "Yeah. I'm scared I will do something to hurt her again, when you are not here. She is so weak, she can't manage by herself, but I am scared."

N: "How did you hurt your wife?"
C: "She asked me to help her get out of bed to go the bathroom. I wanted to scoop her up in my arms and carry her, but she wouldn't hear of it. She says she's gotta walk. The first time she tried to stand up, she started sliding down towards the floor, so I grabbed her with both of my arms around her. I hurt her incision."

N: "What else scares you about your wife's care?"
C: "I don't know anything about her medicines and I have to give them to her, because last night right in front of me, she took her pain pill and then not even 5 minutes later, she reached for the pain pills again. She had no clue she had just taken the pill 5 minutes before. So I took them and I have set up a schedule and I write down when I give her medicines. But I don't know much about the three other bottles she has, and what about the side effects I am supposed to watch for? Let me see . . . Oh, what if she needs help with the colostomy bags? The minute we got home yesterday, the whole thing fell off. She was so exhausted, but she had to get up and take care of it."

N: "So what do you want to do about these things that scare you about caring for your wife—helping her to move, the medications, and colostomy bag?"
C: "Maybe get someone to teach me these things?"

N: "OK, Mr. Kist. You have 2 minutes to get ready for your first lesson. I'll teach you."
C: "Great. Just let me finish here." He looks at his watch and speeds up his movements to deal with the 2-minute limit.

POSTTRAUMATIC STRESS DISORDER

Posttraumatic stress disorder can occur in a person who has witnessed an extraordinarily terrifying and potentially deadly event. After the traumatic event, the person re-experiences all or some of it through dreams or waking recollections and responds defensively to these flashbacks. New behaviors develop related to the traumatic event, such as sleep difficulties, hypervigilance, thinking difficulties, a severe startle response, and agitation (DSM-IV-TR, 2000). This is addressed in detail in Chapter 11.

ACUTE STRESS DISORDER

Acute stress disorder is similar to posttraumatic stress disorder in that the person has experienced a traumatic situation, but the response is more dissociative in nature. The person has a sense that the

> ▶ CLIENT AND FAMILY TEACHING: OCD

- Behavioral and cognitive interventions
- Biologic and psychological treatment approaches
- Importance of maintaining prescribed medication regimen and regular follow-up
- How to manage ritualistic behavior and alternative activities.

event was unreal, thinks he or she is unreal, and forgets some aspects of the event through amnesia, emotional detachment, and a muddled obliviousness to the environment (DSM-IV-TR, 2000).

VICARIOUS TRAUMATIZATION OF CAREGIVERS

Health care professionals can experience the stressful effects of dealing with their clients' traumatic experi-

NURSING CARE PLAN FOR CLIENT WITH ANXIETY

Nursing Diagnosis

> ➤ **Anxiety** (9.3.1)
> *A vague uneasy feeling, whose source is often nonspecific or unknown to the individual.*

ASSESSMENT DATA

- Decreased attention span
- Restlessness, irritability
- Poor impulse control
- Feelings of discomfort, apprehension, or helplessness
- Perceptual field deficits
- Decreased ability to communicate verbally

EXPECTED OUTCOMES

The client will:
- Be free of injury
- Discuss feelings of dread, anxiety, and so forth
- Respond to relaxation techniques with a decreased anxiety level
- Reduce own anxiety level
- Be free of anxiety attacks

IMPLEMENTATION

Nursing Interventions	Rationale
Remain with the client at all times when levels of anxiety are high (severe or panic).	The client's safety is a priority. A highly anxious client should not be left alone—his or her anxiety will escalate.
Move the client to a quiet area with minimal or decreased stimuli. Using a small room or seclusion area may be indicated.	The client's ability to deal with excessive stimuli is impaired. Anxious behavior can be escalated by external stimuli. A smaller room can enhance the client's sense of security. The larger the area, the more lost and panicked the client can become.
Remain calm in your approach to the client.	The client will feel more secure if you are calm and if the client feels you are in control of the situation.

continued on page 287

continued from page 286

Use short, simple, and clear statements.	The client's ability to deal with abstractions or complexity is impaired.
Avoid asking or forcing the client to make choices.	The client's ability to problem solve is impaired. The client may not make sound decisions or may be unable to make decisions at all.
Use of PRN medications may be indicated if the client's level of anxiety is high or if the client is experiencing delusions, disorganized thoughts, and so forth.	Medication may be necessary to decrease the client's anxiety to a level at which he or she can listen to you and feel safe.
Be aware of your own feelings and level of discomfort or anxiety.	Anxiety is communicated interpersonally. Being with the anxious client can raise your own anxiety level.
Encourage the client's participation in relaxation exercises. These can include deep breathing, progressive muscle relaxation, medication, guided imagery, and going (mentally) to a quiet, peaceful place.	Relaxation exercises are effective, nonchemical ways to reduce anxiety.
Teach the client to use relaxation techniques independently.	Independent use of the techniques can give the client confidence in having some conscious control over his or her anxious behavior.
Help the client see mild anxiety as a positive catalyst for change.	A frequent misconception is that anxiety itself is bad and not useful. The client does not need to avoid anxiety per se.

Adapted from Schultz, J. M. & Videbeck, S. L. (1998). Lippincott's manual of psychiatric nursing care plans (5th ed.) Philadelphia: Lippincott-Raven.

ences (Blair & Ramones, 1996; McCann & Pearlman, 1990; Stamm, 1999). Emergency personnel, police officers, firefighters, nurses, physicians, and psychotherapists accumulate these events and the people involved in them and assume that as professionals they "should" be able to handle the effects of these traumatic events. Usually labeled vicarious traumatization of caregivers, stress-related symptoms similar to those of posttraumatic stress disorder can develop through empathic strain, shattered assumptions, stress and fatigue, and countertransference (Crocker, 2000).

 CLINICAL VIGNETTE: OBSESSIVE-COMPULSIVE DISORDER

Sam had just returned home from church. He immediately got undressed and entered the shower. As he showered, he soaped and resoaped his washcloth and rubbed vigorously over every inch of his body. "I can't miss anything! I must get all the germs off," he kept repeating to himself. As he stepped out of the shower, Sam was very careful to step on the clean white bath towel laid on the floor. He folded and refolded the drying towel until it was "just right." Satisfied only for a moment, he took it off the rack and refolded it again and again.

COMMUNITY CARE

Most people with anxiety disorders are encountered in community settings rather than inpatient settings. It is unusual for a nurse to be sent to a person's home to deal specifically with behaviors related to anxiety disorders; rather, the nurse sees these behaviors in clients being treated for other conditions, or in their family members. Formal treatment for people with anxiety disorders usually occurs in community mental health clinics and in the offices of physicians, psychiatric clinical specialists, psychologists, or other mental health counselors. Because the person with an anxiety disorder often believes the sporadic symptoms are related to medical problems, the family practitioner or advanced practice nurse can be the first health care professional to evaluate the person.

Knowledge of community resources will help the nurse guide the client to appropriate referrals for assessment, diagnosis, and treatment. The nurse can add these other health care professionals in the community to the collaborative effort in the treatment process. The nurse can refer the client to a psychiatrist or an advanced practice psychiatric nurse for diagnosis, psychotherapy, and medication. Other community resources such as anxiety disorder groups or self-help groups can provide support and help the client feel less lonely.

SELF-AWARENESS ISSUES

Working with people with anxiety disorders is a different kind of challenge for the nurse. These clients are usually average people in other respects who know that their symptoms are unusual but feel unable to stop them. They experience a high level of frustration and feelings of helplessness and failure. Their lives are out of their control, and they live in fear of the next episode. They go to extreme measures to try to prevent episodes by avoiding people and places where previous events occurred.

It may be difficult for nurses and others to understand why the person cannot simply stop performing the bizarre behaviors interfering with his or her life. Why does the hand-washer whose hands have been painfully scrubbed raw keep on washing his poor sore hands every hour on the hour? Nurses need to understand what and how anxiety behaviors work, not just for client care but to help understand the role anxiety plays in performing nursing responsibilities. Nurses are expected to function at a high level and to avoid allowing their own feelings and needs to hinder the care of their clients. But as emotional beings, nurses are just as vulnerable to stress and anxiety as others, and they have needs of their own.

Nurses may tend to take charge or may feel a need to be admired for helping their clients get better.

INTERNET RESOURCES

Resource	Internet Address
▶ OCD	http://www.mental health.Com /disp20.an05.html
▶ All about OCD	http://www.ocd.mentalhelp.net
▶ Medication for anxiety disorders	http://www.at health.com /nih_medication.html
▶ Obsessive–Compulsive Foundation	http://www.ocfoundation.org
▶ Mood and disorder clinical trials	http://www.emoryclinicaltrials.com
▶ Social phobia fact sheet	http://www.socialphobia.org/fact.html
▶ Surgeon General report, fact sheet, directory, catalog	http://www.surgeongeneral.gov
▶ Anxiolytics	http://www.uams.edu/department of psychiatry/ syllabus/anxiolytics.html

From time to time, nurses should reassess their own motives, values, and performance with peers to ensure they are acting in the best interest of their clients.

Helpful Hints for Working With Clients With Anxiety and Stress-Related Disorders

- Remember that everyone suffers from stress and anxiety from time to time that can interfere with daily life and work.
- Avoid falling into the pitfall of trying to "fix" the client's problems.
- Discuss any uncomfortable feelings with a more experienced nurse for suggestions on how to deal with your feelings toward these clients.

➤ KEY POINTS

- Anxiety is a vague dread that is inconsistent with the situation. Fear is the terror one feels in response to a threatening object.
- There are positive and negative side effects of anxiety. The positive effects produce growth and adaptive change, and the negative effects produce poor self-esteem, fear, inhibition, and anxiety disorders (in addition to other disorders).
- Stress is fear. Everyone experiences stress differently.
- There are four levels of anxiety: mild anxiety (helps us learn, grow, and change), moderate anxiety (increases focus on the alarm, learning is still possible, objective symptoms can be validated), severe anxiety (greatly decreases cognitive function, increases preparation for physical responses, increases space needs), and panic (fight, flight, or freeze response, no learning is possible, the person is attempting to free himself or herself from the discomfort of this high stage of anxiety).
- Defense mechanisms are intrapsychic distortions used by the person to feel more in control. It is believed that these defense mechanisms are overused when a person develops an anxiety disorder.
- Current etiologic theories and studies of anxiety disorders have shown a familial incidence and have implicated the neurotransmitters GABA, norepinephrine, and serotonin.
- In a panic attack, the person feels as if he or she is dying. Symptoms can include palpitations, sweating, tremors, shortness of breath, a sense of suffocation, chest pain, nausea, abdominal distress, dizziness, paresthesias, and vasomotor lability. The person has a fight, flight, or freeze response.
- Panic disorder can occur with or without agoraphobia.
- Primary gain is the relief of anxiety achieved by performing the specific anxiety-reducing behavior. Secondary gain is the attention received from others by having this disorder.
- In phobias, the person is believed to be displacing conflict and anxiety onto some easily avoidable object. Some theorists believe that persons with phobias have a greater external locus of control, whereas normal people feel more of an internal locus of control.
- Specific phobias are cued by a particular object or situation (phobic stimulus).
- A social phobia involves a social interaction that threatens the person.
- Obsessive-compulsive disorder involves recurrent thoughts, ideas, visualizations, and impulses and the ritual behaviors carried out to get rid of the thoughts or reduce anxiety.
- Obsessions are the incessant thoughts; compulsions are the need to act on these thoughts.
- Persons with obsessive-compulsive disorder know that their rituals are unusual, but they feel unable to stop them. This disorder has responded well to tricyclic antidepressants and SSRIs and behavioral therapy. Anxiolytics can be used, but care must be taken with benzodiazepines, which can lead to dependence.
- In a therapeutic relationship, the client can discuss ritualistic behavior without being judged.

Critical Thinking

Questions

1. Because we all have anxiety at times, it is important for nurses to be aware of their own coping mechanisms. Do a self-assessment: What causes you anxiety? What physical, emotional, and cognitive responses occur when you are anxious? What coping mechanisms do you use? Are they healthy? Teach yourself deep-breathing, thought-stopping, and relaxation.

2. How might you respond to someone having a panic attack? How might you handle your own fear?

- Self-awareness about one's anxiety and one's responses to it greatly improves both personal and professional relationships.

REFERENCES

American Psychiatric Association. (2000). *DSM-IV-TR: Diagnostic and statistical manual of mental disorders-Text Revision.* 4th ed. Washington, DC: American Psychiatric Association.

Andreasen, N. C., & Black, D. W. (1995). *Introductory textbook of psychiatry,* 2nd ed. Washington, DC: American Psychiatric Press.

Andrews, M. M., & Boyle, J. S. (1999). *Transcultural concepts in nursing care* (3rd ed.). Philadelphia: Lippincott Williams & Wilkins.

Bandura, A. (1973). *Aggression: a social learning analysis.* Englewood Cliffs, N.J.: Prentice Hall.

Barlow, D. H. (1988). Current models of panic disorder and a view from emotion theory. In A. J. Francis & R. E. Hales (eds.). *American Psychiatric Press review of psychiatry,* Vol 7. Washington, DC: American Psychiatric Press.

Barlow, D. (1993). *Clinical handbook of psychological disorders.* New York: The Guilford Press.

Baxter, L. R., Phelps, M. E., Maziotta, J. C., Schwartz, B. H., & Selin, C. E. (1987). Local cerebral glucose metabolic rates in obsessive and compulsive disorder: a comparison with roles in unipolar depression and normal controls. *Archives of General Psychiatry, 44,* 211–218.

Beck, A. T., & Emery, C. (1985). *Anxiety disorders and phobias: a cognitive perspective.* New York: Basic Books.

Blair, D. T., & Ramones, V. A. (1996). Understanding vicarious traumatization. *Journal of Psychosocial Nursing, 34*(11), 24–30.

Crocker, K. L. (2000). Healing the wounded healers: the impact of vicarious traumatization in caregivers. Continuing education presentation at Nurse Educator 2000, Orlando, Florida, at the MCP Hahnemann University School of Nursing. Jan. 2, 2000.

Emmanuel, N. P., Ware, M. R., Brawman-Minzer, O., Ballenger, J. C., Lydiard, R. B. (1999). Once-weekly dosing of fluoxetine in the maintenance of remission in panic disorder. *Journal of Clinical Psychiatry, 60*(5), 299–301.

Fontaine, K. L. (2000). *Healing practices: alternative therapies for nursing.* Upper Saddle River, N.J.: Prentice-Hall.

Freud, S. (1936). *The problem of anxiety.* New York: W. W. Norton.

Grinspoon, L. (ed.). (1996). Panic attacks and panic disorder, part I. *Harvard Mental Health Letter, 12*(10), 1.

Horwath, E., & Weissman, M. M. (2000). *Anxiety disorders: Epidemiology.* In B. J. Sadock & V. A. Sadock (Eds.). Comprehensive Textbook of Psychiatry, Vol. 1. (7th ed.), pp. 1441–1450. Philadelphia: Lippincott Williams & Wilkins.

Johnson, J. H., & Sarason, I. G. (1978). Life stress, depression and anxiety: internal-external control as a moderator variable. *Journal of Psychosomatic Research, 22,* 205–208.

Kaplan, H. L., Sadock, B. J., & Grebb, J. A. (1994). *Kaplan and Sadock's synopsis of psychiatry,* 7th ed. Baltimore: Williams & Wilkins.

Keltner, N. L., & Folks, D. G. (1997). *Psychotropic drugs,* 2nd ed. Philadelphia: Mosby.

Keltner, N. L., Folks, D. G., Palmer, C. A., & Powers, R. E. (1998). *Psychobiological foundations of psychiatric care.* Philadelphia: Mosby.

Keltner, N. L., Schwecke, L. H., & Bostrom, C. E. (1999). *Psychiatric nursing,* 3rd ed. Philadelphia: Mosby.

Liberthson, R., Sheehan, D. V., King, M. E., & Weyman, A. E. (1986). The prevalence of mitral valve prolapse in patients with panic disorders. *American Journal of Psychiatry, 143,* 511.

Mavissakalian, M., & Michelson, L. (1986). Two-year follow-up of exposure and imipramine treatment of agoraphobia. *American Journal of Psychiatry, 143,* 1106.

McCann, I. L., & Pearlman, L. A. (1990). Vicarious traumatization: a framework for understanding the psychological effects of working with victims. *Journal of Traumatic Stress, 3*(1), 1149–1331.

McEvoy, R. B. (Ed.). (2000). *Facts and comparisons 2000.* St. Louis: Facts and Comparisons, A Wolters Kluwer Company.

Oltmanns, T. F., & Emery, R. E. (1998). *Abnormal psychology,* 2nd ed. Upper Saddle River, N.J.: Prentice-Hall.

Peplau, H. (1952). *Interpersonal relations.* New York: Putnam.

Pitts, F. N., & McClure, J. N. (1967). Lactate metabolism in anxiety neurosis. *New England Journal of Medicine, 277,* 1329–1336.

Reiman, E. M., Raichle, M. E., Robins, E., et al. (1989). Neuroanatomical correlates of a lactate-induced anxiety attack. *Archives of General Psychiatry, 46,* 439.

Schultz, J. M., & Videbeck, S. D. (1998). *Lippincott's manual of psychiatric care plans* (5th ed.). Philadelphia: Lippincott-Raven.

Selye, H. (1956). *The stress life.* St. Louis: McGraw-Hill.

Selye, H. (1974). *Stress without distress.* Philadelphia: J. B. Lippincott.

Spector, R. E. (2000). *Cultural diversity in health and illness,* 5th ed. Upper Saddle River, N.J.: Prentice-Hall Health.

Stamm, B. H. (1999). *Secondary traumatic stress: self-care issues for clinicians, researchers, & educators,* 2nd ed., Towson, Md.: Sidran Press.

Sullivan, G. M., & Coplan, J. D. (2000). Anxiety disorders: Biochemical aspects. In B. J. Sadock & V. A. Sadock (Eds.). *Comprehensive textbook of psychiatry,* Vol. 1 (7th ed.), 1450–1457. Philadelphia: Lippincott Williams & Wilkins.

Sullivan, H. S. (1952). *Interpersonal theory of psychiatry.* New York: W. W. Norton.

Wolpe, J. (1973). *The practice of behavior therapy,* 2nd ed. Oxford: Pergamon.

Yonkers, K. A., & Gurguis, G. (1995). Gender differences in the prevalence and expression of anxiety disorders. In M. V. Seeman (ed.). *Gender & psychopathology.* Washington, DC: American Psychiatric Press.

ADDITIONAL READINGS

Bakker, A., van Dyck, R., Spinhoven, P., van Balkom, A. J. (1999). Paroxetine, clomipramine, & cognitive therapy in the treatment of panic disorder. *Journal of Clinical Psychiatry, 60*(12), 831–838.

Boyd, M. A., & Nihart, M. A. (1998). *Psychiatric nursing: contemporary practice.* Philadelphia: Lippincott.

Garrison, G. D., & Levin, G. M. (2000). Factors affecting prescribing of the newer antidepressants. *Annals of Pharmacotherapeutics, 34*(1), 10.

Goodman, W. K., Price, L. H., Rasmussen, S. A. (1989). The Yale-Brown obsessive-compulsive scale. *Archives of General Psychiatry, 46*, 1000.

Marks, I. M. (1966). Different ages of onset in varieties of phobias. *American Journal of Psychiatry, 123*, 218–221.

McNally, R. J. (1987). Preparedness and phobias. *Psychological Bulletin, 101*, 283–303.

Rachman, S. (1990). The determinants and treatment of simple phobias. *Advances in Behavior Research and Therapy, 12*, 1–12.

van der Kolk, B. A., Boyd, H., Krystal, J., & Greenburg, M. (1984). Posttraumatic stress disorder as a biologically based disorder: implications of the animal model of inescapable shock. In van der Kolk, B. A. (ed.). *Posttraumatic stress disorder: psychological and biological sequelae.* Washington, DC: American Psychiatric Press.

van der Kolk, B. A. (1997). The psychobiology of post-traumatic stress disorder: findings from a community survey. *Journal of Clinical Psychiatry, 58*(9), 16.

Weissman, M. M., Fyer, A. J., Haghighi, F., et al. (1996). Potential panic disorder syndrome: clinical & genetic linkage evidence. *American Journal of Medical Genetics, 2*(1), 24–35.

Chapter Review

Select the best answer for each of the following questions.

1. Louis has become increasingly upset. He is rapidly pacing, hyperventilating, clenching his jaw, wringing his hands, and trembling, has high-pitched random speech, and seems pre-occupied with his thoughts. He is pounding his fist into his other hand as he agitatedly paces. Diagnose his level of anxiety.

   A. Mild

   B. Moderate

   C. Severe

   D. Panic.

2. John likes his environment to be as neat as possible. In fact, he is usually busy arranging items in symmetrical positions. According to Freud, he is displaying fixation in which of the following stages?

   A. Oral

   B. Anal

   C. Genital

   D. Phallic.

3. Sharon "sterilizes" her towels with bleach and hot water in the washing machine. She then wipes every surface she is going to touch with rubbing alcohol and these sterile towels. Today she has been admitted for a ruptured diverticulum and is ambulatory but hooked up to IV medications. What is the appropriate intervention for the first day or two of care in terms of Sharon's need to perform these rituals?

   A. Permit this behavior to continue.

   B. Interrupt her rituals and suggest she do something else.

   C. Order her to stop these rituals.

   D. Educate her about the need to stay in bed and rest instead of cleaning.

4. Taylor is in the school cafeteria line when she feels as if she is suffocating, her heart rate increases, and she has chest pain, sweating, nausea, and dizziness. She runs out of the cafeteria, leaving her books and backpack behind. When you find her outside a few minutes later, she is calming down but is scared something is wrong with her heart. What other disorder do these symptoms indicate?

   A. Posttraumatic stress

   B. Panic

   C. Agoraphobia

   D. Generalized anxiety.

5. Which of the four classes of medications used for panic disorder is considered the safest because of low incidence of side effects and lack of physiologic dependence?

   A. Benzodiazepines

   B. Tricyclics

   C. Monoamine oxidase inhibitors

   D. Selective serotonin reuptake inhibitors.

➤ TRUE-FALSE QUESTIONS

Identify each of the following statements as T (true) or F (false). Correct any false statements.

_____ 1. Some anxiety disorders are related to the use of medications or other substances, traumatic events, or illnesses.

_____

_____ 2. Many victims of head trauma or infections that affect the central nervous system have later developed obsessive-compulsive disorder.

_____

_____ 3. GABA is the amino acid neurotransmitter believed to be dysfunctional in anxiety disorders.

_____

_____ 4. Identical twins have a higher concordance rate of phobias than the general population

_____

➤ FILL-IN-THE-BLANK QUESTIONS

Identify the level of anxiety represented by the following descriptions:

_____ 1. Severe muscle tension, limited perceptual field, frantic

_____ 2. Attentive, impatient, optimal learning level

_____ 3. Flight, fight, or freeze, out of control, irrational

_____ 4. Selective inattention, voice changes, decreased perceptual field

➤ SHORT-ANSWER QUESTIONS

1. Name the four defense mechanism attributed to obsessive-compulsive disorder.

2. Describe systematic desensitization.

➤ CLINICAL EXAMPLE

Mr. Noe has discussed in detail with the community health nurse how his wife cannot be expected to walk 2 to 3 miles a day after her triple-bypass operation because she is afraid to leave the house. He has been taking care of her for the past 13 years, during which time she rarely left the house, and then only with great distress and only accompanied by him. His wife says she gets so anxious she wants to scream and run back in the door if she tries to walk out of it. She believes something terrible will happen to her. She knows this is true because the last time she left the house to go to the doctor she had to have triple-bypass surgery the next day. Mr. Noe takes care of necessary chores outside of the house, attends parents' weekend at their children's colleges, does the grocery shopping, and so forth.

Mrs. Noe has asked the nurse to "figure out how I can get outside and walk every day," but for each suggestion made by the nurse, Mrs. Noe finds some reason it would not work. The nurse is getting frustrated with Mrs. Noe's constant rejection of her suggestions and sternly says, "You haven't the foggiest intention of walking out that door, so why are we doing this?"

1. Rather than giving Mrs. Noe suggestions on how to get her outside to walk, what might be a better plan to suggest to Mrs. Noe?

2. How is Mr. Noe's behavior affecting Mrs. Noe's agoraphobic behaviors? What does the nurse need to explain and recommend to Mr. Noe about his response to her behavior?

3. What other treatments are available for Mrs. Noe?

13 Schizophrenia

Schizophrenia

Learning Objectives

After reading this chapter, the student should be able to:

1. Discuss various theories of the etiology of schizophrenia.

2. Describe the positive and negative symptoms of schizophrenia.

3. Describe a functional assessment for a client with schizophrenia.

4. Apply the nursing process to the care of a client with schizophrenia.

5. Evaluate the effectiveness of antipsychotic medications for clients with schizophrenia.

6. Provide teaching to clients, families, caregivers, and community members to increase knowledge and understanding of schizophrenia.

7. Describe the supportive and rehabilitative needs of clients with schizophrenia who live in the community.

8. Evaluate his or her own feelings, beliefs, and attitudes with regard to clients with schizophrenia.

Key Terms

- Abnormal Involuntary Movement Scale (AIMS)
- akathisia
- alogia
- ambivalence
- anhedonia
- associative looseness
- blunted affect
- catatonia
- command hallucinations
- delusions
- depersonalization
- dystonic reactions
- echolalia
- echopraxia
- extrapyramidal side effects
- flat affect
- flight of ideas
- hallucination
- ideas of reference
- latency of response
- neuroleptics
- neuroleptic malignant syndrome (NMS)
- perseveration
- polydipsia
- psychomotor retardation
- psychosis
- tardive dyskinesia
- thought blocking
- thought broadcasting
- thought insertion
- waxy flexibility
- word salad

Schizophrenia is a disease affecting the brain that causes distorted and bizarre thoughts, perceptions, emotions, movements, and behavior. Schizophrenia cannot be defined as a single illness; rather, it is thought of as a syndrome or disease process that includes many different varieties with varying symptoms, much like the varieties of cancer. For decades, schizophrenia was vastly misunderstood by the public. It was feared as a dangerous and uncontrollable mental disorder, and those with the diagnosis were portrayed as wildly disturbed individuals displaying bizarre behaviors and violent outbursts. Most people believed that persons with schizophrenia needed to be locked away from society and institutionalized. Only recently has the mental health community come to learn and educate the community that schizophrenia is a mental disorder that has a variety of symptoms and presentations and is an illness that can be controlled by medication. Thanks to the increased effectiveness of newer atypical antipsychotic drugs and advances in community-based treatment, many clients can live in the community successfully. Clients whose illness is medically supervised and maintained can often continue to live and sometimes work in the community with community support.

Schizophrenia is usually diagnosed in late adolescence and early adulthood. Only rarely is it manifested in childhood. The peak incidence of onset is 15 to 25 years for men and 25 to 35 years for women (DSM-IV-TR, 2000). The prevalence of schizophrenia is estimated at about 1% of the total population. In the United States, that translates to close to 3 million people who are, have been, or will be affected by the disease. The incidence and the lifetime prevalence are roughly the same throughout the world (Buchanan & Carpenter, 2000).

The symptoms of schizophrenia are divided into two major categories: positive or hard symptoms, which include delusions, hallucinations, and grossly disorganized thinking, speech, and behavior, and negative or soft symptoms, such as flat affect, lack of volition, and social withdrawal or discomfort. The display lists these negative and positive symptoms. The positive symptoms can be controlled by medication, but often the negative signs persist after psychotic symptoms have abated. The negative symptoms often persist over time and present a major barrier to recovery and improved functioning in the client's day-to-day life.

The following are the types of schizophrenia from the DSM-IV-TR 2000. The diagnosis is made according the predominant symptoms:

- Schizophrenia, paranoid type: characterized by persecutory (feeling victimized or spied on) or grandiose delusions, hallucinations, and sometimes by excessive religiosity (delusional religious focus), or hostile and aggressive behavior
- Schizophrenia, disorganized type: characterized by grossly inappropriate or flat affect, incoherence, loose associations, and extremely disorganized behavior

CLINICAL VIGNETTE: SCHIZOPHRENIA

Ricky had come to visit his father and was staying with him in his apartment for a few weeks. Things had gone pretty well for the first week, but Ricky forgot to take his medication for a couple of days. His father knew Ricky wasn't sleeping well at night and he could hear Ricky talking to himself in the next room.

Today when his father was at work, Ricky began to hear some voices outside the apartment. The voices grew louder. They said, "You're no good; you can't do anything right. You can't take care of yourself or protect your dad. We're going to get you both." Ricky grew more frightened and went to the closet where his dad kept his tools and grabbed a hammer and ran outside. When his father came home from work early, Ricky wasn't in the apartment, but his coat and wallet were still there. Ricky's father called a neighbor and they drove around the apartment complex looking for Ricky. They finally found him crouched behind some bushes. Although it was 55 degrees, he was wearing only a T-shirt and shorts and no shoes. Ricky's neighbor called emergency services and they were on the way. Meanwhile, Ricky's father tried to coax Ricky into the car, but Ricky wouldn't come. The voices had grown louder and he was sure it was the devil who had kidnaped his dad and was coming for him too. He saw someone else in the car with his dad. The voices said they would crash the car if he got in. They were laughing at him! He couldn't get into the car; it was only a trap. His dad had tried his best, but he was trapped too. What can I do to protect us from the devil! The voices tell him to use the hammer and destroy the car to finish off the devil. He begins to swing the hammer into the windshield, but someone is holding him back.

The emergency services staff has arrived and they speak quietly and firmly as they remove the hammer from Ricky's hands. They tell Ricky they are taking him to the hospital, where he and his father will be safe. They gently put him on a stretcher with restraints, and his father rides in the emergency van with him to the hospital.

▶ Positive and Negative Symptoms of Schizophrenia

POSITIVE OR HARD SYMPTOMS

Hallucinations: False sensory perceptions or perceptual experiences that do not exist in reality
Delusions: Fixed false beliefs that have no basis in reality
Echopraxia: Imitation of the movements and gestures of another person whom the client is observing
Flight of ideas: Continuous flow of verbalization in which the person jumps rapidly from one topic to another
Perseveration: Persistent adherence to a single idea or topic; verbal repetition of a sentence, word, or phrase, resisting attempts to change the topic.
Associative looseness: Fragmented or poorly related thoughts and ideas
Ideas of reference: False impressions that external events have special meaning for the person
Ambivalence: Holding seemingly contradictory beliefs or feelings about the same person, event, or situation

NEGATIVE OR SOFT SYMPTOMS

Apathy: Feelings of indifference toward people, activities, events
Alogia: Tendency to speak very little or convey little substance of meaning (poverty of content)
Flat affect: Absence of any facial expression that would indicate emotions or mood
Blunted affect: Restricted range of emotional feeling tone, or mood
Anhedonia: Feeling no joy or pleasure from life or any activities or relationships
Catatonia: Psychologically induced immobility, occasionally marked by periods of agitation or excitement; the client seems motionless, as if in a trance
Lack of volition: Absence of will, ambition, or drive to take action or accomplish tasks

- Schizophrenia, catatonic type: characterized by marked psychomotor disturbance, either motionless or excessive motor activity, extreme negativism, mutism, peculiarities of voluntary movement, echolalia, or echopraxia. Motor immobility may be manifested by catalepsy (waxy flexibility) or stupor. The excessive motor activity is apparently purposeless and is not influenced by external stimuli.
- Schizophrenia, undifferentiated type: characterized by mixed schizophrenic symptoms (or other types) along with disturbances of thought, affect, and behavior
- Schizophrenia, residual type: characterized by at least one previous episode but not currently psychotic, social withdrawal, flat affect, looseness of associations.

CLINICAL COURSE

Although the symptoms of schizophrenia are always severe, the long-term course of the disease is not always one of progressive deterioration. The clinical course can vary from patient to patient.

Onset

The onset may be abrupt or insidious, but most clients experience a slow and gradual development of signs and symptoms, such as social withdrawal, unusual behavior, loss of interest in school or work, and often neglect of hygiene. The diagnosis of schizophrenia is usually made when the person begins to display more active positive symptoms of delusions, hallucinations, and disordered thinking (**psychosis**). Regardless of when and how the illness begins and the type of schizophrenia, there are substantial and enduring consequences for most clients and their families.

When and how the illness develops seems to affect the outcome. The age of onset seems to be an important factor in how well the client fares. Those who develop the illness earlier show worse outcomes than those who develop it later. Younger clients display a poorer premorbid adjustment, more prominent negative signs, and more cognitive impairment than do older clients. Those who experience a gradual onset of the disease (about 50%) tend to have both a poorer immediate and a poorer long-term course than those who experience an acute and sudden onset (Buchanan & Carpenter, 2000).

Immediate Course

In the years immediately after the onset of psychotic symptoms, two typical patterns emerge. In one pattern, the client experiences continuous psychosis, with some shift in the severity of symptoms, but never fully recovers from the psychosis. In the other clinical pattern, the client experiences episodes of psychotic symptoms followed by relatively complete recovery from the psychosis between episodes.

Long-Term Course

The intensity of psychosis tends to diminish with age. Many clients with long-term impairment regain some degree of social and occupational functioning. The disease becomes less disruptive to the person's life and easier to manage, but the effects of many years of dysfunction are rarely overcome (Buchanan & Carpenter, 2000). In later life, these clients may live independently or in a structured, family-type setting and may be successful at jobs that have stable expectations in a supportive work environment.

Antipsychotic medications play a crucial role in the course of the disease and the outcome for individual clients. They do not provide a cure for the disorder but are crucial to the successful management of the illness. The more effective the client's response and adherence to these medication regimens, the better the outcome.

RELATED DISORDERS

Other disorders are related to schizophrenia but are distinguished in terms of presenting symptoms and the duration or magnitude of impairment. The DSM-IV-TR (2000) categorizes these disorders as:

- Schizophreniform disorder: The client exhibits the symptoms of schizophrenia, but for less than the 6 months necessary to meet the diagnostic criteria for schizophrenia. There may or may not be impaired social or occupational functioning.
- Schizoaffective disorder: The client exhibits the symptoms of psychosis and at the same time exhibits all the features of a mood disorder, either depression or mania.
- Delusional disorder: The client has one or more nonbizarre delusions—that is, it is a believable idea. Psychosocial functioning is not markedly impaired, and behavior is not obviously odd or bizarre.
- Brief psychotic disorder: The client has a sudden onset of at least one psychotic symptom, such as delusions, hallucinations, or disorganized speech or behavior, that lasts from 1 day to 1 month. The episode may or may not have an identifiable stressor or may follow childbirth.
- Shared psychotic disorder (*folie à deux*): A similar delusion is shared by two people. The person with this diagnosis develops this delusion in the context of a close relationship with someone who has psychotic delusions.

Two other diagnoses, schizoid personality disorder and schizotypal personality disorder, are not psychotic disorders and should not be confused with schizophrenia even though the names sound similar. These two diagnoses are covered in Chapter 16, Personality Disorders.

ETIOLOGY

Whether schizophrenia is an organic disease with underlying physical brain pathology has been an important question for researchers and clinicians for as long as the illness has been studied. In the first half of the 20th century, studies focused on trying to find a particular pathologic structure associated with the disease, largely through autopsy. Such a site was not discovered. In the 1950s and 1960s, the emphasis shifted to examination of psychological and social factors as causative factors. Interpersonal theorists suggested that schizophrenia resulted from dysfunctional relationships in early life and adolescence. One popular theory suggested that schizophrenia resulted from an overly anxious, overly protective, or emotionally cold mother or a distant and controlling father. None of these interpersonal theories was proven, but although newer scientific studies are finding answers in neurologic/neurochemical causes, many people still believe that schizophrenia results from dysfunctional parenting or family dynamics. Many parents or family members of persons diagnosed with schizophrenia agonize over what they did "wrong" or what they could have done to help prevent it (Torrey, 1995).

Newer scientific studies began to demonstrate that schizophrenia is the result of a type of brain dysfunction. In the 1970s, studies began to focus on possible neurochemical causes, and this is still the primary focus of research and theory today. These neurochemical/neurologic theories are supported by the effects of antipsychotic medications, which help control psychotic symptoms, and neuroimaging tools such as computed tomography (CT), which have shown that the brains of persons with schizophrenia are different in structure and function (Gur & Gur, 2000).

The following are the areas of current interest and study.

Biologic Theories

The biologic theories of schizophrenia focus on genetic factors, neuroanatomic and neurochemical factors (structure and function of the brain), and immunovirology (the body's response to exposure to a virus).

GENETIC FACTORS

Most genetic studies have focused on immediate families such as parents, siblings, and offspring to see whether schizophrenia is genetically transmitted or inherited. Few have focused on more distant relatives.

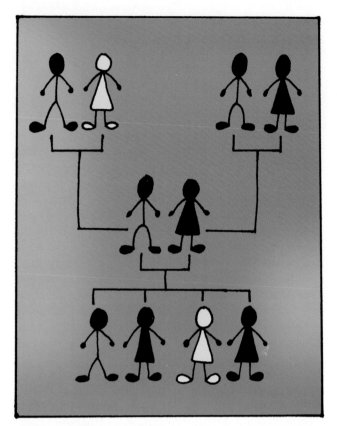

Genetic studies

The most important studies have centered on twin studies, which have demonstrated that identical twins have a 50% risk for the disorder, whereas fraternal twins have only a 15% risk. This indicates that schizophrenia is somewhat inherited. Other important studies have shown that children with one biologic parent with schizophrenia have a 15% risk; this rises to 35% if both biologic parents have schizophrenia. Children whose biologic parents have a history of schizophrenia but who are adopted at birth into a family with no history of schizophrenia still reflect the genetic risk of their biologic parents. All these studies have indicated that there is a genetic risk or tendency for schizophrenia, but this is not the only factor: identical twins have a 50% risk, even though their genes are 100% identical (Cancro & Lehman, 2000).

NEUROANATOMIC AND NEUROCHEMICAL FACTORS

With the development of noninvasive imaging techniques such as CT scans, magnetic resonance imaging (MRI), and positron emission tomography (PET) in the past 25 years, scientists have been able to study the brain structure (neuroanatomy) and activity (neurochemical) of persons with schizophrenia. Studies have demonstrated that persons with schizophrenia have relatively less brain tissue; this could represent a failure in development or a subsequent loss of tissue. CT scans have shown enlarged ventricles in the brain and cortical atrophy. PET studies suggest that there is diminished oxygen and glucose metabolism in the frontal cortical structures of the brain (Fig. 13-1). The research consistently shows decreased brain volume and abnormal brain function in the frontal and temporal areas of persons with schizophrenia. This pathology correlates with the positive signs of schizophrenia (temporal lobe) such as psychosis and the negative signs (frontal lobe) such as lack of volition or motivation and anhedonia. It is unknown whether these changes in the frontal and temporal lobes are due to a failure of these areas to develop properly or whether the areas have been damaged by a virus, trauma, or immune response. Intrauterine influences such as poor nutrition, tobacco, alcohol, and other drugs, and stress are also being studied as possible causes of the pathology found in the brains of persons with schizophrenia (Buchanan & Carpenter, 2000).

Neurochemical studies have consistently demonstrated the existence of alterations in the neurotransmitter systems of the brain in persons with schizophrenia. There seems to be malfunction in the neuronal networks that transmit information by electrical signals from a nerve cell through its axon and across synapses to postsynaptic receptors on other nerve cells. The transmission of the signal across the synapse requires a complex series of biochemical events. Studies have implicated the actions of dopamine, serotonin, norepinephrine, acetylcholine, glutamate, and several neuromodulary peptides.

Currently the most prominent neurochemical theories involve dopamine and serotonin. One prominent theory suggests an excess of dopamine as a causal factor. This theory was developed based on two types of observations. First, drugs that increased activity in the dopaminergic system, such as amphetamine and levodopa, sometimes induced a paranoid psychotic reaction similar to schizophrenia (Egan & Hyde, 2000). Second, drugs blocking postsynaptic dopamine receptors reduce psychotic symptoms; in fact, the greater the ability of the drug to block dopamine receptors, the more effective it is in decreasing schizophrenic symptoms (O'Connor, 1998).

More recently, serotonin has been included among the leading neurochemical factors affecting schizophrenia. The theory regarding serotonin suggests that serotonin has a modulating effect on dopamine, helping to control excess dopamine. Some believe that an excess of serotonin itself plays a role in the development of schizophrenia. Newer atypical antipsychotics such as clozapine (Clozaril) are both dopamine and serotonin antagonists. Drug studies have shown that clozapine can produce a dramatic reduction in psy-

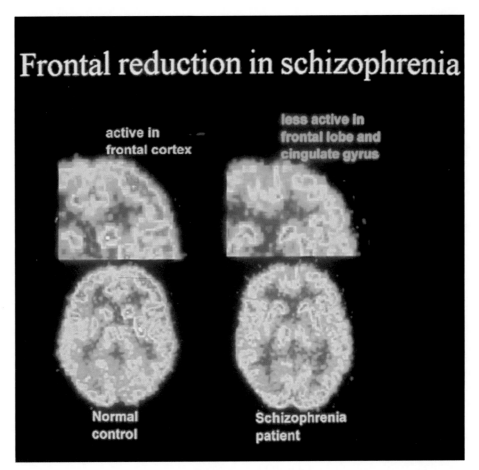

Figure 13-1. *Scan 11.* PET scan with 18F-deoxyglucose shows metabolic activity in a horizontal section of the brain in a control subject (*left*) and in an unmedicated patient with schizophrenia (*right*). Red and yellow indicate areas of high metabolic activity in the cortex; green and blue indicate lower activity in the white matter areas of the brain. The frontal lobe is magnified to show reduced frontal activity in the prefrontal cortex of the patient with schizophrenia. (Courtesy of Monte S. Buchsbaum, MD, The Mount Sinai Medical Center and School of Medicine, New York, New York.)

chotic symptoms and ameliorate the negative signs of schizophrenia (Marder, 2000; O'Connor, 1998).

IMMUNOVIROLOGIC FACTORS

There are popular theories that the altered brain pathology of persons with schizophrenia could be caused by exposure to a virus, or that the body's immune response to a virus could alter brain physiology. Although scientists continue to study this, not many studies have been able to validate these theories (Egan & Hyde, 2000).

Recently researchers have been focusing on infections in pregnant women as a possible origin for schizophrenia. Flu epidemics have been followed a generation later by waves of schizophrenia in England, Wales, Denmark, Finland, and other countries. A re-

cent study published in the *New England Journal of Medicine* reports higher rates of schizophrenia among children born in crowded areas in cold weather, conditions hospitable to respiratory ailments (Mortensen et al., 1999).

CULTURAL CONSIDERATIONS

It is important to be aware of cultural differences when assessing for symptoms of schizophrenia. Ideas that appear to be delusional in one culture, such as beliefs in sorcery or witchcraft, may be common in other cultures. Also, in some cultures, auditory or visual hallucinations, such as seeing the Virgin Mary or hearing God's voice, may be a normal part of religious experiences. The assessment of affect requires sensitivity to differences in eye contact, body language, and acceptable emotional expression; these vary across cultures (DSM-IV-TR, 2000).

In a large study involving 26,400 psychiatric clients, Flaskerud and Hu (1992) found significant differences in the psychiatric diagnoses given to both inpatients and outpatients. African American and Asian clients were diagnosed with schizophrenia more often than whites. Latino clients had fewer diagnoses of schizophrenia than did whites. The study found that these differences in diagnosis could not be attributed to other variables such as sex, age, socioeconomic status, primary language, or expression of psychopathology.

Psychotic behavior observed in countries other than the United States or among particular ethnic groups has been identified as a "culture-bound" syndrome. Although these episodes exist primarily in certain countries, they may be seen in other places as people visit or immigrate to other countries or areas. Mezzich, Lin, and Hughes (2000) summarized some of these psychotic behaviors:

- *Bouffée delirante,* a syndrome found in West Africa and Haiti, involves a sudden outburst of agitated and aggressive behavior, marked confusion, and psychomotor excitement. It is sometimes accompanied by visual and auditory hallucinations or paranoid ideation.
- Ghost sickness is a preoccupation with death and the deceased frequently observed among members of some Native American tribes. Symptoms include bad dreams, weakness, feelings of danger, loss of appetite, fainting, dizziness, fear, anxiety, hallucinations, loss of consciousness, confusion, feelings of futility, and a sense of suffocation.
- *Locura* refers to a chronic psychosis experienced by Latinos in the United States and Latin America. Symptoms include incoherence, agitation, visual and auditory hallucinations, inability to follow social rules, unpredictability, and possible violence.
- *Qi-gong* psychotic reaction is an acute, time-limited episode characterized by dissociative, paranoid, or other psychotic symptoms that occur after participating in the Chinese folk health-enhancing practice of *qi-gong.* Especially vulnerable are persons who become overly involved in the practice.
- *Zar* is an experience of spirits possessing another person seen in Ethiopia, Somalia, Egypt, Sudan, Iran, and other North African and Middle Eastern societies. Afflicted persons may laugh, shout, wail, bang their head on a wall, or be apathetic and withdrawn, refusing to eat or carry out daily tasks. Such behavior is not considered pathologic locally.

Ethnicity may also be a factor in the way a person responds to psychotropic medications. This difference in response is probably due to the person's genetic makeup. Some people metabolize certain drugs more slowly, so the drug level in the bloodstream is higher than desired. African Americans, Caucasians, and Hispanics in the United States appear to require comparable therapeutic doses of antipsychotic medications. However, Asian clients need lower doses of drugs such as haloperidol (Haldol) to obtain the same effects (Kudzma, 1999); therefore, they would be likely to experience more severe side effects if given the traditional or usual doses.

TREATMENT

Psychopharmacology

The primary medical treatment for schizophrenia is psychopharmacology. In the past, electroconvulsive therapy, insulin shock therapy, and psychosurgery were used, but with the discovery of chlorpromazine (Thorazine) in 1952, other treatment modalities have become all but obsolete. Antipsychotic medications, also known as **neuroleptics**, are prescribed primarily for their efficacy in decreasing psychotic symptoms. They do not provide a cure for schizophrenia but are used to manage the symptoms of the disease.

The typical, or older, antipsychotic medications are dopamine antagonists. The newer, or atypical, antipsychotic medications are both dopamine and serotonin antagonists (see Chap. 2). These medications, usual daily dosages, and common side effects are listed in Table 13-1. The typical antipsychotics target the positive signs of schizophrenia, such as delusions, hallucinations, disturbed thinking, and other psychotic symptoms, but have no observable effect on the negative signs. The atypical antipsychotics not only diminish psychotic symptoms, but for many clients they also lessen the negative signs such as lack of volition and motivation, social withdrawal, and anhedonia (Littrell & Littrell, 1998).

Two antipsychotics are available in depot injection forms for maintenance therapy, fluphenazine (Prolixin), in decanoate and enanthate preparations, and haloperidol (Haldol) decanoate (Spratto & Woods, 2000). The vehicle for depot injections is sesame oil, and therefore the medications are slowly absorbed over time into the client's system. The effects of the medications last 2 to 4 weeks, eliminating the need to take oral antipsychotic medication daily (see Chap. 2). The duration of action is 7 to 28 days for fluphenazine and 4 weeks for haloperidol. It may take several weeks of oral therapy with these medications to reach a stable dosing level before the transition to depot injec-

Table 13-1

ANTIPSYCHOTIC DRUGS, USUAL DAILY DOSAGES, AND INCIDENCE OF SIDE EFFECTS

Generic (Trade) Name	Usual Daily Dosage* (mg)	Sedation	Hypotension	EPS	Anticholinergic
TYPICAL ANTIPSYCHOTICS					
Chlorpromazine (Thorazine)	200–1,600	++++	+++	++	+++
Trifluoperazine (Trilafon)	16–32	++	++++	+	
Fluphenazine (Prolixin)	2.5–20	+	+	++++	+
Thioridazine (Mellaril)	200–600	++++	+++	+	+++
Mesoridazine (Serentil)	75–300	++++	++	+	++
Thiothixene (Navane)	6–30	+	+	++++	+
Haloperidol (Haldol)	2–20	+	+	++++	+/0
Loxapine (Loxitane)	60–100	+++	++	+++	++
Molindone (Moban)	50–100	+	+/0	+	++
Perphenazine (Etrafon)	16–32	++	++	+++	+
Trifluoperazine (Stelazine)	6–50	+	+	++++	+
ATYPICAL ANTIPSYCHOTICS					
Clozapine (Clozaril)	150–500	++++	++	+/0	++
Risperidone (Risperdol)	2–8	+++	++	++	+
Olanzapine (Zyprexa)	5–20	++++	+++	+	++
Quetiapine (Seroquel)	150–500		++++	+	+

*Oral dosage only
EPS, extrapyramidal side effects
++++, very significant; +++, significant; ++, moderate; + = mild; +/0 = rare or absent
Adapted from McEvoy, R. B. (Ed.) (2000). *Facts and comparisons 2000*. St. Louis: Facts and Comparisons,
A Wolters Kluwer Company. Spratto, G. R., & Woods, A. L. (2000). *PDR nurse's drug handbook, 2000 edition*.
Montvale, NJ: Medical Economics Company, Inc.

tions can be made. Therefore, these preparations are not suitable for the management of acute episodes of psychosis. They are, however, very useful for clients requiring supervised medication compliance in the long term.

SIDE EFFECTS

The side effects of antipsychotic medications are significant and can range from mild discomfort to permanent movement disorders (Marder, 2000). Because many of these side effects are frightening and upsetting to clients, they are frequently cited as the primary reason why they discontinue or reduce the dosage of their medications. Serious neurologic side effects include extrapyramidal side effects (acute dystonic reactions, akathisia, and parkinsonism), tardive dyskinesia, seizures, and neuroleptic malignant syndrome (discussed below). Nonneurologic side effects include sedation, photosensitivity, and anticholinergic symptoms such as dry mouth, blurred vision, constipation, urinary retention, and orthostatic hypotension. Table 13-2 lists the side effects of antipsychotic medications and appropriate nursing interventions.

Extrapyramidal side effects, reversible movement disorders induced by neuroleptic medication, include dystonic reactions, parkinsonism, and akathisia. **Dystonic reactions** to antipsychotic medications

appear early in the course of treatment and are characterized by spasms in discrete muscle groups such as the neck muscles (torticollis) or eye muscles (oculogyric crisis). Dystonic reactions are extremely frightening and painful for the client. Acute treatment consists of diphenhydramine (Benadryl), given either intramuscularly or intravenously or benzotropin (Cogentin) given intramuscularly. **Parkinsonism** or **neuroleptic-induced parkinsonism** includes shuffling gait, masklike facies, muscle stiffness, and drooling. Treatment of parkinsonism and prevention of further dystonic reactions is achieved with the medications listed in Table 13-3.

Akathisia is characterized by restless movement, pacing, inability to remain still, and the client's report of inner restlessness. Clients are very uncomfortable with these sensations and may stop taking the antipsychotic medication to avoid these side effects. Beta-blockers such as propranolol have been most effective in treating akathisia, and some success has been experienced with benzodiazepines.

Tardive dyskinesia, a late-appearing side effect of antipsychotic medications, is characterized by abnormal, involuntary movements such as lip smacking, tongue protrusion, chewing, blinking, grimacing, and choreiform movements of the limbs and feet. These involuntary movements are embarrassing for clients and may cause them to become more socially isolated. Tardive dyskinesia is irreversible once it has

Table 13-2

SIDE EFFECTS OF ANTIPSYCHOTIC MEDICATIONS AND NURSING INTERVENTIONS

Side Effect	Nursing Intervention
Dystonic reactions	Administer medications as ordered; assess for effectiveness; reassure client if frightened.
Tardive dyskinesia	Assess using tool such as AIMS; report occurrence or increase in score to physician.
Neuroleptic malignant syndrome	Stop all antipsychotic medications; notify physician immediately.
Akathisia	Administer medications as ordered; assess for effectiveness.
Extrapyramidal side effects or neuroleptic-induced parkinsonism	Administer medications as ordered; assess for effectiveness.
Seizures	Stop medication; notify physician; protect client from injury during seizure; provide reassurance and privacy for client after seizure.
Sedation	Caution about activities requiring client to be fully alert, such as driving a car.
Photosensitivity	Avoid sun exposure; when in the sun, wear protective clothing and sun-blocking lotion.
Anticholinergic symptoms	
Dry mouth	Use ice chips or hard candy for relief.
Blurred vision	Assess side effect, which should improve with time; report to physician if no improvement.
Constipation	Increase fluid and dietary fiber intake; may need a stool softener if unrelieved.
Urinary retention	Instruct client to report any frequency or burning with urination; report to physician if no improvement over time.
Orthostatic hypotension	Instruct client to rise slowly from sitting or lying position; wait to ambulate until no longer dizzy or light-headed.

Table 13-3

EFFICACY OF DRUGS USED TO TREAT EXTRAPYRAMIDAL SIDE EFFECTS AND NURSING INTERVENTIONS

Generic Trade Name	Akathisia	Dystonia	Rigidity	Tremor	Nursing Interventions
Benztropine (Cogentin)	2	2	3	2	Increase fluid and fiber intake to avoid constipation; use ice chips or hard candy for dry mouth; assess for memory impairment (another side effect).
Trihexyphenidyl (Artane)	2	3	3	3	
Biperiden (Akineton)	1	3	3	3	
Procyclidine (Kemadrin)	1	3	3	3	
Amantadine (Symmetrel)	3	2	3	2	Use ice chips or hard candy for dry mouth; assess for worsening psychosis (an occasional side effect).
Diphenhydramine (Benadryl)	2	2–3	1	2	Use ice chips or hard candy for dry mouth; observe for sedation.
Diazepam (Valium)	2	1–2	1–2	0–1	Observe for sedation; potential for misuse or abuse.
Lorazepam (Ativan)	2	1–2	1–2	0–1	Observe for sedation; potential for misuse or abuse.
Propranolol (Inderal)	3	0	0	1–2	Assess for palpitations, dizziness, cold hands and feet.

0, no effect; 1, some effect (20% response); 2, moderate effect (20–40% response); 3, good effect (40% response).
McEvoy, R. B. (Ed.). (2000). *Facts and comparisons 2000.* St. Louis: Facts and Comparisons, A Wolters Kluwer Company. *Psychotropic drugs: Fast facts* (3rd ed.). New York: W.W. Norton and Company. Spratto, G. R., & Woods, A. L. (2000). *PDR nurse's drug handbook, 2000 edition.* Montvale, NJ; Medical Economics Company, Inc.

appeared, but progression can be arrested by decreasing or discontinuing the medication. Clozapine (Clozaril), an atypical antipsychotic drug, has not been found to result in this side effect, so it is often recommended for clients who have experienced tardive dyskinesia while taking typical antipsychotic drugs.

It is important to screen clients for late-appearing movement disorders such as tardive dyskinesia. The **Abnormal Involuntary Movement Scale** (AIMS) is used to screen for symptoms of movement disorders. The client is observed in several positions, and the severity of symptoms is rated from 0 to 4. The AIMS can be administered every 3 to 6 months. If the nurse

detects an increased score on the AIMS, indicating increased symptoms of tardive dyskinesia, the physician should be notified so the client's dosage or drug can be changed to prevent advancement of tardive dyskinesia. The AIMS examination procedure is presented in Box 13-1.

Seizures are an infrequent side effect associated with antipsychotic medications. The incidence is 1% in the population of people taking antipsychotics. The notable exception is clozapine, with an incidence of 5%. Seizures may be associated with high doses of the medication. Treatment is a lowered dosage or a different antipsychotic medication.

Box 13-1

➤ ABNORMAL INVOLUNTARY MOVEMENT SCALE (AIMS) EXAMINATION PROCEDURE

Patient identification: _____ Date _____

Rated by: _____

Either before or after completing the examination procedure, observe the patient unobtrusively at rest (e.g., in waiting room).

The chair to be used in this examination should be a hard, firm one without arms.

After observing the patient, he or she may be rated on a scale of 0 (none), 1 (minimal), 2 (mild), 3 (moderate), and 4 (severe) according to the severity of symptoms.

Ask the patient whether there is anything in his/her mouth (i.e., gum, candy, etc.) and if there is to remove it.

Ask patient about the current condition of his/her teeth. Ask patient if he/she wears dentures. Do teeth or dentures bother patient now?

Ask patient whether he/she notices any movement in mouth, face, hands, or feet. If yes, ask to describe and to what extent they currently bother patient or interfere with his/her activities.

0 1 2 3 4	Have patient sit in chair with hands on knees, legs slightly apart, and feet flat on floor. (Look at entire body for movements while in this position.)
0 1 2 3 4	Ask patient to sit with hands hanging unsupported. If male, between legs, if female and wearing a dress, hanging over knees. (Observe hands and other body areas.)
0 1 2 3 4	Ask patient to open mouth. (Observe tongue at rest within mouth.) Do this twice.
0 1 2 3 4	Ask patient to protrude tongue. (Observe abnormalities of tongue movement.) Do this twice.
0 1 2 3 4	Ask the patient to tap thumb, with each finger, as rapidly as possible for 10–15 seconds; separately with right hand, then with left hand. (Observe facial and leg movements.)
0 1 2 3 4	Flex and extend patient's left and right arms. (One at a time.)
0 1 2 3 4	Ask patient to stand up. (Observe in profile. Observe all body areas again, hips included.)
0 1 2 3 4	*Ask patient to extend both arms outstretched in front with palms down. (Observe trunk, legs, and mouth.)
0 1 2 3 4	*Have patient walk a few paces, turn and walk back to chair. (Observe hands and gait.) Do this twice.

Activated movements.

Neuroleptic malignant syndrome (NMS) is a serious and frequently fatal condition seen in persons being treated with antipsychotic medications. It is characterized by muscle rigidity, high fever, increased muscle enzymes (particularly CPK), and leukocytosis (increased leukocytes). It is estimated that 0.1% to 1% of all clients taking antipsychotics develop NMS (O'Connor, 1998). Any of the antipsychotic medications can cause NMS, which is treated by stopping the medication. The client's ability to tolerate other antipsychotic medications after the occurrence of NMS varies, but use of another antipsychotic appears possible in most instances.

Clozapine has the potentially fatal side effect of agranulocytosis (failure of the bone marrow to produce adequate white blood cells). It develops suddenly and is characterized by fever, malaise, ulcerative sore throat, and leukopenia. This side effect may not be manifested immediately but can occur as long as 18–24 weeks after the initiation of therapy. The drug must be discontinued immediately. Clients taking this antipsychotic must have weekly white blood cell counts. Currently, clozapine is dispensed every 7 days only, and evidence of the white cell count is required before a refill is furnished.

Adjunctive Treatment

In addition to pharmacologic treatment, many other modes of treatment can be helpful to the person with schizophrenia. Individual and group therapy, milieu therapy, and family therapy can be instituted for clients in both inpatient and community settings.

Individual and group therapy sessions are often supportive in nature, giving the client an opportunity for social contact and meaningful relationships with other people. Groups that focus on topics of concern such as medication management, use of community supports, and family concerns have also been beneficial to clients with schizophrenia (Fenton & Cole, 1995).

In the acute care setting, a structured environment was found to be more beneficial for the client with schizophrenia than open or unstructured settings (Slately, 1994). The milieu can provide activity groups, resources for resolving conflicts, and opportunities for learning new skills. The nurse can also use music and drawing to ease the client's social withdrawal, decrease anxiety, and promote motivation.

Family education and therapy are known to diminish the negative effects of schizophrenia, thus reducing the relapse rate (McFarlane, 1995). In addition, family members can benefit from a supportive environment that helps them cope with the many difficulties presented when a loved one has schizophrenia.

APPLICATION OF THE NURSING PROCESS

Assessment

Schizophrenia is a clinical syndrome or disease process that affects cognition, perception, emotion, behavior, and social functioning, but it affects each individual differently. The degree of impairment in both the acute or psychotic phase and the chronic or long-term phase varies greatly among individuals; thus, so do the needs of each client and the nursing interventions. The nurse must not make assumptions about the client's abilities or limitations based solely on the medical diagnosis of schizophrenia.

For example, the nurse may care for a client in an acute inpatient setting. The client may appear frightened and is hearing voices (hallucinating), making no eye contact, and mumbling constantly. The nurse would be dealing with the positive or psychotic signs of the disease. Another nurse may encounter a client with schizophrenia in a community setting who is not experiencing psychotic symptoms but rather has a lack of energy for daily tasks and feelings of loneliness and isolation (the negative signs of schizophrenia). Although both clients have the same medical diagnosis, the approach and interventions taken by the nurse would be very different.

HISTORY

The nurse first elicits information about the client's previous history with schizophrenia to establish a baseline of functioning. The nurse asks questions about how the client functioned before the crisis developed, such as "How do you usually spend your time?" and "Can you describe what you do each day?"

The nurse assesses the age of onset of schizophrenia, knowing that poorer outcomes are associated with an earlier age of onset. It is also important to learn the client's previous history of hospital admissions and his or her response to hospitalization.

Assessing Suicidal Ideation. The nurse also assesses the client for previous suicide attempts. Ten percent of all persons with schizophrenia eventually commit suicide. The nurse might ask, "Have you ever attempted suicide?" or "Have you ever heard voices telling you to hurt yourself?"

Assessing Support Systems. It is important for the nurse to assess whether the client has been using current support systems by asking the client or significant others the following questions:

- Has the client kept in contact with family or friends?

- Has the client been to scheduled groups or therapy appointments?
- Does the client seem to run out of money between paychecks?
- Have the client's living arrangements changed recently?

Assessing the Client's Perceptions. Finally, the nurse assesses the client's perception of his or her current situation—that is, what the client believes to be significant events or stressors at the present time. The nurse can assess this by asking, "What do you see as the primary problem now?" or "What do you need help managing now?"

GENERAL APPEARANCE AND MOTOR BEHAVIOR

The appearance may vary widely among different clients with schizophrenia. Some may appear normal in terms of being dressed appropriately, sitting in a chair conversing with the nurse, and exhibiting no strange or unusual postures or gestures. Others may exhibit odd or bizarre behavior. They may appear disheveled and unkempt, with no apparent concern for their hygiene, or they may wear clothing combinations that are strange or inappropriate (for instance, wearing a heavy wool coat and stocking cap in hot weather).

The client's overall motor behavior may also appear odd. The client may be restless and unable to sit still, may exhibit agitation and pacing, or may appear unmoving (**catatonia**). The client may also demonstrate seemingly purposeless gestures (stereotypic behavior) and odd facial expressions such as grimacing. The client may also imitate the movements and gestures of someone he or she is observing (**echopraxia**). These behaviors are likely to be accompanied by rambling speech that may or may not make sense to the listener.

Conversely, the client may exhibit **psychomotor retardation** (a general slowing of all movements). Sometimes the client may be almost immobile, curled into a ball (fetal position). Clients with the catatonic type of schizophrenia can exhibit **waxy flexibility**: they maintain any position in which they are placed, even if the position is awkward or uncomfortable.

The client may exhibit an unusual speech pattern. Two typical patterns are **word salad** (jumbled words and phrases that are disconnected or incoherent, making no sense to the listener) and **echolalia** (repetition or imitation of what someone else says). Speech may be slowed or accelerated in rate and volume: the client may speak in whispers or hushed tones, or may talk loudly or yell. **Latency of response** refers to hesitation before the client responds to questions. This latency or hesitation may last 30 or 45 seconds (Cancro & Lehman, 2000) and usually indicates the client's difficulty with cognition or thought processes. Box 13-2 lists these unusual speech patterns and gives examples.

MOOD AND AFFECT

Clients with schizophrenia report and demonstrate a wide variety of mood and affect. Patients with schizophrenia are often described as having **flat affect**

Box 13-2

▶ UNUSUAL SPEECH PATTERNS OF CLIENTS WITH SCHIZOPHRENIA

Clang associations are ideas that are related to each other based on sound or rhyming rather than meaning.
Example: "I will take a pill if I go up the hill but not if my name is Jill, I don't want to kill."

Neologisms are words invented by the client.
Example: "I'm afraid of grittiz. If there are any grittiz here, I will have to leave. Are you a grittiz?"

Verbigeration is the stereotyped repetition of words or phrases that may or may not have meaning to the listener.
Example: "I want to go home, go home, go home, go home."

Echolalia is the client's imitation or repetition of what the nurse says.
Example: *Nurse:* "Can you tell me how you're feeling?" *Client:* "Can you tell me how you're feeling, how you're feeling?"

Stilted language is use of words or phrases that are flowery, excessive, and pompous.
Example: "Would you be so kind, as a representative of Florence Nightingale, as to do me the honor of providing just a wee bit of refreshment, perhaps in the form of some clear spring water?"

Perseveration is the persistent adherence to a single idea or topic and verbal repetition of a sentence, phrase, or word, even when attempts are made by another to change the topic.
Example: *Nurse:* "How have you been sleeping lately?" *Client:* "I think people have been following me." *Nurse:* "Where do you live?" *Client:* "At my place people have been following me." *Nurse:* "What do you like to do in your free time?" *Client:* "Nothing because people are following me."

Word salad is a combination of jumbled words and phrases that are disconnected or incoherent and make no sense to the listener.
Example: "Corn, potatoes, jump up, play games, grass, cupboard."

(absence of facial expression) or **blunted affect** (exhibiting few observable facial expressions). The typical facial expression is often described as masklike. The affect may also be described as silly, characterized by giddy laughter for no apparent reason. The client may exhibit an inappropriate expression or emotions incongruent with the context of the situation. This incongruence ranges from being mild or subtle to grossly inappropriate. For example, the client may be laughing and grinning while describing the death of a family member or be weeping while talking about the weather.

The client may report feeling depressed and having no pleasure or joy in life (**anhedonia**). Conversely, he or she may report feeling all-knowing and all-powerful and not at all concerned with the circumstance or situation. It is more common for the client to report exaggerated feelings of well-being during episodes of psychotic or delusional thinking and a lack of energy or pleasurable feelings during the chronic or long-term phase of the illness.

THOUGHT PROCESS AND CONTENT

Schizophrenia is often referred to as a thought disorder because that is the primary feature of the disease. Thought process is assessed through verbal communication inferred from what the client says. Thought content is assembled by what the client actually says. In schizophrenia, the client's thought process becomes disordered; the continuity of thoughts and information processing is disrupted (Cancro & Lehman, 2000). The client may suddenly stop talking in the middle of a sentence and remain silent for several seconds to a minute (**thought blocking**). The client may also state he or she believes that others can hear his or her thoughts (**thought broadcasting**) or that others are placing thoughts in the client's mind against his or her will (**thought insertion**).

Clients may also exhibit tangential thinking; the client veers onto unrelated topics, never answering the original question:

Nurse: "How have you been sleeping lately?"
Client: "Oh, I try to sleep at night. I like to listen to music to help me sleep. I really like country-western music best. What do you like? Can I have something to eat pretty soon? I'm hungry."
Nurse: "Can you tell me how you've been sleeping?"

Circumstantiality may be evidenced if the client gives unnecessary details or strays off the topic but eventually provides the requested information:

Nurse: "How have you been sleeping lately?"
Client: "Oh, I go to bed early, so I can get plenty of rest. I like to listen to music or read before bed.

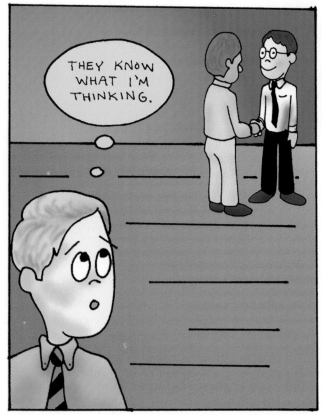

Thought broadcasting

Right now I'm reading a good mystery. Maybe I'll write a mystery someday. But it isn't helping, reading I mean. I have only been getting 2 or 3 hours of sleep at night."

Poverty of content (**alogia**) describes the lack of any real meaning or substance in what the client says:

Nurse: "How have you been sleeping lately?"
Client: "Well, I guess, I don't know, hard to tell."

DELUSIONS

Clients with schizophrenia usually experience **delusions** (fixed, false beliefs that have no basis in reality) in the psychotic phase of the illness. A common characteristic of schizophrenic delusions is the direct, immediate, and total certainty with which the client holds these beliefs. Because the client believes the delusional ideas, he or she will therefore act accordingly. For example, the client with delusions of persecution will probably be suspicious and mistrustful and guarded about disclosing personal information; he or she may check out the room or speak in hushed, secretive tones.

The theme or content of the delusions may vary. Box 13-3 describes the various types of delusions and provides examples. These delusional beliefs are not shaken by external, contradictory information or

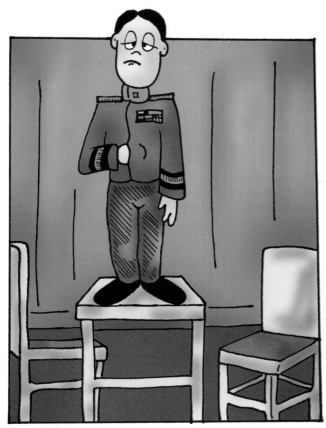

Delusions

> ## TYPES OF DELUSIONS
>
> **Persecutory/paranoid delusions** involve the client's belief that "others" are planning to harm the client or are spying, following, ridiculing, or belittling the client in some way. Sometimes the client cannot define who these "others" are.
> Examples: The client may think that food has been poisoned or that rooms are bugged with listening devices. Sometimes the "persecutor" is the government, FBI, or other powerful organization. Occasionally, specific individuals, even family members, may be named as the "persecutor."
>
> **Grandiose delusions** are characterized by the client's claim to association with famous people or celebrities, or the client's belief that he or she is famous or capable of great feats.
> Examples: The client may claim to be engaged to a famous movie star or related to some public figure, such as claiming to be the daughter of the President of the United States; may claim he or she has found a cure for cancer.
>
> **Religious delusions** often center around the second coming of Christ or another significant religious figure or prophet. These religious delusions appear suddenly as part of the client's psychosis and are not part of his or her religious faith or that of others.
> Examples: Client claims to be the Messiah or some prophet sent from God; believes that God communicates directly to him or her, or that he or she has a "special" religious mission in life or special religious powers.
>
> **Somatic delusions** are generally vague and unrealistic beliefs about the client's health or bodily functions. Factual information or diagnostic testing does not change these beliefs.
> Example: A male client may say that he is pregnant, or a client may report decaying intestines or worms in the brain.
>
> **Referential delusions** or **ideas of reference,** involve the client's belief that television broadcasts, music, or newspaper articles have special meaning for him or her.
> Examples: The client may report that the president was speaking directly to him on a news broadcast, or that special messages are sent through newspaper articles.

facts. If asked why he or she believes such an unlikely idea, the client often replies, "I just know it."

Initially, the nurse assesses the content and depth of the delusion to know what behaviors to expect and to try to establish reality for the client. The nurse must be careful when eliciting information about the client's delusional beliefs not to support or challenge them. The nurse might ask the client to explain what he or she believes, asking questions such as, "Can you explain that to me?" or "Tell me what you're thinking about that."

SENSORIUM AND INTELLECTUAL PROCESSES

One of the hallmark symptoms of schizophrenic psychosis is the presence of **hallucinations** (false sensory perceptions, or perceptual experiences that do not exist in reality). Hallucinations can involve the five senses and bodily sensations. Hallucinations can be threatening and frightening for the client, although less frequently clients report hallucinations as a pleasant experience. Initially, the client perceives hallucinations as real experiences, but at a later point in the illness he or she may recognize them as hallucinations.

Hallucinations are distinguished from illusions, which are misperceptions of actual environmental stimuli. For example, while walking through the woods, a person thinks he sees a snake at the side of the path, but on closer examination, he discovers it is only a curved stick. This is an illusion that was corrected by reality or factual information. Hallucinations have no such basis in reality.

The following are the various types of hallucinations (Cancro & Lehman, 2000):

- *Auditory hallucinations* involve hearing sounds, most often voices, talking to or about the client. There may be one or multiple voices; it may be a familiar or unfamiliar person's voice speaking. Auditory hallucinations are the most common type of hallucination. **Command hallucinations** are voices demanding that the client take action, often to harm himself or herself or others, and are considered dangerous.
- *Visual hallucinations* can involve seeing images that do not exist at all, such as lights or a dead person, or may be a distortion, such as seeing a frightening monster instead of the nurse. These are the second most common type of hallucination.
- *Olfactory hallucinations* involve smells or odors where none exist. It may be a specific scent, such as urine or feces, or more general in nature, such as a rotten or rancid odor. This type of hallucination is often found in clients with dementia, seizures, or cerebrovascular accidents.
- *Tactile hallucinations* refer to sensations such as electricity running through the body or bugs crawling on the skin. Tactile hallucinations are found most often in clients undergoing alcohol withdrawal.
- *Gustatory hallucinations* involve a taste lingering in the mouth, or the sense that food tastes like something else. The taste may be metallic or bitter or may be represented as a specific taste.
- *Cenesthetic hallucinations* involve the client's report that he or she feels bodily functions that are usually undetectable. Examples would be the sensation of urine forming or impulses being transmitted through the brain.
- *Kinesthetic hallucinations* occur when the client is motionless but reports the sensation of bodily movement. Occasionally the bodily movement is something unusual, such as floating above the ground.

During episodes of psychosis, clients are commonly disoriented to time and sometimes place. In the most extreme form of disorientation, **depersonalization**, clients feel detached from their behavior. Although clients can state their name correctly, they feel as if their body belongs to someone else, or that their spirit is detached from their body.

It is difficult to assess the intellectual processes of a client with schizophrenia who is psychotic. The client usually demonstrates poor intellectual functioning as a result of his or her disordered thoughts. However, the nurse should not assume that the client has limited intellectual capacity based on impaired thought processes. It may be that the client cannot focus, concentrate, or pay attention adequately to demonstrate his or her intellectual abilities accurately. Accurate assessments of the client's intellectual abilities are more likely to be obtained when the client's thought processes are clearer.

Clients often have difficulty with abstract thinking and often respond in a very literal way to other people and the environment. For example, when asked to interpret the proverb, "A stitch in time saves nine," the client may explain it by saying, "I need to sew up my clothes." The client may not understand what is being said and can easily misinterpret instructions. This can pose serious problems in medication administration. For example, the nurse may tell the client, "It is always important to take all your medications." The client may misinterpret the nurse's statement and take the entire supply of medication at one time.

JUDGMENT AND INSIGHT

Judgment is frequently impaired in the client with schizophrenia. Because judgment is based on the ability to interpret the environment correctly, it follows that the client with disordered thought processes and environmental misinterpretations will have great difficulty with judgment. At times, the lack of judgment is so severe that the client cannot meet his or her need for safety and protection and places himself or herself in harm's way. This difficulty may range from failing to wear warm clothing in cold weather to failing to seek medical care, even when desperately ill. The client may also fail to recognize needs for sleep, or food.

Insight can also be severely impaired, especially early in the course of the illness, when the client, family, and friends cannot understand what is happening. Over time, some clients can learn about the illness, anticipate problems, and seek appropriate assistance as needed. However, in clients who fail to understand schizophrenia as a long-term health problem requiring consistent management, the disease causes chronic difficulties.

SELF-CONCEPT

Deterioration of the concept of self is a major problem in schizophrenia. The phrase "loss of ego boundaries" describes the client's lack of a clear sense of where his or her own body, mind, and influence end and where those aspects of other animate and inanimate objects begin (Cancro & Lehman, 2000). This lack of ego boundaries is evidenced by depersonalization (detachment from oneself or one's behavior), derealization (environmental objects become smaller or larger, or seem unfamiliar), and ideas of reference. Clients may believe they are fused with another person or object, may not recognize parts of their body as their own, or may fail to know whether they are male or female. These difficulties are the source of many bizarre behaviors, such as public undressing or masturbation, speaking about oneself in the third person, or physically clinging to objects in the environment. Body image distortion may also be present.

ROLES AND RELATIONSHIPS

Social isolation is prevalent in clients with schizophrenia. This is due in part to the positive signs of the disease, such as delusions, hallucinations, and loss of ego boundaries. It is difficult to relate to others when one's concept of self is not clear. Clients also have problems with issues of trust and intimacy, interfering with the ability to establish satisfactory relationships. Low self-esteem, one of the negative signs of schizophrenia, further complicates clients' ability to interact with others and their environment. Clients lack confidence, feel strange or different from other people, and do not believe they are worthwhile people. The result is that clients avoid other people.

The client may experience a great deal of frustration in attempting to fulfill roles in the family and in the community. Success in school or at work can be severely compromised because the client has difficulty thinking clearly, remembering, paying attention, and concentrating and lacks motivation. Clients who develop schizophrenia at younger ages have more difficulties because they did not have the opportunity to be successful in these areas before the illness.

Fulfilling family roles, such as being a son or daughter or sibling, is difficult for the client. Often family members are frightened or embarrassed by the client's behavior or unsure of what to expect if the client's behavior is erratic or unpredictable. Families may also feel guilty or responsible, believing they failed somehow in providing a loving, supportive home life. The client may also feel he or she has disappointed the family because he or she cannot become independent or successful.

PHYSIOLOGIC AND SELF-CARE CONSIDERATIONS

Clients with schizophrenia may have significant self-care deficits. Inattention to hygiene and grooming needs are common, especially during psychotic episodes. The client can become so preoccupied with delu-

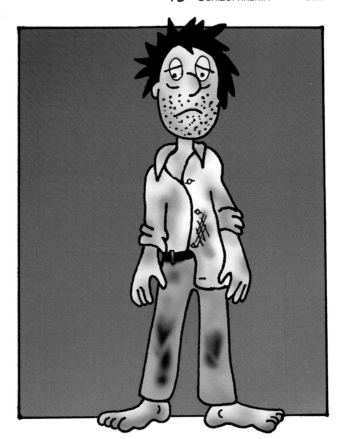

Self-care deficits

sional ideas or hallucinations that he or she fails to perform even basic activities of daily living.

Clients may also fail to recognize sensations such as hunger or thirst, and they may not have an adequate food or fluid intake. This can result in malnourishment and constipation. Constipation is also a common side effect of antipsychotic medications, so the problem becomes even worse. Paranoia or excessive fears that food and fluids have been poisoned are common and may interfere with eating. If the client is agitated and pacing, he or she may be unable to sit down long enough to eat.

Occasionally, clients develop **polydipsia** (excessive water intake), leading to water intoxication. Serum sodium levels can be dangerously low, leading to seizures. Polydipsia is usually seen in clients who have had schizophrenia for many years and have had long-term therapy with antipsychotic medications (May, 1995).

Sleep problems are also common. Clients are stimulated by hallucinations, causing insomnia. Other times, clients are suspicious and believe harm will come to them if they go to sleep. As in other self-care areas, the client may not correctly perceive or acknowledge physical cues such as fatigue.

To assist the client with community living, the nurse assesses daily living skills and functional abilities. Such skills—having a bank account and paying bills, buying food and preparing meals, and using public transportation—are often difficult tasks for the client with schizophrenia. He or she might never have learned such skills or may be unable to accomplish them consistently.

Data Analysis

The assessment data for clients with schizophrenia must be analyzed to determine priorities and establish an effective plan of care. Not all clients will have the same problems and needs, nor is it likely that any individual client will have all the problems that can occur with schizophrenia. There will also be varying levels of family and community support and available services, all of which influence the client's care and outcomes.

The analysis of assessment data generally falls into two main categories: those associated with the positive signs of the disease, and those associated with the negative signs. NANDA nursing diagnoses commonly established based on the assessment of psychotic symptoms or positive signs are:

- Risk for Violence: self-directed or directed at others
- Altered Thought Processes
- Sensory/Perceptual Alterations
- Personal Identity Disturbance
- Impaired Verbal Communication.

NANDA nursing diagnoses based on the assessment of negative signs and functional abilities include:

- Self-care Deficits
- Social Isolation
- Diversional Activity Deficit
- Altered Health Maintenance
- Ineffective Management of Therapeutic Regimen.

Outcome Identification

It is likely that the client with an acute, psychotic episode of schizophrenia will be treated in an intensive setting such as an inpatient hospital unit. During this phase of treatment, the focus of care is on stabilizing the client's thought processes and reality orientation, as well as safety needs. This is also a time to evaluate resources, make referrals, and begin planning for the client's rehabilitation and return to the community.

Examples of outcomes appropriate to the acute, psychotic phase of treatment are:

1. The client will be free of injury to self or others.
2. The client will establish contact with reality.
3. The client will interact with others in the environment.

4. The client will express thoughts and feelings in a safe manner.
5. The client will participate in prescribed therapeutic interventions.

Once the crisis or acute psychotic symptoms have been stabilized, the focus is on developing the client's ability to live as independently and successfully as possible in the community. This usually requires continued follow-up care and participation of the client's family and community support services. Prevention or early recognition and treatment of relapse symptoms is an important part of successful rehabilitation. Dealing with the negative signs of schizophrenia, which are generally not affected by medication, is a major challenge for the client and caregivers.

Examples of treatment outcomes for continued care after acute symptoms have been stabilized are:

1. The client will participate in the prescribed regimen (including medications and follow-up appointments).
2. The client will maintain adequate routines for sleeping and food and fluid intake.
3. The client will demonstrate independence in self-care activities.
4. The client will communicate effectively with others in the community to meet his or her needs.
5. The client will seek or accept assistance to meet his or her needs when indicated.

The nurse must realize the severity of schizophrenia and the profound and sometimes devastating effect it has on the lives of clients and their families. It is equally important to avoid treating the client as a "hopeless case," someone who is no longer capable of having a meaningful and satisfying life. It is not helpful to expect either too much or too little from the client. Careful, ongoing assessment is needed so that appropriate treatment and interventions can address the client's needs and difficulties while helping the client reach his or her optimal level of functioning.

Intervention

PROMOTE SAFETY OF CLIENT AND OTHERS

Safety for both the client and the nurse is the priority when providing care for the client with schizophrenia. The client may be paranoid and suspicious of the nurse and the environment and may feel threatened and intimidated. Although the client's behavior may be threatening to the nurse, the client is also feeling unsafe and may believe his or her well-being to be in jeopardy. Therefore, the nurse must approach the client in a nonthreatening manner. Making demands or being authoritarian will only increase the client's fears. Giving the client an ample amount of personal space usually enhances his or her sense of security.

A fearful or agitated client has the potential to harm himself or herself or others. The nurse must observe for signs of increasing agitation or escalating behavior, such as increased intensity of pacing, loud talking or yelling, and hitting or kicking objects. Interventions to protect the client, nurse, and others in the environment need to be instituted. This may involve medication; moving the client to a quiet, less stimulating environment; and, in extreme situations, the temporary use of seclusion or restraints. See Chapter 10 for a discussion of dealing with anger and hostility and Chapter 14 for dealing with clients who are suicidal.

ESTABLISH A THERAPEUTIC RELATIONSHIP

Establishing trust between the client and nurse also helps allay the fears of a frightened client. Initially, the client may tolerate only 5 or 10 minutes of contact at one time. It takes time to establish a therapeutic relationship, and the nurse must be patient with the client. The nurse should provide explanations that are clear, direct, and easy to understand. Body language should include eye contact but not staring, a relaxed body posture, and facial expressions that convey genuine interest and concern. Telling the client your name and calling the client by name are helpful in establishing trust as well as reality orientation.

The client's response to the use of touch must be carefully assessed. Sometimes gentle touch can convey caring and concern. However, at other times, the client may misinterpret the nurse's touch as threatening and therefore undesirable. As the nurse sits near the client, does he or she move or look away? Is the client frightened or wary of the nurse's presence? If so, that client may not be reassured by touch, but rather might feel frightened or threatened by it.

Therapeutic Communication. Communicating with clients experiencing psychotic symptoms can be difficult and frustrating. The nurse tries to understand and make sense of what the client is saying, but this can be difficult if the client is hallucinating, is withdrawn from reality, or is relatively mute. The nurse must maintain nonverbal communication with the client, especially when verbal communication is not very successful. This involves spending time with the client, perhaps through fairly lengthy periods of silence. The presence of the nurse is a contact with reality for the client and can also demonstrate the nurse's genuine interest and caring to the client. Calling the client by name, making references to the day and time, and commenting on the environment are all helpful ways to continue to make contact with a client who is having problems with reality orientation and verbal communication. Clients who are left alone for long periods of time become more deeply involved in their psychosis, so frequent contact and time spent with the client are important, even if the nurse is unsure that the client is aware of the nurse's presence.

Actively listening to the client is an important skill for the nurse trying to communicate with a client whose verbalizations are disorganized or nonsensical. Rather than dismissing what the client says because it is not clear, the nurse must make efforts to determine the meaning the client is trying to convey. Listening for themes or recurrent statements, asking clarifying questions, and exploring the meaning of the client's statements are all useful techniques to promote increased understanding.

The nurse must let the client know when his or her meaning is not clear. It is never useful to pretend to understand, or just to agree or go along with what the client is saying: this is dishonest and violates the trust relationship between client and nurse.

Nurse: *"How are you feeling today?"* (broad opening statement)

Client: *"Invisible."*

Nurse: *"Can you explain that to me?"* (seeking clarification)

Client: *"Oh, it doesn't matter."*

Nurse: *"I'm interested in how you feel; I'm just not sure I understand."* (offering self/seeking clarification)

Client: *"It doesn't mean much."*

Nurse: *"Let me see if I can understand. Do you feel like you're being ignored, that no one is really listening?"* (verbalizing the implied)

INTERVENTIONS FOR DELUSIONAL THOUGHTS

The client experiencing delusions utterly believes those delusions and cannot be convinced that they are false or untrue. Such delusions have a powerful influence on the client's behavior. For example, if the client's delusion is that he or she is being poisoned, he or she will be suspicious and mistrustful and probably will be resistant to providing information and taking medications.

The nurse must avoid openly confronting the delusion or arguing with the client about the belief. The nurse must also avoid reinforcing the delusional belief by "playing along" with what the client says. It is the nurse's responsibility to present and maintain reality by making simple statements such as, *"I have seen no evidence of that"* (presenting reality) or *"It doesn't seem that way to me"* (casting doubt). As antipsychotic medications begin to have a therapeutic effect, it will be possible for the nurse to discuss the delusional ideas with the client and identify ways in which the delusions interfere with the client's daily life.

The nurse can also help the client to minimize the effects of delusional thinking on his or her life. Distraction techniques, such as listening to music, watching television, writing, or talking to friends, can be useful for the client. Direct action, such as positive self-talk, positive thinking, and ignoring the delusional thoughts, may be beneficial as well (Murphy & Moller, 1993).

INTERVENTIONS FOR HALLUCINATIONS

Intervening with hallucinations requires the nurse to maintain a focus on what is real and to help the client to respond more to reality than to the hallucinations. Initially, the nurse must determine what the client is experiencing—that is, what the voices are saying or what the client is seeing. This will increase the nurse's understanding of the nature of the client's feelings and behavior. In command hallucinations, the client hears voices commanding or directing him or her to do something, often to hurt himself or herself or someone else. For this reason, the nurse must elicit a description of the content of the hallucination so that precautions can be taken to protect the client and others if necessary. The nurse might say, *"I don't hear any voices; what are you hearing?"* (presenting reality/ seeking clarification). This can also help the nurse understand how to relieve the client's fears or paranoia. For example, the client might be seeing ghosts or monster-like images, and the nurse could respond: *"I don't see anything, but you must be frightened. You are safe here in the hospital"* (presenting reality/translating into feelings). This acknowledges the client's feelings of fear but reassures the client that no harm will come to him or her.

Clients do not always report or identify hallucinations. At times the nurse must infer from the client's behavior that hallucinations are occurring. Examples of behavior that often indicate hallucinations include alternately listening and then talking when no one else is present, laughing inappropriately for no observable reason, and mumbling or mouthing words with no audible sound.

A helpful strategy for intervening with hallucinations is to engage the client in a reality-based activity such as playing cards, occupational therapy, or listening to music. It is difficult for the client to pay attention to hallucinations and reality-based activity at the same time, so this technique of distracting the client is often useful.

Teaching the client to talk back to the voices forcefully may also help him or her manage auditory hallucinations (Murphy & Moller, 1993). The client should do this in a relatively private place, rather than in public. Being able to verbalize resistance can help the client feel empowered and capable of dealing with the hallucinations.

COPING WITH SOCIALLY INAPPROPRIATE BEHAVIORS

Clients with schizophrenia often experience a loss of ego boundaries, and this presents difficulties for both themselves and others in their environment and community. Bizarre or strange behaviors that occur include touching others without warning or invitation, intruding into others' living space, talking to or caressing inanimate objects, and a variety of socially inappropriate behaviors such as public undressing, masturbation, or urination. Clients may also approach others and make statements that are provocative, insulting, or sexual in nature. The nurse needs to consider the needs of others as well as the needs of the clients in these situations.

Protecting the client is a primary nursing responsibility, and this includes protecting the client from retaliation by others who might experience the client's intrusions and socially unacceptable behavior. Redirecting the client away from situations or others can interrupt the undesirable behavior and keep the client from further intrusive behaviors. The nurse must also try to protect the client's right to privacy and dignity. Taking the client to his or her room or a quiet area with less stimulation and people is often helpful. Engaging the client in appropriate activities is also indicated. For example, if the client is undressing in front of others, the nurse might say, *"Let's go to your room and you can put your clothes back on"* (encouraging collaboration/redirecting to appropriate activity). If the client is making verbal statements to others, the nurse might ask the client to go for a walk or go to another area to listen to music. The nurse should deal with socially inappropriate behavior in a nonjudgmental and matter-of-fact manner. This means making factual statements with no overtones of scolding or talking to the client as if he or she were a naughty child.

Some behaviors may be so offensive or threatening that others respond by yelling at or ridiculing the client or even taking aggressive action. Although providing physical protection for the client is the first consideration for the nurse, it is also important to help others affected by the client's behavior. Usually the nurse can offer simple and factual statements to others that do not violate the client's confidentiality. The nurse might make statements such as, *"You didn't do anything to provoke that behavior. Sometimes people's illnesses cause them to act in strange and uncomfortable ways. It is important not to laugh at behaviors that are part of someone's illness"* (presenting reality/giving information).

NURSING CARE PLAN   FOR A CLIENT WITH DELUSIONS

Nursing Diagnosis

➤ **Altered Thought Processes** (8.3)
A state in which the individual experiences a disruption in cognitive operations and activities

ASSESSMENT DATA

- Non-reality-based thinking
- Disorientation
- Labile affect
- Short attention span
- Impaired judgment
- Distractibility

EXPECTED OUTCOMES

The client will:
- Be free of injury
- Demonstrate decreased anxiety level
- Interact on reality-based topics

IMPLEMENTATION

Nursing Interventions	Rationale
Be sincere and honest when communicating with the client. Avoid vague or evasive remarks.	Delusional clients are very sensitive about others and can recognize insincerity. Evasive comments or hesitation reinforces mistrust or delusions.
Be consistent in setting expectations, enforcing rules, and so forth.	Clear, consistent limits provide a secure structure for the client.
Do not make promises that you cannot keep.	Broken promises reinforce the client's mistrust of others.
Encourage the client to talk with you, but do not pry or cross-examine for information.	Probing increases the client's suspicion and interferes with the therapeutic relationship. When the client has full knowledge of procedures, he or she is less likely to feel tricked by the staff.
Explain procedures, and try to be sure the client understands the procedures before carrying them out.	When the client has full knowledge of procedures, he or she is less likely to feel tricked by the staff.
Give positive feedback for the client's successes.	Positive feedback for genuine success enhances the client's sense of well-being and helps make nondelusional reality a more positive situation for the client.
Recognize the client's delusions as the client's perception of the environment.	It is important to recognize the client's environmental perceptions to understand the feelings he or she is experiencing.

continued on page 316

continued from page 315

Initially, do not argue with the client or try to convince the client that the delusions are false or unreal.	Logical argument does not dispel delusional ideas and can interfere with the development of trust.
Interact with the client on the basis of real things; do not dwell on the delusional material.	Interacting about reality is healthy for the client.
Engage the client in one-to-one activities at first, then activities in small groups, and gradually activities in larger groups.	The client who is distrustful can best deal with one person initially. Gradual introduction of others when the client can tolerate it is less threatening.
Recognize and support the client's accomplishments (activities or projects completed, responsibilities fulfilled, or interactions initiated).	Recognition of accomplishments can lessen the client's anxiety and the need for delusions as a source of self-esteem.
Show empathy regarding the client's feelings; reassure the client of your presence and acceptance.	The client's delusions can be distressing. Empathy conveys your acceptance of the client and your caring and interest.
Do not be judgmental or belittle or joke about the client's beliefs.	The client's delusions and feelings are not funny to him or her. The client may feel rejected by you or feel unimportant if approached by attempts at humor.
Never convey to the client that you accept the delusions as reality.	You would reinforce the delusion (thus, the client's illness) if you indicated belief in the delusion.
Directly interject doubt regarding delusions as soon as the client seems ready to accept this. Do not argue with the client, but present a factual account of the situation as you see it.	As the client begins to trust you, he or she may become willing to doubt the delusion if you express your doubt.
Attempt to discuss the delusional thoughts as a problem in the client's life; ask the client if he or she can see that the delusions interfere with his or her life.	Discussion of the problems caused by the delusions is a focus on the present and is reality-based.

Adapted from Schultz, J. M. & Videbeck, S. L. (1998). Lippincott's manual of psychiatric nursing care plans *(5th ed.). Philadelphia: Lippincott-Raven.*

The nurse should reassure the client's family that these behaviors are part of the client's illness and are not personally directed at them. Such situations present an opportunity to educate family members about schizophrenia and to help allay their feelings of guilt, shame, or responsibility.

The client should be reintegrated into the treatment milieu as soon as he or she can do so. The client should not feel shunned or punished for inappropri- ate behavior. Limited amounts of stimulation should be introduced gradually. For example, when the client is comfortable and is demonstrating appropriate behavior with the nurse, one or two other people can be engaged in a somewhat structured activity with the client. The client's involvement is gradually increased to small groups and then larger, less structured groups as he or she is able to tolerate the increased level of stimulation without decompensating.

CLIENT AND FAMILY TEACHING

Coping with schizophrenia is a major adjustment for both clients and their families. Understanding the illness, the need for continuing medication and follow-up, and the uncertainty of the prognosis or recovery are key issues. Clients and families need help to cope with the emotional upheaval caused by schizophrenia. See Client and Family Teaching: Schizophrenia for teaching points.

Identifying and managing one's own health needs are primary concerns for everyone, but this is a particular challenge for clients with schizophrenia because their health needs can be complex and their ability to manage them may be impaired. The nurse should help the client to manage his or her illness and health needs as independently as possible. This can be accomplished only through education and ongoing support.

Teaching the client and family members to prevent or manage relapse is an essential part of a comprehensive plan of care. This includes providing factual information about schizophrenia, identifying the early signs of relapse, and teaching health practices to promote physical and psychological well-being. Murphy and Moller (1993) have identified symptom triggers, or factors that increase the risk for relapse, in the areas of the client's health, the environment, and the client's attitudes or behaviors (Box 13-4). Early identification of these risk factors has been found to reduce the frequency of relapse; when relapse cannot be prevented, early identification provides the foundation for interventions to manage the relapse. For example, if the nurse finds that the client is fatigued or lacks adequate sleep or proper nutrition, interventions to promote rest and nutrition may prevent a relapse or minimize its intensity and duration.

Box 13-4

▶ RISK FACTORS FOR RELAPSE

HEALTH RISK FACTORS

- Impaired cause and effect reasoning
- Impaired information processing
- Poor nutrition
- Lack of sleep
- Lack of exercise
- Fatigue
- Intolerable side effects of medication

ENVIRONMENTAL RISK FACTORS

- Financial difficulties
- Housing difficulties
- Stressful changes in life events
- Poor occupational skills, inability to keep a job
- Lack of transportation/resources
- Poor social skills, social isolation, loneliness
- Interpersonal difficulties

BEHAVIOR AND EMOTIONAL RISK FACTORS

- Lack of control, aggressive or violent behavior
- Mood swings
- Poor medication and symptom management
- Low self-concept
- Looks and acts different
- Hopeless feelings
- Loss of motivation

Adapted from Murphy, M. F., & Moller, M. D. (1993). Relapse management in neurobiological disorders: The Moller-Murphy symptom management assessment tool. Archives of Psychiatric Nursing, 7 (4), 1993, p. 230.

▶ CLIENT AND FAMILY TEACHING: SCHIZOPHRENIA

- How to manage illness and prevent relapse
- Importance of maintaining prescribed medication regimen and regular follow-up
- Avoiding alcohol and other drugs
- Self-care and proper nutrition
- Teaching social skills through education, role modeling, and practice
- Counseling and education of family/significant others about the biologic causes and clinical course of schizophrenia and the need ongoing support
- Importance of maintaining contact with community and participating in supportive organizations and care

---

The nurse can use the list of relapse risk factors in a variety of ways. These risk factors can be included in discharge teaching before the client leaves the inpatient setting, so the client and family will know what to watch for and when to seek assistance. The nurse might also use the list when assessing the client in an outpatient or clinic setting, or when working with clients in a community support program. The nurse can also provide teaching to ancillary personnel who may be working with the client so they will know when to contact a mental health professional. Taking medications as prescribed, keeping regular follow-up appointments, and avoiding alcohol and other drugs have been associated with fewer and shorter hospital stays. In addition, clients who can identify and avoid stressful situations are less likely to suffer frequent relapses. Using a list of relapse risk factors is one way to assess the client's progress in the community.

Families experience a wide variety of responses to the illness of their loved one. Some family members might be ashamed or embarrassed or frightened of the client's strange or threatening behaviors. They worry about a relapse. They may feel guilty for having these feelings, or fear for their own mental health or well-being. If the client experiences repeated and profound problems with schizophrenia, the family members may become emotionally exhausted or even alienated from the client, feeling they can no longer deal with the situation. Family members need ongoing support and education, including reassurance that they are not the cause of schizophrenia. Participating in organizations such as the Alliance for the Mentally Ill may help families with their ongoing needs.

Teaching Self-Care and Proper Nutrition. Poor personal hygiene can be a problem for clients when they are experiencing psychotic symptoms and also over the course of the illness as a result of apathy or lack of energy. When the client is psychotic, he or she may pay little attention to hygiene or may be unable to sustain the attention or concentration required to complete grooming tasks. The nurse may need to direct the client through the necessary steps for bathing, shampooing, dressing, and so forth. The nurse should give directions in short, clear statements to enhance the client's ability to complete the tasks. The nurse must allow ample time for grooming and hygiene and should not attempt to rush or hurry the client. The client is encouraged to become more independent as soon as possible—that is, when he or she is better oriented to reality and better able to sustain the concentration and attention needed for these tasks.

If the client has deficits in hygiene and grooming resulting from apathy or lack of energy for tasks, the nurse may vary the approach used to promote the client's independence in these areas. The client is most likely to perform tasks of hygiene and grooming if they become a part of his or her daily routine. Establishing a structure with the client that incorporates his or her preferences has a greater chance of success than if the client waits to decide about hygiene tasks or performs them on a random basis. For example, the client may prefer to shower and shampoo on Monday, Wednesday, and Friday when getting up in the morning. This plan is incorporated into the client's daily routine and becomes a habit. This allows the client to avoid making daily decisions about whether to shower or deciding if he or she feels like showering on a particular day.

Adequate nutrition and fluids are essential to the client's physical and emotional well-being. Careful assessment of the client's eating patterns and preferences allows the nurse to determine whether the client needs assistance in these areas. As with any type of self-care deficit, the nurse provides assistance as long as needed, then gradually promotes the client's independence as soon as he or she can do so.

When the client is in the community, inadequate nutritional intake may also be influenced by factors other than the client's illness, such as lack of money to buy food, lack of knowledge about a nutritious diet, inadequate transportation, or limited abilities to prepare food. A thorough assessment of the client's functional abilities for community living will help the nurse to plan appropriate interventions. See the section below on community-based care.

Teaching Social Skills. Clients may be isolated from others for a variety of reasons. Family or community members may be frightened or embarrassed by the bizarre behavior or statements of the client who is delusional or hallucinating. Clients who are suspicious or mistrustful may avoid contact with others. Other times, clients may lack the social or conversation skills needed to make and maintain relationships with others. Lastly, there is still a stigma attached to mental illness, particularly for persons in whom the positive signs of the illness are not relieved by medication.

The nurse can help the client develop social skills through education, role modeling, and practice. The client may not discriminate between the topics suitable for sharing with the nurse and those suitable for a conversation on a bus. The nurse can help the client learn what are neutral social topics, such as the weather or local events, that are appropriate to any conversation. The client can also benefit from learning that he or she should share certain details of his or her illness, such as the content of delusions or hallucinations, only with a health care provider.

Modeling and practicing social skills with the client can help him or her experience greater success in social interactions. Specific skills, such as eye contact, attentive listening, and taking turns talking, can increase the client's abilities and confidence in socializing. Nursing interventions for clients with schizophrenia are summarized in the display.

Medication Management. Maintaining the medication regimen is vital to the successful outcome for clients with schizophrenia. Failing to take medications as prescribed is one of the most frequent reasons for recurrence of psychotic symptoms and hospital admission (Marder, 2000). Clients who respond well to and maintain an antipsychotic medication regimen may lead relatively normal lives with only an occasional relapse. Those who do not respond well to antipsychotic agents may face a lifetime of dealing with delusional ideas and hallucinations, negative signs, and marked impairment. Many clients find themselves somewhere between these two extremes.

There are many reasons why clients may not maintain the medication regimen. The nurse must

▶ Nursing Interventions for Clients With Schizophrenia

- Promoting safety of client and others and right to privacy and dignity
- Establishing therapeutic relationship by establishing trust:
  Use therapeutic communication (clarifying feelings and statements when speech and thoughts are disorganized or confused).
- Interventions for delusions:
  Do not openly confront the delusion or argue with the client.
  Establish and maintain reality for the client.
  Use distracting techniques.
  Teach the client positive self-talk, positive thinking, and ignoring delusional beliefs.
- Interventions for hallucinations:
  Help present and maintain reality by frequent contact and communication with client.
  Elicit description of hallucination to protect client and others. The nurse's understanding of the hallucination helps him or her know how to calm or reassure the client.
  Engage client in reality-based activities such as card playing, occupational therapy, or listening to music.
- Coping with socially inappropriate behaviors:
  Redirect client away from problem situations.
  Deal with inappropriate behaviors in a nonjudgmental and matter-of-fact manner; give factual statements; do not scold.
  Reassure others that the client's inappropriate behaviors or comments are not his or her fault (without violating client confidentiality).
  Try to reintegrate the client into the treatment milieu as soon as possible.
  Do not make the client feel punished or shunned for inappropriate behaviors.
  Teach social skills through education, role modeling, and practice.
- Client and family teaching (see the display)
- Establishing community support systems and care

determine the barriers to compliance for each patient. Sometimes clients may intend to take their medications as prescribed but have difficulty remembering when and if medications were taken. They may find it difficult to adhere to a routine schedule for medications. There are several methods to help clients remember when to take medications. One is by using a pill box with compartments for days of the week and times of the day. Once the box has been filled, perhaps with assistance from the nurse or case manager, the client often has no more difficulties. It is also helpful to make a chart of all administration times so the client can cross off each time the medications are taken.

Clients may also have practical barriers to medication compliance, such as inadequate funds to obtain expensive medications, lack of transportation, lack of knowledge about how to obtain refills for prescriptions, or inability to plan ahead to get new prescriptions before current supplies run out. All of these obstacles can usually be overcome once they have been identified.

Sometimes clients decide to decrease or discontinue their medications because of uncomfortable or embarrassing side effects. Unwanted side effects are frequently reported as the reason clients stop taking medications (Marder, 2000). There are interventions that can help control some of these uncomfortable side effects (see Table 13-2), such as eating a proper diet and drinking enough fluids, using a stool softener to avoid constipation, sucking on hard candy to minimize dry mouth, or using sunscreen to avoid sunburn. Some side effects, such as dry mouth and blurred vision, improve with time or with lower doses of medication. Medication may be warranted to combat common neurologic side effects such as extrapyramidal side effects or akathisia.

Some side effects, such as those affecting sexual functioning, are embarrassing for the client to report, and the client may confirm the presence of these side effects only if the nurse directly inquires about them. This may require a call to the client's physician or primary provider to obtain a prescription for a different type of antipsychotic.

Sometimes a client discontinues medications because he or she dislikes the idea of taking medications or believes the medications are not needed. The client may have been willing to take the medications when experiencing psychotic symptoms but may believe they are not needed when he or she feels well. By refusing to take the medications, the client may be denying the existence or severity of schizophrenia. These issues of noncompliance are much more difficult to resolve. The nurse can teach the client about schizophrenia, the nature of chronic illness, and the importance of medications in managing symptoms and preventing recurrence. For example, the nurse could say, "This medication helps you think more clearly" or "Taking this medication will make it less likely that you'll hear troubling voices in your mind again."

Even after education, some clients continue to refuse to take medication; they may understand the connection between medication and prevention of relapse only after experiencing a return of psychotic symptoms. A few clients still do not understand the importance of consistently taking medication and even after numerous relapses continue to experience psychosis and hospital admission on a fairly frequent basis.

Evaluation

Evaluation of the plan of care must be considered in the context of each client and family. Ongoing assessment provides data to determine whether the client's individual outcomes were achieved. The client's perception of the success of treatment also plays a part in evaluation. Even if all outcomes are achieved, the nurse must ask whether the client is comfortable or satisfied with the quality of life.

In a global sense, evaluation of the treatment of schizophrenia is based on the following:

- Have the client's psychotic symptoms disappeared? If not, can the client carry out his or her daily life despite the persistence of some psychotic symptoms?
- Does the client understand the prescribed medication regimen? Is he or she committed to adherence to the regimen?
- Does the client possess the necessary functional abilities for community living?
- Are there adequate community resources to help the client live successfully in the community?
- Is there a sufficient after-care or crisis plan in place to deal with recurrence of symptoms or difficulties encountered in the community?
- Are the client and family adequately knowledgeable about schizophrenia?
- Does the client believe he or she has a satisfactory quality of life?

COMMUNITY-BASED CARE

Clients with schizophrenia are no longer hospitalized for long periods of time, but most return to live in the community with support provided by family and support services. Clients may live with family members, independently, or in a residential program such as a group home where they can receive needed services without needing to be admitted to the hospital. Assertive Community Treatment (ACT) programs have shown success in reducing the rate of hospital admission by managing symptoms and medications, assisting clients with social, recreational, and vocational needs, and providing support to clients and their families (McGrew, Wilson, & Bond, 1996). The psychiatric nurse is a member of the multidisciplinary team that works with clients in ACT programs, focusing on the management of medications and their side effects and the promotion of health and wellness (O'Brien, 1998; Wilbur & Arns, 1998). Behavioral home health care is also expanding, with nurses providing care to persons with schizophrenia (as well as other mental illnesses), using the holistic approach to integrate clients into the community (Gibson, 1999;

Rosedale, 1999). Although much has been done to give these clients the support they need to live in the community, there is still a need to increase services to homeless persons and those in prison who have schizophrenia.

Community support programs are often an important link in helping persons with schizophrenia and their families. A case manager may be assigned to the client to provide assistance in handling the wide variety of challenges that face the client in community settings. The client who has had schizophrenia for some time may have a case manager in the community. Other clients may need assistance to obtain a case manager. The nurse may refer the client to a social worker or may directly refer the client to case management services, depending on the type of funding and agencies available in a particular community.

Case management services often include helping the client with housing and transportation, money management, and keeping appointments, as well as socialization and recreation. Although the support of professionals in the community is vital, the nurse must not to overlook the client's need for autonomy and potential abilities to manage his or her own health.

SELF-AWARENESS ISSUES

Working with clients with schizophrenia can present many challenges for the nurse. Suspicious or paranoid behavior on the client's part may make the nurse feel as though he or she is not trustworthy or that his or her integrity is being questioned. The nurse must recognize this type of behavior as part of the illness and not interpret it or respond to it as a personal affront. Taking the client's statements or behavior as a personal accusation only causes the nurse to respond in a defensive manner, which is counterproductive to the establishment of a therapeutic relationship.

The nurse may also feel genuinely frightened or threatened if the client's behavior is hostile or aggressive. The nurse must acknowledge these feelings and take measures to ensure his or her safety. This may involve talking to the client in an open area rather than a more isolated location, or having another staff person present rather than being alone with the client. If the nurse pretends to be unafraid, the client may sense the fear anyway and feel less secure, leading to a greater potential for the client to lose personal control.

As with many chronic illnesses, the nurse may become frustrated if the client is noncompliant with the medication regimen, fails to keep needed appointments, or experiences repeated relapses. The nurse may feel as though a great deal of hard work has been wasted or that the situation is futile or hopeless. Schizophrenia is a chronic illness, and clients may suffer numerous relapses and hospital admissions. The nurse must not take responsibility for the success or failure of treatment efforts or view the client's status as a personal success or failure. Nurses need to look to their colleagues for helpful support and discussion of these self-awareness issues.

Helpful Hints for Working With Clients With Schizophrenia

- Remember that although these clients often suffer numerous relapses and return for repeated hospital stays, they do return to living and functioning in the community. Focusing on the amount of time the client is outside the hospital setting may help decrease the frustration that can result when working with clients with a chronic illness.
- Visualize the client not at his or her worst, but as he or she gets better and symptoms become less severe.
- Remember that the client's remarks are not directed at you personally but are a byproduct of the disordered and confused thinking that these clients experience.

- Discuss these issues with a more experienced nurse for suggestions on how to deal with your feelings and actions toward these clients. You are not expected to have all the answers.

➤ KEY POINTS

- Schizophrenia is a chronic illness requiring long-term management strategies and coping skills. Schizophrenia is a disease of the brain, a clinical syndrome that involves a person's thoughts, perceptions, emotions, movements, and behaviors.
- The effects of schizophrenia on the client may be profound, involving all aspects of the client's life: social interactions, emotional health, and ability to work and function in the community.
- Schizophrenia is conceptualized in terms of positive signs, such as delusions, hallucinations, and disordered thought process, and negative signs, such as social isolation, apathy, anhedonia, and lack of motivation and volition.
- The clinical picture, prognosis, and outcomes for clients with schizophrenia vary widely. Therefore, it is important that each client is

INTERNET RESOURCES

Resource	Internet Address
▶ Internet Mental Health	http://www.mentalhealth.com
▶ Mental Health InfoSource	http://www.mhsource.com/
▶ Mental Health Net	http://www.cmhc.com
▶ National Alliance for the Mentally Ill	http://www.nami.org
▶ Anne Sippi Clinic	http://www.schizophrenia-help.com
▶ Manitoba Schizophrenia Society	http://www.mss.mb.ca
▶ National Alliance for Research on Schizophrenia and Depression	http://www.mhsource.co/narsad.html
▶ Schizophrenia: A Handbook for Families	http://www.mentalhealth.com/bookp40-sc01.html
▶ Schizophrenia Digest	http://www.vaxxine.com/schizophrenia

Critical Thinking

Questions

1. Clients who fail to take medications regularly are often admitted to the hospital repeatedly, and this can become quite expensive. How do you reconcile the client's rights (to refuse treatment or medications) with the need to curtail health care costs that are avoidable?

2. What is the quality of life for the client with schizophrenia who has a minimal response to antipsychotic medications and therefore poor treatment outcomes?

3. If a client with schizophrenia who experiences frequent relapses has a young child, should the child remain with the parent? What factors influence this decision? Who should be able to make such a decision?

4. How does the nurse maintain a positive but honest relationship with a client's family if the client does not respond well to antipsychotic medications?

carefully and individually assessed with appropriate needs and interventions determined.

• Careful assessment of each client as an individual is essential to planning an effective plan of care.

• Families of clients with schizophrenia may experience fear, embarrassment, and guilt in response to their family member's illness. Families must be educated about the disorder, the course of the disorder, and how it can be controlled.

• Failure to comply with treatment and the medication regimen and the use of alcohol and other drugs are associated with poorer outcomes in the treatment of schizophrenia.

• For clients with psychotic symptoms, key nursing interventions include helping to protect the client's safety and right to privacy and dignity, dealing with socially inappropriate behaviors in a nonjudgmental and matter-of-fact manner, helping present and maintain reality for the client by frequent contact and communication, and ensuring appropriate medication administration.

• For the client whose condition is stabilized with medication, key nursing interventions include continuing to offer a supportive, nonconfrontational approach, maintaining the therapeutic relationship by establishing trust and trying to clarify the client's feelings and statements when speech and thoughts

are disorganized or confused, helping to develop social skills by modeling and practicing, and helping to educate the client and family about schizophrenia and the importance of maintaining a therapeutic regimen and other self-care habits.

• Self-awareness issues for the nurse working with clients with schizophrenia include dealing with psychotic symptoms, fear for safety, and frustration with dealing with relapses and repeated hospital admissions.

REFERENCES

American Psychiatric Association. (2000). *DSM-IV-TR: Diagnostic and statistical manual of mental disorders-Text revision* (4th ed.). Washington, DC: American Psychiatric Association.

Buchanan, R. W., & Carpenter, W. T. (2000). Schizophrenia: Introduction and overview. In B. J. Sadock & V. A. Sadock (Eds.). *Comprehensive textbook of psychiatry,* Vol. 1 (7th ed., pp. 1096–1110). Philadelphia: Lippincott Williams & Wilkins.

Cancro, R., & Lehman, H. E. (2000). Schizophrenia: Clinical features. In B. J. Sadock & V. A. Sadock (Eds.). *Comprehensive textbook of psychiatry,* Vol. 1 (7th ed., pp. 1169–1199). Philadelphia: Lippincott Williams & Wilkins.

Egan, M. F., & Hyde, T. M. (2000). Schizophrenia: Neurobiology. In B. J. Sadock & V. A. Sadock (Eds.). *Comprehensive textbook of psychiatry,* Vol. 1 (7th ed., pp. 1129–1147). Philadelphia: Lippincott Williams & Wilkins.

Fenton, W. S., & Cole, S. A. (1995). Psychosocial theories of schizophrenia: Individual, group, and family. In G. O. Goddard (Ed.). *Treatment of psychiatric disorders,* Vol. 1 (2d ed., pp. 988–1018). Washington, DC: American Psychiatric Press.

Flaskerud, J. H., & Hu, L. T. (1992). Racial/ethnic identity and amount and type of psychiatric treatment. *American Journal of Psychiatry, 149*(3), 379–384.

Gibson, D. M. (1999). Reduced hospitalizations and reintegration of persons with mental illness into community living: A holistic approach. *Journal of Psychosocial Nursing, 37*(11), 20–25.

Gur, R. E., & Gur, R. C. (2000). Schizophrenia: Brain structure and function. In B. J. Sadock & V. A. Sadock (Eds.). *Comprehensive textbook of psychiatry,* Vol. 1 (7th ed., pp. 1117–1129). Philadelphia: Lippincott Williams & Wilkins.

Kendler, K. S., & Diehl, S. R. (2000). Schizophrenia: Genetics. In B. J. Sadock & V. A. Sadock (Eds.). *Comprehensive textbook of psychiatry, Vol. 1* (7th ed., pp. 1147–1159). Philadelphia: Lippincott Williams & Wilkins.

Kudzma, E. C. (1999). Culturally competent drug administration. *American Journal of Nursing, 99*(8), 46–51.

Littrell, K. H., & Littrell, S. H. (1998). Emerging applications of newer antipsychotic agents in specific patient populations. *Journal of the American Psychiatric Nurses Association, 4*(4), S42–49.

Marder, S. E. (2000). Schizophrenia: Somatic treatment. In B. J. Sadock & V. A. Sadock (Eds.). *Comprehensive textbook of psychiatry, Vol. 1* (7th ed., pp. 1199–1210). Philadelphia: Lippincott Williams & Wilkins.

May, D. L. (1995). Patient perceptions of self-induced water intoxication. *Archives of Psychiatric Nursing, 9*(5), 295–304.

McEvoy, R. B. (Ed.). (2000). *Facts and comparisons 2000.* St. Louis: Facts and Comparisons, A Wolters Kluwer Company.

McFarlane, E. R. (1995). Families in the treatment of psychotic disorders. *Harvard Mental Health Letter, 12*(4), 4.

McGrew, J. H., Wilson, R. G., & Bond, G. R. (1996). Client perspectives on helpful ingredients of assertive community treatment. *Psychiatric Rehabilitation Journal, 19*(3), 13–21.

Mezzich, J. E., Lin, K., & Hughes, C. C. (2000). Acute and transient disorders and cultural bound syndromes. In B. J. Sadock & V. A. Sadock (Eds.). *Comprehensive textbook of psychiatry,* Vol. 1 (7th ed., pp. 1264–1276). Philadelphia: Lippincott Williams & Wilkins.

Mortensen, P. B., Pedersen, C. B., Westergaard, T., Wohlfahrt, J., Ewald, H., Mors, O., Andersen, P. K., & Melbye, M. (1999). Effects of family history and place and season of birth on the risk of schizophrenia. *New England Journal of Medicine, 340*(8), 603–608.

Murphy, M. F., & Moller, M. D. (1993). Relapse management in neurobiological disorders: The Moller-Murphy symptom management assessment tool. *Archives of Psychiatric Nursing, 7*(4), 226–235.

O'Brien, S. M. (1998). Health promotion and schizophrenia: The year 2000 and beyond. *Holistic Nursing Practice, 12*(2), 38–43.

O'Connor, F. L. (1998). The role of serotonin and dopamine in schizophrenia. *Journal of the American Psychiatric Nurses Association, 4*(4), S30–41.

Rosedale, M. (1999). Managed care opens unlikely doors: Innovations in behavioral home health care. *Home Health Care Management & Practice, 11*(4), 45–48.

Schultz, J. M., & Videbeck, S. L. (1998). *Lippincott's manual of psychiatric nursing care plans* (5th ed.). Philadelphia: Lippincott-Raven.

Slately, A. E. (1994). *Handbook of psychiatric emergencies.* Norwalk, CT: Appleton & Lange.

Spratto, G. R., & Woods, A. L. (2000). *PDR nurse's drug handbook, 2000 edition.* Montvale, NJ: Medical Economics Company, Inc.

Torrey, E. F. (1995). *Surviving schizophrenia: For families, consumers, and providers* (3rd ed.). New York: Harper & Row.

Wilbur, S., & Arns, P. (1998). Psychosocial rehabilitation nurses: Taking our place on the multidisciplinary team. *Journal of Psychosocial Nursing, 36*(4), 33–48.

ADDITIONAL READINGS

Buccheri, R., Yrygstad, L., Kanas, N., Waldron, B., & Dowling, G. (1996). Auditory hallucinations in schizophrenia: Group experience in examining symptom management and behavioral strategies. *Journal of Psychosocial Nursing, 34*(2), 12–25.

Chafetz, L. (1996). The experience of severe mental illness: A life history approach. *Archives of Psychiatric Nursing, 10*(1), 24–31.

Chouvardas, J. (1996). The symbolic and literal in schizophrenic language. *Perspectives in Psychiatric Care, 32*(2), 20–22.

Jaretz, N., & Millsap, L. (1992). Clozapine: Nursing care considerations. *Perspectives in Psychiatric Care, 28*(3), 19–24.

Junginger, J. (1995). Command hallucinations and the prediction of dangerousness. *Psychiatric Services, 46*(9), 911–914.

Postrado, L. T., & Lehman, E. F. (1995). Quality of life and clinical predictors of rehospitalization of persons with severe mental illness. *Psychiatric Services, 46*(11), 1161–1165.

Tuck, I., du Mont, P., Evans, G., & Shupe, J. (1997). The experience of caring for an adult child with schizophrenia. *Archives of Psychiatric Nursing, 11*(3), 118–125.

Chapter Review

Select the best answer for each of the following questions.

1. Which of the following are considered the positive signs of schizophrenia?

   A. Delusions, anhedonia, ambivalence

   B. Hallucinations, illusions, ambivalence

   C. Delusions, hallucinations, disordered thinking

   D. Disordered thinking, anhedonia, illusions.

2. The family of a client with schizophrenia asks the nurse about the difference between typical and atypical antipsychotic medications. The nurse's answer is based on which of the following?

   A. Atypical antipsychotics are newer medications but act in the same ways as typical antipsychotics.

   B. Typical antipsychotics are dopamine antagonists; atypical antipsychotics inhibit the reuptake of serotonin.

   C. Typical antipsychotics have serious side effects; the atypical antipsychotics have virtually no side effects.

   D. Atypical antipsychotics are dopamine and serotonin antagonists; typical antipsychotics are only dopamine antagonists.

3. The nurse is planning discharge teaching for a client taking clozapine (Clozaril). Which of the following is essential to include?

   A. Cautioning the client not to be outdoors in the sunshine without protective clothing

   B. Reminding the client to go to the lab to have blood drawn for a white blood cell count

   C. Instructing the client about dietary restrictions

   D. Giving the client a chart to record a daily pulse rate.

4. The nurse is caring for a client who has been taking fluphenazine (Prolixin) for 2 days. The client suddenly cries out, his neck is twisted to one side, and his eyes appear to have rolled back in the sockets. The nurse finds the following prn medications ordered for the client. Which one should the nurse administer?

   A. Benztropine (Cogentin) 2 mg p.o., BID, prn

   B. Fluphenazine (Prolixin) 2 mg p.o., TID, prn

   C. Haloperidol (Haldol) 5 mg IM, prn extreme agitation

   D. Diphenhydramine (Benadryl) 25 mg IM, prn

5. Which of the following statements would indicate that family teaching about schizophrenia had been effective?

   A. "If our son takes his medication properly, he won't have another psychotic episode."

   B. "I guess we'll have to face the fact that our daughter will eventually be institutionalized."

   C. "It's a relief to find out that we did not cause our son's schizophrenia."

   D. "It is a shame our daughter will never be able to have children."

➤ TRUE-FALSE QUESTIONS

*Identify each of the following statements as T (true)
or F (false). Correct any false statements.*

_____ 1. The inability to experience pleasure is
called alogia.

_____

_____ 2. When the client believes that others are
putting ideas into his or her head, it is
called thought insertion.

_____

_____ 3. The client describing depersonalization
might say, "I feel like I'm outside my body
sometimes."

_____

_____ 4. Imitating the actions of another person is
called echopraxia.

_____

_____ 5. When the client describes fear of leaving
his apartment as well as the desire to get out
and meet others, it is called ambivalence.

_____

_____ 6. One side effect of antipsychotic drugs
that is often treated with benztropine (Cogentin) is tardive dyskinesia.

_____

_____ 7. The client with ideas of reference may believe that the news broadcaster on television sends special messages to him or her.

_____

_____ 8. The client who hesitates 30 seconds before responding to any question is described
as having a poverty of speech content.

_____

➤ FILL-IN-THE-BLANK QUESTIONS

*Identify the type of speech pattern exhibited for each
of the following client statements.*

_____ 1. "Do you have any phletz here?
I like phletz."

_____ 2. "It's time to eat, to eat, to eat."

_____ 3. "Mountains, tigers, pie,
singing, spring."

_____ 4. "Is that clock or a sock, can the
door lock, tick tock."

Give an example of each of the following:

1. Delusion

2. Hallucination

3. Illusion

For each of the following client statements, write a response the nurse might make, and the rationale for the nurse's response.

4. "I can't live in my apartment anymore because it's bugged by the FBI."

5. "Have they told you why I'm here in the hospital?"

6. "I can feel my stomach rotting away."

7. "I must do what God tells me to do."

➤ CLINICAL EXAMPLE

John Jones, 33, has been admitted to the hospital for the third time with a diagnosis of paranoid schizophrenia. John had been taking haloperidol (Haldol) but stopped taking it 2 weeks ago, telling his case manager it was "the poison that is making me sick." Yesterday, John was brought to the hospital after neighbors called the police because he had been up all night yelling loudly in his apartment. Neighbors reported him saying, "I can't do it! They don't deserve to die!" and similar statements.

John appears guarded and suspicious and has very little to say to anyone. His hair is matted, he has a strong body odor, and he is dressed in several layers of heavy clothing, even though the temperature is warm. So far, John has been refusing any offers of food or fluids. When the nurse approached John with a dose of haloperidol, he said, "Do you want me to die?"

1. What additional assessment data does the nurse need to plan care for John?

2. Identify the three priorities, nursing diagnoses, and expected outcomes for John's care, with your rationale for the choices.

3. Identify at least two nursing interventions for the three priorities listed above.

4. What community referrals or supports might be beneficial for John when he is discharged?

Mood Disorders

Learning Objectives

After reading this chapter, the student should be able to:

1. Describe unipolar and bipolar disorders.
2. Assess mood, behaviors, and cognition related to unipolar and bipolar disorders and suicide.
3. Discuss the biologic and psychological theories related to the development of mood disorders.
4. Describe nursing interventions and psychotherapic techniques used with people who have a mood disorder or have suicidal ideation/attempt.
5. Identify self-awareness issues and how to cope with them when dealing with clients with mood disorders or suicidal clients.

Key Terms

anergia

anhedonia (anhedonistic)

anticipatory grieving

asocial behavior

bipolar disorder

circumstantiality

covert cues

diurnal mood variations

dysphoria

electroconvulsive
   therapy (ECT)

euthymic

flight of ideas

grief

hypersomnia

hypertensive crisis

hypomania

insomnia: initial, middle,
   terminal

introjection

kindling

labile emotions

loose associations

mania

mood disorders

no-touch policy

one-to-one suicide
   supervision

overt cues

pressured speech

psychomotor agitation

psychomotor retardation

ruminate

seasonal affective
   disorder (SAD)

suicidal ideation

suicide

suicide lethality
   assessment

tangential speech

tunnel vision

unipolar disorder

Everyone has occasional episodes of feeling sad, low, and tired, with a desire to stay in bed and shut out the world. These episodes are often accompanied by **anergia** (lack of energy), exhaustion, agitation, noise intolerance, and slowed thinking processes that make decisions difficult. However, work, family, and social responsibilities drive most people to go through the motions of their daily routine, even though nothing seems to go right and their irritable mood is obvious to all. These "low periods" pass in a day or so, and energy returns. Fluctuation in mood is so common to the human condition that we think nothing of hearing someone say, "I knew it was going to be a bad day when I slept through the alarm." These occasional "bad days" may be a way for the body to slow down for a system recharge. Sadness in mood can also be a response to misfortunes in our lives. The loss of a friend or relative, financial problems, or the loss of belongings or a job are reasons for a person to grieve.

At the other end of the mood spectrum are episodes of exaggeratedly energetic behavior, with the sure sense that one can take on any task or any relationship. In an elated mood, the person has untiring stamina for work, family, and social events. This feeling of being "on top of the world" also recedes in a few days to a **euthymic** mood of average affect and activity. Happy events stimulate joy and enthusiasm. These mood alterations are normal and do not interfere in any meaningful way with the person's life.

Mood disorders, also known as affective disorders, are pervasive alterations in a person's emotions, manifested by depression or mania. Mood disorders interfere with the person's life. The person is plagued by drastic and long-term sadness, agitation, or elation, accompanied by self-doubt, guilt, and anger, that alters his or her life activities, especially those that involve self-esteem, occupation, and relationships.

Mood disorders are neurobiologic dysfunctions that create altered emotional responses. About 25% of the population will experience some degree of mood disorder in a lifetime. People with mood disorders function within the bounds of reality, except for 9% of this population who become psychotic, with disorganized, bizarre thoughts and actions while in the acute stage of their mood disorder. In people seeking help in primary care settings, depression is more prevalent than hypertension (Montano, 1994).

Mood disorders are not new to humanity. From early history, people have suffered from mood disturbances. Archaeologists have found holes drilled into ancient skulls to relieve the "evil humors" of those suffering from sad feelings and acting strangely. Babylonians and ancient Hebrews believed that overwhelming sadness and extreme behavior were sent to people through the will of God or other divine beings. Biblical notables King Saul, King Nebuchadnezzar, and Moses suffered overwhelming grief of heart, unclean spirit, or bitterness of soul, which are all symptoms of depression. Abraham Lincoln and Queen Victoria had recurrent episodes of depression. Other famous people with mood disorders were writers Virginia Woolf, Sylvia Plath, and Eugene O'Neill; composer George Frideric Handel; former member of the Grateful Dead Jerry Garcia; artist Vincent Van Gogh; philosopher Frederic Nietzsche; newscaster Jim Jensen; TV commentator and host of "60 Minutes" Mike Wallace; and actress Patty Duke (Coffey & Weiner, 1988).

Until the mid-1950s there was no treatment to help the seriously depressed or elated, so people suffered through their altered moods, thinking they were hopelessly weak people to succumb to these devastating symptoms. Family and mental health professionals tended to agree with this assessment, seeing the sufferer as egocentric and only viewing life through a negative lens. It could take up to 2 years for a major depression to subside, and people with bipolar disorder fluctuated between high and low moods. There are still no cures for mood disorders, but there are now effective treatments for both depression and mania.

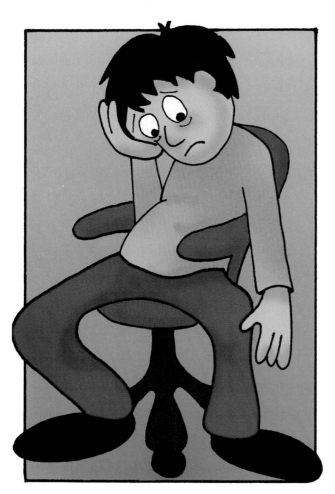

Anergia

CATEGORIES OF MOOD DISORDERS

Mood disorders are separated into two major categories: **unipolar disorder**, which encompasses major depression and dysthymic disorder, during which the person demonstrates the sadness, agitation, and anger of the one extreme mood change of depression, and **bipolar disorder** (formerly known as manic-depressive illness), in which the person's mood cycles between extremes of mania and depression, with periods of normalcy between each extreme, between depression and normalcy, or between mania and normalcy.

Mania is an abnormally elevated mood in which the person is extraordinarily energetic; needs little sleep, rest, or food; has an exaggerated sense of self-importance, inflated self-esteem, poor judgment, increased libido, expanded socialization, high distractibility, and easy irritation; and engages in grandiose behaviors. The high-energy behavior in mania is often exhibited by multiple goal-directed activities, pleasure-seeking, and high-risk behaviors.

The depressive disorders include major depressive disorders, dysthymic disorder, and depressive disorder not otherwise specified. The bipolar disorders include bipolar I disorder, bipolar II disorder, cyclothymic disorder, and bipolar disorder not otherwise specified. This chapter will focus on major depressive disorder and bipolar disorder as the models for discussing the nursing process for mood disorders. There is also a broad discussion of suicide because mood disorders are linked to suicide more than to any other illness, whether psychiatric or medical: depression is present in 80% of those who attempt or commit suicide in the population with diagnosed psychiatric disorders. Suicide is an option to end the helplessness, hopelessness, and internalized anger of mood disorders. The rate of suicide has tripled in the adolescent population (ages 15 to 24) because there is an increased incidence of depression in this population. Men older than 64 have a suicide rate of 38/100,000 compared with the 17/100,000 rate for all men in the United States (Roy, 2000).

RELATED DISORDERS

Mixed anxiety-depressive disorder features a sad (dysphoric) mood that has lasted more than 4 weeks, along with such behaviors as altered sleep, interference with concentration, irritability, fretting, little energy, tearfulness, hypervigilance, pessimism, worthlessness, and anticipation of failure (DSM-IV-TR, 2000). Somatoform disorder and undifferentiated somatoform disorder can be mistaken for mood disorders. In the former, the person has a combination of symptoms affecting multiple areas of the body, including pain and gastrointestinal, sexual, and pseudoneurologic symptoms.

The latter is manifested by at least one unexplained physical symptom. Somatoform disorders are addressed in Chapter 19.

Seasonal affective disorder is a depressive episode that occurs in yearly cycles, tied to the reduction of sunlight in winter months. The person is de-energized, sleeps more, gains weight, loses interest in pleasurable activities, and is cranky. As spring appears, the person regains energy and a pleasant personality, becomes more active, and is less sleepy. Seasonal affective disorder has been called the human equivalent of hibernation.

Grief has symptoms similar to depression and is discussed in Chapter 9.

Two proposed personality disorders (see Chap. 16) that have depressive features are premenstrual dysphoric disorder (mood lability, agitation, anhedonism, fatigue, appetite and sleep changes, interpersonal conflict, physical symptoms, such as engorged breasts, weight gain, and fluid retention, and a sense of feeling overwhelmed in the period between ovulation and menses) and depressive personality disorder (sadness but with fewer symptoms and less impairment than depression; the person can function

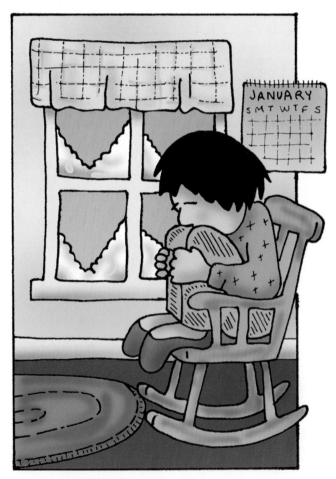

Seasonal affective disorder

near normal, with a great deal of effort, or can have impaired occupational, social, or interpersonal functions) (DSM-IV-TR, 2000).

ETIOLOGY

Mood disorders are believed to reflect dysfunction of the limbic system, hypothalamus, and basal ganglia, structures integral to human emotions. Before the advent of the amazing noninvasive research tools that are now available to observe the most minute areas of body physiology, theories about mood disorders focused on life experiences and how the person chose to respond to them. Did the person learn and grow from positive and negative life experiences, or were the experiences a springboard to depression or mania? Some of these theories had a "blame-the-victim" focus, whereas today's research focuses on the belief that mood disorders are chemical imbalances that are biologic (hormonal, neurologic, or genetic) in nature. The fact that the human body is an incredible tool with self-regulating and self-healing properties that can be aided by the person's will to change is why a combination of psychotherapy and psychotropic drugs is more effective at helping people with mood disorders.

Biologic Theories

GENETIC THEORIES

Genetic studies implicate the transmission of unipolar depression in first-degree relatives, who have twice the risk of the general population (DSM-IV-TR, 2000). Monozygotic twins raised apart have a 54% greater incidence and dizygotic twins have a 24% greater incidence of comorbidity, demonstrating that inherited factors are more important than the environment in which the person has been raised (Kelsoe, 2000).

Comer (1992) discussed the findings of researchers interested in finding genetic links in families with multigenerational high rates of bipolar disorders. These scientists also looked for other family trait distribution patterns (for example, medical conditions or red hair) that may relate to the distribution of bipolar disorder. Researchers of families in Belgium, Italy, and Israel have demonstrated a linkage of bipolar disorder to red/green color blindness and to G6PD deficiency, a medical anomaly transmitted on the X chromosome. Studies of Amish families with multigenerational bipolar disorder compared the DNA from relatives with and without bipolar disease and found a discrepancy in chromosome 11 near the insulin gene and another known gene. Until these studies are replicated, we can draw the conclusion that two different genes are implicated

in bipolar disorders, or that the initial premises of these studies were flawed, so the conclusions drawn were incorrect.

DelBello et al. (1999) discussed indications of a genetic overlap of early-onset bipolar disorder and early-onset alcoholism. He noted that these people have a higher rate of mixed and rapid cycling and a poorer response to lithium, a slower rate of recovery, and more hospital admissions. Mania displayed by these adolescents involves more agitation than elation, and they may respond better to anticonvulsants than to lithium.

NEUROCHEMICAL THEORIES

Neurochemical influences of neurotransmitters (chemical messengers) focus on serotonin and norepinephrine as the two major biogenic amines implicated in mood disorders. Serotonin (5-HT) has many roles in behavior: mood, activity, aggressiveness and irritability, cognition, pain, biorhythms, and neuroendocrine processes (that is, growth hormone, cortisol, and prolactin levels are abnormal in depression). Deficits of serotonin, its precursor tryptophan, or a metabolite (5HIAA) of serotonin found in the blood or cerebrospinal fluid occur in depressed people. Positron emission tomography scans (Fig. 14-1) demonstrate reduced metabolism in the prefrontal cortex, which may promote depression (Tecott, 2000).

Norepinephrine levels may be deficient in depression and increased in mania (Keltner et al., 1997). This catecholamine energizes the body to mobilize during stress and inhibits kindling. **Kindling** is the process by which seizure activity in a specific area of the brain is initially stimulated by reaching a threshold of the cumulative effects of stress, low amounts of electric impulses, or chemicals such as cocaine, which sensitize nerve cells and pathways. These highly sensitized pathways respond by no longer needing the stimulus to induce seizure activity, which now occurs spontaneously. It is theorized that kindling may underlie the cycling of mood disorders as well as addiction. Anticonvulsants inhibit kindling; this may explain their efficacy in the treatment of bipolar disorder (Tecott, 2000).

Dysregulation of acetylcholine and dopamine are also being studied in relation to mood disorders. Mood, sleep, neuroendocrine function, and the electroencephalographic pattern are altered by cholinergic drugs; therefore, acetylcholine seems to be implicated in depression and mania (Table 14-1). The neurotransmitter problem may not be as simple as underproduction or depletion through overuse during stress. Changes in the sensitivity as well as the number of receptors are being evaluated for their roles in mood disorders (Tecott, 2000).

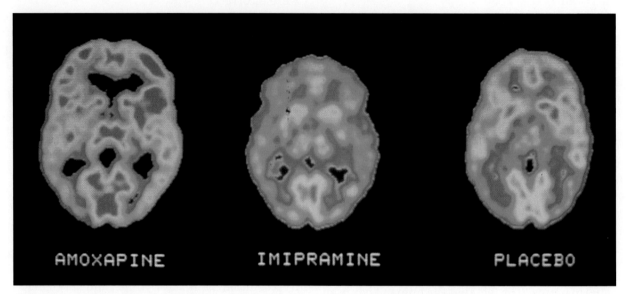

Figure 14-1. Acute effects of antidepressant medications in patients with affective disorder show widespread effects on the cortex that vary dramatically with the medication used. PET scanning is useful in revealing specific patterns of metabolic change in the brain and providing clues to the mechanisms of antidepressant response. (Courtesy of Monte S. Buchsbaum, MD, The Mount Sinai Medical Center and School of Medicine, New York, New York.)

Table 14-1

DRUGS AND CONDITIONS IMPLICATED IN DEPRESSION

DRUGS
Anxiolytics
Antipsychotics
Antivirals (nelfinavir)
Sedative-hypnotics
Antihypertensives (propranolol, reserpine)
Antiparkinsonians (levodopa, amantadine)
Hormones (estrogen, progesterone)
Steroids (cortisone)
Antituberculars (cyloserine)
Immunomodulators (interferon, vincristine, vinblastine)
GI meds (cimetidine, monoctanoin)

PHYSIOLOGIC CONDITIONS
CNS: Alzheimer's, Parkinson's, Huntington's, multiple sclerosis, encephalitis, syphilis, stroke
Electrolyte: sodium, calcium, or potassium excess or deficit
Endocrine: thyroid, parathyroid, or adrenal hormones excess or deficit; glucose tolerance fluctuations; estrogen
Metabolic: deficiencies of thiamine, pyridoxine (B_6), vitamin B_{12}, niacin, vitamin C, iron, folic acid, zinc, protein, vitamin E, magnesium; abnormal fatty acid metabolism; caffeine sensitivity
Collagen: systemic lupus erythematosus, polyarteritis nodosa
Cardiovascular: cardiomyopathy, congestive heart failure, myocardial infarction
Infections: hepatitis, mononucleosis, pneumonia
Others: porphyria

Adapted from Boyd, M. A., & Nihart, M. A. (1998). *Psychiatric nursing: contemporary practice.* Philadelphia: Lippincott.

NEUROENDOCRINE INFLUENCES

Hormonal fluctuations are being studied in relation to depression. Mood disturbances have been documented in persons with endocrine disorders such as those of the thyroid, adrenal, parathyroid, and pituitary. Postpartum hormone alterations have created serious depressions. Premenstrual syndrome involves symptoms of depression along with the physical symptoms of water retention and breast swelling.

Hypothalamic-Pituitary-Adrenocortical Axis. Cortisol levels are increased in many depressed people. In the dexamethasone suppression test (DST), a dose of dexamethasone would suppress the late-afternoon cortisol levels in a person without depression, but would not suppress cortisol levels in many depressed people. This test is not used as a benchmark for depression, however, because the results can be affected by medications and illnesses and are abnormal in only about 50% of depressed people (Hyman & Nestler, 1993).

Hypothalamic-Pituitary-Thyroid Axis. Production by the hypothalamus of thyroid-releasing factor stimulates the anterior pituitary to release thyroid-stimulating hormone, which signals the thyroid gland to work. About one fourth of depressed people have a reduced thyroid-stimulating hormone response to a dose of thyroid-releasing factor. Both hypothyroid and hyperthyroid conditions are related to mood disorders (Charney & Weissman, 1988; Hyman & Nestler, 1993).

BIOLOGIC CYCLES

Yearly patterns are seen in seasonal affective disorder, a depression that occurs when there is less sunlight and remits with increased hours of sun. Light therapy has been successful in the treatment of this disorder. Clients with rapid-cycling bipolar I or bipolar II disorder have four or more mood disturbances in a year. The hormonal shifts induced by lunar cycles can also affect mood, as in premenstrual syndrome. Circadian rhythms are also being researched in relation to **diurnal mood variations** (moods that alter depending on the time of day). During sleep, rapid eye movements start too rapidly and remain too long in depressed people, thus increasing dream time; however, the actual sleep time is decreased and the number of wake periods is increased in depression.

Psychodynamic Theories

Freud (1917) hypothesized that depression stemmed from the rage over abandonment of the infant by the mother through death, emotional detachment, or other absence. This loss of a love object produced insecurity, emptiness, sadness, and anger. This loss occurs in the oral stage of development, when the dependent infant has no conception of individuation from the parent. As an adult, mourners regress to the oral stage and introject their anger about abandonment or unresolved conflicts with the lost object into anger toward themselves. **Introjection** is an unconscious defense mechanism in which a person internalizes the viewpoints and values of the loved object, integrating them into his or her own identity and belief system. The ego is overpowered by the punitive superego. This results in rigidity, with rule-oriented goals that are unrealistic and unattainable, setting the stage for failure.

Freud and Karl Abraham (1927), a member of his study group, realized that the sadness experienced by adults grieving for the death of or separation from a loved one is similar to depression. **Grief** is the normal response to losses of personal relationships, status, health, wealth, occupation, goals, self-esteem, cognitive ability, and other significant objects. Grief that occurs before the loss is **anticipatory grieving**, the mourning that starts, for instance, on receiving the diagnosis of cancer and subsequent loss of health. The object lost can be real or perceived. An example of perceived loss is when an adolescent anticipates loss of love or approval from his parents if he is not selected for the high-school honor society. Contemporary theorists who have studied the grieving process say that the grieving person experiences several discrete stages of grief (Bowlby & Parkes, 1970; Engel, 1964; Kübler-Ross, 1960; Lindemann, 1944); see Chapter 9 for a discussion of these grieving stages. Sadness, agitation, asocial behavior, and sleep changes are some of the grief behaviors the person exhibits until the grieving process lessens and the person returns to adaptive behavior. The chief difference between grief and depression is that grieving is time-limited, usually to 1 or 2 years.

The intrapsychic view of mania is related to fear that the child's increasing autonomy will leave the parent without significance in the child's life. Messages are sent to the child that independence is devalued, so to retain parental approval, the child learns to suppress movement toward autonomy. This conflict creates a double-bind situation for the child, because there are sanctions both for autonomy and the suppression of autonomy. The child responds to the loving side of the parent but grows to hate the controlling side. This love/hate results in ambivalence and depression with a weak ego and an overpowering superego, which in mania is denied. Because mania is the denial of depression, the person with mania is id-dominated, with little manifestation of the superego until the person cycles back toward normalcy or the depressive phase of the bipolar disorder (Gabbard, 2000).

Cognitive Theories

Aaron Beck's (1967*a*, 1967*b*, 1976) theory about the cause of depression relates to depressed people's comprehensively negative thoughts. They view themselves, their world, and their future in a distorted failure mode, repeatedly interpreting experiences as difficult and burdensome and themselves as inconsequential and incompetent.

Social/Environmental Theories

Circumstances such as "ambivalent, abusive, rejecting or highly dependent family relationships" can increase the risk for mood disorders (DSM-IV-TR, 2000). Loss of relationships or an important life role may precede depression. Physical or sexual abuse can be a factor in depression. Social isolation and severely limited finances are implicated in the depression of senior citizens (Boyd & Nihart, 1998).

CULTURAL CONSIDERATIONS

Depression can be masked by other behaviors that are considered age-appropriate, making the disorder difficult to identify and diagnose in certain age groups. Depressed children often appear cranky. They may have school phobia, hyperactivity, learning disorders, failing grades, and antisocial behaviors. Depressed adolescents may engage in substance abuse, join gangs, engage in risky behavior, be underachievers,

or drop out of school. In adults, depression can be signaled by substance abuse, eating disorders, compulsive behaviors such as workaholism and gambling, and hypochondriasis. Elderly people who are cranky and argumentative may actually be depressed.

Many somatic ailments (physiologic ailments) accompany depression. This varies from culture to culture and is more apparent in cultures that believe it is inappropriate to verbalize emotions. For example, Asians who are anxious or depressed are more likely to have somatic complaints of headache or backache or other physical symptoms. Latin cultures complain of "nerves" or headaches; Middle Eastern cultures complain of heart problems (Andrews & Boyle).

MAJOR DEPRESSIVE DISORDER

Major depressive disorder typically involves 2 or more weeks of a sad mood or lack of interest in life activities with at least four other symptoms of depression, such as anhedonia and changes in weight, sleep, energy, concentration, making decisions, self-esteem, and goals. Major depression is twice as common in women and has a 1.5 to 3 times greater incidence in first-degree relatives than in the general population. The incidence of depression decreases with age in women and increases with age in men. Single and divorced people have the highest incidence of depression (Kelsoe, 2000). Depression in prepubertal boys and girls occurs at an equal rate (Keltner et al., 1998).

CLINICAL VIGNETTE: DEPRESSION

"Just get out! I am not interested in food," said Chris to her husband, who had come into their bedroom to invite her to the dinner he and their daughters had prepared. "Can't they leave me alone?" thought Chris to herself as she miserably pulled the covers over her shoulders. Yet she felt guilty about the way she'd snapped at Matt. She knew she'd disparaged their efforts to help, but she couldn't stop.

She was physically and emotionally exhausted. "I can't remember when I felt well . . . maybe last year sometime, or maybe never," she thought fretfully. She'd always worked hard to get things done; lately she could not do anything at all except complain. Kaitlyn, her 13-year-old, accused her of hating everything and everybody, including her family. Chris cringed at her memory of telling Kaitlyn the lingerie she had bought as a 40th birthday present out of her babysitting money "would wash apart on the first washing."

Lissa, age 11, said, "Everything has to be your way, Mom. You scream at us and guilt us out to get your way. You never listen anymore." Matt had long ago withdrawn from her moodiness, acid tongue, and disinterest in sex. One day she overheard Matt tell his brother she was "crabby, agitated, and self-centered and if it wasn't for the girls, I don't know what I'd do. I've tried to get her to go to a doctor, but she says it's all our fault, then she sulks for days. What is our fault? I don't know what to do for her. I feel as if I am living in a minefield and never know what will set off an explosion. I try to remember the love we had together, but her behavior is getting old."

Chris has lost 12 pounds in the past 2 months, has difficulty sleeping, and is hostile, angry, and guilty about it. She has no desire for any pleasure. "Why bother? There is nothing to enjoy. Life is bleak." She feels stuck, worthless, hopeless, and helpless. Hoping against hope, Chris thinks to herself, "I wish I were dead. I'd never have to do anything again."

> ▶ MAJOR SYMPTOMS OF DEPRESSIVE DISORDER

- Depressed mood
- Anhedonism (decreased attention to and enjoyment from previously pleasurable activities)
- Unintentional weight change of 5% or more in a month
- Change in sleep pattern
- Agitation or psychomotor retardation
- Tiredness
- Worthlessness or guilt inappropriate to the situation (possibly delusional)
- Difficulty thinking, focusing, or making decisions
- Hopelessness, helplessness, and/or suicidal ideation. (The degree of hopelessness and helplessness is often used to diagnose the degree of depression.)

Onset and Clinical Course

An untreated episode of depression can last 6 to 24 months before remitting. Fifty to sixty percent of people who have one episode of depression will have another. After a second episode of depression, there is a 70% chance of recurrence. Depressive symptoms can vary from mild to severe. The degree of depression is comparable to the person's sense of helplessness and hopelessness. Some severely depressed people (9%) have psychotic features (DSM-IV-TR, 2000).

Treatment and Prognosis

PSYCHOPHARMACOLOGY

There are three major categories of antidepressants—tricyclic antidepressants (TCAs), monoamine oxidase inhibitors (MAOIs), and selective serotonin reuptake inhibitors (SSRIs)—and some atypical antidepressants. Chapter 2 details biologic treatments. The choice of which antidepressant to use is based on the client's symptoms, age, physical health needs, which drugs have worked or not worked in the past or have worked for a blood relative with depression, and other medications the client is taking.

It is thought that levels of neurotransmitters, especially norepinephrine and serotonin, are decreased in depression. These neurotransmitters are released from the presynaptic neuron to allow them to enter the synapse and link with postsynaptic receptors. Depression results if too few neurotransmitters are released, if they linger too briefly in the synapse, if they are too quickly reabsorbed by the presynaptic neuron that had released them, if the conditions in the synapse do not support neurotransmitter linkage with

postsynaptic receptors, or if the number of postsynaptic receptors has been decreased. The goal is to increase the efficacy of the neurotransmitters that are available and the absorption by the postsynaptic receptors. To do this, antidepressants set up a blockade for the reuptake of norepinephrine and serotonin into their specific nerve terminals, which permits them to linger for a longer time in the synapse and be more available to the postsynaptic receptors, and to increase the sensitivity of the postsynaptic receptor sites (PDR Nurse's Handbook, 1999; Schatzberg & Nemeroff, 1998).

In a client with acute depression with psychotic features, an antipsychotic is used in combination with an antidepressant, especially for TCAs and MAOIs, which have significant lag periods (1 to 4 weeks) before they reach effective levels. Antipsychotics can also be used with SSRIs. The antipsychotic tempers the psychotic features; several weeks into treatment, the client is reassessed to determine whether the antipsychotic can be withdrawn and the antidepressant maintained.

There is increasing evidence that antidepressant therapy should be continued for longer than the 3 to 6 months originally believed necessary, because less recidivism has been found in persons with unipolar depression who receive 18 to 24 months of antidepressant therapy. Antidepressants as a rule should be tapered before being withdrawn.

SSRIs. SSRIs, the newest category of antidepressants (Table 14-2), are effective for most depressions. The action of SSRIs is specific to serotonin reuptake inhibition; they produce fewer sedating, anticholinergic, and cardiovascular side effects, making them safer for use in children and the elderly. SSRIs have low levels of side effects and are relatively safe, and people using these antidepressants are more apt to be compliant with the treatment regimen. Insomnia decreases in 3 to 4 days, appetite returns to a more normal state in 5 to 7 days, and energy returns in 4 to 7 days. In a week to 10 days, mood, concentration, and interest in life improve.

Fluoxetine (Prozac) produces a slightly higher rate of mild agitation and weight loss, but less somnolence. It has a half-life of more than 7 days, which differs from the 25-hour half-life of other SSRIs. It is usually given in the morning. Paroxetine (Paxil) has a slightly higher rate of mild somnolence and constipation but less diarrhea, and it has an antianxiety effect. Sertraline (Zoloft) produces the least anorexia and has somnolence as a side effect. Fluvoxamine (Luvox) produces up to a 40% rate of insomnia (McEvoy, 2000). Mirtazapine (Remeron) has increased appetite and modest weight gain as side effects; this is actually desirable in depressed people who have lost their

Table 14-2

Selective Serotonin Reuptake Inhibitor (SSRI) Antidepressants

Do not take with MAOI antidepressants. Washout period of 2 weeks between MAOI and SSRI. Doses started low, increased slowly. SSRIs should be tapered when therapy completed.

Generic (Brand)	Dose	Nursing Implications
fluoxetine (Prozac)	10–80 mg/day	Headache, nervousness, anxiety, insomnia, nausea, diarrhea, weight loss. Give in AM. If divided dose, give second dose at noon to avoid insomnia. Weigh weekly. Monitor hepatic & renal function tests, monitor potential hyponatremia, loss diabetic control. Monitor rash, hives, fever, leukocytosis, carpal tunnel, arthralgias, edema, respiratory distress, proteinuria. Many drug interactions: warfarin, lithium, phenytoin, TCA, MAOI, Haldol, buspirone, alprazolam, carbamazepine, diazepam.
sertraline (Zoloft)	50–200 mg/day	Agitation, insomnia, headache, dizziness, somnolence, fatigue. Can give in AM or PM. Check fluid and sodium in elderly. Can increase PT, diazepam, MAOI.
paroxetine (Paxil)	10–80 mg/day	Headache, sedation, nausea, dry mouth, constipation, ejaculatory difficulty, seizures, GI hemorrhage. Check fluid and electrolyte balance in aged, weight loss. Drug interactions: cimetidine, antiarrhythmics, phenobarbital, phenytoin, procyclidine, theophylline, warfarin, MAOI.
citalopram (Celexa)	20–40 mg/day	Absorption not affected by food. Dry mouth, sweating, tremors, nausea, flatulence, dyspepsia, somnolence, tachycardia, postural hypotension. Check possible hyponatremia, SIADH.

Adapted from McEvoy, R. B. (Ed.) (2000). *Facts and comparisons 2000.* St. Louis: Facts and Comparisons, A Wolters Kluwer Company.

appetite and lost weight. It is started at higher doses because it is more sedating and has more antihistaminic side effects at the lower doses, which are counteracted at higher doses by the noradrenergic stimulation (Schatzberg & Nemeroff, 1998).

SSRIs can increase the serum levels of lithium, anticonvulsants, antipsychotics, and benzodiazepines. They have less of a lag period than other antidepressants, except for venlafaxine (Effexor), which can maintain an active state for days after being discontinued, and fluoxetine, which can maintain active drug status in the blood for weeks after withdrawal. SSRIs should not be given along with MAOIs because of the risk of the potentially deadly serotonin syndrome (Black et al., 2000).

TCAs. TCAs, introduced for the treatment of depression in the mid-1950s, are the oldest antidepressants. They are used for treatment of depression and reactive depression. They relieve the depressive symptoms of hopelessness, helplessness, anhedonism, inappropriate guilt, suicidal ideation, and daily mood variations (cranky in the morning and better in the evening). Other indications include panic disorder, obsessive-compulsive disorder, and eating disorders. Each TCA has a different degree of efficacy in blocking the activity of norepinephrine and serotonin or increasing the sensitivity of postsynaptic receptor sites. TCAs and heterocyclic antidepressants have a lag period of 10 to

14 days before reaching a serum level that begins to alter symptoms; they take 6 weeks to reach full effect. Because they have a long serum half-life, there is a lag period of 1 to 4 weeks before steady plasma levels are reached and the client's symptoms begin to lessen. They cost less primarily because they have been around longer and generic forms are available.

TCAs are contraindicated in severe impairment of liver function and in myocardial infarction (acute recovery phase). They cannot be given concurrently with MAOIs. Because of their anticholinergic side effects, TCAs must be used cautiously in clients who have glaucoma, benign prostatic hypertrophy, urinary retention or obstruction, diabetes mellitus, hyperthyroidism, cardiovascular disease, renal impairment, or respiratory disorders (Table 14-3).

Overdosage of TCAs occurs over several days and results in confusion, agitation, hallucinations, hyperpyrexia, and increased reflexes. Seizures, coma, and cardiovascular toxicity can occur with ensuing tachycardia, decreased output, depressed contractility, and atrioventricular block. Because many elderly people have concomitant health problems, TCAs are sometimes less appealing to use in the geriatric population than newer types of antidepressants, which have fewer side effects and less drug interactions (PDR Nurse's Handbook, 1999).

The following TCAs are tertiary amines, which produce more blocking of serotonin reuptake.

Table 14-3

TRICYCLIC ANTIDEPRESSANT MEDICATIONS

Tricyclic antidepressants can take 2 or more weeks to reach therapeutic levels. Do not coadminister with MAOI antidepressants.

Generic (Brand)	Dose	Nursing Implications
amitryptyline (Elavil)	Adult: 75–300 mg/day, Geriatric: 10–25 mg hs.	Drowsiness, dizziness, orthostatic hypotension (to decrease, give at h.s.), dry mouth, constipation. Decreases antihypertensives, CNS depress. Check BP: withhold & call MD if change of 10–20 mmHg. Check liver & kidney function test results; Check WBC & diff: possible bone marrow depression. Contraindicated in acute MI, seizure disorders, pregnancy.
clomipramine (Anafranil)	75–300 mg/day in divided doses	Tremor, weight gain. Can increase AST, ALT, prolactin, T_3. Can lower seizure threshhold, can cause neuroleptic malignant syndrome. Check liver function tests. Give with food to reduce GI side effects. Contra-indicated in acute MI, pregnancy, nursing mothers.
doxepin (Sinequan)	Adult: 30–150 mg/day in divided doses or h.s.	Drowsiness, dry mouth, orthostatic hypotension. CNS depression. Contraindicated in acute MI, BPH, glaucoma.
imipramine (Tofranil)	Adult: 75–300 mg/day in divided doses	Sedation, drowsiness, orthostatic hypotension, arrhythmias, heart block, blurred vision, mydriasis, urinary retention. Increased BUN, alk, phos., decreased BG. Give with food. Report gain of 1½–2 lb. In 2–3 days. Check WBC & diff: for bone marrow depression; renal & liver function tests. Check VS, EPS, cholestatic jaundice.
desipramine (Norpramin)	Adult: 75–300 mg/day hs or divided doses.	Same as above.
nortriptyline (Pamelor)	Adult: 25–150 mg/day	Similar to above; fewer cardiac effects; monitor nortriptyline plasma level.

Adapted from McEvoy, R. B. (Ed.) (2000). *Facts and comparisons 2000.* St. Louis: Facts and Comparisons, A Wolters Kluwer Company.

Amitriptyline (Elavil) is taken with food to reduce gastrointestinal distress. It tends to be sedating, so it should be taken at bedtime. It may turn urine a blue-green color. Baseline and intermittent white blood cell counts with differential should be obtained, and the client should be monitored for sore throat and fever, which may indicate bone marrow depression. Blood pressure should be monitored and the drug withheld if there is an increase or decrease in systole of 10 to 20 mmHg. The client should be taught to rise slowly from a recumbent or sitting position to minimize the risk of falls from orthostatic hypotension. Cimetidine increases plasma levels of amitriptyline.

Clomipramine (Anafranil) can cause tremor, elevated liver function tests, and reduced T_3 results. The client should be monitored for seizures and neuroleptic malignant syndrome (fever, sweating, muscle rigidity, labile vital signs, altered level of consciousness, altered mental status, and coma). Fever and sore throat can indicate bone marrow suppression, so a white blood cell count and differential should be obtained.

Doxepin (Sinequan), if used in an oral concentrate, must be diluted with 120 mL of water, milk, or juice. It can be administered at bedtime to reduce daytime sedation.

Imipramine (Tofranil) can create arrhythmias, increase serum bilirubin and alkaline phosphatase levels, and alter levels of blood glucose. Baseline and intermittent complete blood counts with differential and liver and kidney function tests should be obtained. The client should be monitored for fluid and electrolyte status and cholestatic jaundice (aches, pains, chills and fever, yellow skin or sclera, brown urine, chalky stool, itchy skin). It can cause extrapyramidal symptoms in large doses, as well as cardiac arrhythmias, hypotension, respiratory depression, and seizures.

The following TCAs are secondary amines, which produce greater blocking of norepinephrine reuptake.

Desipramine (Norpramin) produces the fewest side effects, especially anticholinergic effects and sedation. It and nortriptyline are the first-line TCAs because of their low side effects. It is usually given in the morning to minimize insomnia, overactivity, and agitation. It can cause heart block, acute glaucoma, and agranulocytosis. Doses are slowly increased to decrease side effects and are slowly decreased to reduce withdrawal symptoms. Smoking decreases its therapeutic action.

Nortriptyline (Pamelor) has fewer side effects and an especially low incidence of orthostatic hypotension. Plasma levels are monitored because there is a narrow range of efficacy. The drug should be withheld if there is a change in blood pressure of 20 mmHg. Nortriptyline can cause stomatitis and acute glaucoma, and it increases the effect of central nervous system depressants.

Protriptyline (Vivactil) is given in the morning to reduce insomnia, overactivity, and agitation. The drug should be withheld if there is a change in systole of 20 mm Hg.

The following are tetracyclic antidepressants.

Amoxapine (Ascendin) may cause extrapyramidal symptoms, tardive dyskinesia, and neuroleptic malignant syndrome, and it can create tolerance in 1 to 3 months. It increases appetite and causes weight gain and cravings for sweets.

Maprotiline (Ludiomil) carries a risk of seizures (especially in heavy drinkers), severe constipation and urinary retention, stomatitis, and other side effects, leading to poor compliance. The drug is started and withdrawn gradually. Central nervous system depressants can increase the effects of this drug.

Atypical Antidepressants. Atypical antidepressants are used when the client has an inadequate response to or side effects from SSRIs (Table 14-4). Atypical antidepressants include venlafaxine (Effexor), bupropion (Wellbutrin), trazodone (Desyrel), and nefazodone (Serzone).

Venlafaxine blocks the reuptake of serotonin, norepinephrine, and dopamine (weakly). It is similar to the TCA clomipramine but has fewer side effects. It is more effective if taken with food to aid absorption. It has a rapid onset of action and a short half-life (5 hours), with a low incidence of anxiety, sexual side effects, dizziness, somnolence, and nausea. Blood pressure should be monitored regularly (McEvoy, 2000).

Bupropion modestly inhibits the reuptake of norepinephrine, weakly inhibits the reuptake of dopamine, and has no effects on serotonin. It produces few side effects, has a two-phase half-life (the first at 1.5 hours and the second at 14 hours), does not cause psychosexual dysfunction or orthostatic hypotension, and is considered safer in terms of cardiovascular side effects. It can increase the seizure risk in people with seizure disorder, head injuries, or bulimia. Headaches, decreased appetite, agitation, weight loss, and insomnia are other side effects. Doses are increased gradually. Bupropion is marketed as Zyban for smoking cessation (Schatzberg & Nemeroff, 1998).

Trazodone is believed to inhibit the uptake of serotonin by brain cells and to increase synapse concentration. It causes moderate orthostatic hypotension, so concomitant use of alcohol and central nervous system depressants should be avoided. Its use is contraindicated in clients recovering from myocardial infarction and receiving electroconvulsive therapy. Giving the drug with food increases absorption. Overdose leads to hypotension, electroencephalographic changes, nausea and vomiting,

Table 14-4

ATYPICAL ANTIDEPRESSANTS

Generic (Brand)	Dose	Nursing Implications
venlafaxine (Effexor, Effexor XR)	25 – 125 mg/bid 33.7 – 225 mg/day	Give with food to increase absorption. Increased BP, P; nausea, vomiting, dry mouth, sweating. Periodic monitoring serum lipids. In renal or liver problems, dose reduced by 25%–50%. Drug interactions: cimetidine, MAOI. Can alter many lab tests: Alk. phosphatase, creatinine, AST, ALT, glucose, lytes, etc.
bupropion (Wellbutrin, Wellbutrin SR)	50 – 100 bid 100 – 300 mg/day	Give with food to decrease n/v. Lowered seizure threshhold. Agitation, restlessness, insomnia, psychosis. Check liver & kidney function, cardiac alterations. Drug interactions: alcohol, amantadine, carbamazepine, fluoxetine, MAOI, retonavir, phenobarbital, phenytoin. May alter taste.
nefazodone (Serzone)	50 – 200 mg/bid	Headache, dizziness, drowsiness. Drug interactions: alprazolam, astemizole, digoxin, MAOI, propanolol, terfenadine, triazolam. Alters results of ALT, AST, LDH, cholesterol, glucose, Hct. Check liver & kidney function. Take prior to meals; food inhibits absorption.

Adapted from McEvoy, R. B. (Ed.) (2000). *Facts and comparisons 2000.* St. Louis: Facts and Comparisons, A Wolters Kluwer Company.

and priapism; respiratory arrest and seizures can occur (McEvoy, 2000).

Nefazodone inhibits the reuptake of serotonin and norepinephrine and has few side effects. Its half-life is 4 hours, and it can be used in clients with liver and kidney disease. It increases the action of certain benzodiazepines (alprazolam, estazolam, and triazolam) and the H_2 blocker terfenadine (McEvoy, 2000).

MAOIs. This class of antidepressants is largely unused today, except by psychiatrists in carefully controlled situations, because of potentially deadly side effects (Table 14-5). The most serious side effect is **hypertensive crisis**, a life-threatening condition that can result when a client taking MAOIs ingests tyramine-containing foods and fluids or other medications, particularly TCAs. Symptoms are occipital headache, hypertension, nausea, vomiting, chills, sweating, restlessness, nuchal rigidity, dilated pupils, fever, and motor agitation. These can lead to hyperpyrexia, cerebral hemorrhage, and death (Box 14-1). MAOIs should **never** be administered with TCAs.

With MAOIs, there is a drug–food interaction related to the degree of tyramine in a food. Tyramine is potentiated 10- to 20-fold by an MAOI, and symptoms can begin 20 to 60 minutes after the client ingests tyramine. For hypertensive crisis, transient antihypertensive agents such as phentolamine mesylate are given to dilate blood vessels and decrease vascular resistance (McEvoy, 2000).

There is a 2- to 4-week lag period before MAOIs reach therapeutic levels. Because of the lag period, adequate washout periods of 5 to 6 weeks are recommended between the time the MAOI is discontinued and another class of antidepressant is started.

Concomitant use of an MAOI and an SSRI can produce serotonin syndrome, which has potentially deadly autonomic and neurologic side effects. It is discussed later in this chapter.

Box 14-1

> ### HYPERTENSIVE CRISIS IN MAOI THERAPY

Hypertensive crisis is a life-threatening condition that results when clients taking MAOI antidepressants ingest food or fluids containing high levels of tyramine. The following are symptoms:

Headache, usually occipital
Pupil dilation
Nausea and vomiting
Photophobia
Nuchal rigidity
Sudden epistaxis
Palpitations
Tachycardia, bradycardia
Diaphoresis
Chest pain
Confusion
Stroke
Sudden hypertension
Death

MAOIs are being re-examined for use in clients who can use them safely, who have shown treatment compliance, and who have refractory depression, panic disorder, social phobias, obsessive-compulsive disorder, posttraumatic stress disorder, bulimia nervosa, resistant generalized anxiety disorder, or premenstrual dysphoria. There may be a resurgence in the use of this category of antidepressants for select clients.

OTHER MEDICAL TREATMENTS AND PSYCHOTHERAPY

Electroconvulsive Therapy. Psychiatrists may use **electroconvulsive therapy** (ECT) to treat depression if the client cannot tolerate the side effects of antidepressants, if many types of antidepressants

---

Table 14-5

MONOAMINE OXIDASE INHIBITOR (MAOI) ANTIDEPRESSANTS

MAOIs oxidize norepinephrine and serotonin. Responsible for antidepressant effect. MAO-B oxidizes tyramine, dopamine, and phenethylamine. Responsible for tyramine's hypertensive effect.

Generic Name (Brand Name)	Dosage Range	Nursing Implications
isocarboxazid (Marplan)	10–30 mg/day	Side effects: drowsiness, dry mouth, overactivity, insomnia, nausea, anorexia, constipation, urinary retention, orthostatic hypotension. Drug interactions: TCAs, SSRs, amphetamines, ephedrine, reserpine, dopamine, levodopa, guanethidine, methyldopa, buspirone, alcohol, meperidine, tyramine.
phenelzine (Nardil)	45–60 mg/day	Same as above. Also used for panic attacks.
tranylcypromine (Parnate)	20–40 mg/day	Same as above. Hypertensive crisis is commonly known as "Parnate–cheese reaction." Helps weight loss.

have been ineffective, or if the client has a health condition that precludes the use of any type of antidepressant. ECT was developed in 1938 by Italian physicists Ugo Cerletti and Lucio Bini, who believed a flawed assumption that schizophrenia and epilepsy could not exist together (Coffey & Weiner, 1990). This belief may have come from the observation that mentally ill people who also had a seizure disorder were better behaved and more compliant with all forms of therapy after a seizure. Bilateral ECT (administering an electric current to both hemispheres of the brain) results in a short period of unconsciousness, generalized seizure, and permanent long-term memory loss. Other side effects of ECT are fractured bones, soft-tissue injuries, and death in about 2/10,000 clients. ECT was later demonstrated to be ineffective in the treatment of schizophrenia (Oltmanns & Emery, 1998).

None of the antidepressants or antipsychotics available in the 1960s could relieve profound depression, but ECT worked. Clients often were willing to pay the price of memory loss to reap the benefit of relief from crippling depression.

Two factors helped make ECT almost obsolete by the mid-1970s. Two books, *One Flew Over the Cuckoo's Nest* by Ken Kesey, and Sylvia Plath's *The Bell Jar,* focused attention on the inappropriate use of ECT as a means of control and punishment of psychiatric inpatients. The second factor was the emergence of newer and more effective psychotropic drugs. In the 1990s, there has been a resurgence in the use of ECT as a viable treatment because the efficacy rate for people with severe or refractory depression is 90% (Murugesan, 1994). It is also effective for rapid-cycling bipolar disorder and major depression with psychotic features.

Today, ECT involves memory assessment before the procedure, medical clearance, laboratory studies, medication, and an informed consent about memory loss. Anesthesia is used. Much like a surgical procedure, the client may receive medications such as atropine to decrease secretions, muscle blockers such as succinylcholine to reduce the risk of bone fractures, and barbiturates such as methohexital for anesthesia. Nail polish, jewelry, hair ornaments, and nonpermanent dental items are removed before the procedure.

Unilateral or bilateral placement of electrodes is used today. Unilateral placement allows the current to pass through only the nondominant side of the brain; this can reduce memory impairment but may be less effective in the treatment of the mood disorder. ECT treatments are administered in a series (for example, three times a week for 6 weeks to 3 months), after which the need for an additional series is assessed.

The post-ECT process is similar to postoperative care, with frequent recording of vital signs, assessment of airway clearance, and prevention of aspiration. After awakening, the client is groggy for a few hours and should not be expected to make significant decisions during this time. There may also be agitation and unsteady gait.

Psychotherapy. A combination of psychotherapy and psychotherapeutic drugs is considered the most effective treatment for depressive disorders (Agency for Health Care Policy and Research Depression Guideline Panel, 1993). There is no one specific type of therapy that is better for the treatment of depression.

Behavioral therapy techniques work toward reshaping the person's behaviors. Shaping is a technique in which a reward is given for specific behaviors. For instance, a depressed person in a formal treatment situation (inpatient or outpatient) would earn points toward a desirable reward by demonstrating proper grooming and attending scheduled programs each day. Modeling behaviors can be done by staff members—for instance, demonstrating a socially acceptable way to disagree with another person without becoming agitated. Positive reinforcement of nondepressive behavior and social skills can be done by giving the person positive feedback for appropriate behavior.

Interpersonal therapy focuses on difficulties in relationships, such as grief reactions, role disputes, and role transitions. For example, a person who as a child never learned how to make and trust a friend outside of the family structure has difficulty establishing a friendship as an adult. Interpersonal therapy helps the person find ways to accomplish this developmental task.

Cognitive therapy concentrates on reframing and invalidating maladaptive assumptions, automatic upsetting thoughts, and illogical magnified thought processes. This model focuses on the person's thoughts, which account for his or her functional attributes.

Psychoanalytic therapy analyzes the person's thoughts, feelings, impulses, desires, fantasies, dreams, actions, words, and childhood experiences to gain insight into the cause of his or her unconscious introjected self-anger.

Family therapy is a general systems view of the family's dysfunctional patterns. The "identified client" is the person who is most sensitive to the spiraling anxiety resulting from the dysfunction and acts as a valve to reduce the family's anxiety by becoming symptomatic. In essence, the identified client unconsciously offers himself or herself as the scapegoat for the family's problems. Each time the family's dysfunction and anxiety increase, the client acts out symptomatically, and the rest of the family can blame their problems on the client's behavior. This pattern repeats itself ineffectively; this is called a first-order change, attempting to do more of the same to fix the problem. The goal of family therapy is to alter one part of the system so that it functions in a healthier manner; in response, the rest of the system changes. This is known as a second-order change (changing the system).

APPLICATION OF THE NURSING PROCESS: DEPRESSION

Assessment

HISTORY

Assessment data can be collected from the client and family or significant others, previous chart information, and others involved in the support or care of the client. There are many words used to describe the symptoms of depression (Box 14-2). For clients with psychomotor retardation, the assessment may require several sessions, because these clients have difficulty connecting words to make a sentence and require more time to construct and verbalize a response. People with psychomotor retardation use one-word responses to yes-or-no questions without expanding on the response. Using open-ended questions might take longer but will elicit more specific assessment data.

Assessing Suicidal Ideation. Many clients with mood disorders, because of their sense of hopelessness and helplessness, have suicidal fantasies. It is a nursing responsibility to ensure the safety of a person who cannot provide for his or her own safety. For all depressed people, it is important to assess for suicidal ideation or suicide attempts. These cues can be overt (open) or covert (hidden). **Overt cues** of suicide are clear, direct statements such as, "I want to kill myself" or "I am going to blow my brains out tonight." Others have more difficulty making such straightforward statements and may try to warn others or ask for help using indirect behaviors or messages. **Covert cues** are more subtle messages about suicide that need to be interpreted (Box 14-3). Some people who have decided on suicide may even appear happy and goal-directed because they have ended the conflicting feelings and finally made a decision. The section on suicide at the end of the chapter provides information on assessment for suicidal ideation and nursing care related to those at risk for suicide.

Assessing the Client's Perception. To assess the client's perception of what the problem is, the nurse asks about the behavioral changes that have occurred: when the changes started, what was going on in the person's life when they started, the length of time the behaviors have existed, and what the client

Box 14-2	
▶ WORDS TO DESCRIBE A DEPRESSED CLIENT	
Actions	**Thoughts and Feelings**
Aggressive	Ambivalent
Agitated	Apathetic
Angry	Anhedonistic
Antagonistic	Ambivalent
Appetite changes	Anxious
Argumentative	Apprehensive
Asocial	Bleak
Blaming	Bitter
Poor concentration	Censured
Distractable	Confused
Disinterested	Dejected
Makes disparaging	Defeated
comments	Defensive
Helpless	Denial
Hostile	Desperate
Inflexible	Despondent
Intolerant	Distressed
Irritable	Feelings of failure
Overdependent	Guilty
Poor hygiene	Hopeless, helpless
Psychomotor agitation	Inadequate
or retardation	Negativism
Reduced spontaneity	Overwhelmed
Sexual lack of interest	Poor self-esteem
Sleep changes	Sad
Speech: quiet,	Shameful
monotonous, slow	Slow, ponderous
Substance abuse	Suicidal
Suicidal ideation	Sure of failure
or actions	Somatic complaints
Tearful	
Unmotivated	
Underachiever	
Unable to make decisions	
Weary	
Worried	
Worthless	

has tried to do about the changes. The nurse must pay attention to the words the client uses to describe his or her mood and behavior.

GENERAL APPEARANCE AND MOTOR BEHAVIOR

Many depressed people look sad; sometimes they just look ill. They are dysphoric, have unpleasant feelings, and cry easily, or they may deny their feelings. Depressed people who are sad have **psychomotor retardation** (slow body movements, slow cognitive processing, and slow verbal interaction). They have

Box 14-3

► COVERT CUES OF SUICIDAL IDEATION

Client Comment	Assessment Questions to Ask
"I just want to go to sleep and not think anymore."	"Specifically just how are you planning to sleep and not think anymore?" "By 'sleep,' do you mean 'die'?" "What is it you do not want to think of anymore?"
"I want it to be all over."	"I wonder if you are thinking of suicide." "What is it you specifically want to be over?"
"It will just be the end of the story."	"Are you planning to end your life?" "How do you plan to end your story?"
"You have been a good friend." "Remember me."	"You sound as if you are saying good-bye. Are you?" "Are you planning to commit suicide?" "What is it you really want me to remember about you?"
"Here is my chess set that you have always admired." "If there is ever any need for anyone to know this, my will and insurance papers are in the top drawer of my dresser."	"What is going on that you are giving away things to remember you by?" "I appreciate your trust. However, I think there is an important message you are giving me. Are you thinking of ending your life?"
"I can't stand the pain anymore."	"How do you plan to end the pain?" "Tell me about the pain." "Sounds like you are planning to harm yourself."
"Everyone will feel bad soon." "I just can't bear it anymore."	"Who is the person you want to feel bad by killing yourself?" "What is it you cannot bear?" "How do you see an end to this?"
"Everyone would be better off without me."	"Who is one person you believe would be better off without you?" "How do you plan to eliminate yourself, if you think everyone would be better off without you?" "What is one way you perceive others would be better off without you?"
Nonverbal change in behavior from agitated to calm, anxious to relaxed, depressed to smiling, hostile to benign, from being without direction to appearing to be goal-directed	"You seem different today. What is this about?" "I sense you have reached a decision. Share it with me."

difficulty connecting their thoughts, need more time to think, and often give up in frustration before being able to complete a thought or task.

MOOD AND AFFECT

The nurse should compare the client's content (words) with his or her process (nonverbal messages). Nonverbal communications are considered more truthful and help the nurse understand the client's level of depression.

Depressed clients may describe themselves as hopeless, helpless, down, or anxious. They are easily frustrated, are angry at themselves, and can be angry at others (DSM-IV-TR, 2000). Others who are depressed are agitated, irritable, crabby, petulant, and easily enraged. Agitated depressed people are said to have **psychomotor agitation** (increased body movements and thoughts), such as pacing, accelerated thinking, and argumentativeness.

Depressed people become **asocial**, withdrawing from social interactions, family and friends, and hobbies. They become **anhedonic** or anhedonistic, losing any sense of pleasure from activities they formerly enjoyed. Typically, they sit alone, staring into space or lost in thought. When addressed, they interact minimally with a few words or a gesture. They are overwhelmed by noise and people who might make demands on them, so they withdraw from the stimulation of interaction with others.

SENSORIUM AND INTELLECTUAL PROCESSES

Concentration and decision making are so reduced that many depressed people have difficulty continuing school or work. In severe depression, the client may be unable to get out of bed or make decisions about what to eat.

JUDGMENT AND INSIGHT

Fatigue and exhaustion (anergia) are common symptoms. Depressed people feel overwhelmed when trying to accomplish even normal activities. They must use a great deal of effort to complete even the simplest task, and they take longer to complete the task.

SELF-CONCEPT

Sense of self-esteem is greatly reduced; clients often use phrases such as "good for nothing" or "just worthless" to describe themselves. They feel guilty about not being able to function and often personalize events or take responsibility for incidents over which they have no control. Depressed people **ruminate** (dwell on and worry about to excess) about past deeds and make harsh negative judgments about themselves. They develop rigid rules and set impossible, inflexible goals, ensuring guilt and anger when they fail to meet them. They believe that others would be better off without them and often contemplate suicide and make suicide attempts.

Depressed people lack energy for activities of daily living, often neglecting regular hygiene and grooming (such as bathing or hair care). Clothing may be dark, drab, and without accent colors or accessories; it may be wrinkled or soiled. Women no longer bother wearing makeup. The appearance of a depressed person reflects his or her low self-esteem and poor sense of self-worth.

ROLES AND RELATIONSHIPS

As noted above, depressed people become asocial and take no pleasure in other people or in activities they formerly enjoyed. They lose interest in sex and have reduced occupational function. They may lose weight because they have no interest in food or eating with others or because they have so little energy. However, some depressed people eat more to compensate for their feelings of emptiness. They especially like carbohydrates and can rapidly gain weight.

PHYSIOLOGIC AND SELF-CARE CONSIDERATIONS

Sleep changes are another common symptom of depression. Usually, the person complains of **middle insomnia** (waking during the night and having difficulty getting back to sleep). Some have **initial in-somnia** (difficulty falling asleep); others awaken too early (**terminal insomnia**). Some depressed people sleep too much (**hypersomnia**) (DSM-IV-TR, 2000).

DEPRESSION RATING SCALES

Some rating scales for depression are completed by the client; others are administered by a mental health professional. These assessment tools, along with evaluation of the client's behavior, thought processes, history, family history, and situational factors, help create a diagnostic picture. Self-rating scales of depressive symptoms include the Zung Self-Rating Depression Scale (Table 14-6), the Beck Depression Inventory, and PRIME-MD (Pfizer). Self-rating scales are used for case-finding in the general public but are not benchmark diagnostic tools (Boyd & Nihart, 1998).

The Hamilton Rating Scale for Depression (1960) is a clinician-rated depression scale that is used like a clinical interview. The clinician rates the range of the client's behaviors, such as depressed mood, guilt, suicide, and insomnia. There is also a section to score diurnal variations, depersonalization (sense of unreality about the self), paranoid symptoms, and obsessions.

Some health maintenance organizations require health care professionals to use a clinician-rated depression scale to diagnose depression and document changes during treatment.

Data Analysis and Planning

Assessment data are analyzed to determine priorities and establish a plan of care. Not all depressed clients have the same problems and needs. Nursing diagnoses commonly established for a depressed person include the following:

- Altered Nutrition: More Than or Less Than Body Requirements
- Anxiety
- Constipation
- Ineffective Individual Coping
- Fatigue
- Hopelessness
- Loneliness
- Powerlessness
- Altered Role Performance
- Self Care Deficit
- Self Esteem Disturbance; Chronic Low
- Sleep Pattern Disturbance: Insomnia, Hypersomnia
- Social Isolation
- Spiritual Distress
- Ineffective Management of Therapeutic Regimen

Table 14-6

ZUNG SELF-RATING DEPRESSION SCALE

Listed below are 20 statements. Please read each one carefully and decide how much of the statement describes how you have been feeling during the past week. Decide whether the statement applies to you for none or a little of the time, some of the time, a good part of the time, or most or all of the time. Mark the appropriate column for each statement.

	None or a Little	Some	Good Part	Most or All
1. I feel downhearted & blue.	1	2	3	4
2. Morning is when I feel the best.	1	2	3	4
3. I have crying spells or feel like it.	1	2	3	4
4. I have trouble sleeping at night.	1	2	3	4
5. I eat as much as I used to.	1	2	3	4
6. I still enjoy sex.	1	2	3	4
7. I notice that I am losing weight.	1	2	3	4
8. I have trouble with constipation.	1	2	3	4
9. My heart beats faster than normal.	1	2	3	4
10. I get tired for no reason.	1	2	3	4
11. My mind is as clear as it used to be.	1	2	3	4
12. I find it easy to do things I used to do.	1	2	3	4
13. I am restless and can't keep still.	1	2	3	4
14. I feel hopeful about the future.	1	2	3	4
15. I am more irritable than usual.	1	2	3	4
16. I find it easy to make decisions.	1	2	3	4
17. I feel that I am useful and needed.	1	2	3	4
18. My life is pretty full.	1	2	3	4
19. I feel that others would be better off if I were dead.	1	2	3	4
20. I still enjoy the things I used to do.	1	2	3	4

Scoring: Each question is rated on a 1–4 scale; questions worded positively are reverse scored. A total score is obtained by summing ratings for each question. The more depressed the respondent, the higher the score. Depressed clients usually have a score of greater than 60.

Zung, W. (1965). A self-rating depression scale. *Archives of General Psychiatry, 12,* 334.

Outcomes

Outcomes for a depressed person relate to the manner in which the depression is manifested—for instance, whether the person is slow or agitated, sleeps too much or too little, or eats too much or too little. Examples of outcomes for a client with the psychomotor retardation form of depression include:

1. The client will eliminate suicidal ideation and/or plans.
2. The client will increase psychomotor activity, including exercise for 10 minutes per day.
3. The client will independently carry out activities of daily living (showering, changing clothing, grooming).
4. The client will list positive attributes to demonstrate increasing self-esteem.
5. The client will socialize with staff and peers.
6. The client will return to occupation or school activities.
7. The client will comply with antidepressant regimen, with re-evaluation visits every 3 months.

8. The client will verbalize symptoms of a recurrence.

Intervention

PROVIDING FOR THE CLIENT'S AND OTHERS' SAFETY

It is a nursing responsibility to ensure the safety of clients with low self-esteem, hopelessness, and helplessness, who often contemplate suicide as a method of escaping from this distress. The nurse should ask the client directly about suicidal thoughts or plans. Contrary to a popular myth, asking about suicide does not give the person the idea of committing suicide; rather, it can give relief and comfort to the person who has had these thoughts but was afraid to tell anyone. The nurse must listen carefully and observe the client's behavior and responses for cues that he or she is not denying or trying to hide thoughts of suicide or even thoughts of harming others. Suicide and depression involve anger turned inward, but anger can also be turned outward to others in the form of assault or

> SUMMARY OF INTERVENTIONS FOR DEPRESSION

- Begin a therapeutic relationship regardless of the client's state of depression
- Ensure safety for clients with low self-esteem
- Listen closely for behavioral cues to suicidal thoughts
- Create a structured and scheduled but non-demanding environment
- Promote independence by encouraging client to perform same activities of daily living. Assist client only when he or she cannot perform them.

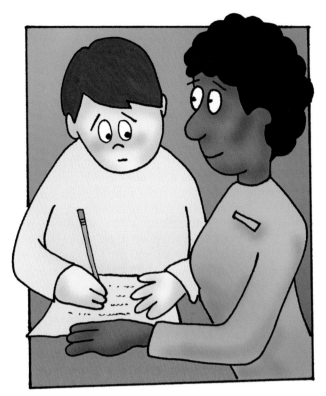

No-suicide contract

homicide, so the nurse must ask if the client plans to hurt others. More details regarding suicide and suicide assessment are presented later in the chapter.

If the client has a suicide plan, the nurse should conduct a **suicide lethality assessment**, also discussed later. Results of the suicide lethality assessment should be reported to the attending physician and treatment team. Hospital or agency policies and procedures are followed for instituting suicide precautions (for instance, removal of harmful items, increased level of supervision).

For clients who have thoughts or plans of suicide, the nurse should establish a **no-suicide contract**, a verbal or written agreement in which the client promises to notify a staff member the moment he or she has thoughts of suicide. Details are presented later in the chapter.

ORIENTING THE CLIENT TO NEW SURROUNDINGS AND STRUCTURING DAILY ACTIVITIES

Orientation to the unit and scheduled activities increases the client's security. Critical pathways provide a framework for the nursing process. Depressed people need a structured and scheduled but nondemanding environment. They need to know what is expected of them, what their day will involve, to whom they should ask questions, and how the treatment process works. They also need to know the rules, legal issues that relate to them, and a brief description of how the unit works.

For example, the nurse can advise the newly admitted client of the following, stopping after each sentence to assess his or her understanding:

"You have been admitted because you are depressed and intended to kill yourself with 30 sleeping tablets that were in your possession. The staff and I will help you stay safe.

Your shoelaces, belt, razor, and other implements that you can use to harm yourself have been taken

away from you and will be returned when you can have them and be safe.

You will meet with your treatment team daily between 9 and 10 AM.

The treatment team consists of the psychiatrist, clinical nurse specialist, social worker, unit nurse, dietitian, occupational therapist, and you.

You will attend a variety of group sessions each morning and afternoon, and one each evening. Visiting hours are from 6 to 8 PM.

Here is a schedule of the daily sessions as well as your copy of the Patient's Bill of Rights for this state. I will be available to answer any questions you have or to read the schedule and rights to you if you would prefer."

PROMOTING A THERAPEUTIC RELATIONSHIP

It is important to have meaningful contact with the depressed client and to begin a therapeutic relationship, regardless of the client's state of depression. Some depressed people are quite open in describing their feelings of sadness, hopelessness, helplessness, or agitation. Depressed people may be unable to sustain a long interaction, so making several shorter visits with the client during each shift helps the nurse to assess the client's status and to establish a therapeutic relationship.

The nurse may find it difficult to interact with a depressed client because he or she empathizes with the client's sadness and depression. To protect himself or herself, the nurse may unconsciously avoid interacting with the depressed client. To avoid this unconscious rejection, the nurse should schedule contacts with the client. Empathized depressed feelings can be relieved by talking to a peer about the relationship with the client as well as the client's treatment plan.

An asocial client with psychomotor retardation (slow speech, slow movement, slow thought processes) may become mute. The nurse should sit beside the client for a few minutes, making occasional remarks. For example:

"Hello, Jonas. I am Barbara, your nurse. I have a few minutes to sit with you. (Pause) The sky is pretty today, but I think we are in for a storm in the next hour."

"Margaret, I have come to spend the next 5 minutes with you before I go to lunch."

Before leaving, tell the client you appreciated sitting with him or her, and the time of your next visit: *"I have enjoyed sitting with you. I will see you around 2:45 PM, when I'll have a few free minutes again."* This can establish a sense of caring and trust, which is essential to the therapeutic relationship.

PROMOTING INDEPENDENCE IN ACTIVITIES OF DAILY LIVING

The ability to perform daily activities is related to the client's level of psychomotor retardation. These levels can change each shift as well as with each event. Encouraging a client to do as much of each task as possible will reduce inappropriate dependence on staff.

To assess the client's ability to perform activities of daily living independently, the nurse should first ask the client to perform the global task. For example:

"Martin, it is time to get dressed. Put on your clothes." (global task)

If client cannot respond to the global request, the task is broken down into smaller segments. For example: *"Martin, choose between your gray or your blue slacks and put on one pair."* The client must still expend some effort to make a choice. The client's reaction helps the nurse assess his or her psychomotor skill, ambivalence, and ability to respond to a concrete message. A depressed person can become easily overwhelmed with a task that has several steps. Success in small, concrete steps can be used as a basis for increasing self-esteem and will build competency for a slightly more complex task the next time.

If the client cannot choose between articles of clothing, the nurse should select a pair of slacks and direct the client to put them on. For example: *"Here are your gray slacks. Put them on."* This still allows the client to participate in dressing. If this is what he is capable of doing at this point in time, this activity

will reduce his dependence on the staff. This is a concrete request, and if the client cannot do this, this gives the nurse information regarding his level of psychomotor retardation.

If the client cannot put his slacks on, the nurse should assist him by saying, *"Let me help you with your slacks, Martin."* The nurse should help the client to dress only when he cannot carry out any of the above steps. This allows the client to do as much as possible for himself and to avoid making dependence on the staff a permanent behavior. The same process can be carried out for eating, taking a shower, and performing routine self-care activities.

Because the client's abilities can quickly change from day to day and even hour to hour, they must be assessed on an ongoing basis. The reason for going through this slow process and assessing the client's abilities each time is related to differences in the speed at which antidepressants take effect; SSRIs and atypical antidepressants have a more rapid onset. This continual assessment takes more time than it would simply to help the client to dress, but it promotes the client's independence and provides dynamic assessment data about the client's psychomotor abilities. Staff members who resist participating in this process should evaluate their own need to have the client remain dependent.

MEDICATION MANAGEMENT

The increased activity and improved mood produced by antidepressants can provide the energy for a suicidal person to carry out the act; thus, suicide risk must be assessed even when the client is receiving an antidepressant.

SSRIs. Serotonin syndrome is a life-threatening problem that occurs when an SSRI interacts with an MAOI (Box 14-4) (Schatzberg & Nemeroff, 1998).

TCAs and Heterocyclics. The common side effects of drowsiness and dizziness can be a problem with TCAs. TCAs can be taken at bedtime to help the person sleep, to maintain daytime productivity, and to avoid dizziness. If gastrointestinal irritation occurs, TCAs can be taken after eating. TCAs decrease the efficacy of antihypertensives; lower the seizure threshold; increase central nervous system depression if taken concurrently with hypnotics, barbiturates, or sedatives; can alter the effects of oral anticoagulants; and can create delirium if given with levodopa. The elderly are at risk for toxicity from TCAs and heterocyclics because they metabolize them more slowly. Cimetidine can increase the plasma levels of these drugs.

Dry mouth, sedation, constipation, and urinary hesitancy may occur; the nurse should monitor input and output and bowel habits. Because of possible

A washout period of at least 3 weeks is necessary between ending one drug and starting another.

MAOIs. Common side effects are dizziness, nausea, vomiting, dry mouth, insomnia, urinary hesitancy, orthostatic hypotension, constipation, weakness, myoclonic jerks, and appetite and weight loss. "Histamine headaches" can occur, usually along with hypotension, diarrhea, salivation, abdominal cramps, and lacrimation. Later in treatment there can be weight gain, carbohydrate craving, sexual performance difficulties, hypoglycemia, cramps, disorientation, peripheral neuropathy, and edema. MAOIs must never be given concurrently with any other category of antidepressant drugs because of the risk of serotonin syndrome. MAOIs can also elevate liver function test results.

Because of the potentially life-threatening effects of hypertensive crisis and serotonin syndrome, clients receiving MAOIs must be able and willing to follow a strict dietary regimen. The client and family should be instructed about which foods have high, medium, or low levels of tyramine and given a list of foods and fluids to avoid and those that should be taken cautiously (Box 14-5). Clients also need to know the symptoms of hypertensive crisis and serotonin syndrome, and emergency measures to take if these occur (withhold the next dose and call the physician). Hypertensive crisis is treated with intravenous phentolamine or the calcium channel blocker nifedipine (given orally); the client can carry the latter for use

orthostatic hypotension, the client should change position and arise slowly.

These drugs can increase intraocular pressure in glaucoma, cause urinary retention in benign prostatic hypertrophy, and produce hyperpyrexia. They should not be abruptly discontinued unless ordered by a physician or an advanced practice nurse.

These drugs should never be administered with MAOIs because they have a highly synergistic effect.

Box 14-4

► SEROTONIN SYNDROME

Serotonin syndrome occurs when there is an inadequate washout period between taking MAOIs and SSRIs or when MAOIs are combined with meperidine. Symptoms of serotonin syndrome include:

- Change in mental state: confusion, agitation
- Neuromuscular excitement: muscle rigidity, weakness, sluggish pupils, shivering, tremors, myoclonic jerks, collapse, muscle paralysis
- Autonomic abnormalities: hyperthermia, tachycardia, tachypnea, hypersalivation, diaphoresis

Adapted from Black, K., Shea, C., Dursun, S., & Kutcher, S. (2000). Selective serotonin reuptake inhibitor discontinuation syndrome: Proposed diagnostic criteria. Journal of Psychiatry and Neuroscience, 25(3), 256–261.

Box 14-5

► DIET CONSIDERATIONS FOR CLIENTS TAKING MAOIs

- To avoid hypertensive crisis, all clients taking MAOIs must avoid foods containing high levels of tyramine.
- Long-term storage of certain foods can increase tyramine levels.
- Tyramine content can vary by brand or batch.

Foods to Eliminate	Cautious Use
Aged cheeses: bleu, Roquefort, Camembert, Brie, cheddar	All other cheeses
Stored long: dairy products	
Processed meats: salami, sausage, pastrami, meat extract, protein supplements	Fresh meats, liver, herring
Processed fish & shrimp paste	
Processed soybean products (tofu, soy sauce)	Raspberries, bananas
Processed: anchovies, pineapple	
Stored long: spinach, nuts, avocado, vinegar, raisins, tomato juice, mushrooms, cucumbers, boiled eggs, wild game, Worcestershire sauce, bread	
Beer, nonalcoholic beer, wine, whiskey, liqueurs	
Yeast products, ginseng	MSG
Soups (esp. miso)	Pizza
Sauerkraut	Caffeine
Stored long: salad dressings	

Adapted from Merriman, S. H. (1999). Monoamine oxidase drugs and diet. Journal of Human Nutrition and Dietetics, 12(1), 21–28.

in emergency situations. Clients also must tell all physicians and dentists who treat them that they are taking an MAOI.

Atypical Antidepressants. This class of antidepressants is well tolerated and less toxic than TCAs, heterocyclics, and MAOIs. It includes venlafaxine, bupropion, and nefazodone.

PROVIDING CLIENT AND FAMILY TEACHING

The client and family must learn how to manage the medication regimen, because the client may need to take these medications for months, years, or even a lifetime. Education promotes compliance. The client should know how often he or she needs to return for monitoring and diagnostic tests.

The client and family should know that treatment outcomes are best when psychotherapy and antidepressants are used in combination. Psychotherapy helps the client explore issues of anger, dependence, guilt, hopelessness, helplessness, object loss, interpersonal issues, and irrational beliefs. The goal is to reverse the client's negative view of the future, improve his or her self-image, and help him or her gain competence and self-mastery.

The nurse can help the client find a psychotherapist through mental health centers that serve the client's residential area. Many mental health centers have sliding payment scales. Mental health centers are listed in the telephone book as well as in information brochures published by county information offices. Directories of advanced practice psychiatric nurses, psychiatrists, psychologists, and psychiatric social workers are available by calling the state organization of each of these disciplines. Because the best outcome involves both psychotherapy and antidepressants, the nurse can help the person find someone who combines both treatment modalities, such as an advanced practice psychiatric nurse or a psychiatrist. Psychologists and psychiatric social workers usually have a cooperative agreement with a psychiatrist to manage their clients' medications.

▶ **CLIENT AND FAMILY TEACHING FOR DEPRESSION**

- Instruct client and family about the action of the prescribed medications.
- Instruct client and family about the side effects of the prescribed medications.
- Instruct client and family about the interactions with other drugs or foods.
- Teach client and family about the importance of keeping appointments for psychotherapy.

Evaluation

A discharge plan is developed that makes use of family and community resources. This includes thorough client and family education about the medication regimen. A person who understands and has had the opportunity to participate in writing his or her treatment plan is more likely to be compliant. The client may be able to remain in the community by using outpatient visits for psychotherapy and medication management, partial hospitalization, or home visits by psychiatric nurses. The client and family should be aware of the criteria for discharge and readmission and should know how to get help assessing the need for readmission. Case managers work with the client and staff to assess, develop, and implement this aspect of care for the person.

BIPOLAR DISORDER

Bipolar disorder I is the label applied to the cyclic mood changes demonstrated by a person who has manic episodes (one pole), periods of profound depression (the second pole), and periods of normal behavior between the two (DSM-IV-TR, 2000). Bipolar disorder was formerly known as manic-depressive illness. During mania, the person is euphoric, grandiose, energetic, and sleepless and has poor judgment and rapid thoughts, actions, and speech.

Whereas a person with unipolar depression has a slow slide into depression that can last for 6 months to 2 years, the person with bipolar disorder cycles between states of depression and normal behavior (bipolar depressed) or mania and normal behavior (bipolar manic), or can run the gamut from mania to normal behavior to depression and back again in repeated cycles (bipolar mixed episodes). Bipolar depression has the same symptoms as unipolar depression, except that the depressive episodes cycle over a period of months and alternate with normal behavior or normal and manic behavior. A person with bipolar mixed episodes alternates between major depressive episodes and manic episodes, but with periods of normal behavior interspersed. Each mood lasts for months before the pattern begins to descend or ascend once again. Figure 14-2 compares unipolar and bipolar disorders, showing the three categories of bipolar cycles.

Bipolar disorder occurs almost equally among men and women. It is more common in highly educated people (Charney & Weissman, 1988). Although sometimes starting in adolescence or after age 50, mania often starts earlier than age 19, when in the space of a few days symptoms escalate, last a few weeks to a few months, and can end just as suddenly as they began.

(text continues on page 354)

NURSING CARE PLAN: DEPRESSION

Nursing Diagnosis

> ### Ineffective Individual Coping
The state in which an individual demonstrates an impairment in adaptive behaviors and problem-solving abilities in meeting life's demands and roles

ASSESSMENT DATA

- Suicidal ideas or behavior
- Slowed mental processes
- Disordered thoughts
- Feelings of despair, hopelessness, and worthlessness
- Guilt
- Anhedonia (inability to experience pleasure)
- Generalized restlessness or agitation
- Sleep disturbances: early awakening, insomnia, or excessive sleeping
- Anger or hostility (may not be overt)
- Rumination
- Sexual dysfunction: diminished interest in sexual activity, inability to experience pleasure
- Fear of intensity of feelings
- Anxiety

EXPECTED OUTCOMES

The client will:
- Be free of self-inflicted harm
- Engage in reality-based interactions
- Express feelings directly with congruent verbal and nonverbal messages
- Express anger or hostility outwardly in a safe manner
- Demonstrate functional level of psychomotor activity
- Demonstrate compliance with and knowledge of medications, if any
- Demonstrate an increased ability to cope with anxiety, stress, or frustration
- Identify a support system in the community

IMPLEMENTATION

Nursing Interventions	Rationale
Provide a safe environment for the client.	Physical safety of the client is a priority. Many common items and environmental situations may be used by the client in a self-destructive manner.
Continually assess the client's potential for suicide.	Depressed clients may have a potential for suicide that may or may not be expressed and that may change with time. You must remain aware of this suicide potential at all times.
Observe the client closely, especially under the following circumstances:	You must be aware of the client's activities at all times when there is a potential for suicide or self-injury:

continued on page 352

continued from page 351

After antidepressant medication begins to raise the client's mood	Risk of suicide increases as the client's energy level is increased by medication.
After any sudden dramatic behavioral change (sudden cheerfulness, relief, freedom from guilt, or giving away personal belongings)	These changes may indicate that the client has come to a decision to commit suicide.
Unstructured time on the unit	Risk of suicide increase when the client's time is unstructured.
Times when the number of staff on the unit is limited	Risk of suicide increases when observation of the client decreases.
Spend time with the client.	Your physical presence is reality.
If the client is ruminating, tell him or her that you will talk about reality or about the client's feelings, but limit the attention given to repeated expressions of rumination.	Minimizing attention and reinforcement may help decrease rumination. Providing reinforcement for reality orientation and expression of feelings will encourage these behaviors.
Initially, assign the same staff members to work with the client whenever possible.	The client's ability to respond to others may be impaired. Limiting the number of new contacts initially will facilitate familiarity and trust. However, the number of people interacting with the client should increase as soon as possible to minimize dependency and to facilitate the client's abilities to communicate with a variety of people.
When approaching the client, use a moderate, level tone of voice. Avoid being overly cheerful.	Being overly cheerful may indicate to the client that other feelings are not acceptable—that being cheerful is the goal or the norm.
Use silence and active listening when interacting with the client. Let the client know that you are concerned and that you consider the client a worthwhile person.	Your presence and use of active listening will communicate your interest and concern. The client may not communicate if you are talking too much. Your silence will convey your expectation that the client will communicate and your acceptance of the client's difficulty with communication.
When first communicating with the client, use simple, direct sentences; avoid complex sentences or directions.	The client's ability to perceive and respond to complex stimuli is impaired.
Avoid asking the client many questions, especially questions that require only brief answers.	Asking questions and requiring only brief answers may discourage the client from communicating or taking responsibility for expressing his or her feelings.

continued on page 353

continued from page 352

Be comfortable sitting with the client in silence. Let the client know you are available to converse, but don't require the client to talk.

Your presence and use of active listening will indicate your interest and concern. Your silence will convey your expectation that the client will communicate and your acceptance of the client's difficulty with communication.

Allow (and encourage) the client to cry. Stay with and support the client if he or she desires. Provide privacy if the client desires and it is safe to do so.

Crying is a healthy way of expressing feelings of sadness, hopelessness, and despair. The client may not feel comfortable crying and may need encouragement or privacy.

Do not cut off interactions with cheerful remarks or platitudes (for example, "No one really wants to die," "Of course life is worth living," or "You'll feel better soon."). Do not belittle the client's feelings. Accept the client's verbalizations of feelings as real, and give support for this ventilation of feelings, especially for expressions of emotions that may be difficult for the client to accept in himself or herself (like anger).

You may be uncomfortable with certain feelings the client expresses. If this is true, it is important for you to recognize this and discuss it with another staff member rather than directly or indirectly communicating your discomfort to the client. Proclaiming the client's feelings to be inappropriate or wrong or otherwise belittling them is detrimental.

Encourage the client to ventilate feelings in whatever way is comfortable—verbal and nonverbal. Let the client know you will listen and accept what is being expressed.

Ventilation of feelings may help relieve feelings of despair, hopelessness, sadness, and so forth. Feelings are not inherently good or bad. You must remain nonjudgmental about the client's feelings and directly express this to the client.

Interact with the client on topics with which he or she is comfortable. Do not probe for information.

Topics that are uncomfortable for the client and probing may be threatening and initially may discourage communication. When trust has been established, the client may be encouraged to discuss more difficult topics.

Teach the client about the problem-solving process: explore possible options, examine the consequences of each alternative, select and implement an alternative, and evaluate the results.

The client may be unaware of a systemic method for solving problems. Successful use of the problem-solving process facilitates the client's confidence in the use of coping skills.

Provide positive feedback at each step of the process. If the client is not satisfied with the chosen alternative, assist the client to select another alternative.

Positive feedback at each step will give the client many opportunities for success and encourage him or her to persist in problem-solving, as well as enhance the client's confidence. The client also can learn to "survive" making a mistake.

Adapted from *Schultz, J. M., & Videbeck, S. L. (1998).* Lippincott's manual of psychiatric nursing care plans *(5th ed.).* Philadelphia: Lippincott-Raven.

CLINICAL VIGNETTE: MANIC EPISODE

"Everyone is stupid! What is the matter? Have you all taken dumb pills? Dumb pills, rum pills, shlummy shlum lum pills!" Mitch screamed as he waited for his staff to snap to attention and get with the program. He had started the "Pickle Barn" 10 years ago and now had a money-making business canning and delivering gourmet pickles.

He knew how to do everything in this place and, running from person to person to watch what each was doing, he didn't like what he saw. It was 8 A.M., and he'd already fired the supervisor, who had been with him for 5 years.

By 8:02 A.M., Mitch had fired six pickle assistants because he did not like the way they looked. Mitch threw pots and paddles at the assistants because they weren't leaving fast enough. Rich, his brother, walked in during this melee and quietly asked everyone to stay, then invited Mitch outside for a walk.

"Are you nuts?" Mitch screamed at his brother. "Everyone here is out of control. I have to do everything." Mitch was trembling, shaking. He hadn't slept in 3 days and didn't need it. The only time he'd left the building in these 3 days was to have sex with any woman who had agreed. He felt euphoric, supreme, able to leap tall buildings in a single bound. He glared at Rich. "I feel good! What are you bugging me for?" He slammed out the door, shrilly reciting, "Rich and Mitch! Rich and Mitch! Pickle king rich!"

Mitch had been stable 10 years ago, when Rich had invested his life savings with Mitch to help buy two tractor-trailers and the large building that housed the pickle barn. Their aunt Jen, who was more like their mother, had then sunk her savings into the business and

building. After one of Mitch's earlier manic episodes, she had taken over the bookkeeping and sales operations and was responsible for expanding their routes to a profitable multistate operation. "Rich and Mitch, Rich and Mitch. With dear old auntie, now we're rich." Mitch couldn't stop talking and speed-walking. Watching Mitch, Rich gently said, "Aunt Jen called me last night. She says you are manic again. When did you stop taking your lithium?"

"Manic? Who's manic? I'm just feeling good. Who needs that stuff? I like to feel good. It is wonderful, marvelous, stupendous. I am not manic," shrieked Mitch as he swerved around to face his brother. Rich, weary and sad, said, "I am taking you to the emergency psych unit. If you do not agree to go, I will have the police take you. I know you don't see this in yourself, but you are out of control and getting dangerous."

Mitch's bipolar disorder had been controlled for years, but Mitch had stopped taking his lithium, stopped seeing the therapist, and stopped being normal. This was the third time in the past year and the sixth time in 3 years Mitch had gone into an acute manic episode, so these episodes were escalating.

Each time Mitch went back on lithium and promised this time he'd stay in treatment, but it seemed to take longer and longer for him to recover and he was never back to the old Mitch. Yesterday Aunt Jen discovered Mitch had ordered another tractor-trailer, placed a "deposit" on a 35-acre estate in Hawaii, and ordered a Jaguar.

Mitch is the real victim of this illness; however, it gets harder and harder for everyone whose life he touches to remember this, since their lives have also been seriously disrupted by Mitch's bipolar disorder.

About a generation ago, the median age of bipolar disorder onset was 32 years. One theory about the declining age of bipolar onset may be related to the cohort effects of cocaine abuse by teenagers (Pliszka et al., 2000). Adolescents are more likely to have psychotic manifestations. Pliszka et al. marked the 1-year prevalence rate of bipolar illness at close to 2%, because half of persons with bipolar illness deny their mania.

Onset and Clinical Course

The diagnosis of a manic episode or mania requires an episode of unusual and incessantly heightened, grandiose, or agitated mood of at least 1 week's duration that includes three or more of the following symptoms: exaggerated self-esteem; sleeplessness; pressured speech; flight of ideas; reduced ability to filter out extraneous stimuli; distractibility; increased number of activities with increased energy; and mul-

tiple, grandiose high-risk activities involving poor judgment with severe consequences, such as going on spending sprees, having sex with strangers, or making impulsive investments.

Clients do not understand how their illness affects others. They often stop taking antimanic drugs because they like the euphoria and feel burdened by the side effects, blood tests, and physician's visits needed to maintain treatment. Family members are concerned and exhausted by their loved one's behavior, often staying up late at night for fear the manic person may do something impulsive and dangerous.

Although manic people prefer to be euphoric and hyperactive, they experience great emotional distress. Those with bipolar disorder are victims of a pervasive illness that affects their life and those of their families forever. The nurse is the health care professional who spends the most time with clients with bipolar illness

UNIPOLAR DISORDER'S GRADUAL DESCENT INTO AND BACK FROM DEPRESSION

CAN LAST 6 TO 24 MONTHS

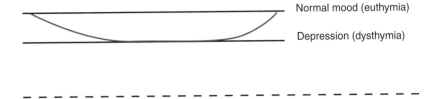

GRAPHIC REPRESENTATION OF CYCLES OF BIPOLAR DISORDER

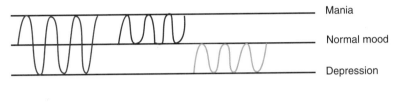

1. Bipolar
   mixed
   or cyclic

2. Bipolar
   manic

3. Bipolar
   depressed

1. Bipolar disorder mixed or cyclic = cycles alternate between periods of depression, back to normal behavior (euthymia) then to mania.

2. Bipolar manic = cycle only alternates between mania and normal (euthymic) behavior.

3. Bipolar depressed = cycle alternates between depression and normal (euthymic) behavior.

Figure 14-2. Unipolar and bipolar disorder timelines

and thus can have the greatest influence on helping them to be compliant with treatment.

Related Disorders

Other disorders that share symptoms with bipolar mood disorders are those related to the use of psychoactive substances, or manic episodes from the ectopic secretion or stimulation of hormones or neurotransmitters from tumors. Endocrine diseases such as hyperthyroidism can produce manic-like psychomotor activity. Agitation and irritability that accompany depression must be evaluated over time to differentiate this from a manic episode.

Treatment and Prognosis

Treatment for bipolar disorder involves a lifetime regimen of bipolar medications, often called antimanic medications, and adherence to the treatment regimen. Psychotherapy is useful in the mildly depressive or the normal portion of the bipolar cycle. It is not useful during acute manic stages, because the person's attention span is brief and little insight can be gained during times of accelerated psychomotor activity (Bouchard, 1999). Psychotherapy in combination with medication can reduce the risk of suicide and injury, provide a source of support to the client and family, and help the client accept the diagnosis and treatment plan (Miklowitz, 1996).

Two major categories of medications are used in bipolar disorder: lithium and anticonvulsants. This

▶ MAJOR SYMPTOMS OF MANIA

• Heightened, grandiose, or agitated mood
• Exaggerated self-esteem
• Sleeplessness
• Pressured speech
• Flight of ideas
• Reduced ability to filter out extraneous stimuli; easily distractible
• Increased number of activities, with increased energy
• Multiple, grandiose high-risk activities, using poor judgment, with severe consequences.

is the only psychiatric disorder in which medications can prevent acute cycles of bipolar behavior. Once thought to help reduce manic behavior only, lithium and these anticonvulsants also protect the person from the effects of bipolar depressive cycles. If a client in the acute stage of mania or depression exhibits psychosis (disordered thinking, as seen in delusions, hallucinations, and illusions), an antipsychotic agent is administered in addition to the bipolar medications. Some clients keep taking both bipolar medications and antipsychotics.

LITHIUM

Lithium is an element, a salt that is contained in the human body, similar to gold, copper, magnesium, manganese, and other trace elements. Once believed to be helpful for bipolar mania only, it was quickly realized that lithium could also partially or completely mute the cycling toward bipolar depression. There is a 70% to 80% response rate in acute mania to lithium therapy. In addition to treating the range of bipolar behaviors, lithium can also stabilize bipolar disorder by reducing the degree and frequency of cycling or eliminating the bipolar behavior (Gold, 1995; Schatzberg & Nemeroff, 1998).

Lithium not only competes for salt receptor sites but also affects calcium, potassium, and magnesium ions, as well as glucose metabolism. Its mechanism of action is unknown, but it is thought to work in the synapse to hasten the destruction of catecholamines (dopamine, norepinephrine), inhibit neurotransmitter release, and decrease the sensitivity of postsynaptic receptors (McEvoy, 2000).

Lithium's action peaks in 30 minutes to 4 hours for regular forms and 4 to 6 hours for the slow-release form (Table 14-7). It crosses the blood–brain barrier and the placenta and is distributed in sweat and breast milk; use is not recommended during pregnancy, because first-trimester developmental abnormalities can occur. The onset of action is 5 to 14 days; with this lag period, antipsychotic agents are carefully used in combination with lithium to reduce symptoms in the acutely manic or acutely depressed client. The half-life of lithium is 20 to 27 hours (McEvoy, 2000).

ANTICONVULSANT DRUGS

Lithium is effective in about 75% of people with bipolar illness. The rest do not respond to lithium treatment or have difficulty taking lithium because of the side effects, problems with the treatment regimen, drug interactions, or medical conditions that contraindicate the use of lithium. Several anticonvulsants traditionally used to treat seizure disorders have proven helpful in stabilizing the moods of persons with bipolar illness. These anticonvulsants are categorized as miscellaneous anticonvulsants. Initially, it was assumed the reason they were effective in bipolar disorder was because anticonvulsants may have

Table 14-7

SYMPTOMS AND INTERVENTIONS OF LITHIUM TOXICITY

Serum Lithium Level	Symptoms of Lithium Toxicity	Treatment
1.5 – 2 mEq/L	Nausea and vomiting, diarrhea, reduction coordination, drowsiness, slurred speech, muscle weakness	Withhold next dose; call physician. Serum lithium levels are ordered and doses of lithium are usually suspended for a few days, or the dose is reduced.
2 – 3 mEq/L	Ataxia, agitation, blurred vision, tinnitus, giddiness, choreoathetoid movements, confusion, muscle fasciculation, hyperreflexia, hypertonic muscles, myoclonic twitches, pruritus, maculopapular rash, movement of limbs, slurred speech, large output of dilute urine, incontinence of bladder of bowel, vertigo	Withhold future doses, call physician, stat serum lithium level. Gastric lavage may be used to remove oral lithium; IV containing saline and electrolytes used to ensure fluid and electrolyte function and maintain renal function.
3.0 – 7.0 mEq/L	Cardiac arrhythmia, hypotension, peripheral vascular collapse, focal or generalized seizures, reduced levels of consciousness from stupor to coma, myoclonic jerks of muscle groups, and spasticity of muscles	All of preceding interventions, plus lithium ion excretion, is augmented with use of aminophylline, mannitol, or urea. Hemodialysis may also be used to remove lithium from the body. Respiratory, circulatory, thyroid, and immune systems are monitored and assisted as needed.

Schatzberg, A. F., & Nemeroff, C. B. (1998). *Textbook of Psychopharmacology,* 2nd ed. Washington, DC: APA;
Wilson, B. A., Shannon, M. T., & Stang, C. L. (1999). *Nurses' drug guide.* Stanford, Conn.: Appleton & Lange.

different actions, similar to the way that diphen-hydramine (Benadryl) works both as an antihistamine to treat allergies and an anticholinergic to treat the extrapyramidal effects of typical antipsychotics (Gold, 1995).

Gold (1995) reported on a National Institute of Health study about the symptoms shared by persons with bipolar disorder and complex partial seizures, including "illusions of significance, jumbled thoughts, altered perceptions of sound and odor intensity, hallucinations of hearing and smell, periods of amnesia, visual distortions of shape and distance, feelings of detachment from the environment, and others." The researchers concluded there may be similarities in the electrical physiology of certain areas of the brain that are delicately altered in both conditions.

Carbamazepine (Tegretol), which had been used for grand mal and temporal lobe epilepsy as well as trigeminal neuralgia, was the first anticonvulsant found to have mood-stabilizing properties, but the threat of agranulocytosis was of great concern. Carbamazepine, chemically similar to the TCAs, has antimanic, antidiuretic, anticholinergic, antiarrhythmic, and antipsychotic effects in addition to its anticonvulsant and antineuralgic ones (McEvoy 2000). Clients taking carbamazepine need to have serum levels of the drug checked regularly to monitor for toxicity and to determine whether the drug has reached therapeutic levels in the serum. Dosage can be titrated by symptoms, especially with the elderly. Baseline and periodic blood counts must also be done to monitor for suppression of blood cells.

Valproic acid (Depakote), also known as divalproex sodium or sodium valproate, is an anticonvulsant used for simple absence and mixed seizures, migraine prophylaxis, and mania. The mechanism of action is unclear. Therapeutic levels are monitored periodically, as are baseline and ongoing periodic liver function tests, including serum ammonia levels and platelet and bleeding times (PDR Nurse's Handbook, 1999).

Clonazepam (Klonopin) is an anticonvulsant and a benzodiazepine (a schedule IV controlled substance) used in simple absence and minor motor seizures, panic disorder, and bipolar disorder. Physiologic dependence can develop with long-term use. A complete blood count with platelets and liver function baseline and periodic tests are required. This drug should be withdrawn slowly during a period of days to weeks to avoid withdrawal symptoms of abdominal and muscle cramps, nausea, vomiting, sweating, tremor, convulsions, or status epilepticus. Symptoms of overdose are drowsiness, somnolence, confusion, irritability, sweating, muscle or abdominal cramps, diminished reflexes, and coma (McEvoy, 2000).

APPLICATION OF THE NURSING PROCESS: BIPOLAR DISORDER

Assessment

HISTORY

Taking a history with a client in the manic phase often proves difficult. The client may jump from subject to subject, making it difficult for the nurse to follow. However, a great deal of information can be gleaned by watching and listening.

GENERAL APPEARANCE AND MOTOR BEHAVIOR

A person in the manic phase is drawn to brightly colored clothing , flashy jewelry, and risky ventures. A woman may wear highly exaggerated makeup, colorful, provocative clothing, and excessive jewelry and hair decorations.

The manic client experiences psychomotor agitation and seems to be in perpetual motion; sitting still is difficult. This continual movement has many ramifications: the person can become exhausted, injury is common and often goes ignored by the client, and the client is too busy to eat or drink, resulting in weight loss and dehydration. Sleep patterns are so disturbed that the person can stay awake for 3 days and feel energetic after only a few hours of sleep (DSM-IV-TR, 2000).

In the manic phase, the person's clothes reflect his or her elevated mood: clothing is brightly colored, flamboyant, attention-getting, and perhaps sexually suggestive. For example, a woman in the manic phase may wear a red-and-yellow flared skirt that swirls around her as she moves and twirls around people. She wears lots of jewelry and hair ornaments; she has even borrowed jewelry and clothing from others until she felt adequately adorned. Her make-up is garish and heavy, with vivid eye shadow, lots of bright lipstick, heavily rouged cheeks, and exaggerated eyeliner. She postures, poses, checks herself in the mirror, and talks to everyone. Female clients often behave seductively, such as "forgetting" to wear underpants and spinning around in a skirt so others will notice.

MOOD AND AFFECT

The person in a manic episode thinks, moves, and talks fast. **Pressured speech**, one of the hallmark symptoms, means unrelentingly rapid and often loud speech, without pauses. A person with pressured speech cannot listen to others and interrupts others. The person ignores verbal and nonverbal cues indicating that others wish to speak and continues with a constant stream of intelligible or unintelligible speech, turning from one listener to another or speaking to no one at all. If interrupted by someone, the manic person often starts over from the beginning. Rapid speech, with rhyming, circumstantiality, and tangential thoughts, is also seen in mania (Box 14-6). Mania is reflected in periods of euphoria, exuberant activity, grandiosity, impulsivity, sleeplessness, and forgetting to eat or stay safe.

THOUGHT PROCESS AND CONTENT

The person's cognitive ability or thinking is confused and jumbled, with thoughts racing one after another, often referred to as **flight of ideas**. The client cannot make connections between concepts and jumps from one subject to another.

Many projects are started at a time, but the manic person cannot carry any to completion. There is little true planning, but the person talks nonstop about plans and projects to anyone and everyone, insisting on the importance of accomplishing these activities. Sometimes he or she tries to enlist the help of someone in one or more of the activities. Risks are not considered, nor are the person's experience, abilities, or resources. These activities are started as they occur in the client's thought processes. At this point, the client may lose his or her job.

Examples of these multiple activities are going on shopping sprees, using credit cards excessively while unemployed and broke, starting several business ventures at once, having promiscuous sex, gambling, taking impulsive trips, embarking on illegal endeavors, making risky investments, talking with multiple people, and speeding (DSM-IV-TR, 2000).

SENSORIUM AND INTELLECTUAL PROCESSES

Clients with mania act out their elation using a variety of attention-getting mechanisms, such as a loud voice, boisterousness, and sexual provocativeness. They butt into everyone else's business, start multiple projects at once, and act omniscient (all-knowing) (Box 14-7). Intellectual functioning is difficult to assess during the manic phase.

JUDGMENT AND INSIGHT

Persons in the manic phase are easily angered and irritated and strike back at what they perceive as censorship by others, because they impose no restrictions on themselves (Fieve, 1995). Their judgment is poor and insight is limited. They believe they are "fine" and have no problems.

SELF-CONCEPT

The manic client often has an elevated sense of self-esteem, believing he or she can accomplish anything. However, this false sense of well-being covers chronic low self-esteem difficulties.

ROLES AND RELATIONSHIPS

Manic people have a great need to socialize but little understanding of their excessive, overpowering, and confrontational social interactions. This need for socialization often winds up in promiscuity. Manic behavior can be acute (with psychotic features of delusions and hallucinations), moderate (demonstrating manic behaviors, but within the bounds of reality), and mild or hypomanic.

The client invades the intimate space and personal business of others. Arguments result when others feel threatened by this boundary invasion. Although the usual mood of the manic person is elation, emotions are unstable and can fluctuate (**labile emotions**) readily between euphoria and hostility. The manic client can become hostile to others, who are perceived to be preventing the manic person from reaching a desired goal. For example, a manic client tells his wife, "You are the most wonderful woman in the world. Give me $50 so I can buy you a ticket to the opera." When she refuses, he snarls and accuses

---

Box 14-6

> ## UNUSUAL SPEECH PATTERNS OF MANIA

Pressured speech: Rapid and accelerated speech, talking very fast without pauses between words and sentences; not listening to anyone else; interrupting others if they try to answer or talk

Flight of ideas: Continuous, rapid, pressured verbalization of many unassociated topics

Rhyming: Use of words, phrases, or sentences that have similar sounds: "I am the man, who is like Dan, the man who can."

Circumstantiality: Use of repetitive, irrelevant descriptions when trying to describe an event, including irrelevant or unrelated actions, thoughts, people involved, places, feelings, needs, and projected reasons

Loose associations: Talking about a number of topics that appear scattered but seem to have some connection to one another

Tangentiality: Describing a situation, losing the train of thought, and jumping to a new unrelated topic; no thoughts or descriptions are completed; constant changing to new topics

Box 14-7

➤ WORDS USED TO DESCRIBE MANIC CLIENT

Actions	Thoughts	Feelings
Acts out thoughts and feelings	Delusions	Amorous
Agitated	Denial	Angered by perceived or real
Aggressive	Disorganized	censure or limits
Argumentative	Distractible	Easily hurt and defensive
Attention-seeking	Fantasies	Elated
Bizarre behaviors and appearance	Flight of ideas	Euphoric
Demanding	Grandiose	Expansive mood
Domineering	Illusions	Grandiose
Dresses in provocative, attention-getting	Irrelevant	Guiltless
attire	Irresponsible	Hedonistic
Eats/drinks little	Jumbled	Hostile
Egocentric	Loose associations	Humorous
Elevated self-esteem	Overwhelmed	Id dominant
Energetic	Parataxic distortions	Impulsive
Frenetic socializing	Poor judgment	Irritable
Indiscriminate sex	Racing thoughts	Labile
Intrusive	Sexually preoccupied	Playful
Makeup: garish, gaudy	Sometimes psychotic	
Multiple activities at one time		
Psychomotor agitation		
Restless		
Risk-taking behavior		
Shameless		
Sleepless		
Speech: rapid, rhyming, circumstantial,		
punning, pressured, flights of ideas; may		
be incoherent		
Spends excessively		
Strikes back easily: physically, verbally		
Uncensored		
Verbigeration		
Witty		

her of being cheap and selfish and may even strike her. Manic persons are id-dominated, unable to delay gratification.

PHYSIOLOGIC AND SELF-CARE CONSIDERATIONS

Because manic clients can go days without sleep or food and not even realize they are hungry or tired, the nurse must provide structure for them. They don't perform hygiene tasks routinely and may ignore their own appearance or hygiene needs.

Data Analysis and Planning

Assessment data are analyzed to determine priorities and establish a plan of care. Nursing diagnoses commonly established are as follows:

- Risk for Violence
- Risk for Injury
- Altered Nutrition: Less Than Body Requirements
- Ineffective Individual Coping
- Noncompliance
- Powerlessness
- Altered Role Performance
- Self Care Deficit
- Self Esteem Disturbance
- Sleep Pattern Disturbance
- Ineffective Management of Therapeutic Regimen

Outcomes

Because of the safety risks that a person in the manic phase takes, safety plays a primary role in care, followed by issues related to self-esteem and socialization. Examples of outcomes appropriate to mania are as follows:

1. The client will be safe and exhibit injury-free behaviors to self and others.
2. The client will get enough sleep.
3. The client will gain self-awareness about potentially dangerous situations (sexually promiscuous behavior, dangerous activities, risky financial and occupational ventures).
4. The client will participate in treatment.
5. The client will take adequate food and fluids.
6. The client will evaluate personal qualities realistically.
7. The client will select one or two goal-directed activities to carry out to completion.
8. The client will interact courteously and appropriately with others.
9. The client will handle conflict politely.
10. The client will eliminate sexual provocativeness from verbal and nonverbal behaviors.

Intervention

PROVIDING FOR THE CLIENT'S AND OTHERS' SAFETY

A primary nursing responsibility is to provide for the physical safety of the client and the safety of those in contact with the client. Persons in the manic phase have little insight into their anger and agitation and how their behaviors affect others. They deny their behavior problems and are easily angered. They often intrude on others' space or appear aggressive in approaching others. The nurse must observe and discuss these behaviors with the client as they occur and empathetically set limits: *"Marsha, please wait until I've finished talking with John instead of interrupting us."*

The client should be told that the staff will not permit the client to harm others or others to harm the client. For the client who feels out of control, the nurse must establish external controls in an empathetic and nonchallenging manner. In the long run, these external controls are comforting to the client, although he or she may respond with aggression. Persons in the manic phase have labile emotions; it is not unusual for a manic person to strike out at a staff member who has set limits in a way the client does not like.

Persons in the manic phase physically and psychologically invade the boundaries of others. It helps to remind the client that others may mistake an overly friendly approach as a threat and try to defend themselves. The nurse can say, *"Getting into John's face to say `good morning' can be scary to him. Greet him from 4 feet away."* This is particularly true if the other client is a paranoid schizophrenic or someone else who has difficulty interpreting the actions of others. Many treatment facilities have a no-touch policy, which means that clients are not allowed to touch one another or staff, and staff will touch clients only when giving treatment and care.

A manic person tends to rely on impulsive, aggressive problem-solving behaviors, but the nurse can help him or her learn new ways of dealing with others. The nurse can role-play with the client socially acceptable ways of getting someone's attention and of disagreeing with someone. It helps to establish a contract with the client to manage distress or conflict in one of the ways practiced in the role-playing.

PROVIDING THERAPEUTIC COMMUNICATION

A manic person has a short attention span, so the nurse should use clear, simple sentences when communicating. The client may not be able to handle lots of information at one time, although he or she gives the appearance of being able to function on many levels at the same time. Information should be broken up into many small segments. It helps to ask the client to repeat the brief message back to ensure he or she has heard and incorporated it.

The client may need to undergo baseline and follow-up laboratory tests. Giving a brief explanation of the purpose of each test allays the person's anxiety. Printed information should be given to reinforce verbal messages, especially those related to rules, schedules, civil rights, treatment, staff names, and patient education.

> ▶ SUMMARY INTERVENTIONS FOR MANIA
>
> - Provide for client's physical safety and safety of those around client.
> - Remind the client to respect distances between self and others.
> - Use short, simple sentences to communicate.
> - Ask the client to identify each person, place, and thing being discussed.
> - Ask the client to decode metaphors, themes, and symbols used in speech.
> - Provide client with a list of daily activities.
> - Ensure that nutritional and fluid balance needs are met.
> - Channel client's need for movement into socially acceptable motor activities.

Channels of communication must be kept open between the client and the nurse, regardless of the client's speech patterns. The manic person's speech may be rapid, circumstantial, rhyming, noisy, or intrusive, with flights of ideas and pressured speech. Such disordered speech indicates the client's thought processes, which are flooded with thoughts, ideas, and impulses. The nurse can say, *"Please speak more slowly. I'm having trouble following you."* This puts the responsibility for the communication difficulty on the nurse rather than blaming the client. This request should be patiently and frequently repeated during the conversation, because the client will return to rapid speech.

The person in the manic phase often uses pronouns when referring to people, making it difficult for the listener to understand who is being discussed and when the conversation has moved on to a new subject. While the client is agitatedly talking, he or she is usually thinking and moving just as quickly, so it is a challenge for the nurse to get a coherent story. The nurse can ask the client to identify each person, place, or thing being discussed.

When the client's speech includes flight of ideas, the nurse can ask the client to explain the relationship between topics—for example, *"How does the size of your shoe relate to the river water's being brown instead of clear?"* The healthier client will describe how he or she made the connection between topics. The nurse listens for and documents themes used in the flight of ideas or incoherent words. Nonverbal messages are also assessed—for example, *"I notice you grimace each time you mention your employer. What does this grimace mean?"* The nurse also assesses and documents the coherence of messages.

The client with pressured speech rarely lets others speak, instead talking nonstop until he or she runs out of steam or just stands there looking at the other person before moving away. The client with pressured speech does not respond to others' verbal or nonverbal signals that indicate a desire to speak. The nurse should not get involved in a power struggle over who will dominate the conversation. Instead, the nurse should be patient, listen for themes and symbols, and compare what the client says with how he or she is saying it (comparing content and process). This can be used to understand underlying messages about the client's needs or feelings.

Again, the nurse asks the client to help decode the metaphors, themes, and symbols included in the rapid, rhyming, circumstantial speech. A client who stops you and says, "I can float like a butterfly and sting like a bee" may mean that he admires the boxer Muhammad Ali, that he is grandiose and euphoric, or that he is warning you that he looks innocuous but has a dangerous side.

STRUCTURING A ROUTINE

The client should be given a list of activities he or she is expected to attend each day. The list should contain only information pertinent to that client; there should be no extraneous information related to other clients or staff. The manic person has difficulty maintaining a single focus; instead, he or she focuses on many irrelevant, tangential issues. Therefore, including irrelevant information on the schedule can confuse the client. After the nurse reviews the list with the client, the client is given a copy so that the nurse does not need to repeat the information. The copy also serves as a resource for the client.

PROVIDING NUTRITION

The client often cannot sit still long enough to eat a meal or drink, so it is a nursing responsibility to ensure that the client's metabolic and fluid balance needs are met. This may be done by providing finger foods, small and frequent containers of fluid, or cans of Ensure that the client can consume as he or she moves. High-calorie, high-protein foods and decaffeinated beverages are recommended. Asking about the client's food and fluid preferences will increase the likelihood that the client will eat and drink these items. The nurse records dietary and fluid intake and output and documents the adequacy of caloric and fluid needs each day or at least three times a week.

ENCOURAGING SLEEP

Little sleep is needed by a person in an acute flare-up of mania. Instead, the person engages in frenetic mental, physical, and emotional activity. The nurse keeps track of the amount of actual sleep and rest the manic person gets. Comfort measures that the person used for sleep at home are assessed, and a quiet atmosphere is provided for rest and sleep. Rest periods are scheduled during the day. The nurse should gently interrupt extended periods of physical activity and use the client's ready distractibility to redirect him or her to a less physically demanding activity.

PROMOTING APPROPRIATE BEHAVIORS

The client needs to be protected from his or her pursuit of socially unacceptable and risky behaviors. The client's need for movement can be directed into socially acceptable large motor activities, such as arranging chairs for a community meeting. In acute mania, the person loses the ability to control his or her behavior and engages in risky behavior. Because an acutely manic person feels extraordinarily powerful, he or she places few restrictions on himself or herself. The person acts out impulsive thoughts, has inflated and grandiose perceptions of his or her abilities, is demanding, and needs immediate gratification. This can affect his or her physical, social, occupational, or financial safety, as well as that of others. For example, a stockbroker who had stopped taking his bipolar medication was in a manic phase and was sure his hunches on three particular stocks would pay off. He convinced four clients to sell all their other stocks to invest in these three companies. At the end of the week, the price of stock in these three companies had fallen so low that the clients had lost all their invested cash. When asked why he thought these three companies were such a sure thing, he answered, "I knew it, but I blew it."

In an acute manic episode, the client loses sexual inhibitions, resulting in provocative and risky behaviors. Clothing may be flashy and tantalizing, with women "forgetting" to wear underpants. The client may engage in repeated, frequent unprotected sex for frivolous reasons: "for cigarettes" or "because he has blue eyes and I am mad at my father for giving me brown eyes." The client may ask staff members or other clients (of the same sex or the opposite sex) for sex, graphically describe sexual acts, or display his or her genitals.

In this stage, the client cannot understand personal boundaries, so it is the staff's role to keep the client in view so they can intervene as necessary. For example, a staff member who sees a client invading the intimate space of other clients can say, *"Jeffrey, I'd appreciate your help in setting up a circle of chairs in the group therapy room."* This large motor activity distracts Jeffrey from his inappropriate behavior, appeals to his need for heightened physical activity, is noncompetitive, and is socially acceptable. The staff's vigilant redirection of the person to a more socially appropriate activity protects the person from the hazards of unprotected sex and reduces the client's embarrassment over these behaviors when he or she returns to normal behavior.

MANAGING MEDICATIONS

Lithium is not metabolized; rather, it is reabsorbed by the proximal tubule and excreted in the urine. Periodic serum lithium levels are needed, so before lithium is instituted, a baseline serum lithium level is obtained. Periodic serum lithium levels are used to monitor the client's safety and to ensure that the dose given has increased the serum lithium level to a treatment level or reduced it to a maintenance level. There is a narrow range of safety between maintenance levels (0.5 to 1 mEq/L), treatment levels (0.8 to 1.5 mEq/L), and toxic levels (1.5 to 2.0 mEq/L) (McEvoy, 2000). The only way to titrate the dose is by evaluating symptoms. Symptoms of lithium overdose

appear as the serum levels increase; the higher the serum lithium level, the greater the chance of symptoms of intoxication or toxicity. Lithium intoxication develops over a period of time. Elderly people can have symptoms of overdose at lower serum levels.

PROVIDING CLIENT AND FAMILY TEACHING

Educating the client about the dangers of sexual promiscuity (disease, rape, pregnancy, arrest) is necessary but goes largely unheeded in the acutely manic client because he or she has little patience and capacity to listen, understand, and see the relevance of this information. The client with euphoria may not see why the behavior is a problem, because he or she believes he or she can do anything with impunity. However, as the person begins to cycle down toward normalcy, sexual acting out lessens and the client becomes educable.

A manic person starts many tasks and creates many goals and tries to carry them out all at the same time. The result is that he or she cannot complete any. The client moves readily between these goals, sometimes obsessing about the importance of one over another, but the goals can quickly change. The client may invest in a business in which he or she has no knowledge or experience, go on spending sprees, impulsively travel, speed, make new "best friends," and take the center of attention in any group. He or she is egocentric and has little concern for others except as listeners, sexual partners, or the means to achieve one of his or her poorly conceived goals.

Education about the cause of bipolar disorder, medication management, ways to deal with behaviors, and potential problems the manic person can encounter is important for the family. Education reduces the guilt, blame, and shame that accompany a family member's mental illness, increases the client's safety, enlarges the support system for the client and the family members as they deal with the client, and promotes compliance. Education takes the "mystery" out of treatment for mental illness, replacing it with a proactive view: this is what we know, this is what can be done, and this is what you can do to help.

Family members often say they know the client has stopped taking his or her medication when, for example, the client becomes more argumentative, talks about buying a Jaguar again, hotly denies anything is wrong, or demonstrates another cue of escalating mania. People sometimes need permission to act on their observations, so a family education session is an appropriate place to give this permission and to set up interventions for various client behaviors.

The client should be taught to adhere to the established dosage of lithium and not to omit doses or change dosage intervals, because these interfere with maintenance of serum lithium levels. The client should know about the many drugs that interact with lithium and should tell each physician he or she consults that he or she is taking lithium. An encephalopathic syndrome (lethargy, weakness, fever, tremors, confusion, and extrapyramidal symptoms) can result from concomitant use of lithium and certain antipsychotics.

When a client taking lithium seems to have an increase in manic be havior, lithium levels should be checked to determine whether there is lithium toxicity. Periodic monitoring of serum lithium levels is necessary to ensure the safety and adequacy of the treatment regimen. Persistent thirst and dilute urine can indicate the need to call a physician and have the serum lithium level checked to see if the dosage needs to be reduced.

Clients and family members should know the symptoms of lithium toxicity and interventions to take, including backup plans if the physician is not immediately available. These should be given in writing and explained to the client.

The client should drink adequate amounts of water (approximately 1 liter per day) and continue with the usual amount of dietary table salt. The client must maintain adequate but not excessive amounts of salt in the diet. Because lithium has a greater affinity for salt receptor sites than sodium chloride, it is more readily "grabbed up" by these receptors, and the person can experience lithium toxicity. Having an adequate amount of sodium chloride in the body fluids will reduce the exclusive reception of lithium by these sites. Too much salt in the diet, because of unusually salty foods or the ingestion of salt-containing antacids, can reduce receptor availability for lithium and increase lithium excretion, so the person is underdosed. If the person becomes dehydrated, there is more lithium in the remaining body fluid. If there is too much water, the lithium is diluted and the dose will be less effective. Monitoring daily weights and the balance between intake and output and checking dependent parts for edema can be helpful in monitoring fluid balance. The physician should be contacted if the client has diarrhea, fever, flu, or any condition that leads to dehydration.

Thyroid function tests are usually ordered as a baseline and every 6 months during treatment with lithium. In 6 to 18 months, a third of the clients taking lithium have an increased level of thyroid-stimulating hormone, which can cause anxiety, labile emotions, and sleeping difficulty. Decreased levels are implicated in fatigue and depression.

Baseline and periodic assessments of renal status are necessary to assess renal function, because most lithium is excreted in the urine. The reduced renal function in the elderly necessitates lower doses. Lithium is contraindicated in people with compro-

mised renal function or urinary retention and those taking low-salt diets or diuretics. Lithium is also contraindicated in persons with brain or cardiovascular damage.

Evaluation

Since there is a higher incidence of suicide in people with mood disorders, evaluation of the ongoing assessment of safety is a necessity. Include data for suicidal ideation, suicide plan, support systems, and new coping techniques, as well as the other nursing diagnoses specific to the individual with mood disorder to provide data for outcome achievement. Both the nurses' evaluative data and the client's perception of success in achieving treatment goals are included.

Evaluation of the treatment of mood disorders includes, but are not limited to:
- Safety issues
- Comparison of mood and affect between start of treatment and present
- Adherence to treatment regimen of medication and psychotherapy
- Changes in client's perception of quality of life
- Achievement of specific goals of treatment, including new coping methods

OTHER MOOD DISORDERS

Dysthymic disorder is a chronic depression in which the person has been depressed more often than not for at least 2 years. It is less debilitating than major depression. SSRIs are effective for this disorder (Comer, 1992; DSM-IV-TR, 2000).

Seasonal affective disorder is a form of depression that is precipitated by decreased exposure to sunlight (normally during the winter); symptoms include reduced energy, decreased activities, increased sleep, and increased appetite, especially for carbohydrates, resulting in weight gain. The higher the latitude in the Northern Hemisphere (fewer daylight hours), the greater the incidence of this disorder. As the hours of daylight increase, depression decreases

> ▶ CLIENT AND FAMILY TEACHING
> FOR THE CLIENT WITH MANIA
> - Teach about the dangers of sexually provocative and promiscuous behavior.
> - Teach about the etiology of bipolar disorder.
> - Teach about medication management.
> - Teach the family ways to handle behaviors.

and the person returns to his or her usual function (DSM-IV-TR, 2000).

In bipolar disorder II, the client demonstrates depression that cycles to normal behavior and at least one episode of hypomanic, but not manic, behavior. **Hypomania** is a condition of expansive or irritable mood similar to mania, but the behaviors are of a lesser degree than mania. The hypomanic phase lasts at least 4 days, with three or more of the following symptoms: grandiosity; decreased sleep; chatty, pressured speech; racing thoughts or flight of ideas; easy distractibility; psychomotor agitation; and foolish, high-risk behaviors (DSM-IV-TR, 2000).

In cyclothymic disorder, the person has hypomanic episodes and mildly depressed episodes during a period of 2 or more years. Essentially, it is a mild form of bipolar disorder: the client's behaviors do not meet the criteria for bipolar disorder I or II (DSM-IV-TR, 2000). DelBello et al. (2000) reported that the person with cyclothymic personality demonstrates many life-disruptive behaviors, such as substance abuse and the inability to sustain a relationship or a job. He or she may not look especially ill but alternates between moderate mania and moderate depression. This disorder is more difficult to diagnose than clearly bi-polar behavior. As a result, the cyclothymic person often does not receive treatment and winds up with more problems than the person with more serious bipolar disease who is treated and has long periods of normal behavior. Cyclothymic disorder is treated with lower doses of lithium.

In bipolar disorder not otherwise specified, the person has rapidly alternating cycles of mild mania and mild depression that occur over days instead of months (DSM-IV-TR, 2000).

Mood disorder due to a general medical condition can be related to the physiologic effects of disequilibrium of any body system—endocrine: increased or decreased function of the thyroid, parathyroid, and adrenal glands; neurologic: head and spinal injuries, cerebrovascular accident, Alzheimer's, Huntington's, and Parkinson's diseases; renal: end-stage renal disease; autoimmune disorders: systemic lupus erythematosus, multiple sclerosis, muscular dystrophy; or malignancies and viruses of any system. There is an increased risk of suicide in persons with this disorder because of the chronic, painful, and incurable aspects of the medical conditions. The onset of this type of depression is related to the onset and diagnosis of the medical condition. Depression can also be related to the use of certain drugs (see Table 14-1).

Substance abuse mood disorder is a mood disorder that occurs secondary to ingesting or withdrawing from such substances as:

- Drugs of abuse: alcohol, cocaine, hallucinogens, amphetamines, inhalants, opioids, sedatives, hypnotics, and anxiolytics

- Prescribed medications: anticonvulsants, analgesics, anticholinergics, antihypertensives, anesthetics, antiparkinsonians, antiulcer drugs, cardiac drugs, contraceptives, muscle relaxants, steroids, and sulfonamides
- Psychotropic drugs: antidepressants, antipsychotics, and benzodiazepines
- Toxic substances: heavy metals, gasoline, paint, propellants from spray cans, correction fluid, and carbon monoxide.

Depending on the nature of the substance and the context in which the symptoms occur, such as during intoxication or withdrawal, the disorder can be manifested by depression, mania, or both (DSM-IV-TR, 2000).

SUICIDE

Suicidal thoughts are common in people with mood disorders, especially depression. **Suicide** is the intentional act of killing oneself. Edwin Shneidman (1963, 1981), a leading suicide researcher, has defined two categories of suicide: direct and indirect. Direct suicides are conscious, voluntary, life-ending acts such as self-immolation (setting oneself on fire), hanging, shooting, poisoning, jumping from a high place, drowning, or suffocation. Indirect suicides are unconscious, hidden desires to die, manifested by chronic risky behaviors such as substance abuse, overeating, indiscriminate sexual activities, noncompliance with the medical regimen, or hazardous sports or occupations.

Attempted suicide is a suicidal act that either failed or was incomplete. In the latter, the person either did not complete the suicidal act because the behavior was a successful cry for help, or the suicidal act was completed but the person was rescued (Roy, 2000). **Suicidal ideation** means the person is having thoughts about killing himself or herself.

Suicide involves the ambivalence of wanting to live and wanting to die. Many fatal accidents are impulsive suicides, but it is impossible to know whether the person who drove into a telephone pole did this intentionally or not. Hence, it is difficult to keep accurate statistics on suicide. There are, however, certain risk factors and behaviors of people who commit suicide. There are also many myths and misconceptions. The nurse must be able to know the facts and warning signs for those at risk for suicide (Box 14-8).

Assessment

POPULATIONS AT RISK

Single people have twice the risk of suicide compared with those who are married. Those who are divorced, widowed, or newly single have a risk more than four times that of married people. Divorced women have a

Box 14-8

➤ MYTHS AND FACTS ABOUT SUICIDE

Myths	Facts
People who talk about suicide never commit suicide.	Suicidal people often send out subtle or not-so-subtle messages that convey their inner thoughts of hopelessness and self-destruction. Both subtle messages (covert cues) and direct messages (overt cues) of suicide should be taken seriously, with appropriate assessments and interventions.
Suicidal people only want to hurt themselves, not others.	While the self-violence of suicide demonstrates anger turned inward, the anger can be directed toward others in a planned or impulsive action. *Physical harm:* Psychotic people may be responding to inner voices that command the individual to kill others before killing the self. A depressed person who has decided to commit suicide with a gun may impulsively shoot the person who tries to grab the gun in an effort to thwart the suicide. *Emotional harm:* Often family members, friends, health care professionals, and even police involved in trying to avert a suicide, or those who did not realize the person's depression and plans to commit suicide, feel intense guilt and shame because of their failure to help, and are "stuck" in a never-ending cycle of despair and grief. Some people, depressed after the suicide of a loved one, will rationalize that suicide was a "good way out of the pain" and plan their own suicide to escape pain. Some suicides are planned to engender guilt and pain in survivors; for example, as someone who wants to punish another for rejecting or not returning love.
There is no way to help someone who wants to kill himself or herself.	Suicidal people have mixed feelings (ambivalent) about their wish to die, wish to kill others, or to be killed. This ambivalence often prompts the cries for help evident in overt or covert cues. Intervention can help the suicidal individual get help from situational supports, choose to live, learn new ways to cope, and move forward in life.
Do not mention the word *suicide* to a person you suspect to be suicidal, since this could give him or her the idea to commit suicide.	Suicidal people have already thought of the idea of suicide and may have begun plans.
Ignoring verbal threats of suicide or challenging a person to carry out his or her suicide plans will reduce the individual's use of these behaviors.	Suicidal gestures are a lethal way to act out. Never should threats be ignored or dismissed and never should a person be challenged to carry out suicidal threats. All plans, threats, gestures or cues should be taken seriously and immediate help given that focuses on the problem about which the person is suicidal. When asked about suicide, it is often a relief for the client to know that his or her cries for help have been heard and that help is on the way.
Once a suicide risk, always a suicide risk.	While it is true that most people who successfully commit suicide have made attempts at least once before, the majority of people with suicidal ideation can have positive resolution to the suicidal crisis. With proper support, finding new ways to resolve the problem helps these individuals become emotionally secure and have no further need for suicide as a way to resolve a problem.

lower suicide rate than divorced men. Women have greater rates of suicide attempts, but men are more successful in carrying out the act because they use more lethal methods. Women tend to use sleeping pills or razors, whereas men shoot or hang themselves or jump off high places (Roy, 2000).

Whites have the highest risk of all cultural groups, committing 72% of all suicides, followed in decreasing order by Native Americans, African Americans, Hispanic Americans, and Asian Americans (Oltmanns & Emery, 1998). Persons older than 65 have the highest rate of suicide. The rate of teenage suicide is increasing at an alarming rate: suicide is now the second leading cause of death for adolescents. This is attributed to the sharp rise in adolescent depression. Other peak suicide times are between ages 30 and 40 (McIntosh, 1992).

Religion plays an important role in suicidal behavior. Those who believe there will be punishment in the afterlife for suicide, such as Catholics, have lower rates of suicide. People who actively practice their religion have lower rates of suicide (Slaby et al., 1986).

The incidence of suicide is higher in the very wealthy or very poor than in the middle class. The greater the degree of hopelessness about the future, the greater the risk of suicide. Occupations having higher rates of suicide are physicians, dentists, attorneys, members of the military, police officers, executives, pharmacists, engineers, and air traffic controllers. Rates are also higher in people living in urban areas, socially mobile persons, migrant workers, students, the gifted, and the elderly.

Persons with the following disorders have higher rates of suicide: mood disorders, substance abuse, schizophrenia, organic brain disorders, personality and panic disorders, and chronic medical conditions. Other high-risk behaviors for suicide include impulsivity, social isolation, and psychosis (Roy, 2000).

A history of previous suicide attempts by a person increases the risk for suicide. The first 2 years after a suicide attempt represent the high-risk period, especially the first 3 months. Those who have a relative who committed suicide are at a higher risk for suicide. One possible rationale is that the relative's suicide offers a sense of "permission" or acceptance of suicide as a method of getting out of a difficult situation. This familiarity and acceptance of suicide is also believed to be part of the rationale behind "copycat suicides" by teenagers, who are greatly influenced by their peers' actions (Roy, 2000).

Most depressed people who have suicidal ideation do not have the energy to implement their suicide plans. The natural energy that accompanies the increased hours of sunlight in spring is believed to explain why most suicides occur in April. Most suicides occur on Monday morning, the time most people return to work (another energy spurt). Research has shown that antidepressant treatment can actually give a depressed person the energy to act on suicidal ideation (Roy, 2000).

WARNINGS OF SUICIDAL INTENT

Most people with suicidal ideation send cues or signals to others about their intent to harm themselves. The nurse should **never** ignore any hint of suicidal ideation, regardless of how trivial or subtle it may seem and regardless of the client's intent or emotional status. Often persons contemplating suicide have ambivalent and conflicting feelings about their desire to die and reach out to others to seek help. For example, a client might say, "I turned on the gas oven last night and didn't light it. I figured it would be an end to my pain, but I couldn't even do that" (Box 14-9).

It is the nurse's responsibility to keep the client safe. Thus, the nurse must identify and assess any cue about suicidal intentions and must directly ask clients who fit the suicide risk profile if they have thoughts or plans of harming themselves. The SAD PERSONS scale (Table 14-8) developed by Patterson (1983) is based on these risk factors and is a helpful mnemonic device for the areas that are important to assess when evaluating for risk of suicide. This scale can be used by any health care professional and is designed to give some sense of when a suicidal person should be admitted to the hospital or, given an adequate support system, can be treated at home.

IMPULSIVITY AND ENGAGING IN RISKY BEHAVIORS

A few people who commit suicide give no warning signs. Some have artfully hidden their distress and their suicide plans; others act impulsively, taking advantage of a situation to carry out the desire to die. Some suicidal people in treatment describe placing themselves in risky or dangerous situations, such as speeding in a blinding rainstorm or when intoxicated. This "Russian roulette" approach to suicide carries a high risk of harm to the person and innocent bystanders as well. It allows the person to feel brave, confronting death over and over and surviving. Other indirect risky or impulsive behaviors in-

---

Box 14-9

> **NURSING ALERT**

Never ignore any suicidal ideation, regardless of how trivial or subtle it may seem and regardless of the client's intent or emotional status.

Table 14-8

SAD PERSONS SUICIDE RATING SCALE

S	Sex	Males have a three times higher rate of suicide because of the more lethal means used to kill themselves.
A	Age	Adolescents, middle age (45), and over 65
D	Depression	25%–30% of the people who attempt suicide have a mood disorder.
P	Previous attempts	50%–80% of successful suicides have attempted to commit suicide at least once before.
E	ETOH	20%–90% of successful suicides are associated with heavy alcohol or drug abuse.
R	Rational thought loss	Psychosis increases the risk of suicide.
S	Social support, lack	Lacking support from relatives, friends, religious practices, and occupational satisfaction increases suicide risk.
O	Organized plan	Method, time, date, place, fantasies of funeral and grieving of significant others
N	No significant other	Single, widowed, divorced, and separated people have a higher risk for suicide.
S	Sickness	Painful, debilitating, terminal illness increases suicide risk.

Points	Intervention Guidelines
0–2	Can stay at home with support of significant others and outpatient treatment
3 or 4	Support of significant others with more intense outpatient care; may consider hospitalization
5 or 6	Hospitalization strongly considered
≥7	Hospitalization recommended

Adapted from Patterson, W. (1983). Evaluation of suicidal patients: the SAD PERSONS scale. *Psychosomatics, 24* (4), 343.

clude overeating, unsafe sex, smoking, anorexia nervosa, drug abuse, drag racing, or bungee jumping.

LETHALITY ASSESSMENT

The suicide lethality assessment can be done by the nurse or any health care professional. The goal is to determine the degree to which the person has planned his or her suicide. This assessment tool follows a "who, what, when, where, how, and how is it that" set of questions to gauge the degree of intention to commit suicide (Box 14-10). The nurse assesses the method, access to the necessary equipment, where and when the suicide is to occur, why the person wants to commit suicide, who the rage is directed toward, and how complete the plan is, including fantasies about the funeral (who will be there and how the client wants each of these people to feel about the suicide). The client's responses are documented and reported to the psychiatrist or other health care provider.

Intervention

AUTHORITATIVE ROLE

Intervention into suicidal ideation or acting out becomes the first priority of nursing care, and the nurse assumes an authoritative role to help the person stay safe. This is a crisis situation in which the person sees few or no alternatives to resolve his or her problems. The nurse can brainstorm with the client and offer suggestions to resolve the problems. After the client has regained equilibrium and has entered into a no-suicide contract, and the desire to commit suicide has been significantly reduced or eliminated, the nurse returns to using therapeutic communication techniques to guide the client to generate and test his or her own resolutions to problems.

SUICIDE PRECAUTIONS

Any item that can be used to commit suicide is removed, such as sharp objects, shoelaces, belts, sheets, pillowcases, extraneous clothing, weapons, flammable liquids, lighters and matches, pencils, pens, medications, and caustic chemicals. The client is not permitted access to high places. Restraints may be needed to prevent the person from hitting the head against the floor or wall.

NO-SUICIDE CONTRACT

A no-suicide contract can be implemented at home as well as in the inpatient treatment setting. In this contract, the client agrees that he or she will notify the staff at the first impulse to harm himself or herself (in the home situation, the caregiver is notified; backup people must be identified if the caregiver is unavailable). The urge to commit suicide may return suddenly, and the client needs to have someone always

(text continues on page 370)

Box 14-10

➤ SUICIDE LETHALITY ASSESSMENT INTERVIEW

Callie, 37, had been seen three times in the past 6 weeks by Dr. Martin in her family practice office for vague neck, back, and abdominal pains. She had been treated with NSAIDs, physiotherapy, and later Percocet, without relief. Laboratory test results and x-rays are normal. During these 6 weeks, Callie has seemed depressed and sad, with labile moods and periods of agitation, and said she felt hopeless and exhausted. At the last checkup, Dr. Martin had jotted a note to herself about a possible psychiatric evaluation for Callie. Today, Callie has a grim smile and seems intense yet less anxious than on previous visits. The nurse feels that something is different and conducts an in-depth emotional assessment of Callie.

Nurse (N): "Dr. Martin will be in shortly, but I have some time to chat with you right now. I am not quite sure I can put my finger on it, but something seems different about you today." (*broad opening*)

Client (C): "Yeah. I have been doing a lot of thinking and have come to some decisions."

N: "Decisions" (*focusing*)

C: *"Oh, uh, just some stuff I have been thinking about."* (Silent, looks down.)

N: (Remains silent and waits with respectful look on face. Waits about 2 minutes.)

C: *"Life is a farce and I am getting out."* (*What: cue of suicidal intent*)

N: "What part of your life is a farce and how are you getting out?" (*focusing*)

C: *"My marriage. I just want it to end."*

N: "What do you want to end, your marriage or your life?" (*connecting two islands of information*)

C: *"Both! My marriage and my life. . . I want to be dead."*

N: "You are thinking of killing yourself." (*consensual validation*)

C: *"Yeah."*

N: "Who else are you thinking of killing?" (*clarifying*)

C: *"Just me."*

N: "How do you plan to kill yourself?" (*focusing*) (*how: identify method and access to equipment to carry out suicide*)

C: *"By shooting myself."*

N: "When have you tried to kill yourself before?" (*placing event in time sequence*)

C: *"Never."*

N. "Where do you have a weapon to use to shoot yourself?" (*clarifying*)

C. *"I've got a gun, my husband's revolver."*

N: "Where is your husband's revolver?" (*focusing*)

C: *"In the attic, in a locked box."*

N: "Where is the key for this locked box?" (*focusing*)

C: *"I have it. I took it off my husband's key ring."*

N: "Where are the bullets for this revolver?" (*focusing*)

C: *"In a separate container in the locked box."*

N: "How do you know how to use a gun?" (*clarifying*)

C: *"I have seen my husband clean and use it. I know enough to get it loaded and get the safety off to fire it."*

N: "Where do you intend to kill yourself?" (*placing plan in time sequence*) (*Ask about where and when suicide will occur*)

C: *"In our bedroom."*

N: "You and your husband's bedroom?" (*clarifying place*)

C: *"Yes."*

N: "When do you plan to carry out your suicide?" (*placing event in time*)

C: *"This afternoon around 3."*

N: "What is significant about 3 PM and killing yourself in your bedroom?" (*connecting islands of information*)

C: *"No one will be home. My brother-in-law who lives with us leaves for work at 2:30 and the kids and my husband get home around 3:30."*

N: "Who else lives with you?" (*clarifying*)

C: *That's all—my husband, two kids, and his brother."*

N: "Whom do you want to find you after you have shot yourself in the bedroom at 3 PM?" (*placing event in sequence*) (*Ask about who the anger is directed toward and why the client wants to hurt this person*)

C: *"My husband."*

N: "What do you want your husband to think as he walks into your bedroom to find you have shot yourself?" (*encouraging description of emotions*)

C: *"I want him to hurt! I want him to know he was wrong to have cheated on me. He said he'd never do it again, but he did. He has had affair after affair. I believed him each time he said he'd never do it again. What a jerk I was. He*

Continued

Box 14-10

> SUICIDE LETHALITY ASSESSMENT INTERVIEW—cont'd

must have laughed his head off each time I bought his line of lies and promises. . . . Life is hopeless. My marriage is a failure. I can't fix it and I can't fix him . . . or me, and I sure can't hide behind denial anymore . . . Would you believe that last month I found him in our bedroom with some strange woman? In our bedroom! Well, from now on, he can just see my brains all over the bedroom, and he'll know he was wrong—dead wrong!"

N: "How has suicide become the only path you see you have?" (*focusing*)

C: *"I've tried everything else."*

N: "What is one thing you have you tried?" (*focusing*)

C: *"I already told you. I believed all of his lies. I tried to be good."*

N: "Define 'being good.'" (*encouraging description of perceptions*)

C: *"Good wife—you know, housekeeper, sex partner, cook, mother to his kids."*

N: "How do you see your being good as fixing your husband's choice to have sex with other women?" (*encouraging description of perceptions*)

C: *"I don't know. It's what my mother said to do when I caught him cheating. 'Be good and he'll love you more.'"*

N: "What about choosing to leave your husband because he was unfaithful to you?" (*encouraging evaluation*)

C: *"Uh . . . I'd never leave him. I couldn't. I have no job skills and the kids are still in grade school."* (Degree of planning related to suicide)

N: "You planned to leave him today in a big way." (*gentle confrontation*)

C: *"Yeah."*

N: "What is the chance your children could be the ones to find you dead in the bedroom?" (*going back to fill in information or questions that have developed; encouraging further contemplation on her plan*)

C: *"Oh! I hadn't thought about the kids finding me. They usually play outside after school. Uh . . . I hadn't . . . (silence)"*

N: "Who would you want to help your husband raise your children after your suicide?" (*encouraging further contemplation on her plan*)

C: *"I don't know . . . I mean, I hadn't thought of that either."*

N: "What are your thoughts and plans related to your funeral?" (*focusing on plan*)

C: *"I have my clothes picked out. Sunday I told my husband that when I died, he should make sure I was laid out in my peach dress. It was the one I got for our 12th anniversary and he had said I looked great in it. He knew the one."*

N: "What did he say when you told him about the peach dress for your funeral?" (*focusing*)

C: *"He told me not to be so dramatic and laughed. I wanted him to choke on his laughter when he saw me in the casket, and I wanted him to picture what he did to me every time he walked in our bedroom and took off his pants."*

N: "What he did to you?"

C: *"What he made me do."*

N: "How do you see your choice to commit suicide as being 'made to' do it by your husband?"

C: *"He' know why he made me do it."*

N: "What would it take to stop you from putting this plan in action?" (*encouraging a plan of action*)

C: *"I don't know. The kids . . . I wasn't thinking of them. I thought I had it worked out, but now it seems . . . agh!"*

N: "You've had lots of emotional burdens and have the right to your own feelings." (*translating into feelings*)

C: *"Yes."*

N: "You were brave to reach out to tell me you were planning to commit suicide today. We, the staff, the doctors, and I, will help you stay safe." (*offering self*) I am going to call the local psychiatric emergency evaluation service, who will send an expert here to the office to talk with you to see what sort of help is needed and is available to you. Dr. Martin has set up this plan for emergency evaluation by an expert for her clients who have thoughts about harming themselves. I'll also stay here with you while you speak to Dr. Martin and the psychiatric evaluator so we can plan how else we can help you to work through this situation. Is this OK with you?" (*offering self*)

C: *'I feel embarrassed and incompetent, but yes, thanks. I never thought I'd tell this to anyone. I don't even know why I kept this appointment today. I . . . uh . . . thanks."*

N: "You're welcome. Which friends or relatives do you consider to be your support system, people you can depend on to help you right now, who I can call to be with you?" (*authoritative plan for action is acceptable in crisis and suicide conditions.*)

C: *"Well, I guess that lets my husband out at this moment. I am angry, disappointed, and hurt by his behavior and do not want to see his face for a while . . . if ever."*

N: "Go on." (*encouraging formulation of a plan of action*)

C. *"Well, my brother-in-law is pretty good. I mean, I talk and he listens and even offers me some good feedback, but he mostly listens. My brother-in-law is my husband's brother. He likes my sister and I think she is sweet on him. They make a good pair and he seems to be happy with one woman, not like his slimy brother."*

Continued

Box 14-10

> ## SUICIDE LETHALITY ASSESSMENT INTERVIEW—cont'd

N: "Which of these two would you like me to contact for you right now, your sister or your brother-in-law?" *(encouraging formulation of a plan of action)*

C: *"My sister, I guess. She is probably at her apartment right now. Here is her phone number."*

N: "You and Dr. Martin and the evaluator will decide exactly how to help you through this crisis. Again, I will be here as you speak to each of these people. I also want to institute a no-suicide contract with you. This involves two things. First, I'll ask your sister to go to your home and remove the locked box with the weapons and ammunition and any other means she can see for you to harm yourself. Is this all right with you? (*authoritative plan of action/ no-suicide contract*)

C: *"Yes. I feel sort of silly, like a child at school who is not trusted to wear her galoshes in the rain."*

N: "I agree, but it is helpful to remove temptation when you are this tempted." *(consensual validation)*

C: *"OK. It's OK. I can see why this has to be done."*

N: "The next part of the no-suicide contract is for you to agree that at the first inkling or perception of wanting to harm yourself, you will immediately notify the person who is there at home with you, or the staff if you are hospitalized, or your therapist, or Dr. Martin. We want you to know you have quick availability to help, as well as a variety of sources of help at any one moment. Before you leave today, I will give both you and your sister a card with Dr. Martin's beeper number. If she is not available, she gives the beeper to me so one of us is available if you can't access others in your support system. Do you agree not to harm yourself and to immediately call someone from your support system at the first recurrence of the thought that you want to hurt yourself?" *(establishing a no-suicide contract)*

C: "Yes. I don't mean to be such trouble."

N: "Just to be sure we are both on the same wavelength, what have you just agreed to do?" *(requesting consensual validation)*

C: "I promise to tell my sister, Dr. Martin, you, or anyone on staff if I am hospitalized if I get these feelings about suicide. I will do this at the first feeling or desire to harm myself. OK. I will."

N: "You have borne a lot of pain alone and now we can help you work through this and grow stronger. Again, we are here to help you, not judge you. Keeping you safe and helping you through a desperate time is what we are here for." *(offering self)*

C: "Yes, thanks."

available for support. A list should be generated of support people who agree to be readily available to the suicidal person.

Most suicidal people adhere to the no-suicide contract because it appeals to their will to live, the flip side of the wish to die. However, it is not a guarantee of safety. The contract is made by the client with input from the nurse or another health care professional. It can also specify a time when the client will be re-evaluated.

SUPPORT SYSTEM LIST

Suicidal people often lack social support systems—relatives, friends, or religious, occupational, and community support groups. This may be the result of the client's asocial behavior associated with the mood disorder, or the fact that the person has moved to a new area because of school, work, a change in family structure, or a change in financial status. The nurse should assess the client's support system and the type of help each person or group can give the client. Mental health clinics, hotlines, psychiatric emergency evaluation services, student health services, church

groups, and self-help groups are part of the community support system.

The nurse should make a list of specific names and agencies that can be called for support; the client's consent should be obtained to avoid breach of confidentiality. Many suicidal people do not have to be admitted to a hospital and can be treated successfully in the community with the help of these support people and agencies.

SUPERVISION

All institutions have policies and procedures related to suicide precautions and supervision. Persons at a high risk for suicide can be admitted to a hospital, where some form of constant supervision is in place. All interventions are explained to the client before they are implemented. The most stringent form of supervision is **one-to-one supervision,** in which one staff person per shift is assigned to be no greater than an arm's length away from the client. The staff person must have the client in visual contact at all times, including when he or she is using the toilet, showering, and having visitors, because it is relatively easy for a person, with proper planning, to commit suicide in a few seconds. In some cases, restraints are used with constant visual supervision. Line-of-sight or eyes-on supervision means the client must always be within visual contact of a staff person, including bathroom and visiting supervision. The suicidal person cannot leave the unit for any reason. All objects that could be harmful are removed, and any objects that visitors bring to the client are searched.

A depressed person with suicidal ideation who looks and acts better after a few weeks of treatment with antidepressants or with increased daylight can be a greater suicide risk than he or she was on admission. The issues related to the wish to die have not been resolved, but the client now has the energy to carry out the suicide plans he or she made while deeply depressed and unable to act. A person with suicidal ideation who has stopped talking about suicide but seems more serene and more goal-directed may not be "getting better" but may have made the decision to kill himself or herself. The serenity comes from making this final decision. Thus, suicide precautions must not be lifted until the order has been written by the psychiatrist. When the order has been written, it is better to ease the precautions gradually and monitor the impact of these changes on the client than to lift them immediately (Box 14-11).

Outcomes

The goals are to keep the person safe and to help him or her to develop new coping skills that do not involve self-harm. Treatment often involves treating the underlying disorder, such as a mood disorder or psychosis, with psychoactive agents. The first outcomes involve the person's safety; later outcomes involve helping the person learn different choices. Examples of outcomes for a suicidal person include:
1. The client will be safe from self-harm and harm to others.

Box 14-11

> ► **Nursing Alert—Antidepressants and Suicidal Ideation**
>
> Depressed people who have suicidal ideation can get the energy to carry out the act after treatment with antidepressants, in the spring when daylight increases, or when depression remits. A depressed person with suicidal ideation who looks and acts better after a few weeks of treatment with antidepressants or with increased daylight can be a greater suicide risk than he or she was on admission.

2. The client will engage in a therapeutic relationship.
3. The client will establish a no-suicide contract.
4. The client will create lists of positive attributes.
5. The client will generate, test, and evaluate realistic plans to address underlying issues.
6. The client will reduce and then extinguish suicidal ideation.
7. The client will verbalize a higher quality of life.

Other outcomes may relate to activities of daily living, sleep and nourishment needs, the need to harm others, and problems specific to the crisis that is driving the person toward suicide.

Family Response

Suicide is the ultimate rejection of family and friends. Implicit in the act of suicide is the message to others that their help was considered incompetent, irrelevant, or unwelcome. Some suicides are done to place blame on a certain person—even to the point of planning how that person will be the one to discover the body. Most are an effort to escape an untenable situation. Even if the person believes his or her suicide was prompted by love for family members, as in the case of someone who commits suicide to avoid lengthy legal battles or to save the family the financial and emotional cost of a lingering death, the family still grieves and may feel guilt, shame, and anger.

Significant others may feel guilty for not knowing how desperate the suicidal person was, ashamed because their help was not sought or trusted and their loved one ended his or her life with a socially unacceptable, often illegal act, and angry about being rejected. Suicide is newsworthy, and there may be whispered gossip and even news coverage. Life insurance companies may not pay survivors' benefits to families of those who kill themselves. Shneidman (1963) found higher death rates among significant others for a year after a family member committed suicide. Also, the one death may spark "copycat suicides" among family members or others, who may feel they have been given permission to do the same. Families can disintegrate after a suicide.

Nurse's Response

When dealing with a client with suicidal ideation or one who has attempted suicide, the nurse's attitude must indicate unconditional positive regard, not for the act but for the person and his or her spiritual desperation. The ideas or attempts are serious signals of the person's desperate emotional state. The nurse must convey the belief that the person can be helped and can grow and change.

Trying to make the client feel guilty for thinking of or attempting suicide is not helpful; this person already feels incompetent, hopeless, and helpless. The nurse should not blame the client or be judgmental when asking about the details of the planned suicide. The nurse must use a nonjudgmental tone of voice and monitor his or her own body language and facial expressions to make sure he or she is not conveying disgust or blame. Suicidal people have **tunnel vision**, meaning they focus solely on their overwhelming feelings of pain and problems and desire to escape. The nurse can help the client see facets of the suicide that he or she had not considered or had denied. For example, pointing out that the client's 7-year-old son may be the one to find him hanging in the garage might start this client thinking about how devastating his suicide would be for the boy.

Shneidman interviewed a woman who was in great pain from burns she suffered when she tried to kill herself by sprinkling lighter fluid over her coat and striking a match. She was saved by a bystander. She said she had never considered the pain involved in burning; instead, she saw it as a way out of her turmoil. Because of her singular focus on death, she could not reason out all the facets of the suicide plan, much less consider alternatives to the problems that plagued her.

Nurses believe that one person can make a difference in another's life. This belief must be conveyed when caring for suicidal people, but nurses must realize that no matter how competent and caring the intervention is, a few clients will still go on to commit suicide. A client's suicide can be devastating to the staff members who treated him or her, especially if the staff members have gotten to know the person and his or her family well over a period of time. Even with therapy, the staff members may end up leaving the health care facility or even the profession.

Legal and Ethical Considerations

Assisted suicide is a topic of national legal and ethical debate, with much attention focused on the court decisions relating to the actions of Dr. Jack Kevorkian, a physician who has participated in numerous assisted suicides. Oregon was the first state to adopt assisted suicide into law and has set up safeguards to prevent indiscriminate assisted suicide. Many people believe it should be legal in any state for health care professionals or family to assist those who are terminally ill and want to die. Others view suicide as against the law of humanity and religion and believe health care professionals should be prosecuted if they assist those who are trying to die. Groups such as the Hemlock Society and people such as Dr. Kevorkian are lobbying for laws to be changed, allowing health care professionals and family members to assist with suicide attempts for the terminally ill. Controversy and emotion continue to surround the issue.

Often nurses must care for people who are terminally or chronically ill and who have a poor quality of life, such as those with the intractable pain of a terminal illness, those with severe disability, and those being kept alive by life-support systems. It is not the nurse's role to decide how long these clients must suffer. It is the nurse's role to provide supportive care for the client and family as they work through the difficult emotional decisions about when these clients should be allowed to die, because persons who have been declared legally dead can be disconnected from life support. Each state has defined legal death and the ways to determine it.

COMMUNITY CARE

Nurses in any area of practice in the community are often the first health care professionals to recognize behaviors consistent with mood disorders. In some cases, a family member may mention his or her distress about the client's withdrawal from activities, difficulty thinking, eating, and sleeping, complaints

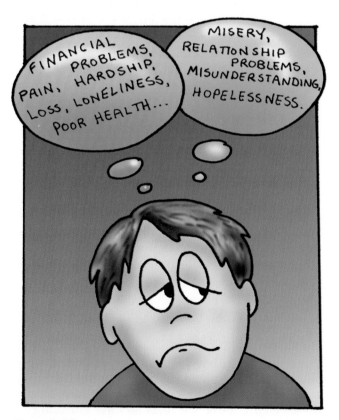

Tunnel vision

of being tired all the time, sadness, and agitation (all symptoms of unipolar depression), or of cycles of euphoria, spending binges, loss of inhibitions, changes in sleep and eating patterns, and loud clothing styles and colors (consistent with the manic phase of bipolar disorder). Documenting and reporting these behaviors can help get these people into treatment. It is estimated that nearly 40% of the population who have been diagnosed with a mood disorder do not get treatment. This may result from the stigma that is still associated with mental disorders, the lack of understanding about the disruption to life that a mood disorder can cause, confusion about treatment choices, or a more compelling medical diagnosis, combined with the reality of a limited amount of time that a health care professional can devote to any one client (Beers et al., 1999).

People with depression can be successfully treated in the community by psychiatrists, psychiatric advanced practice nurses, and primary care physicians. The person with bipolar disorder, however, should be referred to a psychiatrist or psychiatric advanced practice nurse for treatment (Simon, 1998). The physician or nurse who treats a person with bipolar disorder but does not specialize in psychiatry must understand the drug treatment, dosages, desired effects, therapeutic levels, and potential side effects so that he or she can answer questions and promote compliance with treatment (Bouchard, 1999).

Managed care has added another player to the mental health care arena. Psychiatric nurses have become case managers whose goal is to return the client to mental health in the least amount of time and through the least restrictive means. Bily & Snell (1998) identified the benchmarks of the mental health care monitoring process as necessity and appropriateness, provider competence, efficacy, cost-effectiveness, accessibility, safety, and client satisfaction. The rationale for a specific level of care is documented, as well as treatment alternatives.

SELF-AWARENESS ISSUES

Some health care professionals consider suicidal people to be failures, immoral, or unworthy of care. Such a negative and unethical attitude may result from several factors. It may reflect society's negative view of suicide: many states still have laws against suicide, although they are rarely enforced. These health care professionals may feel inadequate and anxious about dealing with a suicidal client (Burgess, 1997), or they may feel discomfort over their own past suicidal ideation or plans that have been suppressed, repressed, or denied. When a person cannot admit that he or she has had such "horrible" thoughts or inclinations and acts out this discomfort in some manner, Sullivan (1953) calls this the "not me" part of the personality. However, most people have had thoughts about "ending it all," even if just for a fleeting moment when life is not going well. The scariness of remembering one's own flirtation with suicide results in anxiety. If this anxiety is not resolved, the staff person can demonstrate avoidance, demeaning behavior, and superiority to a suicidal client. Therefore, to be effective with suicidal clients, the nurse must be aware of his or her own feelings and beliefs about suicide.

Nurses working with depressed clients often empathize with them and begin to feel sad or agitated as well. They may even unconsciously start to avoid contact with such clients to escape such feelings. Nurses must monitor their feelings and reactions closely when dealing with clients with mood disorders to make sure they fulfill their responsibility to establish a therapeutic nurse–client relationship, regardless of the client's mood.

Depressed people also tend to be complainers who reject help. They feel helpless and incompetent, and the nurse can easily become caught up in helping by suggesting ways to fix the problems. Unless the client is in a crisis or is suicidal, the nurse should not try to solve the client's problems. The client often finds some reason why the nurse's solutions would not work: "I have tried that," "It would never work," "I don't have the time to do that," or "You just don't understand." The client's rejection of the nurse's suggestions can make the nurse begin to feel incompetent and to question his or her professional skill. Instead, the nurse should use therapeutic techniques to encourage the client to generate his or her own resolutions to problems. Studies have shown that clients tend to act on plans or solutions they generate rather than those offered by others. Finding their own solutions and acting on them gives clients renewed feelings of competence and self-worth.

In contrast to working with depressed clients, manic clients can be both fun and exhausting because they are so active, chatty, witty, and manipulative. It is easy to overlook their basic needs for food, water, and safety. The grandiose stories may seem humorous, but manic behavior is very serious and can be dangerous to the person and those around him or her.

Helpful Hints for Working With Clients With Mood Disorders

- Remember that the manic person may seem happy, but he or she is suffering inside.
- Put off client teaching until the acute manic phase is resolving.
- Schedule specific short periods of time with a depressed or agitated client to eliminate unconscious avoidance of the client.

INTERNET RESOURCES

Resource	Internet Address
▶ **Cycle of Moods: Bipolar Information Page**	http://www.fotrunecity.com/campus/psychology/781/bipolar
▶ **Emory University Clinical Trials: Mood & Anxiety Disorders**	http://emoryclinicaltrials.com
▶ **Mental Health Disorders: PlanetPsych**	http://www.planetpsych.com/zPsychology_101?Disorders/in
▶ **Bipolar and Other Mood Disorders**	http://www.geocities.com/Hotsprings/4947/moods.html
▶ **Child and Adolescent Mood Disorders**	http://www.mhsource.com/narsad/childhmood.html
▶ **Bipolar Treatment**	http://mhsource.com/bipolar/ect.html
▶ **Manic Depressive Society**	http://www.societymd.org
▶ **Depression Research**	http://mentalhelp.net/depression/research
▶ **Current Opinion in Psychiatry: Journal of World Psychiatry Association**	http://lww.com/store/products?0951-7367
▶ **Bipolar Disorder: Suite 101.com**	http://www.suite101.com/welcome/cfm/mental.health
▶ **Seasonal Affective Disorder**	http://www.ncpamd.com/seasonal.html
▶ **Drug Therapies of Mood Disorders**	http://www.psycom.net/depression.central.drugs.html
▶ **Famous People with Bipolar Disorder**	http://pages.hotbot.com/health/depression/famous_manic
▶ **Guide to Help Patients and Families to Understand Mood Disorders**	http://members.xoom.com/rougesreview

- Do not try to fix the client's problems. Use therapeutic techniques to help him or her find solutions.
- Use a journal to write down feelings of frustration or anger or personal needs to deal with them.
- If a particular client's care is troubling, talk with another professional about the plan of care, how it is being carried out, and how it is working.

➤ KEY POINTS

- Major depression is a unipolar disorder that affects the mood. It robs the person of joy,

Critical Thinking

Questions

1. The charge nurse on a long-term care unit has noticed that the staff member assigned to a particular client with major depression has not approached the client all day, even though one of the interventions planned for this client was to have a consistent staff person spend 5 minutes with her twice per shift. The charge nurse asks why the staff person is ignoring this intervention. The staff person says, "The client hasn't spoken since she was admitted last week, and I get bummed out when I have

to spend time with someone who doesn't even acknowledge me. I go home depressed after spending 5 minutes in her presence, and you want me to do this twice each shift? I'm not going to let this patient pull me down to her level." How can the charge nurse deal with this staff member's response and ensure that the client is getting appropriate care?

2. A 31-year-old client in the manic phase of bipolar disorder has been telling other clients in her partial hospitalization program that she will trade sexual favors for cigarettes. How should the nurse go about assessing why the client has started this behavior? How can the nurse protect the manic client and the other clients?

3. Your 16-year-old son's best friend just dropped off his baseball glove, saying, "Give this to Charlie when he gets home. He has been the best buddy a guy could ever have. You've been cool, too." What do you think is going on with your son's friend? What should you do about this?

4. A client newly diagnosed with bipolar disorder is starting lithium therapy. What baseline assessments must be done before the first dose of lithium? What ongoing assessments accompany lithium therapy? Describe the ongoing documentation needed to assess the client's response to lithium.

self-esteem, and energy and interferes with relationships and occupational productivity. Only 9% of persons with mood disorders exhibit psychosis.

- Symptoms of depression include sadness, lack of interest in previously pleasurable activities, crying, lack of motivation, asocial behavior, and psychomotor retardation (slowed thinking, talking, and movement). Sleep disturbances, somatic complaints, loss of energy, change in weight, and a sense of worthlessness are also seen in unipolar disorders.

- Depression can be masked by agitation, workaholism, substance abuse, risky behaviors, and gambling.

- Studies have found a genetic connection in mood disorders: the incidence of depression is up to three times greater in first-degree relatives; persons with bipolar disorder usually have a blood relative with bipolar disorder.

- A person with bipolar disorder cycles between mania, normalcy, and depression.

The person may also cycle only between mania and normalcy or depression and normalcy.

- A person with mania has a labile mood, is grandiose and manipulative, has high self-esteem, and believes that he or she is capable of anything. The person sleeps little, is always in frantic motion, invades others' boundaries, cannot sit still, and starts many tasks. Speech is rapid and pressured, reflecting the person's rapid thinking, and may be circumstantial and tangential, with features of rhyming punning and flight of ideas. The person shows poor judgment and has little sense of safety needs, thus taking physical, financial, occupational, or interpersonal risks.

- Mood disorders have been shown to be linked to the neurotransmitters serotonin and norepinephrine.

- Kindling involves subclinical seizure activity that once needed a stressor stimulus but that now occurs repeatedly without the need for the stimulus.

- Unipolar disorder is treated with antidepressants. Selective serotonin reuptake inhibitors, the newest type of antidepressants, have the fewest side effects. Tricyclic antidepressants are older, have a longer lag period before reaching adequate serum levels, and are the least expensive.

- Monoamine oxidase reuptake inhibitors are the least used antidepressants because of the risk of hypertensive crisis if the client ingests tyramine-rich foods and fluids. MAOIs also have a lag period before reaching adequate serum levels.

- Lithium is used to treat bipolar disorder. It is helpful for bipolar mania and can partially or completely mute the cycling toward bipolar depression. Lithium is effective in 75% of clients but has a narrow range of safety; thus, ongoing monitoring of serum lithium levels is needed to establish efficacy while avoiding toxicity.

- Lithium has many drug interactions and is contraindicated in several populations: pregnant women; persons with compromised renal function, urinary retention, cardiovascular or brain damage; and persons taking low-salt diets or diuretics. Those taking lithium must have ongoing assessments of renal status and thyroid and liver function tests.

- The person taking lithium must ingest adequate salt and water in the diet to avoid overdosing or underdosing, because lithium salt uses the same postsynaptic receptor sites as sodium chloride does.

- Other antimanic drugs include sodium valproate and carbamazepine (both require baseline and treatment levels to be obtained) and clonazepam, which is also a benzodiazepine.
- For a client with mania, the nurse must monitor food and fluid intake, rest and sleep, and behavior, with a focus of safety, until the antimanic medications can reduce the acute stage of mania and the client can resume responsibility for himself or herself.
- Suicidal ideation means thinking of suicide. Direct suicide is an act designed to end one's life quickly. Indirect suicide is an unconscious, long-term act of life-threatening behavior, such as substance abuse, obesity, indiscriminate sexual activity, hazardous occupations or avocations, or noncompliance with medical treatment.
- Persons with higher rates of suicide than the general population include single people, divorced men, adolescents, the elderly, the very poor or very wealthy, people who live in cities, migrants, students, whites, people with mood disorders, substance abusers, people with medical or personality disorders, and people with psychosis.
- The nurse must be alert to clues to a client's suicidal intent, both overt cues (making threats of suicide) and covert cues (giving away prized possessions, putting his or her life in order, making vague good-byes).
- Conducting a suicide lethality assessment involves determining the degree to which the person has planned his or her death, including time, method, tools, place, person to find the body, reason, and funeral plans.
- Nursing interventions for those at risk of suicide involve keeping the person safe by instituting a no-suicide contract, ensuring close supervision, and removing objects that could be used to commit suicide.
- Some primary nursing responsibilities include reporting any overt or covert suicidal cues, conducting a suicide lethality assessment, establishing a no-suicide contract, and reporting and documentation one's actions.
- Psychiatric nurses have become case managers whose goal is to return the client to mental health in the least amount of time and using the least restrictive means.
- In managed care, the benchmarks of the mental health care monitoring process include necessity and appropriateness, provider competence, efficacy, cost-effectiveness, accessibility, safety, and client satisfaction.

REFERENCES

Abraham, K. (1927). Notes on the psychoanalytic investigation and treatment of manic-depressive insanity and allied conditions. In: *Selected papers on psychoanalysis.* London: Hogarth.

Agency for Health Care Policy and Research Depression Guideline Panel. (1993). *Clinical practice guidelines: depression in primary care.* Publications # 93-0550 & 93-0551. Rockville, Md.: U.S. Dept. of Health and Human Services.

American Psychiatric Association. (2000). *Diagnostic and statistical manual of mental disorders-text revision,* 4th ed. Washington, DC: Author.

Andrews, M. M., & Boyle, J. S. (1999). *Transcultural concepts in nursing care* (3rd ed.). Philadelphia: Lippincott Williams & Wilkins.

Beck, A. (1967a). *Depression: causes and treatment.* Philadelphia: University of Pennsylvania.

Beck, A. (1967b). *Depression: clinical, experimental and theoretical aspects.* New York: Harper & Row.

Beck, A. (1976). *Cognitive therapy and the emotional disorders.* New York: International University.

Beers, M. H., Berkow, R., & Burs, M (Eds.). (1999). *Mood disorders: the Merck manual of diagnosis and therapy,* 17th ed. Whitehouse Station, N.J.: Merck & Co.

Bily, R., & Snell, C. (1998). Caring in a managed care environment—a case study in teamwork. *Journal of Psychosocial Nursing and Mental Health Services, 36*(6), 37–42.

Black, K., Shea, C., Dursun, S., & Kutcher, S. (2000). Selective serotonin reuptake inhibitor discontinuation syndrome: Proposed diagnostic critria. *Journal of Psychiatry and Neuroscience, 25*(3), 256–261.

Bouchard, G. J. (1999). Office management of mania and depression: when patients go to extremes. *Clinician Reviews, 9*(8), 49–71.

Bowlby, J., & Parkes, C. (1970). Separation and loss within the family. In: E. J. Anthony & C. Koupernik (Eds.). *Child in his family.* New York: John Wiley.

Boyd, M. A., & Nihart, M. A. (1998). *Psychiatric nursing: contemporary practice.* Philadelphia: Lippincott.

Charney, E. A., & Weissman, M. M. (1988). Epidemiology of depression and manic syndromes. In A. Georgotas & R. Cancro (Eds.). *Depression and mania.* New York: Elsevier Science Publishing.

Coffey, C. E., & Weiner, R. D. (1990). Electroconvulsive therapy: an update. *Hospital Community Psychiatry 41*(5), 515–521.

Comer, R. J. (1992). *Abnormal psychology.* New York: W. H. Freeman & Co.

DelBello, M. P., Strakowski, S. M., Sax, K. W., McElroy, S. L., Keck, P. E., Jr., West, S. A., & Kmetz, G. F. (1999). Familial rates of affective and substance use disorders in patients with first-episode mania. *Journal of Affective Disorders, 56*(1), 55–60.

Diekstra, R. F. W. (1993). The epidemiology of suicide and parasuicide. *Acta Psychiatrica Scandinavica, 371*(suppl), 9–20.

Engel, G. L. (1964). Grief and grieving. *American Journal of Nursing, 64*(9), 93.

Freud, S. [1917] (1956). Mourning and melancholia. In: *Collected papers,* Vol 4. London: Hogarth.

Gabbard, G. O. (2000). Mood disorders: Psychodynamic aspects. In B. J. Sadock & V. A. Sadock (Eds.). *Comprehensive textbook of psychiatry, Vol. 1* (7th ed., 1328–1338). Philadelphia: Lippincott Williams & Wilkins.

Gold, M. S. (1995). *The good news about depression: breakthrough medical treatments that can work for you.* New York: Bantam Books.

Hamilton, J. (1960). A rating scale for depression. *Journal of Neurology, Neurosurgery, and Psychiatry, 23,* 56.

Hyman, S. E., & Nestler, E. J. (1993). *The molecular foundations of psychiatry.* Washington, DC: APA.

Kaplan, H. I., & Sadock, B. J. (1998). *Synopsis of psychiatry: Behavioral sciences in chemical psychiatry,* 8th ed. Baltimore: Williams & Wilkins.

Kelsoe, J. R. (2000). Mood disorders: Genetics. In B. J. Sadock & V. A. Sadock (Eds.). *Comprehensive textbook of psychiatry, Vol. 1* (7th ed., 1308–1328). Philadelphia: Lippincott Williams & Wilkins.

Keltner, N. L., Folks, D. G., Palmer, C. A., & Powers, R. E. (1998). *Psychobiological foundations of psychiatric care.* Philadelphia: Mosby.

Kübler-Ross, E. (1960). *On death and dying.* New York: Macmillan.

Lindemann, E. (1944). Symptomatology and management of acute grief. *American Journal of Psychiatry, 101,* 141.

McEvoy, R. B. (Ed.). (2000). *Facts and comparisons 2000.* St. Louis: Facts and Comparisons, A Wolters Kluwer Company.

McIntosh, J. L. (1992). Epidemiology of suicide in the elderly. *Suicide and Life-Threatening Behavior, 22*(1), 15–35.

Merriman, S. H. (1999). Monoamine oxidase drugs and diet. *Journal of Human Nutrition and Dietetics, 12*(1), 21–28.

Miklowitz, D. J. (1996). Psychotherapy in combination with drug treatment for bipolar disorder. *Journal of Clinical Psychopharmocology, 16*(2, suppl 1), 56S–66S.

Montano, C. B. (1994). Recognition and treatment of depression in a primary care setting. *Journal of Clinical Psychiatry, 55*(2 suppl), 18–34.

Murphy, G. E. (1994). Suicide and attempted suicide. In: G. Winokur & P. J. Clayton (eds.). *The medical basis of psychiatry,* 2nd ed. Philadelphia: W. B. Saunders.

Murugesan, G. (1994). Electrode placement, stimulus dosing and seizure monitoring during ECT. *Australia & New Zeland Journal of Psychiatry, 28*(4), 657.

Oltmanns, T. F., & Emery, R. E. (1998). *Abnormal psychology,* 2nd ed. Upper Saddle River, N.J.: Prentice-Hall.

Patterson, W. (1983). Evaluation of suicidal patients: the SAD PERSONS scale. *Psychosomatics, 24*(4), 343.

Pliszka, S. R., Sherman, J. O., Barrow, M. V., & Irick, S. (2000). Affective disorder in juvenile offenders: A preliminary study. *American Journal of Psychiatry, 157*(1), 130–132.

Roy, A. (2000). Suicide. In B. J. Sadock & V. A. Sadock (Eds.). *Comprehensive textbook of psychiatry, Vol. 2* (7th ed., 2031–2040). Philadelphia: Lippincott Williams & Wilkins.

Schatzberg, A. F., & Nemeroff, C. B. (1998). *Textbook of psychopharmacology,* 2nd ed. Washington, DC: APA.

Schultz, J. M., & Videbeck, S. L. (1998). *Lippincott's manual of psychiatric nursing care plans* (5th ed.). Philadelphia: Lippincott-Raven.

Shneidman, E. S. (1963). Orientations toward death: subintentioned death and indirect suicide. In: R. W. White (Ed.). *The study of lives.* New York: Atherton.

Shneidman, E. S. (1981). Suicide. *Suicide & Life-Threatening Behavior, 11*(4), 198–220.

Simon, G. E. (1998). Can depression be managed appropriately in primary care? *Journal of Clinical Psychiatry, 59*(suppl 2), 3–8.

Sullivan, H. S. (1953). *The interpersonal theory of psychiatry.* New York: W. W. Norton.

Wilson, B. A., Shannon, M. T., & Stang, C. L. (1999). *Nurses' drug guide.* Stamford, Conn.: Appleton & Lange.

Tecott, L. H. (2000). Monoamine neurotransmitters. In B. J. Sadock & V. A. Sadock (Eds.). *Comprehensive textbook of psychiatry, Vol. 1* (7th ed., 41–50). Philadelphia: Lippincott Williams & Wilkins.

ADDITIONAL READINGS

Cadoret, R. J. (1978). Evidence for genetic inheritance of primary affective disorder in adoptees. *American Journal of Psychiatry, 134,* 463–466.

Freud, S. (1961). *The ego and mechanisms of defense.* New York: International Universities Press.

Jackson, E. N. (1957). *Understanding grief: its roots, dynamics and treatment.* Nashville: Abingdon.

Parkes, C. M. (1972). *Bereavement: studies of grief in adult life.* New York: International Universities Press.

Chapter Review

➤ MULTIPLE-CHOICE QUESTIONS

Select the best answer for each of the following questions.

1. A 45-year-old woman has been pacing and agitated since she was admitted this morning. She is neat, clean, and appropriately dressed, with well-groomed hair. She says she is responsible for her breakup 12 years ago, thinks she is stupid, and knows no one can like her. She yelled at the staff member who asked if she'd like to shower at 11:30 AM. What two behaviors are important to document to track the depth of this client's depression?

    A. Orientation and appearance

    B. Hopelessness and helplessness

    C. Affect and thought processes

    D. Mood and impulse control.

2. Since she refused to shower at 11:30 AM, what is the appropriate next step the staff should take regarding her activities of daily living?

    A. Give her another chance to shower at 6:30 PM, so she can demonstrate her ability to care for herself.

    B. Tell her she will feel better if she showers and changes her clothes.

    C. Leave her alone; she is neat and clean.

    D. Report her refusal to cooperate as an infringement of her daily responsibilities.

3. What are the most common types of side effects from SSRIs?

    A. Dizziness, drowsiness, dry mouth

    B. Convulsions, respiratory difficulties

    C. Diarrhea, weight gain

    D. Jaundice, agranulocytosis.

4. Which class of antidepressants is the treatment of choice for elderly depressed people?

    A. SSRIs

    B. MAOIs

    C. TCA or heterocyclic antidepressants

    D. Atypical antidepressants.

5. Which of the following typifies the speech of a person in the acute phase of mania?

    A. Flight of ideas

    B. Psychomotor retardation

    C. Hesitant

    D. Mutism.

6. What is the rationale for a person taking lithium to have enough water and salt in his or her diet?

    A. Salt dilutes lithium.

    B. Water converts lithium to solute.

    C. Lithium is metabolized in the liver.

    D. Lithium is a salt that has greater affinity for receptor sites than sodium chloride.

7. Identify the serum lithium level for maintenance and safety.

    A. 0.1 to 1.0 mEq/L

    B. 0.5 to 1.5 mEq/L

    C. 10 to 50 mEq/L

    D. 50 to 100 mEq/L.

8. A client says to you, "You are the best nurse I've ever met. I want you to remember me." What is an appropriate response by the nurse?

    A. "Thank you. I think you are special too."

    B. "I suspect you want something from me. What is it?"

    C. "You probably say that to all your nurses."

    D. "Are you thinking of suicide?"

9. A client wears 14 bracelets, 22 necklaces, garish makeup, and bright clothing. When she twirled her skirt in front of the male clients, it was obvious she had no underpants on. The nurse distracts her and takes her to her room to put on underpants. The nurse acted as she did to:

A. Minimize the client's embarrassment about her present behavior.

B. Deter her from dancing.

C. Avoid embarrassing the male clients.

D. Teach her about proper attire.

10. A client at the partial hospitalization program has told you she is desperate to get the money to have a huge birthday bash for herself. She wants everyone to enjoy her birthday. She asks you to help her figure out how to get the money to pay for this event, because she has no job and has reached her limit on her four credit cards. The nurse should:

A. Help her call her credit-card company to see if they will raise her limit.

B. Tell her how great you think she is for wanting to share everything with her peers and the staff.

C. See if there is any money in the coffee account for the program to buy her a cake and soda.

D. Ask her why she feels the need to spend money she does not have to celebrate her birthday.

11. Which of the following can be used in the treatment of bipolar disorder if the client has side effects from taking lithium?

A. Bupropion and clonazepam

B. Mirtazapine and thioridazine

C. Temazepam and tacrine

D. Carbamazepine and valproic acid.

➤ TRUE-FALSE QUESTIONS

Identify each of the following statements as T (true) or F (false). Correct any false statements.

_____ 1. The key difference between symptoms of unipolar depression and bipolar depression is the time cycles of the latter.

_____

_____ 2. Seasonal affective disorder is helped by staying calm in a dark, restful atmosphere.

_____

_____ 3. An agitated person may be manic or depressed.

_____

_____ 4. A person diagnosed with Cushing's syndrome 18 months ago says he has been very sad for the past year. There is no sense documenting this behavior because it is a normal stage of grieving.

_____

_____ 5. People with mania need close monitoring because they are likely to ignore their own safety.

_____

_____ 6. A person who talks about suicide is not likely to do it.

_____

➤ SHORT-ANSWER QUESTIONS

1. Identify four areas that must be included in a patient teaching plan for a client starting lithium treatment.

2. Identify four client statements that would provide covert cues to suicidal ideation.

3. Describe how lithium and anticonvulsant drugs are given for the treatment of mania and how they are titrated.

On her psychiatric rotation, a student nurse who was having marital difficulties selected a client with unipolar depression and psychomotor retardation. After working with this client for a few weeks, she stopped using makeup, began wearing dark clothes, and paid little attention to her grooming. When a concerned faculty member intervened, she said she had been "sad since she started to work with this depressed client who had tried to harm her child." She avoided anything more than a superficial discussion about her behavior. She did admit to selecting this client because she saw her as "a safe person to talk to." She said she had been afraid to talk to a schizophrenic.

Two weeks later the student demonstrated difficulty with succinct thought organization, had little interaction with her peers, and avoided eye contact. Approached again by the faculty member about her deteriorating behavior, the student admitted she was in an unloving marriage, but she said she only had 6 months left in school and could not change how she lived until she graduated. She worked full-time, attended school full-time, took care of a house and family, and believed she could hold things together for 6 months. She refused a referral for free counseling through the student health office or local mental health clinic.

By the end of the semester, she had such difficulty concentrating that she was unsuccessful in meeting her course objectives. She said it was her fear of "going crazy" that precluded her from working with psychotic people. "I didn't want to see myself in them. Instead, I became just like my depressed patient and I can't pull myself out of it." When asked about suicidal ideation, she said, "If I didn't have kids I'd probably consider killing myself, but I could never leave them to be raised by their father. He doesn't pay attention to them."

The student finally agreed to seek help at the mental health clinic. She started taking antidepressants and started psychotherapy. On return to school for the fall semester, her behavior was appreciably better, with a return to her usual energy and affect. The student and the faculty member agreed on a contract to have periodic discussions about her response to clients and her interventions with them. The goals were to help the student avoid personalizing clients' problems, to ensure that personal issues were not affecting her response to her clients, and to discuss client behaviors that she saw or feared in herself and learn to work through these issues.

1. What components should be included in the contract the faculty member set with the student?

2. Identify two nursing diagnoses and expected outcomes for this student.

3. Identify at least two nursing interventions for each priority.

4. How might the other students support their classmate?

Cognitive Disorders

Learning Objectives

After reading this chapter, the student should be able to:

1. Describe the characteristics and risk factors for cognitive disorders.
2. Distinguish between delirium and dementia in terms of symptoms, course, treatment, and prognosis.
3. Apply the nursing process to the care of clients with cognitive disorders.
4. Apply the nursing process to meet the needs of persons who provide care to clients with dementia.
5. Provide education to clients, families, caregivers, and community members to increase knowledge and understanding of cognitive disorders.
6. Evaluate one's own feelings, beliefs, and attitudes with regard to clients with cognitive disorders.

Key Terms

agnosia

Alzheimer's disease

amnestic disorder

aphasia

apraxia

caregiver role strain

confabulation

Creutzfeld-Jakob disease

delirium

dementia

distraction

echolalia

executive functioning

going along

Huntington's disease

Korsakoff's syndrome

palilalia

Parkinson's disease

Pick's disease

reframing

reminiscence therapy

supportive touch

time away

vascular dementia

Cognition involves the brain's ability to process, retain, and use information. Cognitive abilities include reasoning, judgment, perception, attention, comprehension, and memory. These cognitive abilities are essential to a person's ability to make decisions, solve problems, interpret the environment, and learn new information, to name just a few. A cognitive disorder is a disruption or impairment in these higher-level functions of the brain and can have devastating effects on the person's ability to function in daily life, causing him or her to forget family members' names or be unable to perform daily household tasks or manage personal hygiene (Caine & Lyness, 2000).

The primary categories of cognitive disorders are delirium, dementia, and amnestic disorders. These disorders all involve impairment of cognition, but they vary with respect to cause, treatment, prognosis, and effect on the client and family members or caregivers. This chapter will focus on delirium and dementia, with emphasis on the needs of the caregiver.

DELIRIUM

Delirium is a syndrome that involves a disturbance of consciousness accompanied by a change in cognition. Delirium usually develops over a short period of time, sometimes a matter of hours, and fluctuates or changes throughout the course of the day. The client has difficulty paying attention, is easily distracted, is

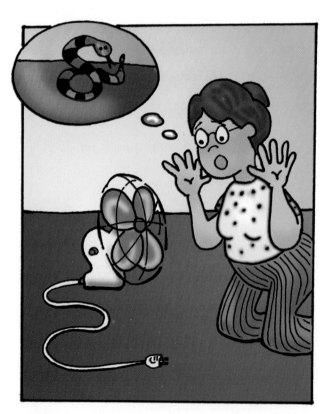

Illusion

disoriented, and may have sensory disturbances such as illusions, misinterpretations, or hallucinations. The banging of a laundry cart in the hallway may be mistaken for a gunshot (misinterpretation), an electrical cord on the floor may appear to be a snake (illusion), or the person may see "angels" hovering above when nothing is there (hallucination). At times, the person also experiences disturbances in the sleep–wake cycle, changes in psychomotor activity, and emotional disturbances such as anxiety, fear, irritability, euphoria, or apathy (DSM-IV-TR, 2000). The accompanying display summarizes the symptoms of delirium.

An estimated 10% to 15% of persons who are in the hospital for general medical conditions are delirious at any given time. Delirium is common in older acutely ill clients. An estimated 30% to 50% of acutely ill geriatric clients become delirious at some time during their hospital stay. Risk factors for the development of delirium include increased severity of physical illness, older age, and baseline cognitive impairment (for example, as seen in dementia; Caine & Lyness, 2000). Children may be more susceptible to delirium, especially when it is related to a febrile illness or certain medications, such as anticholinergics (DSM-IV-TR, 2000).

Cause

Delirium is almost always due to an identifiable physiologic, metabolic, or cerebral disturbance or disease or to drug intoxication or withdrawal. The most common causes of delirium are listed in Box 15-1. Often delirium is due to multiple causes, requiring a careful and thorough physical examination and laboratory tests to pinpoint the causes.

Cultural Considerations

Persons from different cultural backgrounds may not be familiar with the information requested to assess memory, such as the name of former presidents of the United States. Orientation, such as placement and location, may be considered differently in other cultures, and failure to know this information should not be mistaken for disorientation (DSM-IV-TR, 2000). Also, some cultures do not celebrate birthdays, so some people may have difficulty stating their date of birth.

Treatment and Prognosis

The primary treatment for delirium is to identify and treat any causal or contributing medical conditions. Delirium is almost always a transient condition that clears when the underlying causes are successfully treated. However, some causes of delirium, such as head injury or encephalitis, may leave the client with cognitive, behavioral, or emotional impairment, even after the underlying cause resolves.

PSYCHOPHARMACOLOGY

The client with a quiet, hypoactive delirium needs no specific pharmacologic treatment, aside from that indicated for the causative condition. However, many delirious clients show persistent or intermittent psychomotor agitation that can interfere with effective treatment or pose a risk to the client's safety. Sedation to prevent inadvertent self-injury may be indicated. An antipsychotic medication such as haloperidol (Haldol) may be used in doses of 0.5 to 1 mg to decrease agitation. Sedatives and benzodiazepines are avoided because they may worsen the delirium (Caine & Lyness, 2000). The client with impaired liver or kidney function could have difficulty metabolizing or excreting sedatives. The exception is delirium induced by alcohol withdrawal, which is usually treated with benzodiazepines (see Chap. 17).

OTHER MEDICAL TREATMENT

While the underlying causes of the delirium are being treated, the client may also need other supportive physical measures. Adequate, nutritious food and fluid intake will speed recovery. Intravenous fluids or even total parenteral nutrition may be necessary if the client's physical condition has deteriorated and he or she cannot eat and drink.

If the client becomes agitated and threatens to dislodge intravenous tubing or catheters, physical restraints may be necessary so that needed medical treatments can be continued. Restraints are used only when necessary and are kept in place no longer than necessary, because they may increase the client's agitation.

▶ SYMPTOMS OF DELIRIUM

- Difficulty with attention
- Easily distractible
- Disoriented
- May have sensory disturbances such as illusions, misinterpretations, or hallucinations
- Can have sleep–wake cycle disturbances
- Changes in psychomotor activity
- May experience anxiety, fear, irritability, euphoria, or apathy

APPLICATION OF THE NURSING PROCESS: DELIRIUM

The goal of treatment for the client with delirium is to identify and resolve the underlying cause of the delirium. Nursing care focuses on meeting the client's physiologic and psychological needs and maintaining his or her safety. The client's behavior, mood, and level of consciousness can fluctuate rapidly throughout the day. Therefore, the nurse must assess the client continuously to recognize these changes and plan nursing care accordingly.

Box 15-1

> ## MOST COMMON CAUSES OF DELIRIUM

Physiologic or metabolic	Hypoxemia, electrolyte disturbances, renal or hepatic failure, hypo- or hyperglycemia, dehydration, sleep deprivation, thyroid or glucocorticoid disturbances, thiamine or vitamin B_{12} deficiency, vitamin C, niacin, or protein deficiency, cardiovascular shock, brain tumor, head injury, and exposure to gasoline, paint solvents, insecticides, and related substances
Infection	Systemic: sepsis, urinary tract infection, pneumonia Cerebral: meningitis, encephalitis, HIV, syphilis
Drug-related	Intoxication: anticholinergics, lithium, alcohol, sedatives and hypnotics Withdrawal: alcohol, sedatives and hypnotics Reactions to anesthesia, prescription medication or illicit (street) drugs

Compiled from Caine, E. D., & Lyness, J. M. (2000). Delirium, dementia, and amnestic and other cognitive disorders. In B. J. Sadock & V. A. Sadock (Eds.). Comprehensive textbook of psychiatry, Vol. 1 (7th ed., pp. 854–923). Philadelphia: Lippincott Williams & Wilkins, and Ribby, K. J., & Cox, K. R. (1996). Development, implementation, and evaluation of a confusion protocol. Clinical Nurse Specialist, 10(5), 241–247.

Assessment

HISTORY

Because the causes of delirium are often related to a medical illness, alcohol, or other drugs, the nurse obtains a thorough history of these areas. The nurse may need to obtain information from family members if the client's ability to provide accurate data is impaired.

Information about drugs should include prescribed medications, alcohol, illicit drugs, and over-the-counter medications. Although many people may perceive prescribed and over-the-counter medications as relatively safe, combinations of medications or standard doses of medications can produce delirium, especially in the elderly (Mentes, 1995). Box 15-2 lists types of drugs that can cause delirium. Combinations of these drugs significantly increase the risk for delirium.

GENERAL APPEARANCE AND MOTOR BEHAVIOR

The client with delirium often has a disturbance of psychomotor behavior. He or she may be restless and hyperactive, frequently picking at bedclothes or making sudden, uncoordinated attempts to get out of bed. Conversely, the client may have slowed motor behavior, appearing sluggish and lethargic with little movement.

Speech may also be affected, becoming less coherent and more difficult to understand as the delirium worsens. The client may perseverate on a single topic or detail, may be rambling and difficult to follow, or may have pressured speech that is rapid, forced, and usually louder than normal. At times the client may call out or scream, especially at night (Burney-Puckett, 1996).

MOOD AND AFFECT

The client with delirium often has rapid and unpredictable mood shifts. A wide range of emotional responses is possible, such as anxiety, fear, irritability,

---

Box 15-2

> ## DRUGS CAUSING DELIRIUM

Anticonvulsants
Anticholinergics
Antidepressants
Antihistamines
Antipsychotics
Aspirin
Barbiturates
Benzodiazepines
Cardiac glycosides
Cimetidine (Tagamet)
Hypoglycemic agents
Insulin
Narcotics
Propranolol (Inderal)
Reserpine
Thiazide diuretics

Adapted from McEvoy, R. B. (Ed.). Facts and comparisons 2000. St. Louis: Facts and Comparisons, A Wolters Kluwer Company, and Mentes, J. C. A nursing protocol to assess causes of delirium. Journal of Gerontological Nursing, 21(2), 26–30.

anger, euphoria, and apathy. These mood shifts and emotions usually have nothing to do with the client's environment. When the client is particularly fearful and feels threatened, he or she may become combative to defend himself or herself from perceived harm.

THOUGHT PROCESS AND CONTENT

Although the client with delirium has changes in cognition, it is difficult for the nurse to assess these changes accurately and thoroughly. The client's marked inability to sustain attention makes it difficult to assess his or her thought process and content. The content of the client's thoughts is often unrelated to the situation, or speech is illogical and difficult to understand. The nurse may ask how the client is feeling, and he or she will mumble about the weather. Thought processes are often disorganized and make no sense. Thoughts may also be fragmented (disjointed and incomplete). The client may also exhibit delusional thinking, believing that his or her altered sensory perceptions are real.

SENSORIUM AND INTELLECTUAL PROCESSES

The primary, and often initial, sign of delirium is an altered level of consciousness, which is seldom stable and usually fluctuates throughout the day. The client is usually oriented to person but is frequently disoriented to time and place. The client demonstrates a decreased awareness of the environment or situation and instead may focus on irrelevant stimuli, such as the color of the bedspread or the room. The client is also easily distracted by noises, people, or his or her sensory misperceptions.

The client cannot focus, sustain, or shift his or her attention effectively, and there is impaired recent and immediate memory (DSM-IV-TR, 2000). This means the nurse may have to ask questions or provide directions repeatedly; even then, the client may be unable to do what is requested.

The client frequently experiences misinterpretations, illusions, and hallucinations. Misperceptions and illusions are both based on some actual stimulus in the environment: the client may hear a door slam and interpret it as a gunshot, or see the nurse reach for an intravenous bag and think the nurse is about to strike him or her. Examples of common illusions include the client thinking that intravenous tubing or an electrical cord is a snake, or mistaking the nurse for a family member. Hallucinations are most often visual: the client "sees" things for which there is no stimulus in reality, such as an angel or a threatening figure hovering over the bed. Some clients, when more lucid, may be aware that they are experiencing sensory misperceptions. However, others actually believe their misinterpretations are correct and cannot be convinced otherwise.

JUDGMENT AND INSIGHT

The client's judgment is impaired. Clients often cannot perceive potentially harmful situations and cannot act in their own best interest. For example, clients may try repeatedly to pull out intravenous tubing or urinary catheters, causing pain and interfering with the necessary treatment.

Insight depends on the severity of the delirium. The client with mild delirium may recognize that he or she is confused and is receiving treatment and will likely improve. However, the client with severe delirium may have no insight into the current situation.

ROLES AND RELATIONSHIPS

Clients are unlikely to fulfill their roles during the course of the delirium. However, most regain their previous level of functioning and have no longstanding problems with roles or relationships as a result of the delirium.

SELF-CONCEPT

Although delirium has no direct effect on self-concept, the client is often frightened or feels threatened. If the client has some awareness of the situation, he or she may feel helpless or powerless to do anything to change it. If the delirium is due to alcohol or illicit drug use or the overuse of prescribed medications, the client may feel guilt, shame, and humiliation or think, "I'm a bad person; I did this to myself." This would indicate possible long-term problems with self-concept.

PHYSIOLOGIC AND SELF-CARE CONSIDERATIONS

The client with delirium most often experiences a disturbance of the sleep–wake cycle. This may include difficulty falling asleep, daytime sleepiness, nighttime agitation, or even a complete reversal of the usual daytime waking/nighttime sleeping pattern (DSM-IV-TR, 2000). At times, the client may also fail to perceive or ignore internal body cues, such as hunger, thirst, or the urge to urinate or defecate.

Data Analysis

The primary nursing diagnoses for clients with delirium are:

- Risk for Injury
- Acute Confusion.

Additional diagnoses that are commonly selected based on the client assessment are:

- Sensory-Perceptual Alteration
- Altered Thought Processes
- Sleep Pattern Disturbance
- Risk for Fluid Volume Deficit
- Risk for Altered Nutrition: Less Than Body Requirements.

Outcome Identification

Treatment outcomes for clients with delirium may include:

1. The client will be free of injury.
2. The client will demonstrate increased orientation and reality contact.
3. The client will maintain an adequate balance of activity and rest.
4. The client will maintain adequate nutrition and fluid balance.
5. The client will return to his or her optimal level of functioning.

Intervention

PROMOTING THE CLIENT'S SAFETY

Maintaining the client's safety is the priority focus of nursing interventions. Medication should be used judiciously because sedatives may worsen confusion and increase the risk for falls or other injuries (Small, 2000).

The nurse should teach the client to request assistance for activities such as getting out of bed or going to the bathroom. If the client cannot request assistance, close supervision is required to prevent the client from attempting activities he or she cannot perform safely alone. The nurse should respond promptly to the client's call for assistance and check the client at frequent intervals.

If the client is agitated or pulling at intravenous lines or catheters, physical restraints may become necessary. However, the use of restraints may increase the client's fears or feelings of being threatened, so restraints should be used as a last resort. Other strategies should be tried first, such as having a family member stay with the client to reassure him or her.

MANAGING THE CLIENT'S CONFUSION

The nurse should approach the client in a calm manner and speak in a clear, low voice. It is important to give realistic reassurance to the client, such as, *"I know things are upsetting and confusing right now, but your confusion should clear as you get better"* (validating/ giving information). Facing the client while speaking is helpful to capture the client's attention. Explanations should be provided as the client can comprehend, avoiding discussions that are lengthy or too detailed. The nurse should phrase questions or provide directions to the client in short, simple sentences, allowing adequate time for the client to grasp the content of what has been said or to respond to a question. The client should be permitted to make decisions as he or she is able, but the nurse must be careful not to overwhelm or frustrate the client.

The nurse should provide orienting cues when talking with the client, such as calling the client by name and referring to the time of day or the expected activity. For example, the nurse might say, *"Good morning, Mrs. Jones. I see you are awake and look ready for breakfast"* (giving information). It may be necessary to remind the client of the nurse's name and role repeatedly, such as, "My name is Sheila, and I'm your nurse today. I'm here now to walk in the hall with you" (reality orientation). Having orienting objects in the client's room, such as a calendar and clock, is useful in promoting orientation.

Often the use of touch is reassuring to a client and provides a contact with reality. It is important to evaluate each client's response to touch rather than assuming that touch would be welcomed. If the client smiles or draws closer to the nurse when touched, then the client is responding positively to the use of touch. For the client who is fearful, touch may be perceived as threatening rather than comforting, and the client may startle or draw away from the nurse.

Clients with delirium can experience sensory overload, which means there is more stimulation coming into the brain than they can handle. Reducing the stimulation in the environment is helpful because the client is easily distracted and overstimulated. Minimizing environmental noises, including the television or radio, should calm the client. It is also important to monitor the client's response to visitors. Having too many visitors at one time or more than one person talking at a time may increase the client's confusion. The nurse can explain to the visitors that talking quietly, one at a time, will be better tolerated by the client.

The client's room should be well lit to minimize environmental misperceptions. When the client experiences illusions or misperceptions, the nurse corrects the perceptions in a matter-of-fact manner. It is important to validate the client's feelings of anxiety or fear generated by the misperception, but not to reinforce that misperception. For example, if the client hears a loud noise in the hall and asks the nurse, *"Was that an explosion?"* the nurse might respond, *"No, that was a cart banging in the hall. It was really loud, wasn't it? It made me startle a little when I heard it"* (presenting reality/validating feelings).

PROMOTING SLEEP AND PROPER NUTRITION

The nurse needs to monitor the client's sleep and elimination patterns and his or her food and fluid intake. The client may require prompting or assistance to eat and drink adequate amounts of food and fluids. It may be helpful to sit with the client at mealtime or frequently offer fluids. A family member may also be able to help the client improve his or her intake. Assisting the client to the bathroom periodically may be necessary to promote elimination if the client does not make these requests independently.

Promoting a balance of rest and sleep is important if the client is experiencing a sleep pattern disturbance. Discouraging or limiting daytime napping may improve the client's ability to sleep at night. It is also important for the client to have some exercise during the day to promote nighttime sleep. Activities could include sitting in a chair, walking in the hall, or engaging in diversional activities if the client can so.

Evaluation

Usually, successful treatment of the underlying causes of delirium returns the client to his or her previous level of functioning. The client and caregivers or family need to understand what health care practices are necessary to avoid a recurrence of delirium. This may involve monitoring a chronic health condition, careful use of medications, or abstaining from alcohol or other drugs.

> **CLIENT/FAMILY EDUCATION: DELIRIUM**

Monitor chronic health conditions carefully.
Visit physician regularly.
Tell all physicians and health care providers what medications are taken, including over-the-counter medications, dietary supplements, and herbal preparations
Check with physician before taking any non-prescription medication.
Avoid alcohol and recreational drugs.
Maintain a nutritious diet.
Get adequate sleep.
Use safety precautions when working with paint solvents, insecticides, and similar products.

COMMUNITY-BASED CARE

Even when the cause of delirium is identified and treated, the client may not regain all cognitive functions, or problems with confusion may persist. Because delirium and dementia frequently occur together, the client may have dementia. A thorough medical evaluation can confirm the presence of dementia, and appropriate treatment and care can be initiated (see the section that follows).

Once the delirium has cleared and any other diagnoses have been eliminated, it may be necessary for the nurse or other health care professionals to initiate referrals to home health, visiting nurses, or

> **SUMMARY OF NURSING INTERVENTIONS FOR DELIRIUM**

- **Promoting client's safety**
  Teach client to request assistance for activities (getting out of bed, going to bathroom).
  Provide close supervision to ensure safety during these activities.
  Promptly respond to client's call for assistance.
- **Managing client's confusion**
  Speak to client in a calm manner in a clear low voice, using simple sentences.
  Allow adequate time for client to comprehend and respond.
  Allow client to make decisions as much as able.
  Provide orienting verbal cues when talking with client.
  Use supportive touch if appropriate.
- **Controlling environment to reduce sensory overload**
  Keep environmental noise to minimum (television, radio).
  Monitor client's response to visitors; explain to family and friends client may need to visit quietly one on one.
  Validate client's anxiety and fears, but do not reinforce misperceptions.
- **Promoting sleep and proper nutrition**
  Monitor sleep and elimination patterns.
  Monitor food and fluid intake; provide prompts or assistance to eat and drink adequate amounts of flood and fluids.
  Provide periodic assistance to bathroom if client does not make requests.
  Discourage daytime napping to help sleep at night.
  Encourage some exercise during day, like sitting in a chair, walking in hall, or other activities client can manage.

NURSING CARE PLAN FOR A CLIENT WITH DELIRIUM

Nursing Diagnosis

➤ **Acute Confusion** (8.2.2)
The abrupt onset of a cluster of global, transient changes and disturbances in attention, cognition, psychomotor activity, level of consciousness, and/or sleep/wake cycle

ASSESSMENT DATA

- Poor judgment
- Cognitive impairment
- Impaired memory
- Lack of or limited insight
- Loss of personal control
- Inability to perceive harm
- Illusions
- Hallucinations
- Mood swings

EXPECTED OUTCOMES

The client will:
- Be free of injury
- Increase reality contact
- Experience minimal distress related to confusion

IMPLEMENTATION

Nursing Interventions	Rationale
Do not allow the client to assume responsibility for decisions or actions if he or she is unsafe.	The client's safety is a priority. He or she may be unable to discriminate accurately potentially harmful actions or situations.
If limits on the client's behavior or actions are necessary, explain limits, consequences, and reasons clearly, within the client's ability to understand.	The client has the right to be informed of any restrictions and the reasons limits are needed.
Involve the client in making plans or decisions as much as he or she is able to participate.	Compliance with treatment is enhanced if the client is emotionally invested in it.
Give the client factual feedback on his or her misperceptions, delusions, or hallucinations.	The client must be aware of his or her behavior before he or she can take measures to modify that behavior.
In a matter-of-fact manner, convey to the client that others do not share his or her interpretations.	When given feedback in a nonjudgmental way, the client can feel validated for his or her feelings, while recognizing that others do not respond to similar stimuli in the same way.
Assess the client daily or more often if needed for his or her level of functioning.	Clients with organically based problems tend to fluctuate frequently in terms of their capabilities.

continued on page 391

continued from page 390

Allow the client to make decisions as much as he or she is able.

Decision making increases the client's participation and his or her independence and self-esteem.

Assist the client to establish a daily routine, including hygiene, activities, and so forth.

Activities that are routine or part of the client's habits do not require continual decisions about whether or not to perform a particular task.

Adapted from Schultz, J. M., & Videbeck, S. L. (1998). Lippincott's manual of psychiatric nursing care plans (5th ed.). Philadelphia: Lippincott Williams & Wilkins.

a rehabilitation program if the client continues to experience cognitive problems. Various community programs exist to provide care for these persons, such as adult day care or residential care. The client who has ongoing cognitive deficits after an episode of delirium may have difficulties similar to clients with head injuries or mild dementia. The client and family members or caregivers might benefit from support groups to help them deal with the changes in personality and cognitive or motor deficits that remain.

DEMENTIA

Dementia is a mental disorder that involves multiple cognitive deficits, primarily memory impairment and at least one of the following cognitive disturbances: **aphasia** (deterioration of language function), **apraxia** (impaired ability to execute motor functions despite intact motor abilities), **agnosia** (inability to recognize or name objects despite intact sensory abilities), or a disturbance in **executive functioning** (ability to think abstractly and to plan, initiate, se-

CLINICAL VIGNETTE: DEMENTIA

Jack Smith, 74, and his wife Marion, 69, have been living in their home and managing fairly well until lately. The Smiths have two grown children who both live out of town but visit about every 2 months and at holidays and birthdays. Jack has recently had a stroke and entered a rehabilitation facility to try to learn to walk and talk again. Marion wanted to stay at home and wait for his return, but when the children would call to check on her, she would often be crying and confused or frightened. On one visit, they found her looking very tired, dressed in a wrinkled dress that looked soiled. She looked as if she had lost weight and couldn't remember what she had eaten for breakfast or lunch.

Marion's daughter remembered that before her father had the stroke, she noticed that Jack had taken over several routine tasks her mother had always done, such as making the grocery list and planning and helping to cook their meals. Her mother seemed more forgetful and would ask the same questions over and over and often related the same story several times during their visit.

A few weeks after Jack entered the rehab center and Marion was living at home alone, the neighbors found Marion wandering around the neighborhood one morning lost and confused. It was now clear to her children that their mother could not remain in her home alone and take care of herself. It was uncertain how long Jack would need to remain at the rehabilitation center, and they were not sure what his physical capabilities would be when he did return.

Her daughter decided that Marion (and eventually Jack) would come to live with her family. They moved her in with them, but even after getting settled at her daughter's home, Marion continued to be confused and often did not know where she was. She kept asking where Jack was and forgot her grandchildren's names. At times she grew agitated and would accuse them of stealing her purse or other possessions. Later she would always find them. Marion would sometimes forget to go to the bathroom and would soil her clothes. She would forget to brush her hair and teeth and take a bath and often needed help with these activities. When her daughter came home from work in the evening, the sandwich she had made for her mother was often left untouched in the refrigerator. Marion spent much of her time packing her bags to go home and "see Jack."

quence, monitor, and stop complex behavior; DSM-IV-TR, 2000). These cognitive deficits must be sufficiently severe to cause impairment in social or occupational functioning and must represent a decline from the person's previous level of functioning. The accompanying display lists the symptoms of dementia.

Dementia must be distinguished from delirium; if the two diagnoses coexist, the symptoms of dementia remain even when the delirium has cleared. Table 15-1 compares delirium and dementia.

Memory impairment is the prominent early sign of dementia. The client has difficulty learning new material and forgets previously learned material. Initially, recent memory is impaired, such as forgetting where certain objects were placed or forgetting that food is cooking on the stove. In the later stages of dementia, remote memory is affected; the client forgets the names of adult children, his or her lifelong occupation, or even his or her name.

Aphasia usually begins with the inability to name familiar objects or persons, then progresses to speech that becomes vague or empty, with excessive use of terms such as "it" or "thing." The client may exhibit **echolalia** (echoing what is heard) or **palilalia** (repeating words or sounds over and over) (DSM-IV-TR, 2000). Apraxia may cause the client to lose the ability to perform routine self-care activities such as dressing or cooking. Agnosia is frustrating for the client: he or she may look at a table and chairs but be unable to name them. Disturbances in executive functioning are evident as the client loses the ability to learn new material, solve problems, or carry out daily activities such as meal planning or budgeting.

The client with dementia may also underestimate the risks associated with activities or overestimate his or her ability to function in certain situations. For example, the client may cut in front of other drivers, sideswipe parked cars, or fail to slow down when he or she should.

Onset and Clinical Course

When an underlying, treatable cause is not present, the course of dementia is usually progressive. Dementia is often described in stages:

- *Mild*: Forgetfulness is the hallmark of beginning, mild dementia. It exceeds the normal, occasional forgetfulness experienced as part of the aging process. The person has difficulty finding words, frequently loses objects, and begins to experience anxiety about these losses. Occupational and social settings are less enjoyable for the person, and he or she may avoid them. Most people remain in the community during this stage.
- *Moderate*: Confusion is apparent, along with progressive memory loss. The person can no longer perform complex tasks but remains oriented to person and place. Familiar people are still recognized. Toward the end of this stage, the person loses the ability to live independently and requires assistance due to disorientation to time and loss of information such as his or her address and telephone number. The person may remain in the community if adequate caregiver support is available, but some people will move to a supervised living situation.
- *Severe*: Personality and emotional changes occur. The person may be delusional, may wander at night, forgets the names of his or her spouse and children, and requires assistance in activities of daily living (Ribby & Cox, 1996). Most people live in a nursing facility when they reach this stage unless extraordinary support is available in the community.

Cause

There are various causes, although the clinical picture is similar for most of the dementias. Often no definitive diagnosis can be made until a postmortem examination is completed. There is decreased metabolic activity in the brain of the person with dementia (Fig. 15-1), but it is not known whether dementia causes decreased metabolic activity or if decreased metabolic activity results in dementia. A genetic component has been identified for some of the causes of dementia, such as Huntington's disease. Other causes of dementia are related to infections, such as HIV or Creutzfeld-Jakob disease. The most common types of dementia and their known or hypothesized causes are as follows (Caine & Lyness, 2000; DSM-IV-TR, 2000; Small, 2000):

▶ Symptoms of Dementia

- Loss of memory (initial stages, recent memory loss such as forgetting food cooking on the stove; later stages, remote memory loss such as forgetting names of children, occupation)
- Deterioration of language function (forgetting names of common objects such as chair or table, palilalia (echoing sounds), and echoing words that are heard [echolalia])
- Loss of ability to think abstractly and to plan, initiate, sequence, monitor, or stop complex behaviors (loss of executive function): the client loses the ability to perform self-care activities

Table 15-1

Cᴏᴍᴘᴀʀɪsᴏɴ ᴏꜰ Dᴇʟɪʀɪᴜᴍ ᴀɴᴅ Dᴇᴍᴇɴᴛɪᴀ

Indicator	Delirium	Dementia
Onset	Rapid	Gradual and insidious
Duration	Brief (hours to days)	Progressive deterioration
Level of consciousness	Impaired, fluctuates	Not affected
Memory	Short-term memory impaired	Short-, then long-term memory impaired, eventually destroyed
Speech	May be slurred, rambling, pressured, irrelevant	Normal in early stage, progressive aphasia in later stage
Thought processes	Temporarily disorganized	Impaired thinking, eventual loss of thinking abilities
Perception	Visual or tactile hallucinations, delusions	Often absent, but can have paranoia, hallucinations, illusions
Mood	Anxious, fearful if hallucinating; weeping, irritable	Depressed and anxious in early stage, labile mood, restless pacing, angry outbursts in later stages

Adapted from American Psychiatric Association. (2000). *DSM-IV-TR: Diagnostic and statistical manual of mental disorders* (4th ed.). Washington, DC: APA, & Ribby, K. J., & Cox, K. R. (1996). Development, implementation, and evaluation of a confusion protocol. *Clinical Nurse Specialist, 10*(5), 241–247.

- **Alzheimer's disease** is a progressive brain disorder that has a gradual onset but causes an increasing decline in functioning, including loss of speech, loss of motor function, and profound personality and behavioral changes, such as paranoia, delusions, hallucinations, inattention to hygiene, and belligerence. It is evidenced by atrophy of cerebral neurons, senile plaque deposits, and enlargement of the third and fourth ventricles of the brain. The risk of Alzheimer's disease increases with age, and the average duration of the illness from onset of symptoms to death is 8 to 10 years. Dementia of the Alzheimer's type, especially with late onset (after 65 years of age), may have a genetic component. Research has shown linkages to chromosomes 21, 14, and 19 (DSM-IV-TR, 2000).

- **Vascular dementia** has symptoms similar to those of Alzheimer's, but the onset is typically abrupt, followed by rapid changes in functioning, a plateau or leveling-off period,

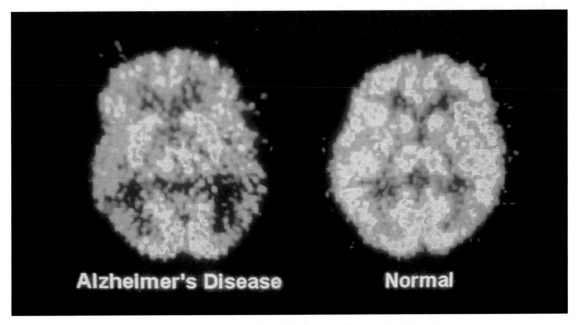

Figure 15-1. Metabolic activity in a subject with Alzheimer's disease (*left*) and in a control subject (*right*). (Courtesy of Monte S. Buchsbaum, MD, The Mount Sinai Medical Center and School of Medicine, New York, New York.)

and then more abrupt changes, another leveling-off period, and so on. Computed tomography (CT scan) or magnetic resonance imaging (MRI) usually shows multiple vascular lesions of the cerebral cortex and subcortical structures as a result of the decreased blood supply to the brain.

- **Pick's disease** is a degenerative disease of the brain that particularly affects the frontal and temporal lobes and results in a clinical picture similar to that of Alzheimer's disease. Early signs include personality changes, loss of social skills and inhibitions, emotional blunting, and language abnormalities. The onset of the disorder is most commonly 50 to 60 years of age, and death occurs in 2 to 5 years.

- **Creutzfeld-Jakob disease** is a central nervous system disorder that typically develops in adults ages 40 to 60 years and involves altered vision, loss of coordination or abnormal movements, and dementia that usually progresses rapidly over the course of a few months. The encephalopathy is caused by an infectious particle that is resistant to boiling, some disinfectants (such as formalin and alcohol), and ultraviolet radiation, but it can be inactivated by pressured autoclaving or bleach.

- Dementia can be due to HIV disease. Dementia and other neurologic problems result from the direct invasion of nervous tissue by HIV and from other illnesses that can be present in AIDS, such as toxoplasmosis or cytomegalovirus. This type of dementia can result in a wide variety of symptoms, ranging from mild sensory impairment to gross memory and cognitive deficits to severe muscle dysfunction.

- **Parkinson's disease** is a slowly progressive neurologic condition characterized by tremor, rigidity, bradykinesia, and postural instability. It results from loss of neurons of the basal ganglia. Dementia has been reported in approximately 20% to 60% of persons with Parkinson's disease and is characterized by cognitive and motor slowing, impaired memory, and impaired executive functioning.

- **Huntington's disease** is an inherited, dominant gene disease that primarily involves cerebral atrophy, demyelination, and enlargement of the ventricles of the brain. Initially, there are choreiform movements that are continuous during waking hours and involve facial contortions, twisting, turning, and tongue movements. Personality

changes are the initial psychosocial manifestations, followed by memory loss, decreased intellectual functioning, and other signs of dementia. The disease begins in the late 30s or early 40s and may last 10 to 20 years or more before death.

- Dementia due to head trauma develops as a direct pathophysiologic consequence of head trauma. The degree and type of cognitive impairment and behavioral disturbances depend on the location and extent of the brain injury. When it occurs in the context of a single injury, this dementia is usually stable rather than progressive. However, repeated head injury (for example, from boxing) may lead to progressive dementia.

An estimated 5 million people in the United States have moderate to severe dementia from various causes (Alzheimer's Association, 1999). The prevalence of dementia rises with age. The estimated prevalence of moderate to severe dementia in persons older than 65 is about 5%. Dementia of the Alzheimer's type is most common type of dementia in North America, Scandinavia, and Europe, whereas vascular dementia is more prevalent in Russia and Japan. Dementia of the Alzheimer's type is more common in women; vascular dementia is more common in men.

Cultural Considerations

For persons from other cultures, the questions used on many assessment tools for dementia may be difficult or impossible to answer, such as the names of former presidents of the United States. The nurse must be aware of the differences in the person's knowledge base to avoid drawing an erroneous conclusion.

The nurse must be aware of different perspectives and beliefs about elderly family members. In many Eastern countries and among Native Americans, elders hold a position of authority, respect, power, and decision making for the family that does not change because they have memory loss or confusion. Other family members may be reluctant, for fear of seeming disrespectful, to make decisions or plans for the elder with dementia. The nurse must work with family members to accomplish goals without making them feel they have betrayed the revered elder.

Treatment and Prognosis

Whenever possible, the underlying cause of dementia is identified so that treatment can be instituted. For example, the progress of vascular dementia, the second most common type of dementia, may be halted with appropriate treatment of the underlying vascular condition (for example, changes in diet, exercise, control of hypertension or diabetes). Improvement of cerebral blood flow may arrest the progress of vascular dementia in some people (Caine & Lyness, 2000).

The prognosis for the progressive types of dementia may vary, as described above, but all involve progressive deterioration of the person's physical and mental abilities until death. Typically, in the latter stages, the client has minimal cognitive and motor function, is totally dependent on the caregiver for daily care, and is unaware of his or her surroundings or the people in the environment. The client may be totally uncommunicative or may make sounds or attempts to verbalize that are unintelligible.

PSYCHOPHARMACOLOGY

For degenerative dementias, no direct therapies have been found to reverse or retard the fundamental pathophysiologic processes (Caine & Lyness, 2000). Levels of numerous neurotransmitters, such as acetylcholine, dopamine, norepinephrine, and serotonin, are decreased in dementia. This has led to attempts at replenishment therapy with acetylcholine precursors, cholinergic agonists, and cholinesterase inhibitors. Tacrine (Cognex), a cholinergic agonist, and donepezil (Aricept), a cholinesterase inhibitor, have shown modest therapeutic effects, slowing the progress of dementia for a period of time (Table 15-2). However, the overall course of the disease remains unaffected. Tacrine causes an elevation of liver enzymes in about 50% of the clients using this medication; therefore, liver function is assessed every 1 to 2 weeks.

Clients with dementia demonstrate a broad range of behaviors that can be treated symptomatically. Doses of medications are one-half to two-thirds lower than usually prescribed (Caine & Lyness, 2000). Antidepressants are effective for significant depressive symptoms. Antipsychotics such as haloperidol (Haldol) may be used to manage psychotic symptoms of delusions, hallucinations, or paranoia. Lithium carbonate, carbamazepine (Tegretol), and valproic acid (Depakote) help to stabilize affective lability and diminish aggressive outbursts. Benzodiazepines are used cautiously because they may cause delirium and can worsen the client's already compromised

cognitive abilities. These medications are discussed in Chapter 4.

SELF-AWARENESS ISSUES

Working with and caring for clients with dementia can be exhausting and frustrating for both the nurse and the caregiver. Teaching is a fundamental role for nurses, but with clients with dementia, teaching can be especially challenging and frustrating. Clients do not retain explanations or instructions, so the nurse must repeat the same things over and over again. The nurse must be careful not to lose patience with these clients and must not give up on them. The nurse may begin to feel that it does no good to repeat instructions or explanations because the client does not understand or remember them. The nurse must discuss these frustrations with others to avoid conveying negative feelings to clients and families, or experiencing professional and personal burnout.

Nurses may get little or no positive response or feedback from clients with dementia. It can be difficult for the nurse to deal with feelings about caring for people who will never "get better and go home." As the dementia progresses, it may seem as if the client is not hearing or responding to anything the nurse does. It is sad and frustrating for the nurse to see clients decline and eventually lose their abilities to manage basic self-care activities and interaction with others. It can be difficult to remain positive and supportive to the client and family when the outcome looks so bleak. In addition, the progressive decline of the client may last months or years, adding to the frustration and sadness. The nurse may need to deal with personal feelings of depression and grief as the dementia progresses; this can be done by discussing the situation with colleagues or even a counselor.

Helpful Hints for Working With Clients With Dementia

- Remember how important it is to provide dignity for the client and family as the client's life ends.

Table 15-2

DRUGS USED TO TREAT DEMENTIA

Name	Dosage Range and Route	Special Considerations
Tacrine (Cognex)	40–160 mg orally per day divided into 4 doses	Monitor liver enzymes for hepatoxic effects. May cause GI upset, flulike symptoms.
Donepezil (Aricept)	5–10 mg orally per day	Monitor for nausea, diarrhea, insomnia. Test stool periodically for GI bleeding.

- Remember that death is the last stage of life. The nurse can provide emotional support for the client and family during this period.
- The caring, patience, and support the nurse offers may go unnoticed by the client but will mean a great deal to the family for a long time.

APPLICATION OF THE NURSING PROCESS: DEMENTIA

This section will focus on caring for clients with progressive dementia, because that is seen most commonly. These guidelines can be used as indicated for clients with dementia that is not progressive.

Assessment

The assessment process may seem confusing and complicated to the client with dementia. He or she may not know, or may forget, the purpose of the interview. The nurse provides simple explanations as often as the client needs them, such as, "I'm asking these questions so the staff can see how your health is." The client may become confused or tire easily, so frequent breaks in the interview may be needed. It helps to ask simple rather than compound questions and to allow the client ample time to answer.

The Folstein Mini-Mental State Exam (Box 15-3) is an example of a short instrument that provides information about the client's ability to recall facts, follow directions, and process abstract information. It does not replace a thorough assessment, but it gives a cursory evaluation of the client's abilities.

HISTORY

The client may be unable to provide an accurate and thorough history of the onset of problems, considering the impairment of recent memory. Interviews with family, friends, or caregivers may be necessary to obtain data.

GENERAL APPEARANCE AND MOTOR BEHAVIOR

The client's ability to carry on meaningful conversation is progressively impaired over time. Aphasia is seen when the client cannot name familiar objects or persons. The client's conversation becomes repetitive, often perseverating on one idea. Eventually, the client's speech may become slurred, followed by a total loss of language function.

The initial finding with regard to motor behavior is the loss of abilities to perform familiar tasks (apraxia), such as dressing or combing one's hair, al-

though the client's actual motor abilities are intact. The client cannot imitate the task when it is demonstrated for him or her. In the severe stage, the client may experience a gait disturbance that makes unassisted ambulation unsafe, if not impossible.

Some clients with dementia show uninhibited behavior, including making inappropriate jokes, neglecting personal hygiene, showing undue familiarity with strangers, or disregarding social conventions for acceptable behavior. This can include the use of profanity or making disparaging remarks about others, when the client had never displayed these behaviors before.

MOOD AND AFFECT

Initially, the client with dementia experiences anxiety and fearfulness over the beginning losses of memory and cognitive functions but may not express these feelings to anyone. The client's mood becomes more labile over time and may shift rapidly and drastically for no apparent reason. Emotional outbursts are common and usually pass quickly. The client may display anger and hostility, sometimes directed at other people. The client begins to demonstrate catastrophic emotional reactions in response to changes in the environment that the client may not accurately perceive or understand, or when the client cannot respond adaptively to a situation. These catastrophic reactions may include verbal or physical aggression, wandering at night, agitation, or other behaviors that seem to indicate a loss of personal control.

The client may display a pattern of withdrawal from the world he or she no longer understands. The client is lethargic, looks apathetic, and pays little attention to the environment or the people in it. He or she appears to lose all emotional affect and appears dazed and listless.

THOUGHT PROCESS AND CONTENT

Initially, the ability to think abstractly is impaired, resulting in loss of the ability to plan, sequence, monitor, initiate, or stop complex behavior (DSM-IV-TR, 2000). The client loses the ability to solve problems or to take action in new situations because he or she cannot think about what to do. The ability to generalize knowledge from one situation to another is lost because the client cannot recognize similarities or differences in situations. These problems with cognition make it impossible for the client to continue working, if he or she is employed. The client's ability to perform tasks such as planning activities, budgeting, or planning meals is lost.

As the dementia progresses, delusions of persecution are common. The client may accuse others of

Box 15-3

➤ FOLSTEIN MINI-MENTAL STATE EXAM

Instructions: Ask all questions in the order listed and score immediately. Record number of total points.

	Maximum Score	Score	Question
Orientation	5	( )	1. Ask the patient to name the year, season, date, day, and month. *(1 point each)*
	5	( )	2. Ask the patient to give his/her whereabouts; state, county, town, street, floor. *(1 point each)*
Registration	3	( )	3. Ask the patient to repeat three unrelated objects that you name. Repeat them and continue to repeat them until all three are learned. *(1 point each)*
Attention & Calculation	5	( )	4. Ask the patient to subtract 7 from 100, stopping after five subtractions, or to spell the word "world" backwards. *(1 point for each correct calculation or letter)*
Recall	3	( )	5. Ask the patient to repeat the three objects previously named. *(1 point each)*
Language	2	( )	6. Display a wrist watch and ask the patient to name it. Repeat this for a pencil. *(1 point each)*
	1	( )	7. Ask the patient to repeat this phrase: "No ifs, ands, or buts!" *(1 point)*
	3	( )	8. Have the patient follow a three-point command, such as "Take a paper in your right hand, fold it in half, and put it on the floor!" *(1 point each)*
	1	( )	9. On a blank piece of paper write "Close your eyes!" Ask the patient to read it and do what it says. *(1 point each)*
	1	( )	10. Ask the patient to write a sentence on a blank piece of paper. It must be written spontaneously. Score correctly if it contains a subject and a verb and is sensible (correct grammar and punctuation are not necessary). *(1 point)*
	1	( )	11. Ask the patient to copy a design you have drawn on a piece of paper (two intersecting pentagons with sides about 1 inch). *(1 point)*
TOTAL SCORE:			*(Maximum score = 30)*

SCORING:	Score of 23 or less	high likelihood of cognitive deficit
	Score of 25–30	normal aging or borderline

Adapted from "Mini-Mental State." A Practical Method for Grading the Cognitive State of Patients for the Clinician. Journal of Psychiatric Research, 12(3):189–198, 1975. The copyright in the Mini Mental State Examination is wholly owned by the MiniMental LLC, a Massachusetts limited liability company.

stealing objects he or she has lost or may believe he or she is being cheated or pursued.

SENSORIUM AND INTELLECTUAL PROCESSES

The client loses intellectual function, which eventually involves the complete loss of his or her abilities. Memory deficits are the initial and essential feature of dementia. Recent and immediate memory is affected first, with an eventual failure to recognize close family members and even oneself. In mild and moderate dementia, the client may make up answers to fill in the memory gaps; this is called confabulation. Agnosia is another hallmark of dementia. Visual spatial relations are lost, often evidenced by the deterioration of the client's ability to write or draw simple objects.

The client's attention span and ability to concentrate are increasingly impaired until the ability to do either is lost. The client has chronic confusion about the environment, other people, and eventually himself or herself. Initially the client is disoriented to time in mild dementia, time and place in moderate dementia, and finally to self as well in the severe stage.

Hallucinations are a common problem. Visual hallucinations are most common and are generally unpleasant. The client is likely to believe the hallucination is reality.

JUDGMENT AND INSIGHT

The client with dementia has poor judgment in light of the cognitive impairment. He or she underestimates risks and unrealistically appraises his or her abilities, resulting in a high risk for injury. The client cannot evaluate situations for risks or danger. For example, he or she may wander outside in the winter wearing only thin nightclothes, not considering this to be a risk.

Insight is limited. Initially, the client may be aware of problems with memory and cognition and may worry that he or she is "losing my mind." However, quite quickly, these concerns over the ability to function diminish, and the client has little or no awareness of the more serious deficits that have developed. It is in this context that the client may accuse others of stealing possessions that have actually been lost or forgotten.

SELF-CONCEPT

Initially, the client may be angry or frustrated with himself or herself for losing objects or forgetting important things. Some clients express sadness at their bodies for getting old and at the loss of functioning that is beginning. Soon, though, the client loses that awareness of self, and it gradually deteriorates until the client can look in a mirror and fail to recognize his or her own reflection.

ROLES AND RELATIONSHIPS

The client's roles and relationships are affected profoundly by dementia. If the client is still employed, work performance suffers even in the mild stage of dementia to the point that work is no longer possible, given the memory and cognitive deficits. The client's role as spouse, partner, or parent deteriorates as the abilities to perform even routine tasks or recognize familiar people are lost. Eventually, the client cannot meet even the most basic needs.

The client's inability to participate in meaningful conversation or social events severely limits relationships. The client quickly becomes confined to the house or apartment, unable to venture out in the world unassisted. Close family members often begin to assume the role of caregiver, which can change previously established relationships. Grown children of the client with dementia experience role reversal—that is, they care for the parent who once cared for them. The spouse or partner may feel as if he or she has lost the previous relationship with the client and now is in the role of custodian for someone who is now a patient.

PHYSIOLOGIC AND SELF-CARE CONSIDERATIONS

Clients with dementia often experience disturbance of the sleep–wake cycle, napping during the daytime and wandering at night. Some clients may ignore internal cues such as hunger or thirst; others have little difficulty with eating and drinking until the dementia is severe. Clients may experience bladder and even bowel incontinence or have difficulty cleaning themselves after elimination. Activities such as bathing and grooming are often neglected. Eventually, clients are likely to require complete care by someone else to meet these basic physiologic needs.

Data Analysis

Many nursing diagnoses can be generated because the effects of dementia on clients are profound; virtually no part of their life is untouched. Nursing diagnoses that are commonly used include the following:

- Risk for Injury
- Sleep Pattern Disturbance
- Risk for Fluid Volume Deficit
- Risk for Altered Nutrition: Less Than Body Requirements
- Chronic Confusion

- Impaired Environmental Interpretation Syndrome
- Impaired Memory
- Impaired Socialization
- Impaired Communication
- Altered Role Performance.

In addition, the nursing diagnoses of Altered Thought Processes and Sensory-Perceptual Alterations would be included for a client with psychotic symptoms. Multiple nursing diagnoses related to the client's physiologic status may also be indicated based on the nurse's assessment, such as alterations in nutrition, hydration, elimination, physical mobility, activity tolerance, and so forth.

Outcome Identification

Treatment outcomes for a client with dementia that is progressive will not involve regaining or maintaining abilities to function. In fact, treatment outcomes need to be revised periodically based on assessment data as the client's overall health status changes. It is common to see outcomes and nursing care that focus on the client's medical condition or deficits. Current literature proposes a focus on psychosocial care that maximizes the client's strengths and abilities for as long as possible. One such model proposed by Taft and colleagues (1997) identifies the therapeutic processes of support, involvement, and validation and the caregiver approach and interventions that can be used with clients with progressive dementia (Box 15-4). The outcomes and interventions that follow are organized according to that model. Treatment outcomes for a client with dementia may include:

1. The client will be free of injury.
2. The client will maintain an adequate balance of activity and rest, nutrition, hydration, and elimination.
3. The client will function as independently as possible, given his or her limitations.
4. The client will feel respected and supported.
5. The client will remain involved in his or her surroundings.
6. The client will interact with others in the environment.

Intervention

Psychosocial models for care of clients with dementia take the approach that each client is a unique person and remains so, even as the progression of the disease blocks the client's ability to demonstrate those unique characteristics. Interventions are based on the belief that the client with dementia has personal strengths. The interventions focus on demonstrating caring, keeping the client involved by relating to the environment and other people, and validating the client's feelings and dignity by being responsive to the client, offering the client choices, and **reframing** (technique in which the nurse offers alternative points of view to explain events) (Taft et al., 1997). This is in contrast to medical models of care that focus on the progressive loss of function and personhood (Tappen et al., 1997).

The following interventions can be used in any setting for a client with dementia. Education for family members caring for the client at home and for professional caregivers in residential or skilled facilities is an essential component of providing safe and

---

Box 15-4

➤ PSYCHOSOCIAL MODEL OF DEMENTIA CARE

Therapeutic Process	Caregiving Approach	Intervention
Support	Social	Empathic caring Supportive touch
Involvement	Social	Providing activities Relating to the environment and others
Validation of client's feelings and dignity	Psychological	Being responsive to client Taking the other's perspective Offering choices Reframing (offering alternative points of view to explain events in the environment)

Taft, L. B., Fazio, S., Seman, D., & Stansell, J. (1997). A psychosocial model of dementia care. Archives of Psychiatric Nursing, 11(1), 18.

▶ SUMMARY OF NURSING INTERVENTIONS FOR DEMENTIA

- **Promoting client's safety and protecting from injury**
  Offer unobtrusive assistance with or supervision of cooking, bathing, or self-care activities.
  Identify environmental triggers to help client avoid them.
- **Promoting adequate sleep, proper nutrition and hygiene, and activity**
  Prepare desirable foods and foods client can self-feed, sitting with client while eating.
  Monitor bowel elimination patterns; intervene with fluids and fiber or prompts.
  Remind client to urinate; provide pads or diapers as needed, checking and changing them frequently to avoid infection, skin irritation, unpleasant odors.
  Encourage mild physical activity such as walking.
- **Structuring environment and routine**
  Encourage client to follow regular routine and habits of bathing and dressing rather than impose new ones.
  Monitor amount of environmental stimulation, and adjust when needed.
- **Providing emotional support**
  Be kind, respectful, calm, and reassuring, and pay attention to client.
  Use supportive touch when appropriate.
- **Promoting interaction and involvement**
  Plan activities geared to client's interests and abilities.
  Reminisce with client about the past.
  If client is nonverbal, remain alert to nonverbal behavior.
  Employ techniques of distraction, time away, going along, or reframing to calm clients who are agitated, suspicious, or confused.

---

supportive care. Examples that apply in a variety of settings are provided.

PROMOTING THE CLIENT'S SAFETY

Safety considerations involve protection from injury, meeting physiologic needs, and managing risks posed by the environment, including internal stimuli such as delusions and hallucinations. The client cannot accurately appraise the environment and his or her abilities and therefore does not exercise normal caution in daily life. For example, the client living at home may forget food cooking on the stove; the client living in a residential care setting may leave for a walk in cold weather without a coat and gloves. Assistance or supervision that is as unobtrusive as possible will protect the client from injury while preserving his or her dignity.

A family member might say, *"I'll sit in the kitchen and talk to you while you make lunch"* (suggesting collaboration) rather than, *"You can't cook by yourself because you might set the house on fire."* In this way, the nurse or caregiver supports the client's desire and ability to engage in certain tasks while providing protection from injury.

The client with dementia may believe that his or her physical safety is jeopardized, and he or she may feel threatened or suspicious and paranoid. These feelings can lead to agitated or erratic behavior that compromises the client's safety. It is important to avoid direct confrontation of the client's fears, as

may be indicated with other clients. The client with dementia may struggle with fears and suspicion throughout the course of the illness. The client's suspicion is often triggered by the presence of strangers, changes in the daily routine, or impaired memory. The nurse must discover and address these environmental triggers rather than confronting the client's paranoid ideas.

For example, if the client reports that his or her belongings have been stolen, the nurse might say, *"Let's go look in your room and see what's there"* and help the client locate the misplaced or hidden items (suggesting collaboration). If the client is in a room with other people and says, *"They're here to take me away!"* the nurse might say, *"Those people are here visiting with someone else. Let's go for a walk and let them visit"* (presenting reality/distraction). The nurse can then take the client to a quieter and less stimulating place, moving the client away from the environmental trigger (Tappen et al., 1997).

PROMOTING ADEQUATE SLEEP AND PROPER NUTRITION, HYGIENE, AND ACTIVITY

The client requires assistance to meet basic physiologic needs. Food and fluid intake needs to be monitored to ensure adequacy. The client may eat poorly, having a limited appetite or being distracted at mealtime. This can be addressed by providing food the client likes, sitting with the client at meals to provide cues to continue eating, having nutritious snacks available whenever the client is hungry, and minimizing noise and undue distraction at mealtime. Clients who have difficulty manipulating utensils may be unable to cut meat or other foods into bite-size pieces. The food should be cut up when it is prepared, not in front of the client, to deflect attention from the client's inability to do so. Food that can be eaten without utensils or finger foods such as sandwiches and fresh fruit may be used.

In contrast, the client may eat too much, even ingesting inedible items. Providing low-calorie snacks, such as carrot and celery sticks, can satisfy the client's desire to chew and eat without unnecessary weight gain.

Enteral nutrition often becomes necessary when the dementia is most severe, although not all families choose to use tube feedings.

Adequate intake of fluids and food is also necessary for proper elimination. The client may fail to respond to cues indicating constipation, so the nurse or caregiver should monitor the client's bowel elimination patterns and intervene with increased fluids and fiber or prompts as needed. Urinary elimination can become a problem if the client does not respond to the urge to void or is incontinent. Reminders to urinate may be helpful when the client is still continent but is not initiating use of the bathroom. Sanitary pads can be used for dribbling or stress incontinence, and adult diapers are indicated for incontinence rather than indwelling catheters. Disposable pads and diapers should be checked frequently and changed promptly when soiled to avoid infection, skin irritation, and unpleasant odors. It is also important to provide good hygiene to minimize these risks.

A balance between rest and activity is an essential component of the daily routine. Mild physical activity such as walking promotes physical health but is not a cognitive challenge. Daily physical activity also helps the client sleep at night. Rest periods should be provided so the client can conserve and regain energy, but extensive daytime napping may interfere with nighttime sleep. The nurse encourages the client to engage in physical activity because the client may not initiate such activities independently, and many clients tend to become sedentary as their cognitive abilities diminish. Clients are often quite willing to participate in physical activities but cannot initiate, plan, or carry out those activities without assistance.

STRUCTURING THE ENVIRONMENT AND ROUTINE

A structured environment and established routines can be reassuring to the client with dementia. Familiar surroundings and routines help eliminate some of their confusion and frustration from memory loss. However, providing routines and structure does not mean forcing the client to conform to the structure of the setting or routines determined by other people. The client should be encouraged to follow his or her usual routine and habits of bathing and dressing rather than imposing new ones. For example, it is important to know whether the client prefers a tub bath or shower, taken at night or in the morning, and to include those preferences in the client's care. Research has shown that attempting to change the client's dressing behavior may even result in physical aggression as the client makes ineffective attempts to resist the unwanted changes (Beck et al., 1997; Potts, Richie, & Kaas, 1996). Monitoring the client's response to daily routines and making needed adjustments are important aspects of care.

The amount of stimulation needs to be monitored and managed based on the client's ability to tolerate stimulation. Generally, the client can tolerate less stimulation when he or she is fatigued, hungry, or stressed. Also, with the progression of dementia, the client's tolerance for environmental stimuli decreases. As this tolerance diminishes, the client will need a quieter environment, with fewer people and less noise or distraction.

PROVIDING EMOTIONAL SUPPORT

The therapeutic relationship between the client and nurse involves "empathic caring" (Tappen et al., 1997), which includes being kind, respectful, calm, and reassuring and paying attention to the client. These are the same qualities used with many different clients in a variety of settings. In most situations, clients give positive feedback to the nurse or caregiver, but clients with dementia often seem to ignore the nurse's efforts and may even respond with negative behavior such as anger or suspicion. This makes it more difficult for the nurse or caregiver to sustain caring behavior with these clients. However, nurses and caregivers must maintain all the qualities of the therapeutic relationship, even when the client does not seem to respond.

Because of their disorientation and memory loss, clients with dementia often become anxious and require a great deal of patience and reassurance (Tappen et al., 1997). Reassurance can be conveyed by approaching the client in a calm, supportive manner, as if the nurse and the client are a team—a "we can do it together" approach. The nurse should reassure the client that he or she knows what is happening and can take care of things when the client is confused and cannot do so. For example, if the client is confused about getting dressed, the nurse might say, "I'll be glad to help you with that shirt. I'll hold it for you while you put your arms in the sleeves" (offering self/suggesting collaboration).

Supportive touch is effective with many clients. Touch can provide reassurance and convey caring when words may not be understood. Holding the hand of the client who is tearful and sad, and tucking the client into bed at night are examples of ways to use supportive touch. As with any use of touch, the nurse must evaluate each client's response to touch. Clients who respond positively to the nurse's touch will smile or move closer toward the nurse. Others may feel threatened by physical touch and look frightened or pull away from the nurse, especially if the touch is sudden or unexpected, or if the client misperceives the nurse's intent.

PROMOTING INTERACTION AND INVOLVEMENT

In a psychosocial model of dementia care, the nurse or caregiver plans activities that reinforce the client's identity and keep him or her engaged and involved in the business of living (Taft et al., 1997). These activities should be tailored to the client's interests and abilities and should not be just routine group activities that "everyone is supposed to do." For example, the client with an interest in history may enjoy documentary programs on television, or the client who likes music may enjoy singing. The client often needs the involvement of another person to sustain attention in the activity and to enjoy the activity more fully. Clients who have long periods without anything to engage their interest are more likely to become restless and agitated. Clients engaged in activities are more likely to be calm and less likely to become restless and agitated.

Reminiscence therapy (thinking about or relating personally significant past experiences) is an effective intervention for clients with dementia (Nugent, 1995; Rentz, 1995). Rather than lamenting that the client is "living in the past," family and caregivers are encouraged to engage in reminiscing with the client. Reminiscing uses the client's remote memory, which is not affected as severely or quickly as recent or immediate memory. Photo albums may be useful in stimulating remote memory, and they provide a focus on the client's past. Sometimes clients like to reminisce about local or national events and talk about their role or what they were doing at the time. In addition to keeping the client involved in the business of living, reminiscence can also build self-esteem as the client talks about accomplishments. Active listening, asking questions, and providing cues to continue will promote the successful use of reminiscence.

Clients have increasing problems interacting with others as the dementia progresses. Initially, verbal language is present, but it may be difficult to understand as words are lost or the content becomes vague. The nurse must listen carefully to the client and try to determine the meaning behind what is being said. The nurse might say, *"Are you trying to say you want to use the bathroom?"* or *"Did I get that right, you are hungry?"* (seeking clarification). It is also important not to interrupt the client or try to finish his or her thoughts. If the client becomes frustrated when the nurse cannot understand his or her meaning, the nurse might say, *"Can you show me what you mean or where you want to go?"* (assisting to take action).

When verbal language becomes less coherent, the nurse should remain alert to the client's nonverbal behavior. When nurses or caregivers consistently work with a particular client, they develop the ability to determine the client's meaning through nonverbal behavior. For example, if the client becomes restless, it may indicate that he or she is hungry if it is close to mealtime, or tired if it is late in the evening. Sometimes it is not possible to determine exactly what the client is trying to convey, but the nurse can still be responsive to the client's feelings. For example, if a client is pacing and looks upset but cannot indicate what is bothering him or her, the nurse might say, *"You look worried. I don't know what's the matter, but let's go for a walk together"* (making an observation/ offering self).

Interacting with clients with dementia often means dealing with thoughts and feelings that are not based in reality but arise from the client's suspicion or chronic confusion. Rather than attempting to explain reality or allay suspicious or angry feelings, it is often useful to employ the techniques of distraction, time away, or going along to reassure the client (Tappen et al., 1995). Distraction involves shifting the client's attention and energy to a more neutral topic. For example, the client may display a catastrophic reaction to the current situation, such as jumping up from dinner and saying, *"My food tastes like poison!"* The nurse might intervene with distraction by saying, *"Can you come to the kitchen with me and find something you'd like to eat?"* or *"You can leave that food. Can you come and help me find a good program on television?"* (redirection/ distraction). The client often calms down when his or her attention is directed away from the triggering situation.

Time away involves leaving the client for a short period of time, then coming back to him or her to re-engage in interaction. For example, the client may get angry and yell at the nurse for no discernible reason. The nurse can leave the client for a short period of time, perhaps 5 or 10 minutes, and then return to the client without making reference to the previous outburst. The client may have little or no memory of the incident and may be pleased to see the nurse on his or her return.

Going along means providing emotional reassurance to the client without correcting his or her misperception or delusional idea. The nurse does not engage in the client's delusional ideas or reinforce them, but nor does he or she deny or confront their existence. For example, the client may be fretful, repeatedly saying, *"I'm so worried about the children. I hope they're OK,"* speaking as though her adult children were small and needed protection. The nurse could reassure the client by saying, *"There's no need to worry; the children are just fine"* (going along), which is likely to have a calming effect on the client. The nurse has effectively responded to the client's worry without addressing the reality of the client's concern. Going along is a specific intervention for clients with dementia and should not be used for clients experiencing delusions who are expected to improve.

The nurse can use reframing techniques to offer the client different points of view or explanations for situations or events that occur. Because of their perceptual difficulties and confusion, clients frequently interpret environmental stimuli as threatening. Loud noises often frighten and agitate them. For example, one client may interpret another's yelling as a direct personal threat. The nurse can provide an alternative explanation, such as, *"That lady has a lot of family problems, and she yells sometimes because she's frustrated"* (reframing). The client with dementia is often reassured by this alternative explanation and becomes less frightened and agitated (Taft et al., 1997).

Evaluation

Treatment outcomes are constantly changing as the disease progresses. For example, in the early stage of dementia, maintaining independence for the client may mean the client gets dressed with minimal assistance. Later on, the client may keep some independence by selecting what foods to eat. In the late stage of dementia, maintaining independence may be accomplished when the client wears his or her own clothing rather than an institutional nightgown or pajamas.

The nurse must assess the client for changes as they occur and revise the outcomes and interventions as needed. When the client is cared for at home, this includes providing ongoing education to family members and caregivers while supporting them as the client's condition worsens. See the sections below on the role of the caregiver and community-based care.

AMNESTIC DISORDERS

Amnestic disorders are characterized by a disturbance in memory that is due to the direct physiologic effects of a general medical condition or the persisting effects of a substance, such as alcohol or other drugs (DSM-IV-TR, 2000). The memory disturbance is sufficiently severe to cause marked impairment in social or occupational functioning and represents a significant decline from the previous level of functioning. Confusion, disorientation, and attentional deficits are common. Persons with amnestic disorders are similar to those with dementia with respect to memory deficits, confusion, and problems with attention, but they do not have the multiple cognitive deficits seen in dementia, such as aphasia, apraxia, agnosia, and impaired executive functions.

Several medical conditions can cause brain damage and result in an amnestic disorder—for example, stroke or other cerebrovascular events, head injury, and neurotoxic exposures, such as carbon monoxide poisoning, chronic alcohol ingestion, and vitamin B_{12} or thiamine deficiency. Alcohol-induced amnestic disorder results from a chronic thiamine or vitamin B deficiency called **Korsakoff's syndrome**. Box 15-5 lists common causes of amnestic disorders.

The main difference between dementia and amnestic disorders is that once the underlying medical cause is treated or removed, the client's condition no longer deteriorates.

Treatment and Prognosis

Treatment of amnestic disorders focuses on eliminating the underlying cause and rehabilitating the client, including the prevention of further medical problems. Some amnestic disorders may improve over

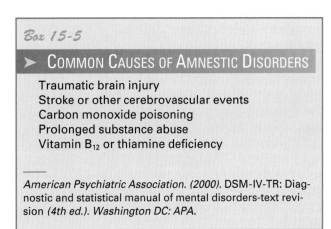

Box 15-5

▶ COMMON CAUSES OF AMNESTIC DISORDERS

Traumatic brain injury
Stroke or other cerebrovascular events
Carbon monoxide poisoning
Prolonged substance abuse
Vitamin B_{12} or thiamine deficiency

American Psychiatric Association. (2000). DSM-IV-TR: Diagnostic and statistical manual of mental disorders-text revision (4th ed.). Washington DC: APA.

time once the underlying cause is stabilized. Other clients may have persistent impairment of memory and attention problems, with minimal improvement; this can occur in cases of chronic alcohol ingestion or malnutrition. Treatment for clients with Korsakoff's syndrome involves abstinence from alcohol. Treatment for the client with amnestic disorder due to a stroke involves rehabilitation and reduction of risk factors for another stroke. Clients with acute-onset amnestic disorder due to a stroke or traumatic brain injury often recover most of their memory with time.

Nursing Diagnoses and Interventions

Nursing diagnoses and interventions are similar to those used when dealing with the memory loss, confusion, and impaired attention abilities of clients with dementia or delirium (see the display on nursing interventions for dementia).

COMMUNITY-BASED CARE

At least half of all nursing home residents have Alzheimer's disease or some other illness that causes dementia. In addition, for every person with dementia in a nursing home, there are two or three with similar impairments being cared for in the community by some combination of family members, friends, and paid caregivers (Tappen et al., 1997).

Programs and services for clients with dementia and their families have increased with the growing awareness of Alzheimer's disease, the increasing numbers of elderly persons in the United States, and the fund-raising efforts for education by celebrities and even the family of former president Ronald Reagan. Home care is available through home health agencies, public health, and visiting nurses. These services offer assistance with bathing, food preparation, transportation, among others. Periodic assessment by the nurse ensures that the level of care provided is appropriate to the client's current needs.

Adult day care centers provide supervision, meals, support, and recreational activities in a group setting. The client may attend the center a few hours a week or full-time on weekdays if needed. Respite care offers in-home supervision for the client so that family members or caregivers can run errands or have social time of their own.

Residential facilities are available for clients who do not have in-home caregivers or whose needs have progressed beyond the care that could be provided at home. These clients usually require assistance with activities of daily living, such as eating and taking medications. Clients in a residential facility are often referred for skilled nursing home placement as the dementia progresses.

Referrals for community-based services can be initiated by the physician, nurse, or family. Families can contact the local public health department or the department of human or social services listed in the phone book. If the client has been admitted to the hospital, social services can also assist in making an appropriate referral.

ROLE OF THE CAREGIVER

Most family caregivers are women (72%) who are either adult daughters (29%) or wives (23%). Husbands account for 13% of all caregivers. The trend toward caring for family members with dementia at home is due to the high costs of institutional care, dissatisfaction with institutional care, and difficulty locating suitable placements for clients with behaviors that are sometimes disruptive and difficult to manage (Small, 2000). Family members identify many other reasons for becoming a primary caregiver, including the desire to reciprocate for past assistance, love and affection, family values or loyalty, duty or obligation, and avoiding feelings of guilt (Carruth, 1996).

The caregiver needs to know about dementia and the care the client requires, which will continually change as the disease progresses. The caregiver may also be dealing with other family members who may or may not be supportive of the caregiver, or who may have differing expectations. Many caregivers have other demands on their time, such as their own family, career, or personal life. The caregiver must deal with his or her feelings of loss and grief as the client's health continually declines (Liken & Collins, 1993).

Caring for a client with dementia can be emotionally and physically exhausting and stressful. Caregivers may need to make drastic changes in their own life to provide care for the family member, such as quitting a job. Caregivers may have young children to care for as well. They often feel exhausted and as if they are "on duty" 24 hours a day. Caregivers caring for a parent may have difficulty acting as a parent to their mother or father (role reversal). They may feel uncomfortable or depressed about having to bathe, feed, or change diapers for their parent.

Role strain is identified when the demands of providing care threaten to overwhelm the caregiver. Indications of role strain include constant fatigue that is unrelieved by rest, increased use of alcohol or other drugs, social isolation, inattention to personal needs, and the inability or unwillingness to accept

▶ Caregiver Education: Dementia

- To help clients cope with memory loss and confusion, encourage them to follow their usual routine and habits of bathing, and dressing rather than imposing new ones.
- Because safety from injury is a risk for clients with dementia, caregivers should encourage as much independence as possible for the client in performing self-care responsibilities but should provide support when engaging in potentially dangerous activities such as cooking or bathing. For example, sit in the kitchen and chat with the client while he or she is cooking, or sit outside the door while the client is bathing rather than doing it for him or her.
- Clients who are bored, alone, and not engaged in any activities tend to become more agitated and irritable. Try to encourage clients to participate in activities that are of interest.
- Clients with dementia frequently believe their physical safety is jeopardized and may feel threatened or suspicious and paranoid. These feelings can lead to agitated or erratic behavior and compromise the client's safety. Avoid direct confrontation of the client's fears or paranoia, but try to anticipate and eliminate the environmental triggers that cause them, such as the presence of strangers, changes in the daily routine, or impaired memory.
- Monitor food and fluid intake to ensure clients are getting adequate fluid and nutrition because these clients often eat poorly, have a limited appetite, are distracted at mealtime, or do not respond to normal cues when thirsty. Independence in eating and drinking should be encouraged as much as possible. Try to avoid feeding the client until this becomes necessary. Sit with the client at meals to provide cues to continue eating, try to minimize noise and undue distraction, prepare desirable and nutritious snacks and food that the client can eat without the use of utensils, such as sandwiches or fresh fruit.
- Promote proper bowel elimination patterns by giving increased fluids and fiber or prompts as needed. Remind the client to urinate, but try to avoid initiating use of the bathroom. For clients who are incontinent, sanitary pads or adult diapers should be used but should be checked frequently and changed promptly when soiled to avoid infection, skin irritation, and unpleasant odors.
- Promote an adequate balance of rest and activity in the client's daily routine by encouraging and assisting clients to engage in mild physical activity such as walking, which helps the client feel better, stimulates bowel elimination, and helps the client sleep better at night. Clients need to rest during the day at intervals but should be discouraged from extensive daytime napping, which may interfere with adequate sleep at night.
- Monitor chronic health problems carefully, have the client visit a physician regularly, and inform all physicians and health care providers about all medications taken, including over-the-counter medications, dietary supplements, and herbal preparations.
- Check with the physician before taking any non-prescription preparation, and make sure the client avoids alcohol and recreational drugs.
- Monitor your own health and needs for socialization, recreation, and respite from the caregiver role to avoid or diminish caregiver role strain.

help from others. The caregiver may feel unappreciated by other family members, as indicated by statements such as, "No one ever asks how *I* am!" (Small, 2000). In some situations, role strain can be a factor in the neglect or abuse of the client with dementia (see Chap. 11).

Supporting the caregiver is an important component of providing care to clients with dementia at home. The caregiver needs to have an ongoing relationship with a knowledgeable health professional; the client's physician can make referrals to other health care providers. Depending on the situation, that person may be a nurse, care manager, or social worker. This person can provide information, support, and assistance during the time that home care is provided. The caregiver needs education about dementia and the type of care the client needs. The caregiver should use the interventions previously discussed to promote the client's well-being, deal with deficits and limitations, and maximize the quality of the client's life. Because the care needed by the client changes as the dementia progresses, this education by the nurse, care manager, or social worker is an ongoing process.

The caregiver needs an outlet for dealing with his or her own feelings. Support groups are available that can help the caregiver express feelings of frustration, sadness, anger, guilt, or ambivalence, all of which are common. Attending a support group regularly also means the caregiver has time that is focused on him or her by people who understand the many demands of caring for a family member with dementia. The client's physician can provide information about support groups, and the local chapter

NURSING CARE PLAN FOR A CLIENT WITH DEMENTIA

Nursing Diagnosis

➤ **Impaired Memory** (8.3.1)
The state in which an individual experiences a temporary or permanent inability to remember or recall bits of information or behavioral skills

ASSESSMENT DATA

- Inability to recall factual information or events
- Inability to learn new material or recall previously learned material
- Inability to determine if a behavior was performed
- Agitation or anxiety regarding memory loss

EXPECTED OUTCOMES

The client will:
- Respond positively to memory cues
- Demonstrate decreased agitation or anxiety
- Use long-term memory effectively as long as it remains intact

IMPLEMENTATION

Nursing Interventions	Rationale
Provide opportunities for reminiscence or recall of past events. This can be done on a one-to-one basis or in a small group.	Long-term memory remains intact even after the client begins to lose recent memory function. Reminiscence is usually an enjoyable activity for the client.
Encourage the client to use written cues such as a calendar, lists, or a notebook.	Written cues decrease the client's need to recall appointments, activities, and so on without assistance.
Keep environmental changes to a minimum. Determine practical and convenient locations for the client's possessions, and return items to this location after use. Establish a usual routine of activities and alter the routine only when necessary.	There is less demand on memory function when structure is incorporated into the client's environment and daily routine.
Provide single-step instructions for the client when instructions are needed.	Clients with memory impairment cannot remember multi-step instructions.
Provide verbal connections between implements and their functions rather than assuming the client will know what is expected of him or her. For example, "Here is a washcloth to wash your face," "Here is a spoon you can use to eat your dessert."	Giving the client an implement while stating its related function is an approach that compensates for memory loss.

continued on page 407

continued from page 406

Integrate reminders of previous events into current interactions, such as, "Earlier you put some clothes in the washing machine. It's time to put them in the dryer."

Providing links with previous behaviors helps the client make connections that he or she may not be able to make independently.

Increase assistance with tasks as needed, but do not rush to do things for the client that he or she can still do independently.

It is important to maximize independent function and to assist the client unobtrusively when memory function has deteriorated further.

Use a matter-of-fact approach when assuming tasks the client can no longer perform. Do not allow the client to work unsuccessfully at any given task for an extended period of time.

It is important to preserve the client's dignity and minimize his or her frustration with progressive memory loss.

Adapted from Schultz, J. M., & Videbeck, S. L. (1998). Lippincott's manual of psychiatric nursing care plans *(5th ed.). Philadelphia: Lippincott-Raven.*

of the National Alzheimer's Disease Association is listed in the phone book. Area hospitals and public health agencies can also help the caregiver locate community resources.

The caregiver should be able to seek and accept assistance from other people or agencies. Often caregivers think that others may not be able to provide care as well as they do, or say they will seek help when they "really need it." Caregivers must maintain their own well-being and not wait until they are exhausted before seeking relief. Sometimes family members disagree about care for the client. The primary caregiver may feel as if other family members should volunteer to help without being asked, but other family members feel that the primary caregiver chose to take on the responsibility and do not feel obligated to help out on a regular basis. Whatever the feelings are among family members, it is important for them all to express their feelings and ideas and participate in caregiving according to their own expectations. Many families need assistance to reach this type of compromise.

Finally, the caregiver needs support for maintaining a personal life. He or she needs to continue to socialize with friends and engage in leisure activities or hobbies, not focus solely on the care of the client. The caregiver who is rested and happy and has his or her own needs met is better prepared to manage the rigorous demands of the caregiver role. Most caregivers need to be reminded to take care of themselves; this is not a selfish act but is really in the best interest of the client in the long run.

➤ KEY POINTS

- Cognitive disorders involve disruption or impairment in the higher functions of the brain and include delirium, dementia, and amnestic disorders.
- Delirium is a syndrome involving a disturbance in consciousness and changes in cognition. It is usually caused by an underlying, treatable medical condition such as physiologic or metabolic imbalances, infections, nutritional deficits, medication reactions or interactions, drug intoxication, or alcohol withdrawal.
- The primary goals in the nursing care of clients with delirium are protection from injury, management of confusion, and meeting the physiologic and psychological needs of the client.
- Dementia is a disease involving memory loss and multiple cognitive deficits, such as language deterioration (aphasia), motor impairment (apraxia), or inability to name or recognize objects (agnosia).
- Dementia is usually progressive, beginning with prominent memory loss (mild stage) and confusion and loss of independent functioning (moderate), followed by total disorientation and loss of functioning (severe).
- Medications used to treat dementia, tacrine and donepezil, slow the progress of the disease for about 6 months. Other medications given to clients with dementia, such

INTERNET RESOURCES

Resource	Internet Address
▶ Alzheimer web	http://dsmallpc2.path.unimelb.edu.au/ad.html
▶ Alzheimer's Disease Education and Referral	http://www.alzheimers.org/
▶ Support and education for patients, caregiver, doctors, and others	http://candid.ion.ucl.ac.uk
	http://www.Alzheimers.com
	http://mayo/common/htm/alzheimers/htm
▶ National Alzheimer's Association	http://www.alz.org
▶ Minneapolis Geriatric Research, Education and Clinical Center (GRECC)	http://www.integritycomm.com/grecc/home.htm
▶ Alzheimer's page, Washington University, St. Louis, MO	http://www.biostat.wustl.edu/alzheimers/submit/caregiv.html

as antipsychotics, antidepressants, or benzodiazepines, help manage symptoms but do not affect the course of dementia.

- A psychosocial model for providing care for people with dementia addresses the client's needs for safety, structure, support, interpersonal involvement, and social interaction.

Critical Thinking

Questions

1. The nurse is working in a long-term care setting with clients with dementia. One of the ancillary staff makes a joke about a client in the client's presence. The nurse tells the staff person that is unacceptable behavior. The staff person replies, "Oh, he can't understand what I'm saying, and besides, he was laughing too. What's the big deal?" How should this nurse respond?

2. A client is newly diagnosed with dementia in the early stages. Can the client make decisions about advance medical directives? Why or why not? At what point in the progression of dementia can the client no longer make quality-of-life decisions?

- Many persons with dementia receive care at home rather than in institutional settings such as nursing homes. Caregivers must be educated and given assistance in caring for clients with dementia.

- Often the care of clients with dementia falls on a caregiver, such as a spouse or son or daughter. This caregiver role can be physically and emotionally exhausting and stressful, contributing to caregiver role strain.

- To deal with the exhausting demands of the caregiver role, family caregivers need ongoing education and support from a health care professional such as a nurse, social worker, or case manager.

- Caregivers need to learn how to meet the client's physiologic and emotional needs and protect him or her from injury. These areas include monitoring the client's health, avoiding alcohol and recreational drugs, ensuring adequate nutrition, scheduling regular check-ups, getting adequate rest, promoting activity and socialization, and helping the client maintain independence as much as possible.

- The therapeutic relationship with clients with dementia is supportive and protective and recognizes the client's individuality and dignity.

REFERENCES

Alzheimer's Association Mid-Iowa Chapter. (1999). Des Moines, IA.

American Psychiatric Association. (2000). *DSM-IV-TR: Diagnostic and statistical manual of mental disorders-text revision* (4th ed.). Washington, DC: American Psychiatric Association.

Beck, C., Heacock, P., Mercer, S. O., Walls, R. C., Rapp, C. G., & Vogelpohl, T. S. (1997). Improving dressing behavior in cognitively impaired nursing home residents. *Nursing Research, 46*(3), 126–132.

Burney-Puckett, M. (1996), Sundown syndrome: Etiology and management. *Journal of Psychosocial Nursing, 34*(5), 40–43.

Caine, E. D., & Lyness, J. M. (2000). Delirium, dementia, and amnestic and other cognitive disorders. In B. J. Sadock & V. A. Sadock (Eds.). *Comprehensive textbook of psychiatry, Vol. 1* (7th ed., pp. 854–923). Philadelphia: Lippincott Williams & Wilkins.

Carruth, A. K. (1996). Motivating factors, exchange patterns, and reciprocity among caregivers of parents with and without dementia. *Research in Nursing & Health, 19*, 409–419.

Liken, M. A., & Collins, C. E. (1993). Grieving: Facilitating the process for dementia caregivers. *Journal of Psychosocial Nursing, 31*(1), 21–26.

Maxmen, J. S., & Ward, N. G. (1995). *Psychotropic drugs: Fast facts* (2nd ed.). New York: W. W. Norton & Co.

McEvoy, R. B. (Ed.). (2000). *Facts and comparisons 2000.* St. Louis: Facts and Comparisons, A Wolters Kluwer Company.

Mentes, J. C. (1995). A nursing protocol to assess causes of delirium. *Journal of Gerontological Nursing, 21*(2), 26–30.

"Mini-Mental State." A Practical Method for Grading the Cognitive State of Patients for the Clinician. *Journal of Psychiatric Research, 12*(3):189–198, 1975. The copyright in the Mini Mental State Examination is wholly owned by the MiniMental LLC, a Massachusetts limited liability company. For information about how to obtain permission to use or reproduce the Mini Mental State Examination, please contact John Gonsalves, Jr., Administrator of the MiniMental LLC, at 31 St. James Avenue, Suite 1, Boston, Massachusetts 02116-(617)587-4215.

Nugent, E. (1995). Try to remember: Reminiscence as a nursing intervention. *Journal of Psychosocial Nursing, 33*(11), 7–11.

Potts, H. W., Richie, M. F., & Kaas, M. J. (1996). Resistance to care. *Journal of Gerontological Nursing, 22*(11), 11–16.

Rentz, C. A. (1995). Reminiscence: A supportive intervention for the person with Alzheimer's disease. *Journal of Psychosocial Nursing, 33*(11), 15–20.

Ribby, K. J., & Cox, K. R. (1996). Development, implementation, and evaluation of a confusion protocol. *Clinical Nurse Specialist, 10*(5), 241–247.

Schultz, J. M., and Videbeck, S. D. (1998). *Lippincott's manual of psychiatric nursing care plans* (5th ed.). Philadelphia: Lippincott-Raven.

Small, G. W. (2000). Alzheimer's disease and other dementias. In B. J. Sadock & V. A. Sadock (Eds.). *Comprehensive textbook of psychiatry, Vol. 2* (7th ed., pp. 3068–3085). Philadelphia: Lippincott Williams & Wilkins.

Taft, L. B., Fazio, S., Seman, D., & Stansell, J. (1997). A psychosocial model of dementia care: Theoretical and empirical support. *Archives of Psychiatric Nursing, 11*(1), 13–20.

Tappen, R. M., Williams-Burgess, C., Edelstein, J., Touhy, T., & Fishman, S. (1997). Communicating with individuals with Alzheimer's disease: Examination of recommended strategies. *Archives of Psychiatric Nursing, 11*(5), 249–256.

SUGGESTED READINGS

Dellasega, C., & Cutezo, E. (1994). Strategies used by home health nurses to assess the mental status of homebound elders. *Journal of Community Health Nursing, 11*(3), 129–138.

Kolanowski, A. M., & Whall, A. L. (1996). Life-span perspective of personality in dementia. *Image, 28*(4), 315–320.

Kozak-Campbell, C., & Hughes, A. M. (1996). The use of functional consequences theory in acutely confused hospitalized elderly. *Journal of Gerontological Nursing, 22*(1), 27–36.

Neelon, V. J., Champagne, M. T., Carlson, J. R., & Funk, S. G. (1996). The NEECHAM confusion scale: Construction, validation, and clinical testing. *Nursing Research, 45*(6), 324–330.

Schofield, I. (1997). A small exploratory study of the reaction of older people to an episode of delirium. *Journal of Advanced Nursing, 25*, 942–952.

Chapter Review

MULTIPLE-CHOICE QUESTIONS

Select the best answer for each of the following questions.

1. The nurse is talking with a woman who is worried that her mother has Alzheimer's disease. The nurse knows that the first sign of dementia is:

   A. Disorientation to person, place, or time

   B. Memory loss that is more than ordinary forgetfulness

   C. Inability to perform self-care tasks without assistance

   D. Variable with different people.

2. The nurse has been teaching a caregiver about donepezil (Aricept). The nurse knows that teaching has been effective by which of the following statements?

   A. "Let's hope this medication will stop the Alzheimer's disease from progressing any further."

   B. "It is important to take this medication on an empty stomach."

   C. "I'll be eager to see if this medication makes any improvement in concentration."

   D. "This medication will slow the progress of Alzheimer's disease for a while."

3. When teaching a client about tacrine (Cognex), the nurse will include which of the following?

   A. Taking tacrine can increase the risk for elevated liver enzymes.

   B. Tacrine causes agranulocytosis in some clients.

   C. The most common side effect is skin rash.

   D. It has no known serious side effects.

4. Which of the following statements by the caregiver of a client newly diagnosed with dementia requires further intervention by the nurse?

   A. "I will remind Mother of things she has forgotten."

   B. "I will keep Mother busy with favorite activities as long as she can participate."

   C. "I will try to find new and different things to do every day."

   D. "I will encourage Mother to talk about her friends and family."

5. A client with dementia is attempting to remove the intravenous tubing from his arm, saying to the nurse, "Get off me! Go away!" The client is experiencing which of the following?

   A. Delusions

   B. Hallucinations

   C. Illusions

   D. Disorientation.

➤ TRUE-FALSE QUESTIONS

Identify each of the following statements as T (True) or F (False). Correct any false statements.

_____ 1. When a client cannot think of the word he or she is looking for, it is called confabulation.

_____

_____ 2. An example of agnosia would be a client looking at a coat but calling it a table.

_____

_____ 3. Apraxia refers to the client's inability to make a decision.

_____

_____ 4. The nurse would expect that a client with aphasia could not make any vocal sounds.

_____

_____ 5. Palilalia refers to the repetition of words or sounds.

_____

_____ 6. The alcohol-induced amnestic disorder called Korsakoff's syndrome indicates a deficiency in protein.

_____

_____ 7. The ability to plan and execute complex behaviors is part of executive functioning of the brain.

_____

_____ 8. Echolalia refers to the imitation of another person's behavior.

_____

➤ FILL-IN-THE-BLANK QUESTIONS

Identify each of the following behaviors as occurring primarily in delirium *or* dementia.

_____ Change in level of consciousness

_____ Sudden, acute confusion

_____ Loss of long-term memory

_____ Tactile hallucinations

_____ Slurred speech

_____ Loss of language abilities

_____ Change in personality traits

_____ Chronic confusion.

Describe each of the following interventions for a client with dementia, and give an example.

Distraction

Time away

Going along

Reminiscence

➤ CLINICAL EXAMPLE

Martha Smith, a 79-year-old widow with Alzheimer's disease, was admitted to a nursing home. The disease has progressed over the past 4 years to the point that she can no longer live alone in her own house. Martha has poor judgment and no short-term memory. She had stopped paying bills, preparing meals, or cleaning her home. She had become increasingly suspicious of her visiting nurse and home health aide, finally refusing to allow them in the house.

After her arrival at the facility, Martha has been sleeping poorly, frequently wandering from her room in the middle of the night. She seems agitated and afraid in the dining room at mealtimes, is eating very little, and has lost weight. If left alone, Martha would wear the same clothing day and night and would not attend to her personal hygiene.

1. What additional assessments would the nurse want to make to plan care for this client?

2. What nursing diagnoses would the nurse identify for this client?

3. Write an expected outcome and at least two interventions for each of the nursing diagnoses.

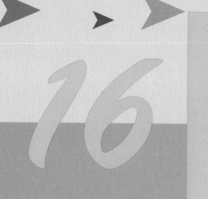

16 Personality Disorders

Learning Objectives

After reading this chapter, the student should be able to:

1. Describe personality disorders in terms of the client's difficulty in perceiving, relating to, and thinking about himself or herself, others, and the environment.

2. Discuss factors thought to influence the development of personality disorders.

3. Apply the nursing process to the care of clients with personality disorders.

4. Provide education to clients, families, and community members to increase their knowledge and understanding of personality disorders.

5. Evaluate one's own feelings, attitudes, and responses to clients with personality disorders.

Key Terms

antisocial personality disorder

avoidant personality disorder

borderline personality disorder

character

cognitive restructuring

confrontation

decatastrophizing

dependent personality disorder

depressive personality disorder

dysphoric

histrionic personality disorder

limit-setting

narcissistic personality disorder

no self-harm contract

obsessive-compulsive personality disorder

paranoid personality disorder

passive-aggressive personality disorder

personality

personality disorders

positive self-talk

schizoid personality disorder

schizotypal personality disorder

temperament

thought-stopping

time-out

Personality can be defined as an ingrained, enduring pattern of behaving and relating to oneself and others that includes one's perceptions, attitudes, and emotions regarding oneself and the world. These behaviors and characteristics are consistent across a broad range of situations and are not easily changed. People are usually not consciously aware of their personality. Many factors influence one's personality: some stem from our biologic and genetic makeup, and others are acquired as one develops and interacts with the environment and other people.

Personality disorders are diagnosed when a person's personality traits become inflexible and maladaptive and significantly interfere with how the person functions in society or cause the person emotional distress. Personality disorders are not usually diagnosed until adulthood, when one's personality is more completely formed, but these maladaptive patterns of behavior can often be traced back to adolescence or early childhood. Although there can be a great deal of variance among clients with personality disorders, for many there is significant impairment in fulfilling family, academic, employment, and other functional roles.

The diagnoses are made when the person exhibits enduring patterns of behavior that deviate from the expectations of the culture in two or more of the following areas:

- Ways of perceiving and interpreting oneself, other people, and events (cognition)
- Range, intensity, lability, and appropriateness of emotional response (affect)
- Interpersonal functioning
- Ability to control impulses or express behavior at the appropriate time and place (impulse control).

Personality disorders are longstanding because personality characteristics are not easily changed. This means that clients with personality disorders continue to behave in their same familiar ways, even when these behaviors cause them difficulties or distress. There is no specific medication that alters a person's personality, and therapy designed to help the client make changes is often long term, with very slow progress. Some people with personality disorders believe their problems stem from other people or the world in general, not recognizing that their own behavior is causing difficulties. For these reasons, people with personality disorders are difficult to treat; this may be frustrating for the nurse and other caregivers, as well as family and friends. There are also difficulties in diagnosing and treating clients with personality disorders because of similarities and subtle differences between the categories or types. There is often overlap between types, and many people with personality disorders also have coexisting major mental illness.

CATEGORIES OF PERSONALITY DISORDERS

The *Diagnostic and Statistical Manual of Mental Disorders-Text Revision* (DSM-IV-TR, 2000) lists personality disorders in a separate and distinct category from other major mental illnesses. They are on axis II of the multiaxial classification system (see Chap. 1). The DSM-IV-TR classifies personality disorders into "clusters," or categories based on the predominant or identifying features of the disorders (Box 16-1):

- Cluster A includes people whose behavior appears odd or eccentric and includes paranoid, schizoid, and schizotypal personality disorders.
- Cluster B includes people who appear dramatic, emotional, or erratic and includes antisocial, borderline, histrionic, and narcissistic personality disorders.
- Cluster C includes people who appear anxious or fearful and includes avoidant, dependent, and obsessive-compulsive personality disorders.

Box 16-1

➤ DSM-IV PERSONALITY DISORDER CATEGORIES

Cluster A: Individuals whose behavior appears odd or eccentric (paranoid, schizoid, and schizotypal personality disorders)

Cluster B: Individuals who appear dramatic, emotional, or erratic (antisocial, borderline, histrionic, and narcissistic personality disorders)

Cluster C: Individuals who appear anxious or fearful (avoidant, dependent, and obsessive-compulsive personality disorders)

Proposed personality disorder categories: depressive and passive-aggressive personality disorders

Adapted from American Psychiatric Association. (2000). DSM-IV-TR: Diagnostic and statistical manual of mental disorders-text revision *(4th ed.). Washington DC: APA.*

Two disorders that are not official personality disorders but are being studied for inclusion as personality disorders (they are included in the DSM-IV-TR) are depressive and passive-aggressive personality disorders.

In psychiatric settings, nurses most often encounter clients with borderline and antisocial personality disorders. Thus, these two disorders will be the primary focus of this chapter. Clients with borderline personality disorder are often hospitalized because their emotional instability may lead to self-inflicted injuries. Clients with antisocial personality disorder may enter a psychiatric setting as part of a court-ordered evaluation or as an alternative to jail.

There will be a brief discussion of the other personality disorders. Most clients with these other personality disorders are not treated in acute care settings for the primary diagnosis of the personality disorder. Nurses may encounter clients with personality disorders in any health care setting or in the psychiatric setting because the client is already hospitalized for another major mental illness.

ONSET AND CLINICAL COURSE

Personality disorders are relatively common, occurring in 10% to 13% of the general population. The incidence is even higher for persons in lower socioeconomic groups or unstable or disadvantaged populations. Fifteen percent of all psychiatric inpatients have a primary diagnosis of personality disorder. Forty percent to 45% of those with a primary diagnosis of major mental illness also have a coexisting personality disorder that significantly complicates treatment. In mental health outpatient settings, the incidence of personality disorder is 30% to 50% (Cloninger & Svrakic, 2000). Clients with personality disorders have a higher death rate, especially as a result of suicide; they also have higher rates of suicide attempts, accidents, and emergency room visits and increased rates of separation, divorce, and involvement in legal proceedings regarding child custody (Gunderson & Phillips, 1995).

Personality disorders have been highly correlated with criminal behavior (70% to 85% of criminals have personality disorders), alcoholism (60% to 70% of alcoholics have personality disorders), and drug abuse (70% to 90% of those who abuse drugs have personality disorders) (Gunderson & Phillips, 1995).

People with personality disorders are often described as "treatment-resistant." This is not surprising, considering that personality characteristics or patterns of behavior are deeply ingrained. It is difficult to make changes in one's personality; if they do occur, they evolve slowly. This slow course of treatment can be very frustrating for family and friends as well as health care providers.

Another barrier in treatment arises because these people often do not perceive their dysfunctional or maladaptive behaviors as a problem—indeed, sometimes these behaviors are a source of pride to the person. For example, a person who is belligerent or aggressive may perceive himself or herself as having a strong personality and being someone who can't be taken advantage of or pushed around. These people often do not see the need to change their behavior and may view changes as a threat.

The difficulties associated with personality disorders persist throughout young and middle adulthood but tend to diminish in the 40s and 50s. Those with antisocial personality disorder are less likely to engage in criminal behavior, but problems with substance abuse and disregard for others' feelings persist. People with borderline personality disorders tend to demonstrate decreased impulsive behavior, increased adaptive behavior, and more stable relationships by age 50. This increased stability and decreased problem behavior can occur even without treatment. Some personality disorders, such as schizoid, schizotypal, paranoid, avoidant, and obsessive-compulsive, tend to remain consistent throughout the person's life (DSM-IV-TR, 2000).

CAUSE

Genetic Factors

Personality develops through the interaction of hereditary dispositions and environmental influences (Cloninger & Svrakic, 2000). Genetic differences account for about half of the variances in temperament traits. **Temperament** corresponds to the biologic processes of sensation, association, and motivation that underlie the integration of skills and habits based on emotion (Cloninger & Svrakic, 2000). The four temperament traits are harm avoidance, novelty seeking, reward dependence, and persistence. People have a genetic predisposition for each of these four traits of temperament that affects their automatic responses to certain situations. These response patterns are ingrained by age 2 to 3 years.

Persons with high harm avoidance exhibit fear of uncertainty, social inhibition, shyness with strangers, rapid fatigability, and pessimistic worry in anticipation of problems. Those with low harm avoidance are carefree, energetic, outgoing, and optimistic. High harm-avoidance behaviors result in maladaptive inhibition and excessive anxiety. Low harm-avoidance behaviors may result in unwarranted optimism and unresponsiveness to potential harm or danger.

A high novelty-seeking temperament results in someone who is quick-tempered, curious, easily bored, impulsive, extravagant, and disorderly. He or she may become easily bored and distracted with daily life, is prone to angry outbursts, and may be fickle in relationships. The person low in novelty seeking is slow-tempered, stoical, reflective, frugal, reserved, orderly, and tolerant of monotony; he or she may adhere to a routine of activities.

Reward dependence defines how persons respond to social cues. Persons high in reward dependence are tender-hearted, sensitive, sociable, and socially dependent. They may become overly dependent on the approval of others and readily take on the ideas or wishes of others without regard for their own beliefs or desires. Persons with low reward dependence are practical, tough-minded, cold, socially insensitive, irresolute, and indifferent to being alone; social withdrawal, detachment, aloofness, and disinterest in others can result.

Highly persistent people are hard-working, persevering, and ambitious overachievers who respond to fatigue or frustration as a personal challenge. They may persevere even when the situation dictates they should change or stop what they are doing. People with low persistence are inactive, indolent, unstable, and erratic. They tend to give up easily when frustrated, and they rarely strive for higher accomplishments.

These four temperament traits are genetically independent dimensions that occur in all possible combinations (Cloninger & Svrakic, 2000). Some of the descriptions above of high and low levels of temperament traits correspond closely with the descriptions of the various personality disorders.

Psychosocial Factors

Although temperament is largely inherited, character is influenced by social learning, culture, and random life events unique to each person (Cloninger & Svrakic, 2000). **Character** is developed over time as one comes into contact with people and situations and confronts challenges, producing concepts about the self and the external world. Three major character traits have been distinguished: self-directedness,

cooperativeness, and self-transcendence (Cloninger & Svrakic, 2000). When fully developed, these character traits define a mature personality.

Self-directedness defines the extent to which a person is responsible, reliable, resourceful, goal-oriented, and self-confident. Self-directed people are realistic and effective and can adapt their behavior to achieve goals. People who are low in self-directedness are blaming, helpless, irresponsible, and unreliable and cannot set and pursue meaningful goals.

Cooperativeness refers to the extent to which a person sees himself or herself as an integral part of human society. Highly cooperative persons are described as empathic, tolerant, compassionate, supportive, and principled. Low-cooperativeness people are self-absorbed, intolerant, critical, unhelpful, revengeful, and opportunistic—that is, they look out for themselves without regard for the rights and feelings of others.

Self-transcendence describes the extent to which a person considers himself or herself to be an integral part of the universe as a whole. Self-transcendent people are spiritual, unpretentious, humble, and fulfilled. These traits are helpful when dealing with suffering, illness, or death. People who are low in self-transcendence are practical, self-conscious, materialistic, and controlling. Such people may have difficulty accepting suffering, loss of control, personal and material losses, and death.

Character matures in a stepwise manner in stages from infancy through late adulthood. Chapter 3 discusses psychological development according to Freud, Erikson, and others. Each stage has an associated developmental task that must be performed for the mature development of the personality. Failure to complete a developmental task jeopardizes the person's ability to achieve future developmental tasks. For example, if the tasks of basic trust is not achieved in infancy, mistrust results and subsequently interferes with the achievement of all future tasks. Box 16-2 summarizes Erikson's developmental tasks.

Box 16-2

> ### ERIKSON'S DEVELOPMENTAL TASKS

Birth to 18 months	Develop basic trust in mother figure and generalize it to others
18 months to 3 years	Gain self-control and independence in the environment
3 to 6 years	Develop a sense of purpose, ability to initiate and direct own activities
6 to 12 years	Achieve self-confidence from significant others, peers, acquaintances
12 to 20 years	Integrate previous tasks into a secure sense of self
20 to 30 years	Form an intense, lasting relationship to another person, cause, institution, or creative effort
30 to 65 years	Achieve life goals, concern for welfare of future generations
65 to death	Derive meaning from own life, positive sense of self-worth

A person's experiences with family, peers, and others in the world can have a significant impact on his or her psychosocial development. Social education in the family creates an environment that can support or oppress specific character development. For example, a family environment where cooperation with others (compassion, tolerance) is not demonstrated or valued does not support development of that trait in children. Likewise, the person who has nonsupportive or difficult peer relationships when growing up has difficulty relating to others and forming satisfactory relationships.

In summary, personality develops in response to inherited dispositions (temperament) and environmental influences (character), experiences unique to each person. Personality disorders result when the combination of temperament and character development produces maladaptive, inflexible ways of viewing oneself, coping with the world, and relating to others.

CULTURAL CONSIDERATIONS

Judgments about personality functioning must take into account the person's ethnic, cultural, and social background (DSM-IV-TR, 2000). Members of minority groups, immigrants, political refugees, or people from different ethnic backgrounds may display guarded or defensive behavior as a result of language barriers or previous negative experiences; this should not be confused with paranoid personality disorder. People with religious or spiritual beliefs such as clairvoyance, speaking in tongues, or evil spirits as a cause of disease could be misinterpreted as having a schizotypal personality disorder.

There is also a difference in how some cultural groups view avoidance or dependent behavior, particularly for women. An emphasis on deference, passivity, and politeness should not be confused with the traits of a dependent personality disorder. Cultures that value work and productivity may produce citizens with a strong emphasis in these areas, and this should not be confused with obsessive-compulsive personality disorder.

Certain personality disorders, such as antisocial and schizoid personality disorders, are most often diagnosed in men. Borderline and histrionic personality disorders are more often diagnosed in women. Social stereotypes about typical gender roles and behaviors can influence diagnostic decisions if clinicians are not aware of such biases (Cloninger & Svrakic, 2000).

TREATMENT

Several treatment strategies are used with clients with personality disorders, based on the type and severity of the disorder or the amount of distress or functional impairment the client experiences. Combinations of medication and group and individual therapy are more likely to be effective than any single treatment (Cloninger & Svrakic, 2000). However, not all people with personality disorders seek treatment, even when significant others in their lives urge them to do so. Typically, persons with paranoid, schizoid, schizotypal, narcissistic, and passive-aggressive personality disorders are least likely to engage in or remain in treatment of any kind. These people see their problems as caused by others rather than due to their own behavior.

Psychopharmacology

Pharmacologic treatment of clients with personality disorders focuses on treatment of the client's symptoms rather than the particular subtype of personality disorder. The four symptom categories that underlie personality disorders are aggression and behavioral dysfunction, affective symptoms and mood dysregulation, anxiety, and cognitive-perceptual distortions, including psychotic symptoms. These four symptom categories relate to the underlying temperaments that distinguish the DSM-IV-TR clusters of personality disorders: high novelty seeking and cluster B disorders correspond to the target symptoms of impulsiveness and aggression; high harm avoidance and cluster C disorders correspond to the categories of anxiety and depression symptoms; and low reward dependence and cluster A disorders correspond to the categories of affective dysregulation, detachment, and cognitive disturbances (Soloff, 1998).

Several types of aggression have been described in people with personality disorders. Aggression may occur in impulsive persons (some with a normal electroencephalogram, some with an abnormal one), in persons who exhibit predatory or cruel behavior, or in persons with organic-like impulsivity, poor social judgment, and emotional lability (Cloninger & Svrakic, 2000). Lithium, anticonvulsant mood stabilizers, and benzodiazepines are most often used to treat aggression. Low-dose neuroleptics may be useful in modifying predatory aggression.

Mood dysregulation symptoms include emotional instability, emotional detachment, depression, and dysphoria. Emotional instability and mood swings respond favorably to lithium, carbamazepine (Tegretol), valproate (Depakote), or low-dose neuroleptics such as haloperidol (Haldol). Emotional detachment, cold and aloof emotions, and disinterest in social relations often respond to selective serotonin reuptake inhibitors (SSRI antidepressants) or atypical antipsychotics, such as risperidone (Risperdal), olanzapine (Zyprexa), and quetiapine (Seroquel). Atypical depression is often treated with SSRIs or monoamine oxidase inhibitor antidepressants (MAOIs), or low-dose antipsychotic medications (Soloff, 1998).

Anxiety seen with personality disorders may be chronic cognitive anxiety, somatic anxiety, or severe acute anxiety. Chronic, ever-present anxiety responds to SSRI and MAOI antidepressants, as does chronic somatic anxiety, or anxiety manifested by multiple physical complaints. Episodes of acute, severe anxiety are best treated with MAOI antidepressants or low-dose antipsychotic medication.

Cognitive-perceptual disturbances include magical thinking, odd beliefs, illusions, suspiciousness, ideas of reference, and low-grade psychotic symptoms. These chronic, low-level, psychotic-like symptoms usually respond to low-dose antipsychotic medications (Cloninger & Svrakic, 2000).

Table 16-1 summarizes drug choices for various target symptoms of personality disorders. These drugs, including side effects and nursing considerations, are discussed in detail in Chapter 2.

Individual and Group Psychotherapy

The type of therapy that is helpful to clients with personality disorders varies according to the type and severity of their symptoms and the particular disorder. Inpatient hospitalization is usually indicated when safety issues are a concern—for example, a person with borderline personality disorder who has suicidal ideas or engages in self-injury. Otherwise, hospitalization is not useful and may even result in dependence on the hospital and staff.

Individual and group psychotherapy goals for clients with personality disorders focus on building trust, teaching basic living skills, providing support, decreasing distressing symptoms such as anxiety, and improving interpersonal relationships (Cloninger & Svrakic, 2000). Relaxation or meditation techniques can help manage anxiety for clients with cluster C personality disorders. Improvement in basic living skills through the relationship with a case manager or therapist can improve the functional skills of persons with schizotypal and schizoid personality disorders.

Table 16-1

DRUG CHOICES FOR SYMPTOMS OF PERSONALITY DISORDERS

Target Symptom	Drug of Choice
Aggression/impulsivity	
Affective aggression (normal)	Lithium
	Anticonvulsants
	Low-dose antipsychotics
Predatory (hostility/cruelty)	Antipsychotics
	Lithium
Organic-like aggression	Cholinergic agonists (donepezil)
	Imipramine (Tofranil)
Ictal aggression (abnormal)	Carbamazepine (Tegretol)
	Diphenylhydantoin (Dilantin)
	Benzodiazepines
Mood dysregulation	
Emotional lability	Lithium
	Carbamazepine (Tegretol)
	Antipsychotics
Atypical depression/dysphoria	MAOIs
	SSRIs
	Antipsychotics
Emotional detachment	SSRIs
	Atypical antipsychotics
Anxiety	
Chronic cognitive	SSRIs
	MAOIs
	Benzodiazepines
Chronic somatic	MAOIs
	SSRIs
Severe anxiety	MAOIs
	Low-dose antipsychotics
Psychotic symptoms	
Acute and psychosis	Antipsychotics
Chronic and low-level psychotic-like symptoms	Low-dose antipsychotics

Adapted from Cloninger, C. R., & Svrakic, D. M. (2000). Personality disorders. In B. J. Sadock & V. A. Sadock (Eds.). *Comprehensive textbook of psychiatry*, Vol. 2 (7th ed., pp. 1723–1764). Philadelphia: Lippincott Williams & Wilkins.

Assertiveness training groups can assist persons with dependent and passive-aggressive personality disorders to have more satisfying relationships with others and to build self-esteem.

Cognitive-behavioral therapy has been particularly helpful for clients with personality disorders (Linehan, 1993). Several cognitive restructuring techniques are used to change the way the client thinks about himself or herself and others—for example, thought stopping, where the client stops negative thought patterns; positive self-talk, which is designed to change the client's negative messages to himself or herself; and decatastrophizing, which teaches the client to view life events more realistically, not as cat-

astrophes. Examples of these techniques are presented later in this chapter.

Table 16-2 summarizes the symptoms of and nursing interventions for personality disorders.

APPLICATION OF THE NURSING PROCESS: ANTISOCIAL PERSONALITY DISORDER

Antisocial personality disorder is characterized by a pervasive pattern of disregard for and violation of the rights of others, with central characteristics of deceit and manipulation of others. This pattern has also been referred to as psychopathy, sociopathy, or

Table 16-2

SUMMARY OF SYMPTOMS AND NURSING INTERVENTIONS FOR PERSONALITY DISORDERS

Personality Disorder	Symptoms/Characteristics	Nursing Interventions
Paranoid	Mistrust and suspicions of others, guarded, restricted affect	Serious, straightforward approach; teach client to validate ideas before taking action; involve client in treatment planning
Schizoid	Detached from social relationships; restricted affect; involved with things more than people	Improve client's functioning in the community; assist client to find case manager
Schizotypal	Acute discomfort in relationships; cognitive or perceptual distortions; eccentric behavior	Develop self-care skills; improve community functioning; social skills training
Antisocial	Disregard for rights of others, rules, and laws	Limit-setting; confrontation; teach client to solve problems effectively and manage emotions of anger or frustration
Borderline	Unstable relationships, self-image, and affect; impulsivity; self-mutilation	Promote safety; help client cope and control emotions; cognitive restructuring techniques; structure time; teach social skills
Histrionic	Excessive emotionality and attention-seeking	Teach social skills; provide factual feedback about behavior
Narcissistic	Grandiose; lack of empathy; need for admiration	Matter-of-fact approach; gain cooperation with needed treatment; teach client any needed self-care skills
Avoidant	Social inhibitions; feelings of inadequacy; hypersensitive to negative evaluation	Support and reassurance; cognitive restructuring techniques; promote self-esteem
Dependent	Submissive and clinging behavior; excessive need to be taken care of	Foster client's self-reliance and autonomy; teach problem-solving and decision-making skills; cognitive restructuring techniques
Obsessive-compulsive	Preoccupation with orderliness, perfectionism, and control	Encourage negotiation with others; assist client to make timely decisions and complete work; cognitive restructuring techniques
Depressive	Pattern of depressive cognitions and behaviors in a variety of contexts	Assess self-harm risk; provide factual feedback; promote self-esteem; increase involvement in activities
Passive-aggressive	Pattern of negative attitudes and passive resistance to demands for adequate performance in social and occupational situations	Help client to identify feelings and express them directly; assist client to examine own feelings and behavior realistically

Clinical Vignette: Antisocial Personality Disorder

Steve found himself in the local jail again after being arrested for burglary. Steve had told the police it wasn't breaking and entering; he had his friend's permission to use his parents' home, but they'd just forgotten to leave the key. Steve has a long juvenile record of truancy, fighting, and marijuana use, which he blames on "having the wrong friends." This is his third arrest, and Steve claims the police are picking on him ever since an elderly lady in the community gave him $5,000 when he was out of work. He intends to pay her back when his ship comes in. Steve's wife of 3 years left him recently, claiming he couldn't hold a decent job and was running up bills they couldn't pay. Steve was tired of her nagging and was ready for a new relationship anyway. He wishes he could win the lottery and find a beautiful girl to love him. He's tired of people demanding that he grow up, get a job, and settle down. They just don't understand that he's got more exciting things to do than that.

dyssocial personality disorder. This disorder occurs in about 3% of the general population and is three to four times more common in men than women. In prison populations, about 50% of prisoners have a diagnosis of antisocial personality disorder. Antisocial behaviors tend to peak in the 20s and diminish significantly after age 45 (DSM-IV-TR, 2000).

Assessment

Clients are skillful at deceiving others, so during assessment it helps to check and validate information from other sources.

HISTORY

The onset of antisocial personality disorder is in childhood or adolescence, although the formal diagnosis is not made until age 18. Childhood histories of enuresis, sleepwalking, and syntonic acts of cruelty are characteristic predictors that the disorder will develop. In adolescence, the client may have engaged in lying, tru-

ancy from school, vandalism, sexual promiscuity, and use of drugs and alcohol. Families have high rates of depression, substance abuse, antisocial personality disorder, poverty, and divorce. The client's childhood is often marked by erratic, neglectful, harsh, or even abusive parenting (Gunderson & Phillips, 1995).

GENERAL APPEARANCE AND MOTOR BEHAVIOR

The client's appearance is often normal; he or she may be quite engaging and even charming. Depending on the circumstances of the interview, the client may exhibit signs of mild or moderate anxiety, especially if the assessment was arranged by another person or agency.

MOOD AND AFFECT

Clients often display false emotions chosen to suit the occasion or to work to his or her advantage. For example, a client who is forced to seek treatment instead of going to jail may appear engaging or try to evoke sympathy by sadly relating a story of his or her "terrible childhood." The client's actual emotions are quite shallow.

These clients cannot empathize with the feelings of others, which allows them to exploit others without guilt or remorse. Usually they feel remorse only if they are caught breaking the law or exploiting someone.

THOUGHT PROCESS AND CONTENT

Clients do not experience disordered thoughts, but their view of the world is narrow and distorted. They tend to believe that others are governed by coercion and personal profit, just as they themselves are. They view the world as a cold and hostile place and therefore can rationalize their own behavior. Clichés such as, "It's a dog-eat-dog world" represent the way they believe the world to be. Clients believe they are only taking care of themselves, because no one else will.

> ### Symptoms of Antisocial Personality Disorder
>
> - Violation of the rights of others
> - Lack of remorse for behavior
> - Shallow emotions
> - Lying
> - Rationalization of own behavior
> - Poor judgment
> - Impulsivity
> - Irritability and aggressiveness
> - Lack of insight
> - Thrill-seeking behaviors
> - Exploitation of people in relationships
> - Poor work history
> - Consistent irresponsibility

SENSORIUM AND INTELLECTUAL PROCESSES

The client is oriented, has no sensory-perceptual alterations, and has an average or above-average IQ.

JUDGMENT AND INSIGHT

The client generally exercises poor judgment for a variety of reasons. The client pays no attention to the legality of his or her actions and does not take morals or ethics into account when making decisions. The client's behavior is primarily determined by what he or she wants, and the need is perceived as immediate. In addition to seeking immediate gratification of needs, the client is also impulsive. This impulsivity ranges from simple failure to use normal caution (waiting for a green light to cross a busy street) to the extreme of thrill-seeking behaviors such as driving recklessly on residential streets.

The client lacks insight and almost never sees his or her actions as the cause of his or her problems. It is always someone else's fault: some source external to the client is responsible for his or her situation or behavior.

SELF-CONCEPT

Superficially, the client appears confident, self-assured, and accomplished, perhaps even flip or arrogant. The client feels fearless, disregards his or her own vulnerability, and usually believes he or she cannot be caught in the lies, deceit, or illegal actions. The client may be described as egocentric (believing the world revolves around himself or herself), but actually the client's self is quite shallow and empty, devoid of personal emotions. The client cannot make a realistic appraisal of his or her own strengths and weaknesses.

ROLES AND RELATIONSHIPS

The client manipulates and exploits those around him or her. Relationships are viewed as serving the needs of the client and are pursued only for his or her personal gain. The client never thinks about the repercussions to others of his or her actions. For example, a client is caught scamming an elderly person out of her entire life savings. The client's only comment when caught is, "Can you believe that's all the money I got? I was cheated! There should have been more."

Clients are often involved in many relationships, sometimes simultaneously. They may marry and have children, but they cannot sustain long-term commitments. They are usually unsuccessful as a spouse or parent and leave other people abandoned and disappointed. They may readily obtain employment with their skillful use of superficial social skills, but over time they have a poor work history. This may be due to absenteeism, theft, or embezzlement, or they may simply quit because they were bored with working.

Data Analysis

People with antisocial personality disorder generally do not seek treatment voluntarily unless they perceive some personal gain. For example, the client may choose a treatment setting as an alternative to jail or to gain sympathy from an employer, citing stress as a reason for absenteeism or poor job performance. Inpatient treatment settings are not necessarily effective for these clients and may, in fact, bring out their worst qualities.

Nursing diagnoses commonly used when working with clients with antisocial personality disorder include:

- Ineffective Individual Coping
- Altered Role Performance
- Risk for Violence.

Outcome Identification

The focus of treatment is often based in behavioral changes. Although it is unlikely to affect the client's view of the world and others or his or her insight, it is possible for the client to make changes in behavior. Treatment outcomes may include:

1. The client will demonstrate nondestructive ways to express feelings and frustration.
2. The client will identify ways to meet his or her own needs that do not infringe on the rights of others.
3. The client will achieve or maintain satisfactory role performance (e.g., at work, as a parent).

Intervention

THERAPEUTIC RELATIONSHIP AND PROMOTING RESPONSIBLE BEHAVIOR

The nurse must provide structure in the therapeutic relationship, identifying acceptable and expected behaviors and being consistent in those expectations. The nurse must minimize the client's attempts to manipulate and control the relationship.

Limit-setting is an effective technique that involves three steps: stating the behavioral limit (describing the unacceptable behavior), identifying the consequences that will occur if the limit is exceeded, and identifying the behavior that is expected or desired. Consistent limit-setting in a matter-of-fact, non-

> **NURSING INTERVENTIONS FOR THE CLIENT WITH ANTISOCIAL PERSONALITY DISORDER**
>
> • Promoting responsible behavior
>   Limit-setting
>   State the limit.
>   Identify consequences of exceeding the limit.
>   Identify expected or acceptable behavior.
>   Consistent adherence to rules and
>   treatment plan
>   Confrontation
>   Point out problem behavior.
>   Keep client focused on self.
> • Helping clients solve problems and control
>   emotions
>   Effective problem-solving skills
>   Decreased impulsivity
>   Expressing negative emotions, such as anger
>   or frustration
>   Taking time out from stressful situation
> • Enhancing role performance
>   Identifying barriers to role fulfillment
>   Decreasing or eliminating use of drugs and
>   alcohol.

judgmental manner is crucial to the success of this technique. For example, the client may approach the nurse in a flirtatious manner and attempt to gain personal information. The nurse would use limit-setting by saying, *"It is not acceptable for you to ask personal questions. If you continue to do that, I will terminate our interaction. This time needs to be used to work on solving your job-related problems."* The nurse should not become angry and respond to the client in a harsh or punitive manner (Stravynski et al., 1994).

Confrontation is another technique designed to manage manipulative or deceptive behavior. The nurse points out the client's problematic behavior while remaining neutral and matter-of-fact; the nurse avoids responding to the client in an accusatory manner. Confrontation can also be used to keep the client focused on the topic and in the present. The nurse can keep the focus on the client's behavior rather than his or her attempts to justify the behavior (Stravynski et al., 1994). For example:

Nurse: *"You've said you're interested in learning to manage angry outbursts, but you have missed the last three group meetings."*

Client: *"Well, I can tell no one in the group likes me. Why should I bother?"*

Nurse: *"The group meetings are designed to help you and the others, but you can't work on issues if you're not here."*

HELPING CLIENTS SOLVE PROBLEMS AND CONTROL EMOTIONS

The client with antisocial personality disorder has an established pattern of reacting impulsively when confronted with problems. The nurse can teach the client problem-solving skills and help the client practice those skills. Problem-solving skills include identifying the problem, exploring alternative solutions and the related consequences, choosing and implementing an alternative, and evaluating the results. Although the client has the cognitive ability to solve problems, he or she needs to learn a step-by-step approach to dealing with problems. For example, the client's car isn't running, so he stopped going to work. The problem is transportation to work, and alternative solutions might be taking the bus, asking a coworker for a ride, getting the car fixed, and so forth. The nurse can help the client discuss the various options and choose one so that he can go back to work.

Managing emotions, especially anger and frustration, can be a major problem. When the client is calm and not upset, the nurse can encourage him or her to identify sources of frustration, how the client responded to the frustration, and the consequences of those actions. In this way, the nurse can help the client to anticipate stressful situations and learn ways to avoid negative consequences in the future. Taking a time-out, or leaving the area and going to a neutral place to regain internal control, is often a helpful strategy for the client. This helps the client avoid impulsive reactions and angry outbursts when in an emotionally charged situation, regain control of his or her emotions, and engage in constructive problem-solving.

ENHANCING ROLE PERFORMANCE

The nurse should help the client identify specific problems at work or home that are barriers to success in fulfilling his or her roles. Assessing the client's use of alcohol and other drugs is essential when examining role performance, because many clients use or abuse these substances. The client tends to blame others for his or her failures and difficulties, and the nurse must redirect the client from blaming others to examining the source of his or her problems realistically. Referrals to vocational or job programs may be indicated.

Evaluation

The effectiveness of treatment is evaluated based on attainment of outcomes or some progress in these areas. If the client can maintain a job with acceptable performance, meet basic family responsibilities, and avoid committing illegal or immoral acts, then treatment has been successful.

APPLICATION OF THE NURSING PROCESS: BORDERLINE PERSONALITY DISORDER

Borderline personality disorder is characterized by a pervasive pattern of unstable interpersonal relationships, self-image, and affects and marked impulsivity. About 2% to 3% of the general population has borderline personality disorder, and it is five times more common in those with a first-degree relative with the diagnosis. Borderline personality disorder is the most common personality disorder found in clinical settings. It is three times more common in women than men. Under stress, transient psychotic symptoms are common. Eight percent to 10% of persons with this diagnosis commit suicide, and many more suffer permanent damage from self-mutilation (self-inflicted injury such as cutting or burning; DSM-IV-TR, 2000). Typically, recurrent self-mutilation is a cry for help, an expression of intense anger or helplessness, or a form of self-punishment. It is also a means to block emotional pain by inducing physical pain. The client believes he or she is still alive if he or she can experience physical pain in the face of emotional numbing of feelings.

Working with the client with borderline personality disorder can be frustrating. The client may be clinging and asking for help one minute, then angry and acting out, rejecting all offers of help, the next. The client attempts to manipulate staff to gain immediate gratification of needs and at times will sabotage his or her own treatment plan by purposely failing to do what has been agreed on. The client's labile mood, unpredictability, and diverse behaviors can make it seem as if the staff is always "back to square one" with the client.

Assessment

HISTORY

Many of these clients report disturbed early relationships with their parents, often beginning at age 18 to 30 months. Commonly, these clients' early attempts at achieving independence developmentally were met with punitive responses from parents or threats of withdrawal of parental support and approval. In 50% of clients, parental alcoholism and physical or sexual abuse were present. Clients tend to use transitional objects extensively, such as a teddy bear, and this may continue into adulthood. The transitional object is often a favorite item from childhood, when the client felt safe, such as a pillow, blanket, or doll.

GENERAL APPEARANCE AND MOTOR BEHAVIOR

Clients experience a wide range of dysfunction, from severe to mild, and their initial behavior and presentation may vary widely, depending on their present status. When dysfunction is severe, the client may appear disheveled and may be unable to sit still, or may display very labile emotions. In other cases, the initial appearance and motor behavior may seem normal. The client seen in the emergency room threatening suicide or self-harm may look close to being out of control, whereas a client seen in an outpatient clinic may appear fairly calm and rational.

CLINICAL VIGNETTE: BORDERLINE PERSONALITY DISORDER

Sally had been calling her therapist all day, ever since their session this morning. But the therapist hadn't called her back, even though all her messages said this was an emergency. She was sure her therapist was angry at her and was probably going to drop her as a client. Then she'd have no one; she'd be abandoned by the only person in the world she could talk to. Sally was upset and crying as she began to run the razor blade across her arm. As the blood trickled out, she began to calm down. Then her therapist called and asked what the problem was. Sally was sobbing as she told her therapist that she was cutting her arm because the therapist didn't care anymore, that she was abandoning Sally just like everyone else in her life—her parents, her best friend, every man she had a relationship with. No one was ever there for her when she needed them.

> ## SYMPTOMS OF BORDERLINE PERSONALITY DISORDER

- Fear of abandonment, real or perceived
- Unstable and intense relationships
- Unstable self-image
- Impulsivity or recklessness
- Recurrent self-mutilating behavior, or suicidal threats or gestures
- Chronic feelings of emptiness and boredom

- Labile mood
- Irritability
- Polarized thinking about self and others ("splitting")
- Impaired judgment
- Lack of insight
- Transient psychotic symptoms such as hallucinations demanding self-harm.

MOOD AND AFFECT

The client's pervasive mood is **dysphoric**, involving unhappiness, restlessness, and malaise. The client often reports intense feelings of loneliness, boredom, and frustration and feels "empty." He or she rarely experiences periods of satisfaction or well-being. Although there is a pervasive depressed affect, the client's affect is unstable and erratic. The client may become irritable, even hostile or sarcastic, and complain of episodes of panic anxiety. Intense emotions such as anger and rage are experienced but are rarely expressed in a productive or useful way. The client usually is hypersensitive to others' emotions, which can easily trigger emotional reactions in the client. Minor changes may precipitate a severe emotional crisis—for example, when an appointment must be changed from one day to the next. It is common for the client to experience major emotional trauma when the therapist takes a vacation.

THOUGHT PROCESS AND CONTENT

The client's thinking about himself or herself and others is often polarized and extreme, sometimes referred to as splitting. Other people are adored and idealized, even after a brief acquaintance, then quickly devalued if they do not meet the client's expectations in some way. The client has excessive and chronic fears of abandonment, even in normal situations, reflecting his or her intolerance of being alone. The client may also engage in obsessive ruminating about almost anything, without regard to the relative importance of the issue.

The client may experience dissociative episodes (periods of wakefulness when one is unaware of one's actions). Self-harm behaviors often occur during these dissociative episodes, although other times the client may be fully aware of injuring himself or herself. As stated earlier, under extreme stress, the client may develop transient psychotic symptoms, such as delusions or hallucinations.

SENSORIUM AND INTELLECTUAL PROCESSES

The client's intellectual capacities are intact, and the client is fully oriented to reality. The exception is when transient psychotic symptoms occur; during this time, reports of auditory hallucinations encouraging or demanding self-harm are most common. These symptoms usually abate when the stress is relieved. Many clients also report flashback episodes of previous abuse or trauma. These experiences are consistent with posttraumatic stress disorder, which is common in clients with borderline personality disorder.

JUDGMENT AND INSIGHT

The client frequently reports behaviors consistent with impaired judgment and lack of care and concern for safety, such as gambling, shoplifting, and reckless driving. Decisions are made impulsively based on emotions rather than facts.

The client has difficulty accepting responsibility for meeting needs outside of a relationship. Life's problems and failures are seen as a result of the shortcomings of others. Because others are always to blame, the client's insight is limited. A typical reaction to a problem situation is, "I wouldn't have gotten into this mess if so-and-so had been there."

SELF-CONCEPT

The client has an unstable view of himself or herself that shifts dramatically and suddenly. The client may appear needy and dependent one moment and angry, hostile, and rejecting the next. Sudden changes in opinions and plans about career, sexual identity, values, and types of friends are often seen. The client views himself or herself as inherently bad or evil and often reports feeling as if he or she doesn't really exist at all.

Suicidal threats, gestures, and attempts are common. Self-harm and mutilation behaviors, such as cutting, punching, or burning, are common. These behaviors must be taken very seriously because these clients are at increased risk for completed suicide, even if numerous previous attempts have not been life-threatening. These self-inflicted injuries cause the client much pain and often require extensive treatment; some result in massive scarring or permanent disability, such as paralysis or loss of mobility from injury to nerves, tendons, and other essential structures.

ROLES AND RELATIONSHIPS

Clients hate being alone, but their erratic, labile, and sometimes dangerous behaviors often isolate them from other people. Relationships are unstable, stormy, and intense, a cycle that repeats itself again and again. These clients have extreme fears of abandonment and have difficulty believing a relationship still exists once the person is away from them. Clients engage in many desperate types of behavior, even suicide attempts, to gain or maintain relationships. Their feelings for others are often distorted, erratic, and inappropriate. For example, they may view someone they have only met once or twice as their best and only friend or the "love of my life." If another person does not immediately reciprocate their feelings, they may feel rejected, become hostile, and declare them to be their enemy. These erratic changes in emotion can occur in the space of an hour. Often these situations precipitate self-mutilating behavior, and occasionally clients may attempt to harm others physically.

Clients usually have a history of poor school and work performance due to constant changing of career goals and shifts in identity or aspirations, preoccupation with maintaining relationships, and fear of real or perceived abandonment. Clients lack the concentration and self-discipline to follow through on sometimes mundane tasks associated with work or school.

PHYSIOLOGIC AND SELF-CARE CONSIDERATIONS

In addition to suicidal and self-harm behavior, the client may also engage in bingeing (excessive overeating) and purging (self-induced vomiting), abuse of alcohol and other drugs, unprotected sex, or reckless behavior, such as driving while intoxicated. The client usually has difficulty sleeping.

Data Analysis

Nursing diagnoses for clients with borderline personality disorder may include:

- Risk for Suicide
- Risk for Self-Mutilation
- Ineffective Individual Coping
- Social Isolation.

Outcome Identification

Treatment outcomes may include:
1. The client will be safe and free of significant injury.
2. The client will not harm others or destroy property.
3. The client will demonstrate increased control of impulsive behavior.
4. The client will take appropriate steps to meet his or her own needs.
5. The client will identify acceptable ways to meet dependency needs.
6. The client will verbalize greater satisfaction with relationships.

Interventions

Clients with borderline personality disorder are often involved in long-term psychotherapy, addressing issues of family dysfunction and abuse. The nurse is most likely to have contact with these clients in times of crisis, when they are exhibiting self-harm behaviors or transient psychotic symptoms. Brief hospitalizations are often used to manage these difficulties and stabilize the client's condition.

▶ NURSING INTERVENTIONS FOR THE CLIENT WITH BORDERLINE PERSONALITY DISORDER

- Promoting client's safety
  - No self-harm contract
  - Safe expression of feelings and emotions
- Helping client cope and control emotions
  - Identifying feelings
  - Journal entries
  - Moderating emotional responses
  - Decreasing impulsivity
  - Delaying gratification
- Cognitive restructuring techniques
  - Thought-stopping
  - Decatastrophizing
- Structuring time
- Teaching social skills
- Teaching effective communication skills
- Therapeutic relationship
  - Limit-setting
  - Confrontation

PROMOTING THE CLIENT'S SAFETY

The physical safety of the client is always a priority. Nurses must always seriously consider suicidal ideation with the presence of a plan, access to means for enacting the plan, and self-harm behaviors and institute appropriate interventions (see Chap. 14). Clients often experience chronic suicidality, or ongoing, intermittent ideas of suicide that occur over months or years. The challenge for the nurse, in concert with the client, is to determine when the suicidal ideas are likely to be translated into action.

The client's self-harm urges may be enacted by cutting, burning, or punching himself or herself, sometimes causing permanent physical damage. Self-injury can occur when a client is enraged, when he or she experiences dissociative episodes or psychotic symptoms, or for no readily apparent reason. Helping the client avoid self-injury can be difficult when antecedent conditions vary greatly. Sometimes the client may discuss the self-harm urges with the nurse if he or she feels comfortable doing so. The nurse must remain nonjudgmental when discussing this topic with the client. The nurse can encourage the client to engage in a **no self-harm contract**, in which the client promises to try to keep from harming himself or herself and to report to the nurse when he or she is losing control. The nurse should emphasize that the no self-harm contract is not a promise to the nurse, but rather an agreement with oneself to be safe. This distinction is critical to avoid blurring the boundaries between the nurse and the client (Dycoff et al., 1996).

When the client is relatively calm and thinking clearly, it is helpful for the nurse to explore self-harm behavior. Sensational aspects of the injury are avoided; the focus is on identifying the client's mood and affect, his or her level of agitation and distress, and the circumstances surrounding the incident. In this way, the client can begin to identify trigger situations, moods, or emotions that precede self-harm and use more effective coping skills to deal with the trigger issues.

If the client does injure himself or herself, the injury and need for treatment should be assessed in a calm, matter-of-fact manner. Lecturing or chastising the client is punitive and has no positive effect on self-harm behaviors. Deflecting attention from the actual physical act is usually desirable.

PROMOTING THE THERAPEUTIC RELATIONSHIP

Regardless of the clinical setting, the nurse must provide structure and limit-setting in the therapeutic relationship. In a clinic setting, this may mean seeing the client for scheduled appointments of a predetermined length rather than whenever the client appears, demanding the nurse's immediate attention. In the hospital setting, the nurse would plan to spend a specific amount of time with the client to work on issues or coping strategies rather than giving the client exclusive access when he or she has had an outburst. Limit-setting and confrontation techniques, described earlier, are also helpful.

ESTABLISHING BOUNDARIES IN RELATIONSHIPS

Clients have difficulty maintaining satisfying interpersonal relationships. Personal boundaries are unclear, and clients often have unrealistic expectations of relationships. Erratic patterns of thinking and behaving often alienate them from others. This may be true for professional relationships as well as those with family and friends. The client can easily misinterpret the nurse's genuine interest and caring as a personal friendship, and the nurse may feel flattered by the client's compliments. The nurse must be quite clear about establishing the boundaries in the therapeutic relationship, ensuring that neither the client's nor the nurse's boundaries are violated. For example:

Client: *"You're better than my family and the doctors. You understand me better than anyone else."*

Nurse: *"I'm interested in helping you get better, just as the other staff are."* (establishing boundaries)

TEACHING EFFECTIVE COMMUNICATION SKILLS

It is important to teach the client basic communication skills, such as eye contact, active listening, taking turns talking, validating the meaning of another's communication, and using "I" statements ("I

> ▶ **CLIENT/FAMILY TEACHING FOR BORDERLINE PERSONALITY DISORDER**
>
> - Teaching social skills
>   - Maintaining personal boundaries
>   - Realistic expectations of relationships
> - Teaching time structuring
>   - Making written schedule of activities
>   - Making a list of solitary activities to combat boredom
> - Teaching self-management through cognitive restructuring
>   - Decatastrophizing situation
>   - Thought-stopping
>   - Positive self-talk
> - Assertiveness techniques, such as "I" statements
> - Use of distraction, such as walking or listening to music

think . . . ," "I feel . . . ," "I need . . ."). The nurse can model these techniques and engage in role-playing with the client. The nurse should ask how the client feels when interacting and should give feedback about nonverbal behavior, such as, "I notice you were looking at the floor when discussing your feelings."

HELPING THE CLIENT TO COPE AND CONTROL EMOTIONS

Clients often react to situations with extreme emotional responses without actually recognizing their feelings. The nurse can help the client identify his or her feelings and learn to tolerate the feelings without an exaggerated response such as destruction of property or self-harm. Keeping a journal often helps the client gain awareness of his or her feelings. The nurse can review the client's journal entries as a basis for discussion.

Another aspect of emotional regulation is decreasing impulsivity and learning to delay gratification. When the client has an immediate desire or request, he or she must learn that it is not reasonable to expect it will be granted without delay. The client can use distraction, such as taking a walk or listening to music, to deal with the delay, or he or she can think about ways to meet the need for himself or herself. The client can write in his or her journal about the feelings that occur when gratification is delayed.

RESHAPING THINKING PATTERNS

Clients view everything, people and situations, in terms of extremes—totally good or totally bad. **Cognitive restructuring** is a technique useful in changing patterns of thinking by helping the client to recognize when negative thoughts and feelings occur and to replace them with positive patterns of thinking. **Thought-stopping** is a technique that can be used to alter the process of negative or self-critical thought patterns such as, "I'm dumb, I'm stupid, I can't do anything right." When the thoughts begin, the client may actually say, "Stop!" in a loud voice to help stop the negative thoughts from continuing. Later, more subtle means such as forming a visual image of a stop sign will be a cue to interrupt the negative thoughts. The client then learns to replace recurrent, negative thoughts of worthlessness with more positive thinking such as **positive self-talk**, in which the client reframes negative thoughts into positive ones: "I made a mistake, but it's not the end of the world. Next time, I'll know what to do" (Linehan, 1993).

Decatastrophizing is a technique that involves learning to assess situations realistically rather than always assuming a catastrophe will happen. The nurse asks, "So what is the worst thing that could happen?" or "How likely do you think that is?" or "How do you suppose other people might deal with that?" or "Can you think of any exceptions to that?". In this way, the client must consider other points of view and actually think about the situation; in time, he or she may become less rigid and inflexible in his or her thinking (Loughrey et al., 1997).

STRUCTURING THE CLIENT'S DAILY ACTIVITIES

Feelings of chronic boredom and emptiness, fear of abandonment, and intolerance of being alone are common problems. The client is often at a loss about how to manage unstructured time, becomes more unhappy and ruminative, and may engage in frantic and desperate behaviors to change the situation, such as self-harm. Minimizing unstructured time by planning activities can help the client manage time alone. The client can make a written schedule that includes appointments, shopping, reading the paper, or going for a walk. The client is more likely to follow the plan if it is in written form. This can also help the client to plan ahead to spend time with other people, instead of frantically calling others when in distress. The written schedule also allows the nurse to help the client engage in more healthful behaviors such as exercise, planning meals, and cooking nutritious food.

Evaluation

As with any personality disorder, changes may be small and occur slowly over time. The degree of functional impairment of clients with borderline personality disorder may vary widely. Clients with severe impairment may be evaluated in terms of their ability to be safe and refrain from self-injury. Other clients may be employed and have fairly stable interpersonal relationships. Generally, when clients experience fewer crises less frequently over time, treatment has been effective.

OTHER CLUSTER A PERSONALITY DISORDERS

Paranoid Personality Disorder

CLINICAL PICTURE

Paranoid personality disorder is characterized by a pervasive mistrust and suspiciousness of others. The person interprets the actions of others as potentially harmful to himself or herself. During periods of stress, transient psychotic symptoms may develop. The incidence is estimated to be 0.5% to 2.5% of the

(*text continues on page 432*)

NURSING CARE PLAN   MANIPULATIVE BEHAVIOR

Nursing Diagnosis

➤ **Ineffective Individual Coping** (5.1.1.1)
Impairment of adaptive behaviors and problem-solving abilities of a person in meeting life's demands and roles

ASSESSMENT DATA

- Denial of problems or feelings
- Lack of insight
- Inability or refusal to express emotions directly (especially anger)
- Dishonesty
- Anger or hostility
- Superficial relationships with others
- Somatic complaints
- Seductive behavior or sexual acting out
- Preoccupation with other clients' problems ("playing therapist") or with staff members to avoid dealing with his or her own problems
- Intellectualization or rationalization of problems
- Dependency
- Manipulation of staff or family
- Attempting to gain special treatment or privileges

EXPECTED OUTCOMES

The client will:
- Express feelings directly, verbally and nonverbally
- Participate in the treatment program, activities, and so forth
- Communicate directly and honestly with staff and other clients about himself or herself
- Develop or increase feelings of self-worth
- Demonstrate decreased manipulative, attention-seeking, or passive-aggressive behaviors
- Demonstrate independence from the hospital environment and staff
- Demonstrate increased responsibility for himself or herself
- Demonstrate increased feelings of self-worth
- Demonstrate appropriate interactions with others
- Demonstrate problem-solving skills when dealing with situations or others

IMPLEMENTATION

Nursing Interventions	Rationale
State the limits and the behavior you expect from the client. Do not debate, argue, rationalize, or bargain with the client.	Specific limits let the client know what is expected from him or her. Arguing, bargaining, justifying, and so forth interject doubt and undermine the limit.
Be consistent, not only with this particular client, but also with all other clients; that is, do not insist that this client follow a rule, while excusing another client from the same rule.	Consistency provides structure and reinforces limits. Making exceptions undermines limits and encourages manipulative behavior.

continued on page 430

continued from page 429

Enforce all policies or regulations. Without apologizing, point out reasons for not bending the rules.

Institutional regulations provide a therapeutic structure. Apologizing for regulations undermines this structure and encourages manipulative behavior.

Be direct and use confrontation with the client if necessary; however, be sure to examine your own feelings. Do not react to the client punitively or in anger.

You are a role model of appropriate behavior and self-control. There is no justification for punishing a client. Remember, the client is acceptable as a person regardless of his or her behaviors, which may or may not be acceptable.

Do not discuss yourself, other staff members, or other clients with this client.

Your relationship with the client is professional. Sharing personal information about yourself or others is inappropriate and can be used in a manipulative way.

Set limits on the frequency and length of interactions with the client, particularly those with therapists significant to the client. Set definite and limited appointment times with therapists (like Thursday, 2:00 to 2:30 PM), and allow interactions only at those times.

Setting and maintaining limits can help decrease attention-seeking behaviors and reinforce appropriate behaviors.

Do not attempt to be popular, liked, or the "favorite staff member" of this client.

It is not necessary or particularly desirable for the client to like you personally. A professional relationship is based on the client's therapeutic needs, not personal feelings.

Do not accept gifts from the client or encourage a personal dependency relationship.

Maintaining your professional role is therapeutic for the client. Your acceptance of personal gifts from the client may foster manipulative behavior. (For example, the client may expect that you will grant special favors.)

Withdraw your attention from the client if he or she begins saying that you are "the only staff member I can talk to . . ." or "the only one who understands" and so forth; confront the client with the idea that this is not a desirable situation. Emphasize the importance of the milieu in his or her therapy.

It is important that the client establish and maintain trust relationships with a variety of people, staff, and other clients. If you are "the only one," the client may be too dependent or may be flattering you as a basis for manipulation.

Discuss the client's perceptions and feelings (eg, anger, hurt, feelings of being rejected or unworthy) about being denied special privileges. Encourage the client's expression of those feelings.

The client's ability to identify and express feelings is impaired. You can help the client, especially with emotions that may be uncomfortable for him or her. The client may not be used to accepting limits.

continued on page 431

continued from page 430

Discuss the client's behavior with him or her in a nonjudgmental manner, using examples in a non-threatening way.	Providing nonjudgmental feedback can help the client to acknowledge problems and develop insight.
Help the client identify the results and the dynamics of his or her behavior and relationships. (You might say, "You seem to be . . ." or "What effect do you see . . .?")	Reflection and feedback can be effective in increasing the client's insight.
Encourage the client to express feelings.	Appropriate expression of feelings is a healthy, adult behavior.
In your interactions with the client, emphasize expression of feelings rather than intellectualization.	The client may use intellectualization as a way of avoiding feelings and dealing with his or her emotions.
Be kind but firm with the client. Make it clear that limits and caring are not mutually exclusive, that you set and maintain limits because you care, that the client can feel hurt from someone who cares about him or her, that caring and discipline are not opposites.	The client is acceptable as a person regardless of his or her behaviors, which may or may not be acceptable. Because you care about the client's well-being, you set and maintain limits to encourage the client's growth and health.
Involve the client in care planning to assess his or her motivation and establish goals, but do not allow the client to dictate the terms of therapy or treatment (for example, what type of therapy, which therapists, length and frequency of interactions). Involve the client in the full treatment program.	Including the client in planning his or her care can encourage the client's sense of responsibility for his or her health. Allowing the client to dictate his or her care may encourage manipulation by the client.
Give attention and support when the client exhibits appropriate behavior—attends activities, expresses feelings, and so forth.	Positive feedback provides reinforcement for the client's growth and can enhance self-esteem. It is essential that the client be supported in positive ways and not given attention only for unacceptable behaviors.
Teach the client a step-by-step approach to solving problems: identifying problems, exploring alternatives, evaluating consequences of alternatives, and making a decision.	The client may be unaware of a logical process for examining and resolving problems.
Teach the client social skills. Describe and demonstrate specific skills, such as eye contact, attentive listening, nodding, and so forth. Discuss the types of topics that are appropriate for social conversation, such as the weather, news, local events, and so forth.	The client may have little or no knowledge of social interaction skills. Modeling provides a concrete example of the desired skills.

continued on page 432

continued from page 431

Set and maintain limits on seductive or sexual behavior that is inappropriate or unacceptable.	The client may use seductive behavior (that is familiar to him or her) to approach others, particularly if he or she lacks appropriate social skills. The use of sexual or seductive behavior also may be manipulative.

Adapted from Schultz, J. M., & Videbeck, S. L. (1998). Lippincott's manual of psychiatric nursing care plans *(5th ed.). Philadelphia: Lippincott-Raven.*

general population, and it is more common in men than women. Data about prognosis and long-term outcomes are limited because persons with paranoid personality disorders do not readily seek or remain in treatment (DSM-IV-TR, 2000).

Clients appear aloof and withdrawn and may remain a considerable physical distance from the nurse, viewing this as necessary for their protection. Clients may also appear guarded or hypervigilant, surveying the room and its contents and looking behind furniture or doors, and generally appears alert for any impending danger. They may choose to sit near the door to have ready access to an exit, or with their back against the wall to prevent anyone from sneaking up behind them. They may have a restricted affect, unable to demonstrate warm or empathic emotional responses such as, "You look nice today" or "I'm sorry you're having a bad day." Their mood may be labile, quickly changing from quietly suspicious to angry or hostile, and responses may become sarcastic for no apparent reason. Thoughts, thought processing, and content are distorted by the constant mistrust and suspicion that clients feel toward others and the environment. Clients frequently see malevolence in the actions of others when none exists. They may spend a disproportionate amount of time examining and analyzing the behavior and motives of others to discover hidden and threatening meanings. Clients often feel attacked by others and may devise elaborate plans or fantasies for protection.

Clients use the defense mechanism of projection, blaming other people, institutions, or events for their own difficulties. It is common for clients to blame the government for personal problems. For example, a client who gets a parking ticket may say it is part of a plot by the police to drive him out of the neighborhood. He may engage of fantasies of retribution or devise elaborate and sometimes violent plans to get even.

Although most clients do not carry out such plans, there is a potential danger.

Conflict with authority figures on the job is a common problem; clients may even resent being given directions for work by a supervisor. Paranoia may extend to feelings of being singled out for menial tasks, being treated as stupid, or being more closely monitored than other employees.

NURSING INTERVENTIONS

It is difficult to form an effective working relationship with a paranoid or suspicious client. The nurse must remember that the client takes everything seriously and is particularly sensitive about the reactions and motivation of others. Therefore, the nurse must approach the client in a formal and business-like manner, refraining from social chitchat or jokes. Being on time, keeping commitments, and being particularly straightforward are essential to the success of the nurse–client relationship.

Because the client needs to feel in control, it is important to involve him or her in formulating a plan of care. Ask the client what he or she would like to accomplish in concrete terms, such as minimizing problems at work or getting along with others. The client is more likely to engage in the therapeutic process if he or she believes he or she has something to gain from it. One of the most effective interventions is helping the client learn to validate ideas before taking action; however, this requires the client to trust and listen to one person. The rationale behind this intervention is that the client can avoid problems if he or she can refrain from taking action until he or she has validated his or her ideas with another person. This helps the client refrain from acting on paranoid ideas or beliefs and start basing decisions and actions on reality-based information.

Schizoid Personality Disorder

CLINICAL PICTURE

Schizoid personality disorder is characterized by a pervasive pattern of detachment from social relationships and a restricted range of expression of emotions in interpersonal settings. It occurs in approximately 0.5% to 7% of the general population and is more common in men than women. Persons with a schizoid personality disorder avoid treatment much as they avoid other relationships, unless there is a significant change in their life circumstances (DSM-IV-TR, 2000).

The client displays a constricted affect and little, if any, emotion. The client is aloof and indifferent, appearing emotionally cold and uncaring or unfeeling. No leisure or pleasurable activities are reported, because the client rarely experiences enjoyment. Even under stress or adverse circumstances, the client's response appears passive and disinterested. There is marked difficulty experiencing and expressing emotions, particularly feelings of anger or aggression. Oddly, the client does not report feeling distressed over this lack of emotion; it is more distressing to family members. The client usually has a rich and extensive fantasy life, although he or she may be reluctant to reveal that information to the nurse or anyone else. The ideal relationships that occur in the client's fantasies are rewarding and gratifying, in stark contrast to real-life experiences. The fantasy relationship often includes someone the client has met only briefly. However, the client can distinguish the fantasies from reality, and no disordered or delusional thought processes are evident.

The client is generally accomplished intellectually and is often involved with computers or electronics in hobbies or work. He or she may spend long hours solving puzzles or mathematical problems, although these pursuits are seen as useful or productive rather than fun.

The client may be indecisive and lack any future life goals or direction. He or she sees no need for planning life and really has no aspirations. The client has little opportunity to exercise judgment or decision-making skills because he or she rarely engages in these activities. Insight might be described as impaired, at least by the social standards of others: the client does not see his or her situation as a problem and does not understand why his or her lack of emotion or social involvement is troubling to others. The client is self-absorbed and is a loner in almost all aspects of daily life. Given an opportunity to engage with another person, the client will decline. The client is also indifferent to either praise or criticism and is relatively unaffected by the emotions or opinions of others. There is also a dissociation from or an absence of bodily or sensory pleasures. For example, the client experiences no pleasure or has little reaction to beautiful scenery or a sunset or a walk on the beach.

The client has a pervasive lack of desire for involvement with others in all aspects of life. He or she does not have or desire friends, rarely dates or marries, and has little or no sexual contact. The client may have some connection with a person who is a first-degree relative, often a parent. The client may remain in the parental home well into adulthood if he or she can maintain adequate separation and distance from other family members. The client has few social skills, is oblivious to the social cues or overtures of others, and does not engage in social conversation. He or she may have success in vocational areas, provided the job requires little contact with others and is valued by the client, such as computers or electronics.

NURSING INTERVENTIONS

Nursing interventions focus on improved functioning in the community. If the client needs housing or a change in living circumstances, the nurse can make referrals to social services or appropriate local agencies for assistance. The nurse can help agency personnel find suitable housing that will accommodate the client's desire and need for solitude. For example, the client with a schizoid personality disorder would function best in a board and care facility, where meals and laundry service are provided but little interaction is required. Facilities designed to promote socialization through group activities would be less desirable.

If the client has an identified family member as his or her primary relationship, the nurse must ascertain whether that person can continue in that role. If that person cannot, the client may need to establish at least a working relationship with a case manager in the community. The case manager can then help the client obtain services and health care, help manage finances, and so on. The client has a greater chance of success if he or she can relate his or her needs to one person instead of neglecting important areas of daily life.

Schizotypal Personality Disorder

CLINICAL PICTURE

Schizotypal personality disorder is characterized by a pervasive pattern of social and interpersonal deficits marked by acute discomfort with and reduced capacity for close relationships, as well as cognitive or perceptual distortions and eccentricities of behavior. About 3% to 5% of the population has schizotypal personality disorder, and it is slightly more common in men than women. These persons may experience transient psychotic episodes in response to extreme stress. An estimated 10% to 20% of persons with schizotypal personality disorder go on to develop schizophrenia (DSM-IV-TR, 2000).

The client often has an odd appearance that causes others to notice him or her. Clothes are ill-fitting, do not match, and may be stained or dirty. The client may be unkempt and disheveled. He or she may wander aimlessly without any purpose, at times becoming preoccupied with some detail of the environment. Speech is coherent but may be loose, digressive, or vague. The client often provides unsatisfactory answers to questions, being unable to specify or describe information in a clear manner. He or she frequently uses words incorrectly, making his or her speech sound bizarre. For example, in response to a question about sleeping habits, the client might respond, "Sleep is slow, the REMs don't flow." The client has a restricted range of emotions—that is, he or she lacks the ability to experience and express a full range of emotions, such as anger, happiness, and pleasure. The client's affect is often flat and sometimes is silly or inappropriate to the situation.

Cognitive distortions include ideas of reference, magical thinking, odd or unfounded beliefs, and a preoccupation with parapsychology, such as ESP and clairvoyance. Ideas of reference usually involve the client's belief that events have special meaning for him or her; however, these ideas are not firmly fixed and delusional, as may be seen in clients with schizophrenia. In magical thinking, which is normal in small children, the client believes he or she has special powers—that by thinking about something, he or she can make it happen. In addition, sometimes the client may express ideas that indicate paranoid thinking and suspiciousness, usually about the motives of other people.

The client feels a great deal of anxiety around other people, especially if they are unfamiliar. This does not improve with time or repeated exposures; rather, the anxiety may intensify. This is due to the client's belief that the anxiety is warranted because strangers cannot be trusted. The client does not view his or her anxiety as a problem that arises due to a threatened sense of self. Interpersonal relationships are troublesome for the client, and therefore there may be only one significant relationship, usually with a first-degree relative. The client may remain in his or her parents' home well into the adult years. The client has a limited capacity for close relationships, even though he or she may be unhappy being alone.

The client cannot respond to normal social cues and hence cannot engage in superficial conversation. The client may have skills that could be useful in a vocational setting, but he or she is not often successful in employment without support or assistance. Mistrust of others, bizarre thinking and ideas, and unkempt appearance can make it difficult for the client to get and keep jobs.

NURSING INTERVENTIONS

The focus of nursing care for clients with schizotypal personality disorder is development of self-care and social skills and improved functioning in the community. Clients should be encouraged to establish a daily routine for hygiene and grooming. Having a daily routine is important, rather than relying on the client's ability to decide when hygiene and grooming tasks are necessary. It is useful for the client to have an appearance that is not bizarre or disheveled, because stares or comments from others can increase the client's discomfort. Because these clients are uncomfortable around other people, and this is not likely to change, the nurse must help the client to function in the community with a minimum of discomfort. It may help to ask the client to prepare a list of people in the community with whom he or she must have contact, such as a landlord, store clerk, or pharmacist. The nurse can then role-play interactions that the client would have with each of these people, allowing the client to practice making clear and logical requests to obtain services or conduct personal business. Because face-to-face contact is more uncomfortable, the client may be able to make written requests or use the telephone for business when possible. Social skills training may help the client to talk clearly with others and reduce bizarre conversation. It helps to identify one person with whom the client can discuss unusual or bizarre beliefs, such as a social worker or family member. Given an acceptable outlet for these topics, the client may be able to refrain from having these conversations with people who might react negatively to the bizarre comments.

OTHER CLUSTER B PERSONALITY DISORDERS

Histrionic Personality Disorder

CLINICAL PICTURE

Histrionic personality disorder is characterized by a pervasive pattern of excessive emotionality and attention-seeking. It occurs in 2% to 3% of the general population and 10% to 15% of the clinical population and is seen more often in women than men. Treatment is usually sought for depression, unexplained physical problems, and difficulties in relationships (DSM-IV-TR, 2000).

The client's tendency to exaggerate the closeness of relationships or to dramatize relatively minor occurrences can result in unreliable data. The client's speech is usually colorful, full of superlative adjectives, and presented in a theatrical fashion. It becomes apparent, however, that although colorful and entertaining, descriptions may be vague and lack detailed information. The client's overall appearance is normal, although he or she may be overdressed for a clinical interview, such as wearing an evening dress and high heels. The client is overly concerned with impressing others by his or her appearance and spends inordinate amounts of time, energy, and money to this end. The client's dress and flirtatious behavior is not limited to social situations or relationships but is seen in occupational and professional settings as well. The nurse may feel he or she is being charmed or even seduced by the client.

The client is emotionally expressive, gregarious, and effusive. Emotions are often expressed with inappropriate exaggeration, such as, "He is the most wonderful doctor! He is so fantastic! He has changed my life!" to describe a physician the client may have seen once or twice. However, the client cannot specify why the doctor is viewed so highly. Expressed emotions, although colorful, are insincere and shallow; this is readily apparent to others, but not the client. The client experiences rapid shifts in moods and emotions and may be laughing uproariously one moment and sobbing the next. This rapid shifting of intense emotions may seem phony or forced to the observer. The client is self-absorbed and focuses most of his or her thinking on himself or herself, with little or no thought about the needs of others. The client is highly suggestible and will agree with almost anyone to gain attention. He or she expresses strong opinions very firmly, but because they are based on little evidence or facts, the opinions often shift under the influence of someone the client is trying to impress.

The client is uncomfortable when he or she is not the center of attention and goes to great lengths to gain that status. The client uses his or her physical appearance and dress to gain attention. At times the client may fish for compliments in unsubtle ways, fabricate unbelievable stories, or create a public scene to turn the focus of attention to himself or herself. The client may even faint, become ill, or fall to the floor to gain attention. The client brightens considerably when given attention after some of these behaviors, leaving others to feel they have been used. Any comment or statement that is seen as uncomplimentary or unflattering may produce a strong response, such as a temper tantrum or crying outburst.

The client tends to exaggerate the intimacy of relationships. Almost all acquaintances are referred to as "dear, dear friends." The client may embarrass family members or friends by flamboyant and inappropriate public behavior, such as hugging and kissing someone who has just been introduced, or sobbing uncontrollably over a minor incident. The client may ignore old friends if someone new and interesting has been introduced. Persons with whom the client has relationships often describe themselves as being used, manipulated, or exploited shamelessly by the client for his or her personal gain.

The client may have a wide variety of vague physical complaints or may relate exaggerated versions of physical illness. These episodes usually center around the attention the client received (or failed to receive) when they occurred rather than any particular physiologic concern.

NURSING INTERVENTIONS

The nurse should give the client feedback about his or her social interaction with others, including manner of dress and nonverbal behavior. Feedback should focus on appropriate alternatives, not merely criticism. For example, the nurse might say, *"When you embrace and kiss another person on first meeting them, they may interpret your behavior in a sexual manner. It would be more acceptable to stand at least 2 feet away from them and shake hands."*

It may also help to discuss social situations to explore the client's perceptions of the reactions and behavior of others. Teaching the client social skills and role-playing those skills in a safe, nonthreatening environment can help the client gain confidence in his or her ability to interact with others. The nurse must be specific in describing and modeling these social skills, including establishing eye contact, active listening, and respect for personal space. It also helps to outline the topics of discussion that are appropriate for casual acquaintances, for closer friends or family, and for the nurse only.

The client may be quite sensitive to discussing self-esteem and may respond with exaggerated emotions. It is important to explore the client's personal strengths and assets, giving the client specific feedback about positive characteristics. Encouraging the client to use assertive communication, such as "I" statements, may promote self-esteem and help the client to get his or her needs met in a more appropriate manner. The nurse must convey confidence in the client's abilities in a genuine manner.

Narcissistic Personality Disorder

CLINICAL PICTURE

Narcissistic personality disorder is characterized by a pervasive pattern of grandiosity (in fantasy or behavior), a need for admiration, and a lack of empathy. It occurs in 1% to 2% of the general population and 2% to 16% of the clinical population. Fifty percent to 75% of persons with this diagnosis are male. Narcissistic traits are common in adolescence and do not necessarily indicate that a personality disorder will develop in adulthood. Individual psychotherapy is the most effective treatment, and hospitalization is rare unless comorbid conditions exist for which the client requires inpatient treatment (DSM-IV-TR, 2000).

The client may display an arrogant or haughty attitude. He or she lacks the ability to recognize or empathize with the feelings of others. The client may express envy of others and begrudge others any recognition or material success, believing it should rightfully be his or hers. The client tends to disparage, belittle, or discount the feelings of others. The client's grandiosity may be overtly expressed, or he or she may quietly expect to be recognized for his or her perceived greatness. The client is often preoccupied with fantasies of unlimited success, power, brilliance, beauty, or ideal love. These fantasies reinforce the client's

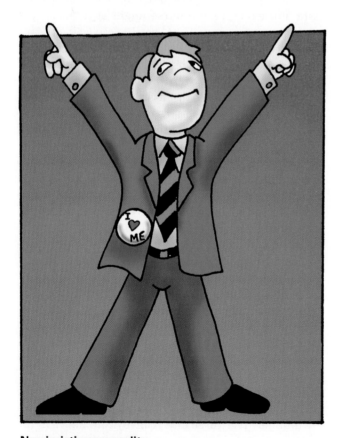

Narcissistic personality

sense of superiority. The client may ruminate about long-overdue admiration and privilege and compare himself or herself favorably with famous or privileged people.

Thought-processing abilities are intact, but insight is limited or poor. Clients believe themselves to be superior and special and are unlikely to consider that their behavior has any relation to their problems: the problem is viewed as the fault of others.

The client's underlying self-esteem is almost always fragile and vulnerable, and he or she is hypersensitive to criticism and needs the constant attention and admiration of others. The client often displays a sense of entitlement (unrealistic expectation of special treatment or automatic compliance with wishes). He or she may believe that only special or privileged people can appreciate his or her unique qualities or are worthy of his or her friendship. The client expects special treatment from others and is often puzzled or even angry when this does not occur. Relationships are often formed and exploited to elevate the client's own status. The client assumes that others are totally concerned about his or her welfare. The client discusses his or her own concerns in lengthy detail, with no regard for the needs and feelings of others, and often becomes impatient or contemptuous of others who talk about their own needs and concerns.

In the work setting, the client may experience some success because he or she is ambitious and confident. However, there are often difficulties because the client has trouble working with others (whom he considers to be inferior) and has limited ability to accept criticism or feedback. The client is also likely to believe that he or she is underpaid and underappreciated or should have a higher position of authority, even though he or she is not qualified to do so.

NURSING INTERVENTIONS

The client with narcissistic personality disorder can present one of the greatest challenges to the nurse. The nurse must use self-awareness skills to avoid the anger and frustration that can be engendered by the client's behavior and attitude. The client may behave in a rude and arrogant manner, may be unwilling to wait, and may be harsh and critical of the nurse. The nurse must not internalize such criticism or take the client's behavior personally. The goal is to gain the client's cooperation with other treatment as indicated. Teaching about the client's comorbid medical or psychiatric condition, the medication regimen, and any needed self-care skills is done in a matter-of-fact manner. Limits should be set on rude or verbally abusive behavior, and the nurse should explain what is expected from the client.

OTHER CLUSTER C PERSONALITY DISORDERS

Avoidant Personality Disorder

CLINICAL PICTURE

Avoidant personality disorder is characterized by a pervasive pattern of social discomfort and reticence, low self-esteem, and hypersensitivity to negative evaluation. It occurs in 0.5% to 1% of the general population and 10% of the clinical population and is equally common in men and women. Clients are good candidates for individual psychotherapy (DMS-IV-TR, 2000).

The client is likely to report being overly inhibited as a child, often avoiding unfamiliar situations and people with an intensity beyond that expected at age-appropriate developmental stages. This inhibition may have continued throughout the client's upbringing, contributing to low self-esteem and social alienation. The client is apt to be anxious and may fidget in the chair and make poor eye contact with the nurse. The client may be reluctant to ask questions or make requests. He or she may appear sad in addition to being anxious. The client describes being shy, fearful, socially awkward, and easily devastated by real or perceived criticism. His or her usual response to these feelings is to become more reticent and withdrawn.

The client has very low self-esteem. He or she is hypersensitive to the negative evaluation of others and readily believes he or she is inferior to others. The client is reluctant do anything perceived as risky, which for this client is almost anything. The client is fearful and convinced that he or she will make a mistake, be humiliated, or embarrass himself or herself and others. Because the client is unusually fearful of rejection, criticism, shame, or disapproval, he or she tends to avoid situations or relationships that may result in these feelings. The client usually has a strong desire for social acceptance and human companionship: he or she wishes for closeness and intimacy but fears possible rejection and humiliation. These fears hinder socialization, making the client seem awkward and socially inept and reinforcing the client's beliefs about himself or herself. The client may need excessive reassurance of guaranteed acceptance before he or she is willing to risk forming a relationship.

The client may report some success in occupational roles because he or she is so eager to please or win a supervisor's approval. However, the client's shyness, awkwardness, or fear of failure may prevent him or her from seeking jobs that might be more suitable or challenging or rewarding. For example, the client may reject a promotion and continue to remain in an entry-level position for years, even though he or she is well qualified to advance.

NURSING INTERVENTIONS

The client requires much support and reassurance from the nurse. In the nonthreatening context of the relationship, the nurse can help the client explore positive aspects of himself or herself, positive responses from others, and possible reasons for the client's self-criticism. Helping the client practice self-affirmations and positive self-talk may be useful in promoting self-esteem. Other cognitive restructuring techniques, such as reframing and decatastrophizing (described previously), can enhance self-worth. The nurse can teach the client social skills and help him or her practice these skills in the safety of the nurse–client relationship. Although the client has many social fears, those are often counterbalanced by his or her desire for meaningful social contact and relationships. The nurse must be careful and patient with the client and not expect him or her to rush into implementation of social skills too rapidly.

Dependent Personality Disorder

CLINICAL PICTURE

Dependent personality disorder is characterized by a pervasive and excessive need to be taken care of that leads to submissive and clinging behavior and fears of separation. These behaviors are designed to elicit caretaking from others. It occurs in as much as 15% of the population and is seen three times more often in women than men. The disorder runs in families and is most common in the youngest child. Persons with dependent personality disorder often seek treatment for anxious, depressed, or somatic symptoms (DSM-IV-TR, 2000).

Clients are frequently anxious and may be mildly uncomfortable. They are often pessimistic and self-critical, and their feelings are easily hurt by others. They commonly report feeling unhappy or depressed; this is most likely associated with the actual or threatened loss of support from another. They are excessively preoccupied with unrealistic fears of being left alone to care for themselves. They believe they would fail on their own, so keeping or finding a relationship occupies a great deal of their time. They have a tremendous amount of difficulty making decisions, no matter how minor. They seek advice and repeated reassurances about all types of decisions, from what to wear to what type of job to pursue. Although they can make judgments and decisions, they lack the confidence to do so.

Clients perceive themselves as unable to function outside of a relationship with someone who can tell them what to do. They are very uncomfortable and feel helpless when alone, even if the current relationship is intact. They have difficulty initiating projects or completing simple daily tasks independently. They believe that they needs someone else to assume responsibility for them, a belief that far exceeds what is age- or situation-appropriate. They may even fear gaining competence because it would mean an eventual loss of support from the person on whom they depend. They may do almost anything to sustain a relationship, even if it is of poor quality. This includes doing unpleasant tasks, going places they dislike, or in extreme cases, tolerating abuse. Clients are reluctant to express disagreement for fear of losing the other person's support or approval; they may even consent to engage in activities that are wrong or illegal to avoid that loss.

When the client does experience the end of a relationship, he or she urgently and desperately seeks another. The unspoken motto of the client seems to be, "Any relationship is better than none at all."

NURSING INTERVENTIONS

The nurse must help the client express feelings of grief and loss over the end of a relationship while fostering the client's sense of autonomy and self-reliance. Helping the client identify his or her strengths and needs is more helpful than the client's overwhelming belief that "I can't do anything alone!" Cognitive restructuring techniques such as reframing and decatastrophizing may be beneficial.

The client may need assistance in daily functioning if he or she has little or no past success in this area. Included are such things as planning menus, doing the weekly shopping, budgeting money, balancing a checkbook, paying bills, and so forth. Careful assessment to determine areas of need is essential. Depending on the client's abilities and limitations, referral to agencies for services or assistance may be indicated.

The nurse may also need to teach the client problem-solving and decision-making skills and help apply them to daily life. The nurse must refrain from giving advice about problems or making decisions for the client, even though the client may ask the nurse to do so. The nurse can help the client explore problems, serve as a sounding board for discussion of alternatives, and provide support and positive feedback for the client's efforts in these areas.

Obsessive-Compulsive Personality Disorder

CLINICAL PICTURE

Obsessive-compulsive personality disorder is characterized by a pervasive pattern of preoccupation with orderliness, perfectionism, mental and interpersonal control, and orderliness at the expense of flexibility, openness, and efficiency. This disorder occurs in about 1% to 2% of the population, affecting twice as many men as women. This rises to 3% to

10% in clients in mental health settings. There is an increased incidence in oldest children and people in professions involving facts, figures, or a methodical focus on detail. These people often seek treatment because they recognize that their life is pleasureless or they are experiencing problems with work or relationships. Clients frequently benefit from individual therapy (DSM-IV-TR, 2000).

The client's demeanor is formal and serious, and questions are answered with precision and much detail. The client often reports feeling the need to be perfect beginning in childhood. He or she was expected to be good and do the right thing to win the parents' approval. Expressing emotions or asserting independence was probably met with harsh disapproval and emotional consequences. The client's emotional range is usually quite constricted. He or she has difficulty expressing emotions, and the emotions that are expressed are rigid, stiff, and formal, lacking spontaneity. The client can be very stubborn and reluctant to relinquish control, making it difficult for him or her to be vulnerable to others by expressing feelings. The client's affect is also restricted: he or she usually appears anxious and fretful, or stiff and reluctant to reveal underlying emotions.

The client is preoccupied with orderliness and tries to maintain order in all areas of life. The client strives for perfection as though it were attainable and is preoccupied with details, rules, lists, and schedules to the point that he or she often misses "the big picture." The client becomes absorbed in his or her own perspective, believes he or she is right, and does not listen carefully to others, having already dismissed what the other person is saying. The client checks and rechecks the details of any project or activity; often the project is never completed because the client is "trying to get it right." The client has problems with judgment and making decisions—specifically, actually reaching a decision. The client considers and reconsiders alternatives, and the desire for perfection keeps the client from reaching a decision. Rules or guidelines are interpreted literally, and the client cannot be flexible or modify decisions based on circumstances. The client prefers to have written rules to govern each and every activity at work. The client's insight is limited, and he or she is often oblivious to the fact that his or her behavior is a source of annoyance and frustration to others. If confronted with this annoyance, the client is stunned, unable to believe others "don't want me to do a good job."

This client has low self-esteem and is always harsh, critical, and judgmental of himself or herself, believing that he or she "could have done better," regardless of how well the job has been done. Praise and reassurance from others does not change this belief. The client is burdened by extremely high and unattainable standards and expectations. Although no one could live up to these expectations, the client feels guilty and worthless for being unable to achieve them. The client tends to evaluate himself or herself and others based solely on deeds or actions, without regard for personal qualities.

The client has a great deal of difficulty in relationships and has few friends and little social life. He or she does not express warm or tender feelings to others; attempts to do so are very stiff and formal and may sound insincere. For example, if a significant other expresses love and affection, this client's typical response might be, "The feeling is mutual."

If the client is married or has children, these relationships are often difficult because the client may be harsh and unrelenting in these roles. For example, the client is probably frugal, does not give gifts or want to discard old items, and insists that those around him or her do the same. Shopping for something new to wear may seem frivolous and wasteful. The client cannot tolerate lack of control and hence may organize family outings to the point that no one enjoys them. These types of behaviors can cause daily strife and discord in family life.

At work, the client may experience some success, particularly in fields when precision and attention to detail are seen as desirable qualities. However, the client may miss deadlines while trying to achieve perfection or may fail to make needed decisions while searching for more data. The client fails to make timely decisions because he or she is always striving for perfection. This client has difficulties working collaboratively with others, preferring to "do it myself" so it is done correctly. If the client does accept help from others, he or she may give such detailed instructions and watch the other person so closely that coworkers are insulted and annoyed and refuse to work with him or her. New situations and compromise are also difficult for the client, given his or her excessive need for routine and control.

NURSING INTERVENTIONS

The nurse may be able to help the client view decision-making and completion of projects from a different perspective. Rather than striving for the goal of perfection, the client can set a goal of completing the project or making the decision by a specified deadline. Helping the client to accept or tolerate less-than-perfect work or decisions that are made on time may alleviate some of the client's difficulties at work or home. The client may benefit from cognitive restructuring techniques. The nurse can ask, "What is the worst that could happen?" or "How might your boss (or your wife) see this situation?" These questions may challenge some of the client's rigid and inflexible thinking.

Encouraging the client to take risks, such as letting someone else plan a family activity, may improve the client's relationships with others. Practicing negotiation with family or friends may also help the client relinquish some of his or her need for control.

OTHER RELATED DISORDERS

The following two disorders, depressive personality disorder and passive-aggressive disorder, are under study to be included as personality disorders. They are currently listed and described in the DSM-IV-TR.

Depressive Personality Disorder

CLINICAL PICTURE

Depressive personality disorder is characterized by a pervasive pattern of depressive cognitions and behaviors that occurs in a variety of contexts. It occurs equally in men and women and occurs more often in people with relatives who have major depressive disorders. People with depressive personality disorders often seek treatment due to their distress and generally have a favorable response to antidepressant medications (DSM-IV-TR, 2000).

Although the client with depressive personality disorder may seem to have similar behavior characteristics as the client with major depression, such as moodiness, brooding, joylessness, and pessimism, the disorder is much less severe. The client with depressive personality disorder usually does not experience the severity and long duration of major depression, nor the hallmark symptoms of sleep disturbances, loss of appetite, recurrent thoughts of death, and total disinterest in all activities. Major depressive episode is discussed in Chapter 14.

The client has a sad, gloomy, or dejected affect. Persistent feelings of unhappiness, cheerlessness, and hopelessness are expressed, regardless of the situation. The client often reports the inability to experience joy or pleasure in any activity; he or she cannot relax and does not display a sense of humor. The client may experience feelings of anger that are repressed, or left unsaid. The client broods and worries over all aspects of daily life. Thinking is negative and pessimistic, and the client rarely sees any hope for improvement in the future. He or she views this pessimism as "being realistic." Regardless of positive outcomes in a given situation, negative thinking continues. The client's judgment or decision-making skills are usually intact but dominated by pessimistic thinking; the client often blames himself or herself or others unjustly for situations beyond one's control.

The client's self-esteem is quite low, with feelings of worthlessness and inadequacy, even when he or she has been successful. Self-criticism often leads to punitive behavior and feelings of guilt or remorse. The client may appear overtly quiet and passive, preferring to follow others rather than being a leader in any work or social situation. Although clients feel dependent on the approval of others, they tend to be overly critical of others and are quick to reject others first. This client, who needs and wants the approval and attention of others, actually drives others away, which reinforces his or her feelings of being unworthy of anyone's attention.

NURSING INTERVENTIONS

When working with clients who report depressed feelings, it is always important to assess whether there is risk for self-harm. If the client expresses suicidal ideation or has urges for self-injury, the nurse must provide interventions and plan care as indicated (see Chap. 14).

The nurse should explain that the client must take action to feel better rather than waiting to feel better. Becoming involved in activities or engaging with others provides opportunities to interrupt the client's cyclical, negative thought patterns.

Giving the client factual feedback, rather than general praise, reinforces the client's attempts to interact with others and gives specific, positive information about improved behaviors. An example of general praise is, *"Oh, you're doing so well today."* This statement does not identify specific positive behaviors. Allowing the client to identify specific positive behaviors often helps to promote self-esteem. An example of specific praise is, *"You talked to Mrs. Jones for 10 minutes, even though it was difficult. I know that took a lot of effort."* This statement gives the client a clear message about what specific behavior was effective and positive—the client's ability to talk to someone else.

Cognitive restructuring techniques such as thought-stopping or positive self-talk (discussed previously) can also enhance self-esteem. The client is taught to recognize negative thoughts and feelings and learn new, positive patterns of thinking about himself or herself.

It may be necessary to teach the client effective social skills, such as eye contact, attentive listening, and topics that are appropriate for initial social conversation (eg, the weather, current events, local news). Even if the client knows these social skills, it is important to practice them, first with the nurse and then with others. Practicing with the nurse is initially less threatening for the client. Another simple but effective technique is to help the client practice

giving others compliments. This requires the client to identify something positive rather than negative in others. Giving compliments to others also promotes receiving compliments in return, which further enhances positive feelings.

Passive-Aggressive Personality Disorder

CLINICAL PICTURE

Passive-aggressive personality disorder is characterized by a pervasive pattern of passive resistance to demands for adequate social and occupational performance and a negative attitude. It occurs in 1% to 3% of the general population and 2% to 8% of the clinical population. It is thought to be slightly more prevalent in women than men (DSM-IV-TR, 2000).

The client may appear cooperative, even ingratiating, or sullen and withdrawn, depending on the circumstances. The client's mood may fluctuate rapidly and erratically, and he or she may be easily upset or offended. The client may alternate between hostile self-assertion, such as stubbornness or fault-finding, and excessive dependence, expressing contrition and guilt. There is a pervasive attitude that is negative, sullen, and defeatist. The client's affect may be sad or angry. The client's negative attitude influences thought content: the client perceives and anticipates difficulties and disappointment where none exist. The client has a negative view of the future, believing that nothing good ever lasts. His or her ability to make judgments or decisions is often impaired. The client is frequently ambivalent and indecisive, preferring to allow others to make decisions that the client will then criticize. Insight is also limited: the client tends to blame others for his or her own feelings and misfortune. Rather than accepting reasonable responsibility for the situation, the client may alternate blaming behavior with exaggerated remorse and contrition.

The client experiences intense conflict between dependence on others and his or her desire for assertion. Self-confidence is low despite the bravado shown. The client may complain that he or she is misunderstood and unappreciated by others and may report feeling cheated, victimized, and exploited. Clients habitually resent, oppose, and resist demands to function at a level expected by others. This opposition occurs most frequently in work situations but can also be evident in social functioning. The resistance is expressed by procrastination, forgetfulness, stubbornness, and intentional inefficiency, especially in response to tasks assigned by authority figures. The client may also obstruct the efforts of coworkers by failing to do his or her share of the work. In social or family relationships, the client may play the role of the martyr who "sacrifices everything for others," or he or she may be aggrieved and misunderstood. These behaviors in relationships are sometimes effective in manipulating others to do as the client wishes, without the client needing to make a direct request.

The client often has a variety of vague or generalized somatic complaints and may even adopt a sick role. The client then can be angry or bitter, complaining that "no one can figure out what's wrong with me. I just have to suffer. It's my bad luck!"

NURSING INTERVENTIONS

The nurse may encounter a great deal of resistance from the client in identifying feelings and expressing them directly. Often clients do not recognize that they feel angry and may express that anger in indirect ways. The nurse can help the client examine the relationship between feelings and subsequent actions. For example, the client may intend to complete a project at work but then procrastinates, forgets, or becomes "ill" and misses the deadline, or the client may intend to participate in a family outing but becomes ill, forgets, or "has an emergency" when it is time for the outing. By focusing on the client's behavior, the nurse can help the client see what is so annoying or troubling to other people. The nurse can also help the client learn appropriate ways to express feelings directly, especially negative feelings such as anger. Methods such as having the client write about the feelings or role-play are effective. However, if the client is unwilling to engage in this process, the nurse cannot force him or her to do so.

COMMUNITY-BASED CARE

Caring for clients with personality disorders occurs primarily in community-based settings. Acute psychiatric settings such as the hospital are useful for safety concerns for short periods of time. The nurse will use skills in dealing with clients with personality disorders in clinics, outpatient settings, doctors' offices, and many medical settings. Often the personality disorder is not the focus of attention; rather, the client may be seeking treatment for a physical condition.

Most people with personality disorders are treated in group or individual therapy settings, community support programs, or self-help groups. Others will not seek treatment for their personality disorder but may be treated for a major mental illness. Wherever the nurse encounters clients with personality disorders, including in his or her own life, the interventions discussed in this chapter can prove useful.

SELF-AWARENESS ISSUES

Because clients with personality disorders take a long time to change their behaviors, attitudes, or coping skills, nurses working with them can easily become frustrated or angry. These clients continually test the limits or boundaries of the nurse–client relationship with attempts at manipulation. These feelings of anger or frustration need to be discussed with colleagues to help the nurse recognize and cope with his or her own feelings.

The overall appearance of clients with personality disorders can be misleading. Unlike clients who are psychotic or severely depressed, clients with personality disorders look as though they are capable of functioning more effectively. The nurse can easily but mistakenly believe the client simply lacks motivation or the willingness to make changes, and may feel frustrated or angry. It is easy for the nurse to think, "Why does the client continue to do that? Can't he see it only gets him into difficulties?" This reaction is similar to what the client has probably received from others in his or her life.

Clients with personality disorders also challenge the ability of therapeutic staff to work as a team. For example, clients with antisocial or borderline personalities often manipulate staff members by attempts at splitting staff—that is, causing staff to disagree or contradict each other in terms of the limits of the client's treatment plan. This can be quite disruptive to the treatment team. In addition, team members may have differing opinions about individual clients. One staff member may believe that the client needs assistance, but another staff member may believe the client is overly dependent. Ongoing communication among staff is necessary to remain firm and consistent about expectations for clients.

Helpful Hints for Working With Clients With Personality Disorders

- Talking to colleagues about feelings of frustration will help you deal with your emotional responses so you can be more effective with clients.
- Clear, frequent communication with other health care providers can help diminish the client's manipulation.
- Do not take undue flattery or harsh criticism personally; it is a result of the client's personality disorder.
- Set realistic goals, remembering that behavior changes in clients with personality disorders take a long time. Progress can be very slow.

INTERNET RESOURCES

Resource	Internet Address
▸ **Personality disorders**	http://www.focusas.com/Personality Disorders.html
▸ **Borderline personality disorder**	http://www.mental-health-matters.com/borderline.html
	http://members.aol.com/BPDCentral/index.html
▸ **Schizoid personality disorder**	http://www.grohol.com/sx30.html
▸ **Avoidant personality disorder**	http://www.geocities.com/HotSprings13764
▸ **Schizotypal personality disorder**	http://www.mentalhealth.com/dis/p20-pe03.html
▸ **Histrionic personality disorder**	http://www.mentalhealth.com/dis/p20-pe06.html

➤ KEY POINTS

- People with personality disorders have traits that are inflexible and maladaptive and cause either significant functional impairment or subjective distress.
- Personality disorders are relatively common and are diagnosed in early adulthood, although some behaviors are evident in childhood or adolescence.
- Rapid or substantial changes in personality are unlikely. This can be a primary source of frustration for family members, friends, and health care professionals.

Critical Thinking

Questions

1. Where do you see yourself in relation to the four types of temperament (harm avoidance, novelty seeking, reward dependence, and persistence)?
2. What has been the most significant influence on your development as a person?
3. There is a significant correlation between the diagnosis of antisocial personality disorder and criminal behavior. The DSM-IV-TR includes "violation of the rights of others" in the definition of this disorder. Is this personality disorder more a social than a mental health problem? Why?

- Schizotypal personality disorder is characterized by social and interpersonal deficits, cognitive and perceptual distortions, and eccentric behavior.
- Persons with paranoid personality disorders are suspicious, mistrustful, and threatened by others.
- Persons with depressive personality disorder are sad, gloomy, and negative, experience no pleasure, and tend to brood or ruminate about their lives.
- Schizoid personality disorder includes marked detachment from others, restricted emotions, indifference, and fantasy.
- Persons with antisocial personality disorder often appear glib and charming, but they are suspicious, insensitive, and uncaring and often exploit others for their own gain.
- Persons with borderline personality disorder have markedly unstable mood, affect, self-image, interpersonal relationships, and impulsivity and often engage in self-harm behavior.
- Persons with obsessive-compulsive personality disorder are preoccupied with orderliness, perfection, and interpersonal control at the expense of flexibility, openness, and efficiency.
- Histrionic personality disorder is characterized by excessive emotionality and dramatic, attention-seeking, and seductive or provocative behavior.
- Narcissistic personality disorder is characterized by grandiosity, need for admiration,

lack of empathy for others, and a sense of entitlement.

- Avoidant personality disorder is characterized by social discomfort and reticence in all situations, low self-esteem, and hypersensitivity to negative evaluation.
- Dependent personality disorder is characterized by a pervasive and excessive need to be taken care of that leads to submissive and clinging behaviors and fears of separation and abandonment.
- Persons with passive-aggressive personality disorder demonstrate passive resistance to demands for adequate social and occupational performance and negativity and often play the role of a martyr.
- Nurses working with clients with personality disorders must address with colleagues their feelings of anger and frustration and must avoid being manipulated by clients.
- The therapeutic relationship is crucial in caring for clients with personality disorders. Nurses can help clients identify their feelings and dysfunctional behaviors and develop appropriate coping skills and positive behaviors. Therapeutic communication and role-modeling help promote appropriate social interactions, which help improve interpersonal relationships.
- Several therapeutic strategies are effective when working with clients with personality disorders. Cognitive restructuring techniques such as thought-stopping, positive self-talk, and decatastrophizing are useful, as are self-help skills and skills to help the client function better in the community.
- Psychotropic medications are prescribed for clients with personality disorders based on the type and severity of symptoms the client experiences in the following categories: aggression and impulsivity, mood dysregulation, anxiety, and psychotic symptoms.
- Clients with borderline personality disorder often have self-harm urges that are enacted by cutting, burning, or punching themselves, sometimes causing permanent physical damage. The nurse can encourage the client to enter into a no self-harm contract, in which the client promises to try to keep from harming himself or herself and to report to the nurse when he or she is having self-harm urges.
- Nurses need to use self-awareness skills to minimize client manipulation and deal with feelings of frustration.

REFERENCES

American Psychiatric Association. (2000). *DSM-IV-TR: Diagnostic and statistical manual of mental disorders-text revision* (4th ed.). Washington DC: American Psychiatric Association.

Cloninger, C. R., & Svrakic, D. M. (2000). Personality disorders. In B. J. Sadock & V. A. Sadock (Eds.). *Comprehensive textbook of psychiatry*, Vol. 2 (7th ed., pp. 1723–1764). Philadelphia: Lippincott, Williams & Wilkins.

Dycoff, D., Goldstein, L., & Schacht-Levine, L. (1996). The investigation of behavioral contracting in patients with borderline personality disorder. *Journal of the American Psychiatric Nurses Association, 2*(3), 71–78.

Gunderson, J. G., & Phillips, K. A. (1995). Personality disorders. In H. I. Kaplan & B. J. Sadock (Eds.). *Comprehensive textbook of psychiatry*, Vol. 1, (6th ed., pp. 1425–1461). Baltimore: Williams & Wilkins.

Linehan, M. M. (1993). *Cognitive-behavioral treatment of borderline personality disorder*. New York: The Guilford Press.

Loughrey, L., Jackson, J., Molla, P., & Wobbleton, J. (1997). Patient self-mutilation: When nursing becomes a nightmare. *Journal of Psychosocial Nursing, 35*(4), 30–34.

Schultz, J. M., & Videbeck, S. L. (1998). *Lippincott's manual of psychiatric nursing care plans* (5th ed.). Philadelphia: Lippincott-Raven.

Soloff, P. H. (1998). Algorithms for the treatment of personality dimensions: Symptom-specific treatments for cognitive-perceptual, affective, and impulsive-behavioral dysregulation. *Bulletin of the Meninger Clinic, 62*(2), 195–215.

Stravynski, A., Belisle, M., Marcoullier, M., et al. (1994). The treatment of avoidant personality disorder by social skills training in the clinic or in real-life setting. *Canadian Journal of Psychiatry, 39*(8), 377–383.

ADDITIONAL READINGS

Arntz, A., Dietzel, R., & Dressen, L. (1999). Assumptions in borderline personality disorder: Specificity, stability, and relationship with etiological factors. *Behaviour Research and Therapy, 37*, 545–557.

Atre-Vaidya, N., & Hussain, S. M. (1999). Borderline personality disorder and bipolar mood disorder: Two distinct disorders of a continuum? *Journal of Nervous & Mental Diseases, 187*(5), 313–315.

Barstow, D. G. (1995). Self-injury and self-mutilation: Nursing approaches. *Journal of Psychosocial Nursing, 33*(2), 19–22.

Boyarsky, B. K., Perone, L. A., Lee, N. C., & Goodman, W. K. (1991). Current treatment approaches to obsessive-compulsive disorder. *Archives of Psychiatric Nursing, 5*(5), 166–175.

Chengappa, K. N. R., Ebeling, T., Kang, J. S., Levine, J., & Prepally, H. (1999). Clozapine reduces severe self-mutilation and aggression in psychotic patients with borderline personality disorder. *Journal of Clinical Psychiatry, 6*(7), 477–483.

Clark, L. A., & Watson, D. (1999). Personality disorder, and personality disorder: Toward a more rational conceptualization. *Journal of Personality Disorders, 13*(2), 142–151.

Cremin, D., Lemmer, B., & Davison, S. (1995). The efficacy of a nursing challenge to patients: Testing a new intervention to decrease self-harm behavior in severe personality disorder. *Journal of Psychiatric and Mental Health Services, 2*(4), 237–246.

Dickey, C. C., et al. (1999). Schizotypal personality disorder and MRI abnormalities of temporal lobe gray matter. *Biological Psychiatry, 45*, 1393–1402.

Erzurum, V. Z., & Varcelotti, J. (1999). Self-inflicted burn injuries. *Journal of Burn Care & Rehabilitation, 20*(1), 22–24.

Faye, P. (1995). Addictive characteristics of the behavior of self-mutilation. *Journal of Psychosocial Nursing, 33*(6), 36–39.

Green, H., & Ugarriza, D. N. (1995). The stably unstable borderline personality disorder: History, theory, and nursing intervention. *Journal of Psychosocial Nursing, 33*(1), 26–30.

Hampton, M. D. (1997). Dialectical behavior therapy in the treatment of persons with borderline personality disorder. *Archives of Psychiatric Nursing, 11*(2), 96–101.

Hollander, E. (1999). Managing aggressive behavior in patients with obsessive-compulsive disorder and borderline personality disorder. *Journal of Clinical Psychiatry, 60*, 38–44.

Hoover, S. D., & Norris, J. (1996), Validation study for impaired personal boundaries, proposed nursing diagnosis. *Nursing Diagnosis, 7*(4), 147–151.

Hueston, W. J., Werth, J., & Mainous, A. G. (1999). Personality disorder traits: Prevalence and effects on health status in primary care patients. *International Journal of Psychiatry in Medicine, 29*(1), 63–74.

Joyce, A. L., McCallum, M., & Piper, W. E. (1999). Borderline functioning, work, and outcome in intensive evening treatment. *International Journal of Group Psychotherapy, 49*(3), 343–368.

Langdon, R., & Coltheart, M. (1999). Mentalising, schizotypy, and schizophrenia. *Cognition, 71,* 43–71.

Links, P. S., Heslegrave, R., & van Reekum, R. (1999). Impulsivity: The core of borderline personality disorder. *Journal of Personality Disorders, 13*(1), 1–9.

Miller, S. A., & Davenport, N. C. (1996). Increasing staff knowledge and improving attitudes toward patients with borderline personality disorder. *Psychiatric Services, 47*(5), 533–535.

Millon, T. (1981). *Disorders of personality: DSM-III: Axis II.* New York: John Wiley & Sons.

Millon, T. (1996). *Disorders of personality: DSM-IV and beyond.* New York: John Wiley & Sons.

Nehls, N. (1999). Borderline personality disorder: The voice of patients. *Research in Nursing & Health, 22,* 285–293.

Phillips, K. A., & Gunderson, J. G. (1999). Depressive personality disorder: Fact or fiction? *Journal of Personality Disorders, 13*(2), 128–134.

Roller, B., & Nelson, V. (1999). Group psychotherapy treatment of borderline personalities. *International Journal of Group Psychotherapy, 49*(3), 369–385.

Ryder, A. G., & Bagby, R. M. (1999). Diagnostic variability or depressive personality disorder: Theoretical and conceptual issues. *Journal of Personality Disorders, 13*(2), 99–117.

San Blise, M. L. (1995). Everything I learned, I learned from patients: Positive radical reframing. *Journal of Psychosocial Nursing, 33*(12), 18–25.

West, M., Rose, M., & Sheldon-Keller, A. (1994). Assessment of patterns of insecure attachment in adults and application to dependent and schizoid personality disorders. *Journal of Personality Disorders, 8*(3), 249–256.

Wetzler, S., & Morey, L. C. (1999). Passive-aggressive personality disorder: The demise of a syndrome. *Psychiatry, 62,* 49–59.

Chapter Review

Select the best answer for each of the following questions.

1. When working with a client with a paranoid personality disorder, the nurse would use which of the following approaches?

   A. Cheerful

   B. Friendly

   C. Serious

   D. Supportive.

2. Which of the following underlying emotions is commonly seen in a passive-aggressive personality disorder?

   A. Anger

   B. Depression

   C. Fear

   D. Guilt.

3. Cognitive restructuring techniques include all of the following except:

   A. Decatastrophizing

   B. Positive self-talk

   C. Reframing

   D. Relaxation.

4. Transient psychotic symptoms that occur with borderline personality disorder are most likely treated with which of the following?

   A. Anticonvulsant mood stabilizers

   B. Antipsychotics

   C. Benzodiazepines

   D. Lithium.

5. Clients with a histrionic personality disorder are most likely to benefit from which of the following nursing interventions?

   A. Cognitive restructuring techniques

   B. Improving community functioning

   C. Providing emotional support

   D. Teaching social skills.

➤ TRUE-FALSE QUESTIONS

Identify each of the following statements as T (true) or F (false). Correct any false statements.

_____ 1. Character is the part of personality that is inherited.

_____ 2. The client with a schizoid personality disorder would benefit from having a variety of social contacts in the community.

_____ 3. Identifying appropriate, expected behavior is an important part of limit-setting.

_____ 4. Clients with personality disorders can be expected to make steady, rapid progress in group therapy.

_____ 5. A client with obsessive-compulsive personality disorder usually has no problem meeting deadlines at work.

_____ 6. The client with narcissistic personality disorder is usually motivated to seek treatment to improve social relationships.

_____ 7. Clients with dependent personality disorder have difficulties making decisions and solving problems.

_____ 8. Clients with borderline personality disorder may engage in self-mutilation behavior as a means of dealing with intense emotions.

➤ FILL-IN-THE-BLANK QUESTIONS

Identify the personality disorder that is described in each of the following.

_____ Unstable relationships, affect, and self-image

_____ Disregard for the rights of others

_____ Detachment from social relationships, restricted affect

_____ Social inhibitions, feelings of inadequacy

➤ SHORT-ANSWER QUESTIONS

Describe the behavior associated with each of the following temperament traits.

Harm avoidance: High

Harm avoidance: Low

Novelty seeking: High

Novelty seeking: Low

Reward dependence: High

Reward dependence: Low

Persistence: High

Persistence: Low

➤ CLINICAL EXAMPLE

Susan Marks, age 25, is diagnosed with borderline personality disorder. She has been attending college sporadically but has only 15 completed credits and has no real career goal. She is angry because her parents have told her she must get a job and support herself. Last week, she met a man in the park and fell in love with him on their first date. She has been calling him repeatedly, but he will not return her calls. Declaring that her parents have deserted her and her boyfriend doesn't love her anymore, she slashes her forearms with a sharp knife. She then calls 911, stating, "I'm about to die! Please help me!" She is taken by ambulance to the emergency room and is admitted to the inpatient psychiatry unit.

1. Identify two priority nursing diagnoses that would be appropriate for Susan on her admission to the unit.

2. Write an expected outcome for each of the identified nursing diagnoses.

3. List three nursing interventions for each of the identified nursing diagnoses.

4. What community resources or referrals would be beneficial for Susan?

Substance Abuse

Surveys conducted by the National Institute for Mental Health estimate that in the United States, about 14% of the adult population meet the criteria for an alcohol-related disorder, and 6.2% of adults meet the criteria for a substance-related disorder other than alcohol or tobacco (Jaffe, 2000*c*). These figures do not include adolescents, whose increasing use of alcohol and other drugs is a national concern. A survey of 12- to 17-year-olds by the Substance Abuse and Mental Health Services Administration indicated that 9% had used an illicit substance and 18.8% had consumed alcohol in the month before the survey (1997). The actual prevalence of substance abuse is difficult to determine precisely because many people meeting the criteria for diagnosis do not seek treatment, and surveys conducted to estimate prevalence are based on self-reported data that may not be accurate.

Substance use/abuse and related disorders have become a national health problem. The cost of substance use and related disorders is estimated to be $144 billion per year in terms of health care and job loss (Galanter & Kleber, 1994). This figure includes the cost of related problems such as increased HIV infection and AIDS from intravenous drug use but does not include the health care costs related to tobacco. Fifty percent of motor vehicle fatalities are estimated to be related to alcohol.

The number of babies suffering the physiologic and emotional consequences of prenatal exposure to alcohol or drugs (for example fetal alcohol syndrome, "crack babies") is increasing at alarming rates. Chemical abuse also results in an increased incidence of violence, including domestic abuse, homicide, and child abuse and neglect. These rising statistics regarding substance abuse do not bode well for future generations.

Studies have shown that half of all persons seeking treatment for alcohol-related disorders have at least one parent who is or was an alcoholic (Finfgeld, 1997). Many people who are in treatment programs as adults report having their first drink of alcohol as a young child, before the age of 10. This first drink was often a taste of the drink of a parent or family member. With the increasing rates of use being reported among young people today, this problem seems to be spiraling out of control unless great strides can be made through programs for prevention, early detection, and effective treatment.

TYPES OF SUBSTANCE ABUSE

Many substances can be used and abused; some of them can be legally obtained, and some are illegal. This discussion will include alcohol and prescription medications as substances that can be abused. Abuse of more than one substance is termed **polysubstance abuse**. The DSM-IV-TR lists 11 diagnostic classes of substance abuse:

- Alcohol
- Amphetamines or similarly acting sympathomimetics
- Caffeine
- Cannabis
- Cocaine
- Hallucinogens
- Inhalants
- Nicotine
- Opioids
- Phencyclidine (PCP) or similarly acting drugs
- Sedatives, hypnotics, or anxiolytics.

The DSM-IV-TR also categorizes substance-related disorders into two groups: those that include disorders of abuse and dependence, and substance-induced disorders such as intoxication, withdrawal, delirium, dementia, psychosis, mood disorder, anxiety, sexual dysfunction, and sleep disorder.

In this chapter, the specific symptoms of intoxication, overdose, withdrawal, and detoxification are described for each substance, with the exception of caffeine and nicotine. Although caffeine and nicotine abuse can cause significant physiologic health problems and can result in substance-induced disorders such as sleep disorders, anxiety, and withdrawal, treatment of these two substances is usually not viewed as falling into the mental health arena. **Intoxication** is use of a substance that results in maladaptive behavior, and **withdrawal syndrome** refers to the negative psychological and physical reactions that occur when use of the substance ceases or is dramatically decreased. **Detoxification** is the process of safely withdrawing from a substance. The treatment of other substance-induced disorders such as psychosis and mood disorders is discussed in depth in separate chapters.

Substance abuse can be defined as using a drug in a way that is inconsistent with medical or social norms and despite negative consequences. The DSM-IV-TR makes a distinction between substance abuse and dependence for purposes of medical diagnosis. Substance abuse denotes problems in social, vocational, or legal areas of the person's life, whereas substance dependence also includes problems associated with addiction, such as tolerance, withdrawal, and unsuccessful attempts to stop using the substance. This distinction between abuse and dependence is frequently viewed as unclear and unnecessary (Jaffe, 2000*c*) because clinical decisions are not affected by the distinction once withdrawal or detoxification has been completed. Hence, the terms substance abuse and substance dependence or chemical dependence can be used interchangeably. In this chapter, the term substance use is used to include both abuse and dependence; it is not meant to refer to the occasional or one-time user.

ONSET AND CLINICAL COURSE

Much of the research on substance use has focused on alcohol because it is legal and more widely used; thus, more is known about its effects. The prognosis for alcohol use in general is unclear because usually only those seeking treatment are studied.

The early course of alcoholism typically begins with the first episode of intoxication between the ages of 15 and 17 years (Schuckit, 2000), and the first evidence of minor alcohol-related problems is seen in the late teens. These events do not differ significantly from the experiences of people who do not go on to develop alcoholism. A pattern of more severe difficulties for people with alcoholism begins to emerge in the middle 20s to the middle 30s, such as the alcohol-related breakup of a significant relationship, an arrest for public intoxication or driving while intoxicated, evidence of alcohol withdrawal, early alcohol-related health problems, or significant interference with functioning at work or school. During this time, the person experiences his or her first **blackout**, an episode during which the person continues to function but has no conscious awareness of his or her behavior at the time, nor any memory of the behavior later.

The later course of alcoholism, when the person's functioning is definitely affected, is often characterized by periods of abstinence or temporarily controlled drinking. Abstinence may occur after some legal, social, or interpersonal crisis, and the person may then set up rules about drinking, such as drinking only at certain times or only drinking beer. This period of temporarily controlled drinking soon leads to an escalation of alcohol intake, more problems, and a subsequent crisis. The cycle is repeated again and again (Schuckit, 2000).

For many, substance use is a chronic illness characterized by remissions and relapses to former levels of use (Jaffe, 2000c). The highest rates for successful recovery are for people who abstain from substances, are highly motivated to quit, and have a past history of life success (that is, satisfactory experiences in coping, work, relationships, and so forth). Although an estimated 60% to 70% of people in alcoholism treatment remain sober after 1 year (Schuckit, 2000), this may be an optimistic estimate, because most relapses occur during the second year after treatment.

Evidence shows that some people with alcohol-related problems can moderate or quit drinking on their own without a treatment program; this is called **spontaneous remission** (Finfgeld, 1997). The abstinence may be in response to a crisis or a promise to a loved one. Whatever the reason, spontaneous remission can occur in as many as 20% of alcoholics, although it is highly unlikely that persons in the later stage of alcoholism can recover without treatment (Schuckit, 2000).

Poor outcomes have been associated with an earlier age of onset, longer periods of substance use, and the coexistence of a major psychiatric illness. With extended use, there is greater risk of mental and physical deterioration and infectious disease, such as HIV infection and AIDS, hepatitis, and tuberculosis, especially for persons with a history of intravenous drug use. In addition, persons addicted to alcohol and drugs have a rate of suicide that is 20% higher than that of the general population.

RELATED DISORDERS

Substance-induced disorders such as anxiety, mood disorders, and dementia are discussed in other chapters—for instance, Chapter 15 discusses delirium, which may be seen in severe alcohol withdrawal. A clinical care plan for a client receiving treatment for substance abuse is featured near the end of this chapter. The effects on adults who grew up in a home with an alcoholic parent are discussed later, as are the special needs of clients with a dual diagnosis of substance use and a major psychiatric disorder.

ETIOLOGY

The exact causes of drug use, dependence, and addiction are not known, but a variety of factors are thought to contribute to the development of substance-related disorders (Jaffe, 2000c). Much of the research on biologic and genetic factors has been done on alcohol abuse, but psychological, social, and environmental studies have examined other drugs as well.

Biologic Factors

The children of alcoholic parents are at higher risk for developing alcoholism and drug dependence than are children of nonalcoholic parents (Jaffe, 2000c). This increased risk is due in part to environmental factors, but there is evidence that genetic factors are important as well. Several studies of twins have shown a higher rate of concordance (when one twin has it, the other twin gets it) among identical than fraternal twins. Adoption studies have shown higher rates of alcoholism in sons of biologic fathers with alcoholism than those of nonalcoholic biologic fathers. These studies lead theorists to describe the genetic component of alcoholism as a genetic vulnerability that is then influenced by a variety of social and environmental factors. Prescott and Kendler (1999) found that 48% to 58% of the variation in causes of alcoholism was due to genetics, with the remainder due to environmental influences.

Neurochemical influences on substance use patterns have been studied primarily in animal research (Jaffe, 2000c). The ingestion of mood-altering substances stimulates dopamine pathways in the limbic system, producing pleasant feelings or a "high," which is a reinforcing, or positive, experience. Distribution of the substance throughout the brain alters the balance of neurotransmitters that modulate pleasure, pain, and reward responses. Researchers have proposed that some people have an internal alarm that limits the amount of alcohol consumed to one or two drinks, so that the person feels a pleasant sensation but goes no further. People without this internal signaling mechanism experience the high initially but continue to drink until central nervous system depression is marked and they are intoxicated.

Social and Environmental Factors

Cultural factors, social attitudes, peer behaviors, laws, and cost and availability all influence initial and continued use of substances (Jaffe, 2000c). In general, substances that carry less social disapproval, such as alcohol and cannabis, are used by younger experimenters; drugs such as cocaine and opioids, which are more costly and rate higher disapproval, are used at a later age. Consumption of alcohol increases in areas where availability increases and decreases in areas where cost has risen due to increased taxation. The social use of cannabis, although illegal, is viewed by many as not very harmful; some even advocate legalizing the use of marijuana for social purposes. Urban areas where cocaine and opioids are readily available also have high crime rates, high unemployment, and substandard school systems, resulting in high rates of cocaine and opioid use and low rates of recovery. Thus, environment and social customs can influence a person's use of substances.

Psychological Factors

In addition to the genetic links to alcoholism, family dynamics are thought to play a part. Children of alcoholics are four times as likely to develop alcoholism (Schuckit, 2000). Some theorists believe that inconsistency in the parent's behavior, poor role modeling, and lack of nurturing pave the way for the child to adopt a similar style of maladaptive coping, stormy relationships, and substance abuse. Others hypothesize that even children who abhorred their family life are likely to abuse substances as adults because they lack adaptive coping skills and cannot form successful relationships (Tweed & Ryff, 1996).

Alcohol can be used as a coping mechanism or a way to relieve stress and tension, increase feelings of power, and decrease psychological pain. However, high doses of alcohol actually increase muscle tension and nervousness (Schuckit, 2000).

CULTURAL CONSIDERATIONS

Attitudes toward substance use, patterns of use, and physiologic differences to substances vary in different cultures. Muslims do not drink alcohol, but wine is an integral part of Jewish religious rites. Some Native American tribes use peyote, a hallucinogen, in religious ceremonies. It is important to be aware of such beliefs when assessing whether a substance abuse problem exists.

Certain ethnic groups have genetic traits that either predispose them to or protect them from developing alcoholism. For instance, **flushing**, a reddening of the face and neck due to increased blood flow, has been linked to variants of genes for enzymes involved in alcohol metabolism. Even small amounts of alcohol can produce flushing, which may be accompanied by headaches and nausea. The flushing reaction is highest among people of Asian ancestry (National Institute on Alcohol Abuse and Alcoholism, 2000).

Another genetic difference between ethnic groups is found in other enzymes involved in metabolizing alcohol in the liver. Variations have been found in the structure and activity levels of the enzymes among Asians, African Americans, and whites. One enzyme found in people of Japanese descent has been associated with faster elimination of alcohol from the body. Other enzyme variations are being studied to determine what effect they may have on the metabolism of alcohol among various ethnic groups (National Institute on Alcohol Abuse and Alcoholism, 2000).

Statistics for individual tribes vary, but alcohol abuse overall plays a part in the five leading causes of death for Native Americans (motor vehicle crashes, alcoholism, cirrhosis, suicide, and homicide). Among tribes with high rates of alcoholism, an estimated 75% of all accidents are alcohol-related (National Institute on Alcohol Abuse and Alcoholism, 2000).

TYPES OF SUBSTANCES AND TREATMENT

The classes of mood-altering substances have some similarities and differences in terms of intended effect, intoxication effects, and withdrawal symptoms, but treatment approaches after detoxification are quite similar. This section presents a brief overview of seven classes of substances and the effects of intoxication, overdose, withdrawal, and detoxification, highlighting important elements of which the nurse should be aware.

Alcohol

INTOXICATION AND OVERDOSE

Alcohol is a central nervous system depressant that is rapidly absorbed into the bloodstream. Initially, the effects are relaxation and loss of inhibitions. With intoxication, there is slurred speech, unsteady gait, lack of coordination, and impaired attention, concentration, memory, and judgment. Some people become aggressive or display inappropriate sexual behavior when intoxicated. The person who is intoxicated may experience a blackout.

An overdose, or excessive alcohol intake in a short period of time, can result in vomiting, unconsciousness, and respiratory depression. This combination can result in aspiration pneumonia or pulmonary obstruction. Alcohol-induced hypotension can lead to cardiovascular shock and death. Treatment of an alcohol overdose is similar to that for any central nervous system depressant: gastric lavage or dialysis to remove the drug, and support of respiratory and cardiovascular functioning in an intensive care unit. The administration of central nervous system stimulants is contraindicated (Lehne, 1998). The physiologic effects of repeated intoxication and long-term use are listed in Box 17-1.

WITHDRAWAL AND DETOXIFICATION

Symptoms of withdrawal usually begin 4 to 12 hours after cessation or marked reduction of alcohol intake. Symptoms include coarse hand tremors, sweating, elevated pulse and blood pressure, insomnia, anxiety, and nausea or vomiting. Severe or untreated withdrawal may progress to transient hallucinations, seizures, or delirium, called delirium tremens (DTs). Alcohol withdrawal usually peaks on the second day and is over in about 5 days (DSM-IV-TR, 2000). This can vary, however, and it may take 1 to 2 weeks.

> ### Box 17-1
> ### ► PHYSIOLOGIC EFFECTS OF LONG-TERM ALCOHOL USE
> - Cardiac myopathy
> - Wernicke's encephalopathy
> - Korsakoff's psychosis
> - Pancreatitis
> - Esophagitis
> - Hepatitis
> - Cirrhosis
> - Leukopenia
> - Thrombocytopenia
> - Ascites

Because alcohol withdrawal can be life-threatening, detoxification needs to be accomplished under medical supervision. If the client's withdrawal symptoms are mild and he or she can abstain from alcohol, he or she can be safely treated at home. For withdrawal that is more severe, or for clients who cannot abstain during detoxification, a short admission of 3 to 5 days is the most common setting for detoxification. Some psychiatric units may also admit clients for detoxification, but this is less common.

Safe withdrawal is usually accomplished with the administration of benzodiazepines such as diazepam (Valium), chlordiazepoxide (Librium), or lorazepam (Ativan) to suppress the withdrawal symptoms. The amount of medication needed and the frequency of administration are determined by the client's vital signs and the presence and severity of withdrawal symptoms. Often, a protocol is used that is based on an assessment tool such as the Global Assessment of Alcohol Withdrawal (Box 17-2). For example, the protocol may indicate Valium 10 mg po to be given every 1 to 2 hours for a diastolic blood pressure of more than 90 mmHg, a pulse greater than 100, a temperature greater than 100°F, or a global assessment score of 6 to 10. Higher doses are ordered for higher blood pressure, pulse, or global assessment scores.

 CLINICAL VIGNETTE: DETOXIFICATION

John is a 62-year-old man admitted at 5 AM Monday for an elective knee replacement surgery. The surgical procedure, including the anesthetic, went smoothly. John was stabilized in the recovery room in about 3 hours. His blood pressure was 124/82, temperature 98.8°F, pulse 76, respirations 16. John was alert, oriented, and verbally responsive, so he was transferred to a room on the orthopedic unit.

By 10 PM, John is agitated, sweating, and saying, "I have to get out of here!" His blood pressure is 164/98, pulse 98, and respirations 28. His surgical dressing is dry and intact and he has no complaints of pain. The nurse talks with John's wife and asks about his usual habits of alcohol consumption. John's wife says he consumes three or four drinks each evening after work and has beer or wine with dinner. John did not report his alcohol consumption to his doctor before surgery. John's wife says, "No one ever asked me about how much he drank, so I didn't think it was important."

Box 17-2

➤ GLOBAL ASSESSMENT OF ALCOHOL WITHDRAWAL

NAUSEA AND VOMITING

"Do you feel sick to your stomach? Have you vomited? Observation. Document 0–7
0 - no nausea or vomiting
1 - mild nausea w/no vomiting
2 -
3 -
4 - intermittent nausea w/dry heaves
5 -
6 -
7 - constant nausea, frequent dry heaves and vomiting

TREMOR

Arms extended and fingers spread apart. Observation. Document 0–7.
0 - no tremor
1 - not visible, but can be felt fingertip to fingertip
2 -
3 -
4 - moderate, w/arms extended
5 -
6 -
7 - severe, even with arms not extended

PAROXYSMAL SWEATS

Observation. Document 0–7
0 - no sweat visible
1 - barely perceptible sweating, palms moist
2 -
3 -
4 - beads of sweat obvious on forehead
5 -
6 -
7 - drenching sweats

ANXIETY

"Do you feel nervous?"
Observation. Document 0–7
0 - no anxiety, at ease
1 - mildly anxious
2 -
3 -

4 - moderately anxious, or guarded, so anxiety is inferred
5 -
6 -
7 - equivalent to acute panic states, as seen in severe delirium or acute schizophrenic states

AGITATION

Observation. Document 0–7
0 - normal activity
1 - somewhat more than normal activity
2 -
3 -
4 - moderately fidgety and restless
5 -
6 -
7 - paces back and forth, constant thrashing about

TACTILE DISTURBANCES

"Have you any itching, pins and needles, burning or numbness or bugs crawling on or under your skin?" Document 0–7
0 - none
1 - very mild itching, pins & needles, etc.
2 - mild itching, etc.
3 - moderate itching, etc.
4 - moderately severe hallucinations.
5 - severe hallucinations
6 - extremely severe hallucinations
7 - continuous hallucinations

AUDITORY DISTURBANCES

"Are you more aware of sounds around you? Are they harsh? Do they frighten you? Are you hearing things that you know are not there?" Observation. Document 0–7
0 - not present
1 - very mild harshness or ability to frighten
2 - mild harshness or ability to frighten
3 - moderate harshness or ability to frighten
4 - moderately severe hallucinations

5 - severe hallucinations
6 - extremely severe hallucinations
7 - continuous hallucinations

VISUAL DISTURBANCES

"Does the light appear to be too bright? Is the color different? Does it hurt your eyes? Are you seeing anything that is disturbing to you? Are you seeing things that you know are not there?" Document 0–7
0 - not present
1 - very mild sensitivity
2 - mild sensitivity
3 - moderate sensitivity
4 - moderately severe hallucinations
5 - severe hallucinations
6 - extremely severe hallucinations
7 - continuous hallucinations

HEADACHE, FULLNESS IN HEAD

"Does your head feel different? Does it feel like there is a band around your head?" Do not rate dizziness or light-headedness, rate severity. Document 0–7
0 - not present
1 - very mild
2 - mild
3 - moderate
4 - moderately severe
5 - severe
6 - very severe
7 - extremely severe

ORIENTATION AND CLOUDING OF SENSORIUM

"What day is this? Where are you?" Observation. Document 0–4
0 - oriented and can do serial additions
1 - cannot do serial additions or is uncertain about dates
2 - disoriented for date by no more than 2 calendar days
3 - disoriented by more than 2 calendar days
4 - disoriented for place and/or person

Sedatives, Hypnotics, and Anxiolytics

INTOXICATION AND OVERDOSE

This class of drugs includes all central nervous system depressants. The intensity of the effect depends on the particular drug. The effects of the drugs, symptoms of intoxication, and withdrawal symptoms are similar to those of alcohol. This class includes barbiturates, nonbarbiturate hypnotics, and anxiolytics, particularly benzodiazepines. Benzodiazepines and barbiturates are the most frequently abused drugs in this category (Ciraulo & Sarid-Segal, 2000). In the usual prescribed doses, these drugs cause drowsiness and reduce anxiety, which is the intended purpose. Intoxication symptoms include slurred speech, lack of coordination, unsteady gait, labile mood, impaired attention or memory, and even stupor and coma.

Benzodiazepines alone, taken orally in overdose, are rarely fatal, but the person will be lethargic and confused. Treatment includes gastric lavage followed by ingestion of activated charcoal and a saline cathartic; dialysis can be used if symptoms are severe (Lehne, 1998). The client's confusion and lethargy will improve as the drug is excreted.

Barbiturates, in contrast, can be lethal when taken in overdose. They can cause coma, respiratory arrest, cardiac failure, and death. Treatment in an intensive care unit is required, using lavage or dialysis to remove the drug from the system and to support respiratory and cardiovascular function.

WITHDRAWAL AND DETOXIFICATION

The onset of withdrawal symptoms depends on the half-life of the drug (see Chap. 2). Medications whose actions typically last about 10 hours, such as lorazepam, produce withdrawal symptoms in 6 to 8 hours; longer-acting medications such as diazepam may not produce withdrawal symptoms for a week (DSM-IV-TR, 2000). The withdrawal syndrome is characterized by symptoms that are the opposite of the acute effects of the drug—that is, autonomic hyperactivity (increased pulse, blood pressure, respirations, and temperature), hand tremor, insomnia, anxiety, nausea, and psychomotor agitation. Seizures and hallucinations occur only rarely in severe benzodiazepine withdrawal (Ciraulo & Sarid-Segal, 2000).

Detoxification from sedatives, hypnotics, and anxiolytics is often managed medically by tapering the amount of the drug the client receives over a period of days or weeks, depending on the drug and the amount the client had been using. **Tapering**, or administering decreasing doses of a medication, is essential with barbiturates to prevent coma and death, which will occur if the drug is stopped abruptly. For example, when tapering the dosage of a benzodiazepine, the client may be given Valium 10 mg four times a day; the dose is decreased every 3 days, and the number of times a day the dose is given is also decreased, until the client is safely withdrawn from the drug.

Stimulants (Amphetamines, Cocaine, Others)

Stimulants are drugs that stimulate or excite the central nervous system. Although the DSM-IV-TR categorizes amphetamines, cocaine, and central nervous system stimulants separately, the effects, intoxication, and withdrawal symptoms of these drugs are virtually identical. For our purposes, they are grouped together.

Stimulants have limited clinical use (with the exception of stimulants used to treat attention deficit hyperactivity disorder; see Chap. 18) and a high potential for abuse. Amphetamines ("uppers") were popular in the past; they were used by people who wanted to lose weight or stay awake. Cocaine, an illegal drug that has virtually no clinical use in medicine, is highly addictive and is a popular recreational drug because of the intense and immediate feeling of euphoria it produces.

INTOXICATION AND OVERDOSE

Intoxication from stimulants develops rapidly; effects include the high or euphoric feeling, hyperactivity, hypervigilance, talkativeness, anxiety, grandiosity, hallucinations, stereotypic or repetitive behavior, anger, fighting, and impaired judgment. Physiologic effects include tachycardia, elevated blood pressure, dilated pupils, perspiration or chills, nausea, chest pain, confusion, or cardiac arrhythmias. Overdoses of stimulants can result in seizures and coma; deaths are rare (Jaffe, 2000a). Treatment with chlorpromazine (Thorazine), an antipsychotic, controls hallucinations, lowers blood pressure, and relieves nausea (Lehne, 1998).

WITHDRAWAL AND DETOXIFICATION

Withdrawal from stimulants occurs within a few hours to several days after cessation of the drug and is not life-threatening. Marked dysphoria is the primary symptom and is accompanied by fatigue, vivid and unpleasant dreams, insomnia or hypersomnia, increased appetite, and psychomotor retardation or agitation. Marked withdrawal symptoms are referred to as "crashing"; the person may experience depressive symptoms for several days, including suicidal ideation. Stimulant withdrawal is not treated pharmacologically.

Cannabis (Marijuana)

Cannabis sativa is the hemp plant, which is widely cultivated for its fiber, used to make rope and cloth, and for its seeds, used to make oil. It has become widely known for its psychoactive resin (Macfadden & Woody, 2000). This resin contains more than 60 substances, called cannabinoids, of which delta-9-tetrahydrocannabinol (THC) is thought to be responsible for most of the psychoactive effects. Marijuana refers to the upper leaves, flowering tops, and stems of the plant; hashish is the dried resinous exudate from the leaves of the female plant. Cannabis is most often smoked in cigarettes ("joints"), but it can be eaten.

Cannabis is the most widely used illicit substance in the United States. Research has shown that cannabis has short-term effects of lowering intraocular pressure, but it is not approved for the treatment of glaucoma. It has also been studied for its effectiveness in relieving the nausea and vomiting associated with cancer chemotherapy and the anorexia and weight loss of AIDS. Currently, two cannabinoids, dronabinol (Marinol) and nabilone (Cesamet), have been approved for treating nausea and vomiting from cancer chemotherapy (Voth & Schwartz, 1997).

INTOXICATION AND OVERDOSE

Cannabis begins to act less than 1 minute after inhalation. Peak effects usually occur in 20 to 30 minutes and last at least 2 to 3 hours. Users report a high feeling similar to that of alcohol, lowered inhibitions, relaxation, euphoria, and increased appetite. Symptoms of intoxication include impaired motor coordination, inappropriate laughter, impaired judgment and short-term memory, and distortions of time and perception. Anxiety, dysphoria, and social withdrawal may occur in some users. Physiologic effects, in addition to increased appetite, include conjunctival injection (bloodshot eyes), dry mouth, hypotension, and tachycardia. Excessive use of cannabis may produce delirium or rarely cannabis-induced psychotic disorder, both of which are treated symptomatically. Overdoses of cannabis do not occur (Macfadden & Woody, 2000).

WITHDRAWAL AND DETOXIFICATION

Although some people have reported withdrawal symptoms of muscle aches, sweating, anxiety, and tremors, no clinically significant withdrawal syndrome is identified (Lehne, 1998).

Opioids

Opioids are popular drugs of abuse because they desensitize the user to both physiologic and psychological pain and induce a sense of euphoria and well-being. Opioid compounds include both potent prescription analgesics such as morphine, meperidine (Demerol), codeine, hydromorphone, oxycodone, methadone, oxymorphone, hydrocodone, and propoxyphene, and illegal substances such as heroin and normethadone. Persons who abuse opioids spend a great deal of their time obtaining the drugs and often engage in illegal activity to get them. Health care professionals who abuse opioids often write prescriptions for themselves or divert prescribed pain medication for patients to themselves (DSM-IV-TR, 2000).

INTOXICATION AND OVERDOSE

Opioid intoxication develops soon after the initial euphoric feeling; symptoms include apathy, lethargy, listlessness, impaired judgment, psychomotor retardation or agitation, dilated pupils, drowsiness, slurred speech, and impaired attention and memory. Severe intoxication or opioid overdose can lead to coma, respiratory depression, pupillary constriction, unconsciousness, and death. Administration of naloxone (Narcan), an opioid antagonist, is the treatment of choice because it reverses all signs of opioid toxicity. Naloxone is given every few hours until the opioid level drops to a nontoxic level; this process may take days (Lehne, 1998).

WITHDRAWAL AND DETOXIFICATION

Opioid withdrawal develops when drug intake ceases or is markedly decreased, or it can be precipitated by the administration of an opioid antagonist. Initial symptoms are anxiety, restlessness, aching back and legs, and cravings for more opioids (Jaffe & Jaffe, 2000). Symptoms that develop as withdrawal progresses include nausea, vomiting, dysphoria, lacrimation, rhinorrhea, sweating, diarrhea, yawning, fever, and insomnia. Symptoms of opioid withdrawal cause significant distress but do not require pharmacologic intervention to support life or bodily functions. Short-acting drugs such as heroin produce withdrawal symptoms in 6 to 24 hours; the symptoms peak in 2 to 3 days and gradually subside in 5 to 7 days. Longer-acting substances such as methadone may not produce significant withdrawal symptoms for 2 to 4 days, and the symptoms may take 2 weeks to subside. Methadone can be used as a replacement for the opioid, and the dosage is then decreased over a 2-week period. Substitution of methadone during detoxification reduces symptoms to no worse than a mild case of flu (Lehne, 1998). Withdrawal symptoms such as anxiety, insomnia, dysphoria, anhedonia, and drug craving may persist for weeks or months.

Hallucinogens

Hallucinogens are substances that distort the user's perception of reality and produce symptoms similar to psychosis, including hallucinations (usually visual) and depersonalization. Hallucinogens also cause increased pulse, blood pressure, and temperature, dilated pupils, and hyperreflexia. Examples of hallucinogens are mescaline, psilocybin, lysergic acid diethylamide (LSD), and "designer drugs" such as Ecstasy. Phencyclidine (PCP), developed as an anesthetic, is included in this section because it acts similarly to hallucinogens.

INTOXICATION AND OVERDOSE

Hallucinogen intoxication is marked by a variety of maladaptive behavioral or psychological changes: anxiety, depression, paranoid ideation, ideas of reference, fear of losing one's mind, and potentially dangerous behavior such as jumping out a window in the belief that one can fly (Abraham, 2000). Physiologic symptoms include sweating, tachycardia, palpitations, blurred vision, tremors, and lack of coordination. PCP intoxication often involves belligerence, aggression, impulsivity, and unpredictable behavior.

Toxic reactions to hallucinogens (except PCP) are primarily psychological; overdoses as such do not occur. These drugs are not a direct cause of death, although fatalities have occurred from accidents, aggression, and suicide. Treatment of toxic reactions is supportive. Psychotic reactions are best managed by isolation from external stimuli, using physical restraints if necessary for the safety of the client and others. PCP toxicity can include seizures, hypertension, hyperthermia, and respiratory depression. Medications are used to control seizures and blood pressure, cooling devices such as a hyperthermia blanket are used, and mechanical ventilation is used to support respirations (Lehne, 1998).

WITHDRAWAL AND DETOXIFICATION

No withdrawal syndrome has been identified for hallucinogens, although some people have reported a craving for the drug. Hallucinogens can produce flashbacks, a transient recurrence of perceptual disturbances like those experienced with hallucinogen use. These episodes occur even after all traces of the hallucinogen are gone and may persist for a few months up to 5 years.

Inhalants

Inhalants are a diverse group of drugs, including anesthetics, nitrates, and organic solvents, that are inhaled for their effects. The most common substances in this category are aliphatic and aromatic hydrocarbons found in gasoline, glue, paint thinner, and spray paint. Less frequently used halogenated hydrocarbons include cleaners, correction fluid, spray can propellants, and other compounds containing esters, ketones, and glycols (DSM-IV-TR, 2000). Most of the vapors are inhaled from a rag soaked with the compound, from a paper or plastic bag, or directly from the container. Inhalants can cause significant brain damage, peripheral nervous system damage, and liver disease.

INTOXICATION AND OVERDOSE

Inhalant intoxication involves dizziness, nystagmus, lack of coordination, slurred speech, unsteady gait, tremor, muscle weakness, blurred vision; stupor and coma can occur. Significant behavioral symptoms are belligerence, aggression, apathy, impaired judgment, and inability to function. Acute toxicity causes anoxia, respiratory depression, vagal stimulation, and arrhythmias. Death may occur from bronchospasm, cardiac arrest, suffocation, or aspiration of the compound or vomitus (Crowley, 2000). Treatment consists of supporting respiratory and cardiac functioning until the substance is removed from the body. There are no antidotes or specific medications to treat inhalant toxicity.

WITHDRAWAL AND DETOXIFICATION

There are no withdrawal symptoms or detoxification procedures for inhalants as such, although frequent users report psychological cravings. People who abuse inhalants may suffer from persistent dementia or inhalant-induced disorders such as psychosis, anxiety, or mood disorders, even if the inhalant abuse ceases. These disorders are all treated symptomatically (Crowley, 2000).

TREATMENT AND PROGNOSIS

Current treatment modalities are based on the concept of alcoholism (and other addictions) as a medical illness that is progressive, chronic, and characterized by remissions and relapses (Jaffe, 2000c). Until the 1970s, organized treatment programs and clinics for substance abuse were scarce. Before the illness of addiction was fully understood, most of society and even the medical community viewed chemical dependency as a personal problem; the user was advised to "pull yourself together" and "get control of your problem." A noted exception, the Hazelden Clinic in Minnesota, was founded in 1949; because of its success, many programs are based on the Hazelden model of treatment.

Today, treatment for substance use is available in a variety of community settings, not all of which involve health professionals. Alcoholics Anonymous (AA) was founded in the 1930s by alcoholics. This self-help group developed the **12-step program** model for recovery (Box 17-3), which is based on the philosophy that total abstinence is essential and that alcoholics need the help and support of others to maintain sobriety. Key slogans reflect the ideas in the 12 steps, such as "one day at a time" (approach sobriety one day at a time), "easy does it" (don't get frenzied about daily life and problems), and "let go and let God" (turn your life over to a higher power). Each new member has a sponsor who helps the new member. Once sober, a member can be a sponsor for another person.

Regular attendance at meetings is emphasized. Meetings are available daily in larger cities and at least weekly in smaller towns or rural areas. AA meetings may be "closed" (only those who are pursuing recovery can attend) or "open" (anyone can attend). Meetings may be educational, with a featured speaker; other meetings simply offer the opportunity for members to tell about their battles with alcohol and to ask the others for help staying sober.

Many treatment programs, regardless of the setting, use the 12-step approach and emphasize participation in AA. They also include individual counseling and a wide variety of groups. Group experiences involve education about substances and their use, problem-solving techniques, and cognitive techniques to identify and modify faulty ways of thinking. An overall theme is coping with life, stress, and other people without the use of substances.

Although traditional treatment programs and AA have been successful for many people, they are not effective for everyone. Some object to the emphasis on God and spirituality; others do not respond to the confrontational approach and being labeled an alcoholic or an addict. Women and minorities have reported feeling overlooked or ignored by an essentially "white, male, middle-class" organization. Treatment programs have developed to meet these needs, such as Women for Sobriety (exclusively for women) and Rational Recovery (treatment program that does not include AA or its tenets). There are also self-help support groups for gay, lesbian, and non-Christian members.

The 12-step concept of recovery has been used for other drugs as well. Such groups include Narcotics Anonymous; Al-Anon, a support group for spouses, partners, and friends of alcoholics; and AlaTeen, a group for children of parents with substance problems. This same model has been used in self-help groups for people with gambling problems and eating disorders. National addresses for these groups are listed in Box 17-4.

Treatment Settings and Programs

Clients being treated for intoxication and withdrawal or detoxification are encountered in a wide variety of medical settings, from the emergency room to the outpatient clinic. Clients needing medically supervised detoxification are often treated on medical units in the hospital setting and then referred to an appropriate outpatient treatment setting when they are medically stable.

Extended or outpatient treatment is provided by health professionals in a variety of settings, including clinics or centers offering day and evening programs, halfway houses, residential settings, or special chemical dependency units in hospitals. Generally, the type of setting for treatment is selected based on the

---

Box 17-3

➤ TWELVE STEPS OF ALCOHOLICS ANONYMOUS

1. We admitted that we were powerless over alcohol, that our lives had become unmanageable.
2. Came to believe that a Power greater than ourselves could restore us to sanity.
3. Made a decision to turn our wills and lives over to the care of God as we understood Him.
4. Made a searching and fearless moral inventory of ourselves.
5. Admitted to God, to ourselves, and to another human being the exact nature of our wrongs.
6. Were entirely ready to have God remove all these defects of character.
7. Humbly asked Him to remove our shortcomings.
8. Made a list of all persons we had harmed, and became willing to make amends to them all.
9. Made direct amends to such people whenever possible, except when to do so would injure them or others.
10. Continued to take personal inventory and when we were wrong promptly admitted it.
11. Sought through prayer and meditation to improve our conscious contact with God as we understood Him, praying only for knowledge of His will for us and the power to carry that out.
12. Having had a spiritual awakening as a result of these steps, we tried to carry this message to alcoholics and to practice these principles in all our affairs.

client's needs as well as his or her insurance coverage. For example, for someone who has limited insurance coverage, is working, and has a supportive family, the outpatient setting may be chosen first because it is less expensive, the client can continue to work, and the family can provide support. If the client cannot remain sober during outpatient treatment, then inpatient treatment may be required. Clients with repeated treatment experiences may need the structure of a halfway house, with a gradual transition into the community.

Pharmacologic Treatment

Pharmacologic treatment in substance abuse has two main purposes: to permit safe withdrawal from alcohol, sedative/hypnotics, and benzodiazepines and to prevent relapse. Table 17-1 summarizes drugs used in substance abuse treatment. For clients whose primary substance is alcohol, vitamin B_1 (thiamine) is often prescribed to prevent or treat Wernicke's syndrome or Korsakoff's syndrome, neurologic conditions that can result from heavy alcohol use. Cyanocobalamin (vitamin B_{12}) and folic acid are often prescribed for clients with nutritional deficiencies.

Alcohol withdrawal is usually managed with a benzodiazepine anxiolytic agent, which is used to suppress the symptoms of abstinence. The most commonly used benzodiazepines are diazepam, chlordiazepoxide, and lorazepam. These medications can be administered on a fixed schedule around the clock during withdrawal. However, giving these medications on an as-needed basis according to symptom parameters is just as effective and results in a speedier withdrawal (Lehne, 1998).

Disulfiram (Antabuse) may be prescribed to help deter clients from drinking. If a client taking disulfiram drinks alcohol, a severe adverse reaction occurs, with flushing, a throbbing headache, sweating, nausea, and vomiting. In severe cases, severe hypo-tension, confusion, coma, and even death may result (see Chap. 2). The client must also avoid a wide variety of products that contain alcohol, such as cough syrup, lotions, mouthwash, perfume, aftershave, vinegar, and vanilla and other extracts. The client must read product labels carefully because any product containing alcohol can produce symptoms.

Methadone, a potent synthetic opiate, is used as a substitute for heroin in some maintenance programs. The client takes one daily dose of methadone, which meets the physical need for opiates but does not produce cravings for more. Methadone does not produce the high associated with heroin. The client has essentially substituted his or her addiction to heroin for an addiction to methadone; however, methadone is safer because it is legal, is controlled by a physician, and is available in tablet form. The client avoids the risks of intravenous drug use, the high cost of heroin (which often leads to criminal acts), and the questionable content of street drugs.

Levomethadyl is a narcotic analgesic whose only purpose is the treatment of opiate dependence. It is used in the same manner as methadone.

Naltrexone (ReVia) is an opioid antagonist often used to treat overdose. It blocks the effects of any opioids that might be ingested, thereby negating the effects of using more opioids. It has also been found to reduce the cravings for alcohol in abstinent clients, although research is in the early stages (Freed & York, 1997). Acamprosate, which modulates neurotransmission of GABA and NMDA, has been used with some success in the United Kingdom to decrease alcohol cravings and maintain abstinence, but it is not yet available in the United States (Swift, 1999).

Clonidine (Catapres) is an alpha-2-adrenergic agonist used to treat hypertension. It is given to clients with opiate dependence to suppress some of the effects of withdrawal or abstinence. It is most effective against nausea, vomiting, and diarrhea but produces modest relief from muscle aches, anxiety,

Table 17-1

DRUGS USED FOR SUBSTANCE ABUSE TREATMENT

Drug	Use	Dosage	Nursing Considerations
diazepam (Valium)	Alcohol withdrawal	5–20 mg every 3–4 hours prn	Monitor vital signs and global assessments for effectiveness; may cause dizziness or drowsiness
chlordiazepoxide (Librium)	Alcohol withdrawal	50–100 mg, repeat in 2–4 hours if necessary; not to exceed 300 mg/day	Monitor vital signs and global assessments for effectiveness; may cause dizziness or drowsiness
disulfiram (Antabuse)	Maintain abstinence from alcohol	500 mg/day for 1–2 weeks, then 250 mg/day	Teach client to read labels to avoid products with alcohol
methadone (Dolophine)	Maintain abstinence from heroin	Up to 120 mg/day for maintenance	May cause nausea and vomiting
levomethadyl (ORLAAM)	Maintain abstinence from opiates	60–90 mg 3 times a week for maintenance	Do not take drug on consecutive days; take-home doses are not permitted
naltrexone (ReVia, Trexan)	Blocks the effects of opiates; reduces alcohol cravings	350 mg/week, divided into 3 doses for opiate-blocking effect; 50 mg/day for up to 12 weeks for alcohol cravings	Client may not respond to narcotics used to treat cough, diarrhea, or pain; take with food or milk; may cause headache, restlessness, or irritability
clonidine (Catapres)	Suppresses opiate withdrawal symptoms	0.1 mg every 6 hours prn	Take blood pressure before each dose, withhold if client is hypotensive
bromocriptine (Parlodel)	Diminish cocaine cravings	0.5–1.5 mg/day	May cause dizziness or drowsiness; take with food
thiamine (vitamin B_1)	Prevent or treat Wernicke-Korsakoff syndrome in alcoholism	100 mg/day	Teach client about proper nutrition
Folic acid (folate)	Treat nutritional deficiencies	1–2 mg/day	Teach client about proper nutrition; urine may be dark yellow
Cyanocobalamin (vitamin B_{12})	Treat nutritional deficiencies	25–250 mcg/day	Teach client about proper nutrition

Adapted from Lehne, R. A. (1998). *Pharmacology for nursing* (3rd ed.). Philadelphia: W. B. Saunders; Spratto, G. R., & Woods, A. L. (2000). *PDR nurse's drug handbook.* Montvale, NJ: Medical Economics Co.

and restlessness. Clonidine does not diminish cravings for opiates (Lehne, 1998).

Bromocriptine (Parlodel) is a dopamine agonist often used to treat clients with Parkinson's disease. It is sometimes prescribed for clients with cocaine dependence to decrease cravings and help maintain abstinence, but it is not considered highly effective (Lehne, 1998).

Dual Diagnosis

The client with both substance abuse and another psychiatric illness is said to have a **dual diagnosis**. Dual diagnosis clients who have schizophrenia or schizoaffective or bipolar affective disorder present the greatest challenge to health care professionals. It is estimated that 50% of persons with a substance abuse disorder also have a mental health diagnosis

(Jaffe, 2000*c*). Traditional methods of treatment for major psychiatric illness or primary substance abuse often have little success in these clients for the following reasons:

- Clients with a major psychiatric illness may have impaired abilities to process abstract concepts; this is a major barrier in substance abuse programs.
- Substance use treatment emphasizes avoidance of all psychoactive drugs. This may not be possible for the client who needs psychotropic drugs to treat his or her mental illness.
- The concept of "limited recovery" is more acceptable in the treatment of psychiatric illnesses, but substance abuse has no limited recovery concept.
- The notion of lifelong abstinence, which is central to substance use treatment, may

seem overwhelming and impossible to the client who lives "day to day" with a chronic mental illness.

- The use of alcohol and other drugs can precipitate psychotic behavior, making it difficult for professionals to identify whether symptoms are due to active mental illness or substance abuse.

It has been suggested that dual diagnosis clients present challenges that cannot be met in either traditional setting. Only a few units specialize in the treatment of dual diagnosis clients, and their work is demanding, with a high rate of recidivism (Jerrell & Ridgely, 1995). Research and funding are needed to develop more effective methods of treatment.

SELF-AWARENESS ISSUES

The nurse must examine his or her beliefs and attitudes about substance abuse. A history of substance use in the nurse's own family can strongly influence his or her interaction with clients. The nurse may be overly harsh and critical, telling the client that he or she should "realize how you're hurting your family." Conversely, the nurse may unknowingly act out old family roles and engage in enabling behavior, such as sympathizing with the client's reasons for using substances. Examining one's own substance use or the use by close friends and family may be difficult and unpleasant but is necessary if the nurse is to have therapeutic relationships with clients.

The nurse might also have different attitudes about various substances of abuse. For example, a nurse may have empathy for the client who is addicted to prescription medication but might be disgusted by the client who uses heroin or other illegal substances. It is important to remember that the treatment process and underlying issues of substance abuse, remission, and relapse are quite similar, regardless of the substance.

Many clients experience periodic relapses. For some, being sober is a life-long struggle. The nurse may become cynical or pessimistic when clients return for multiple attempts at substance use treatment. Such thoughts as "he deserves health problems if he keeps drinking" or "she should expect to get hepatitis or HIV infection if she keeps doing IV drugs" are a signal that the nurse has some self-awareness problems that will prevent him or her from working effectively with clients and their families.

Helpful Hints for Working With Clients and Families With Substance Abuse Problems

- Remember that substance abuse is a chronic, recurring disease for many people, just like diabetes or heart disease. Even though clients look like they should be able to control their substance abuse easily, they cannot without assistance and understanding.
- Examine substance abuse problems in your own family and friends, even though it may be painful. Recognizing your own background, beliefs, and attitudes is the first step toward managing those feelings effectively so they do not interfere with the care of clients and families.
- Approach each treatment experience with an open and objective attitude. The client may be successful in maintaining abstinence after his or her second or third (or more) treatment experience.

CLINICAL VIGNETTE: TREATMENT

Sam, age 38, is married with two children. Sam's father was an alcoholic, and his childhood was chaotic. His father was seldom around for Sam's school activities or family events, and when he was present, his drunken behavior spoiled the occasion. When Sam graduated from high school and left home, he vowed he would never be like his father.

Initially, Sam had many hopes and dreams about becoming an architect and raising a family with love and affection, and he pictured himself as a devoted and loving spouse. But he'd had some bad luck. He got into trouble for underage drinking in college, and his grades slipped because he missed classes after celebrating with his friends. Sam believes life has treated him unfairly—after all, he only has a few beers with friends to relax. Sometimes he overdoes it and he drinks more than he intended—but doesn't everybody? Sam's big plans for the future are on hold.

Today, Sam's boss told him he would be fired if he was late or absent from work in the next 30 days. Sam tells himself that the boss is being unreasonable; after all, Sam is an excellent worker, when he's there. The last straw was when Sam's wife told him she was tired of his drinking and irresponsible behavior. She threatened to leave if Sam did not stop drinking. Her parting words were, "You're just like your father!"

APPLICATION OF THE NURSING PROCESS

It can be difficult to identify persons with substance use problems. Substance use typically includes the use of defense mechanisms, especially **denial**. The client may directly deny having any problems, or may minimize the extent of problems or his or her actual substance use. In addition, the nurse may come into contact with clients with substance problems in a variety of settings unrelated to mental health. The client may come to a clinic for treatment of medical problems related to alcohol use, or the client may develop withdrawal symptoms while in the hospital for surgery or an unrelated condition. The nurse must be alert to the possibility of substance use in these situations and prepared to recognize their existence and make appropriate referrals.

Several screening instruments are available that can be used in any setting. The CAGE questionnaire (Box 17-5) is simple and easy to remember and use (Ewing, 1984). Answering "yes" to one or more of the four questions indicates a need for further assessment of substance use problems. The questions can be modified for any substance.

The Alcohol Use Disorders Identification Test (AUDIT) is a useful screening device to detect hazardous drinking patterns that may be precursors to full-blown substance use disorders (Bohn et al., 1995). This tool (Box 17-6) promotes recognition of problem drinking in the early stage, when resolution without formal treatment is more likely (Finfgeld, 1997). Early detection and treatment are associated with more positive outcomes.

Detoxification is the initial priority. A nursing care plan for the client in alcohol withdrawal is in-

cluded at the end of this chapter. Priorities for individual clients will be based on their physical needs and may include safety, nutrition, fluids, elimination, and sleep. The remainder of this section will focus on care of the client being treated for substance abuse after detoxification.

Assessment

HISTORY

The client may report a chaotic family life, with a parent or other family members with substance abuse problems, although this is not always the case. The client generally describes some kind of crisis that precipitated entry into treatment, such as physical problems or development of withdrawal symptoms while being treated for another condition. Usually other people are involved in the client's decision to seek treatment, such as an employer threatening loss of a job, or a spouse or partner threatening loss of a relationship. Rarely does the client decide to seek treatment independently, with no outside influence.

GENERAL APPEARANCE AND MOTOR BEHAVIOR

The client's appearance and speech may be normal, or he or she may appear anxious, tired, and disheveled if he or she has just completed a difficult course of detoxification. The client may appear physically ill, depending on his or her overall health status and any health problems resulting from substance use. Most clients are somewhat apprehensive about treatment, may resent being in treatment, or feel pressured by others to be there. This may be the first time in a long time that the client has had to deal with any difficulty without the help of a psychoactive substance.

MOOD AND AFFECT

Wide ranges of mood and affect are possible. Some clients are sad and tearful, expressing guilt and remorse for their behavior and circumstances. Others may be angry and sarcastic or quiet and sullen, unwilling to talk to the nurse. Irritability is common because the client is newly free of substances. The client may be pleasant and seemingly happy, appearing unaffected by the situation, especially if he or she is still in denial about the substance use.

THOUGHT PROCESS AND CONTENT

Clients are likely to minimize their substance use, blame others for their problems, and rationalize their behavior. They may think they cannot survive with-

---

Box 17-5

► CAGE QUESTIONNAIRE

If the client answers "yes" to one of the following questions, this calls for further inquiry:
- Have you ever felt you ought to **C**ut down on your drinking?
- Have people **A**nnoyed you by criticizing your drinking?
- Have you ever felt bad or **G**uilty about your drinking?
- Have you ever had a drink first thing in the morning to steady your nerves or get rid of a hangover (**E**ye-opener)?

Adapted from Ewing, J. A. (1984). Detecting alcoholism: The CAGE questionnaire. JAMA, 252, 1902–1907. © American Medical Association.

Box 17-6

> ## ALCOHOL USE DISORDER IDENTIFICATION TEST (AUDIT)

The following questionnaire will give you an indication of the level of risk associated with your current drinking pattern. To accurately assess your situation, you will need to be honest in your answers. This questionnaire was developed by the World Health Organization, and is used in many countries to assist people to better understand their current level of risk in relation to alcohol consumption.

1. How often do you have a drink containing alcohol? (0) Never, (1) Monthly or less, (2) 2 to 4 times a month, (3) 2 to 3 times a week, (4) 4 or more times a week.
2. How many standard drinks do you have on a typical day when you are drinking? (0) 1 or 2, (1) 3 or 4, (2) 5 or 6, (3) 7 to 9, (4) 10 or more.
3. How often do you have six or more drinks on one occasion? (0) Never, (1) Less than monthly, (2) Monthly, (3) Weekly, (4) Daily or almost daily.
4. How often during the last year have you found that you were not able to stop drinking once you had started? (0) Never, (1) Less than monthly, (2) Monthly, (3) Weekly, (4) Daily or almost daily.
5. How often during the past year have you failed to do what was normally expected of you because of drinking? (0) Never, (1) Less than monthly, (2) Monthly, (3) Weekly, (4) Daily or almost daily.
6. How often during the last year have you needed a drink in the morning to get yourself going after a heavy drinking session? (0) Never, (1) Less than monthly, (2) Monthly, (3) Weekly, (4) Daily or almost daily.
7. How often during the last year have you had a feeling of guilt or remorse after drinking? (0) Never, (1) Less than monthly, (2) Monthly, (3) Weekly, (4) Daily or almost daily.
8. How often during the last year have you been unable to remember what happened the night before because you had been drinking? (0) Never, (1) Less than monthly, (2) Monthly, (3) Weekly, (4) Daily or almost daily.
9. Have you or someone else been injured as a result of your drinking? (0) Never, (1) Less than monthly, (2) Monthly, (3) Weekly, (4) Daily or almost daily.
10. Has a relative, a doctor, or other health worker been concerned about your drinking or suggested that you cut down? (0) No, (2) Yes, but not in the last year, (4) Yes, during the last year.

Adapted from Babor, T., de la Fuente, J. R., Saunders, J., Grant. (1992). Alcohol Use Disorders Identification Test (AUDIT): Guidelines for use in primary health care. World Health Organization, Geneva. Used with permission. Bohn, Babor & Kranzler (1995)

> ## SYMPTOMS OF SUBSTANCE ABUSE

- Denial of problems
- Minimizes use of substance
- Rationalization
- Blaming others for problems
- Anxiety
- Irritability
- Impulsivity
- Feelings of guilt and sadness, or anger and resentment
- Poor judgment
- Limited insight
- Low self-esteem
- Ineffective coping strategies
- Difficulty expressing genuine feelings
- Impaired role performance
- Strained interpersonal relationships
- Physical problems such as sleep disturbances and inadequate nutrition

out the substance, or may express no desire to do so. They may focus their attention on finances, legal issues, or employment problems as their main source of difficulty, rather than their substance use. They may believe they can quit "on their own" if they wanted to, and continue to deny or minimize the extent of the problem.

SENSORIUM AND INTELLECTUAL PROCESSES

Clients are generally oriented and alert, unless they are experiencing lingering effects of withdrawal. Intellectual abilities are intact unless the client has experienced neurologic deficits from long-term alcohol use or inhalant use.

JUDGMENT AND INSIGHT

The client is likely to have exercised poor judgment, especially while under the influence of the substance.

The client's judgment may still be affected: he or she may behave impulsively, such as leaving treatment to obtain the substance of choice. Insight is usually limited regarding substance use. The client may have difficulty acknowledging his or her behavior while using, or may not see loss of jobs or relationships as connected to the substance use. The client may still believe that he or she can control the substance use.

SELF-CONCEPT

The client generally has low self-esteem, which may be expressed directly or may be covered with grandiose behavior. The client does not feel adequate to cope with life and stress without the substance and is often uncomfortable around others when not using. The client often has difficulty identifying and expressing true feelings, having in the past preferred to escape feelings and avoid any personal pain or difficulty with the help of the substance.

ROLES AND RELATIONSHIPS

Clients have usually experienced many difficulties with social, family, and occupational roles. Absenteeism and poor work performance are common. Often, family members have told the client that the substance use was a concern, and it may have been the subject of family arguments. Relationships in the family are often strained. The client may be angry at family members who were instrumental in bringing him or her to treatment or who threatened loss of a significant relationship.

PHYSIOLOGIC CONSIDERATIONS

Many clients have a history of poor nutrition (using rather than eating) and sleep disturbances that persist beyond detoxification. The client may have liver damage from drinking alcohol, hepatitis or HIV infection from intravenous drug use, or lung or neurologic damage from using inhalants.

Data Analysis

Each client has nursing diagnoses specific to his or her physical health status. These may include:
- Altered Nutrition: Less Than Body Requirements
- Risk for Infection
- Risk for Injury
- Diarrhea
- Fluid Volume Excess
- Activity Intolerance
- Self-Care Deficits.

Nursing diagnoses commonly used when working with clients with substance use include:

- Ineffective Denial
- Altered Role Performance
- Altered Family Processes: Alcoholism
- Ineffective Individual Coping.

Outcome Identification

Treatment outcomes for clients with substance use may include:
1. The client will abstain from alcohol and drug use.
2. The client will express feelings openly and directly.
3. The client will verbalize acceptance of responsibility for his or her own behavior.
4. The client will practice nonchemical alternatives to deal with stress or difficult situations.
5. The client will establish an effective aftercare plan.

Intervention

HEALTH TEACHING FOR CLIENT AND FAMILY

The client and family members need facts about the substance, its effects, and recovery. Myths and misconceptions such as the following must be dispelled:
- "It's a matter of will power."
- "I can't be an alcoholic if I only drink beer or on weekends."
- "I can learn to use drugs socially."
- "I'm OK now; I could handle using once in a while."

Education about relapse is important. Family members and friends should be aware that the client who begins to revert to old behaviors, returns to substance-using acquaintances, or thinks he or she can "handle myself now" is at a high risk for relapse, and

---

> ### ▶ CLIENT AND FAMILY TEACHING:
> ### CLIENTS WITH SUBSTANCE ABUSE
>
> - Substance abuse is an illness.
> - Dispel myths about substance abuse.
> - Abstinence from substances is not a matter of will power.
> - Any alcohol, whether beer, wine, or liquor, can be an abused substance.
> - Prescribed medication can be an abused substance.
> - Feedback from family about a return to previous maladaptive coping mechanisms is vital.
> - Continued participation in an aftercare program is important.

they need to take action. Whether the client plans to attend a self-help group or has other resources, a specific plan for continued support and involvement after treatment increases the client's chances for recovery.

FAMILY ISSUES

Alcoholism (and other substance abuse) is often called a family illness. All of those who have a close relationship with a person who abuses substances suffer emotional, social, and sometimes physical anguish.

Codependence is a maladaptive coping pattern on the part of family members or others that results from a prolonged relationship with the person who uses substances (Beattie, 1987). Codependence is characterized by poor relationship skills, excessive anxiety and worry, compulsive behaviors, and resistance to change. These dysfunctional behavior patterns are learned as family members try to adjust to the behavior of the substance user. Codependent behaviors (sometimes called enabling behaviors) seem helpful on the surface but actually help perpetuate the substance use—for example, a wife who continually calls in to report that her husband is sick when he is really drunk or hungover. Although this appears to be helpful, it really just helps him continue to avoid the consequences of his behavior and continue abusing.

There may be dramatic shifts in roles, such as when a child actually looks out for or takes care of a parent. Codependent behaviors have also been identified in health care professionals when they make excuses for a client's behavior or do things for clients that they can do for themselves.

An adult child of an alcoholic is someone who was raised in a family where one or both parents were addicted to alcohol and who has been subjected to the many dysfunctional aspects associated with parental alcoholism (Ackerman, 1987). In addition to being at high risk for alcoholism and eating disorders, children of alcoholics often develop an inability to trust, an extreme need to control, an excessive sense of responsibility, and denial of feelings that persist into adulthood. Many people growing up in a home with parental alcoholism believe their problems will be solved when they are old enough to leave home and escape the situation. However, they may begin to have problems in relationships, low self-esteem, and excessive fears of abandonment or insecurity as adults. They may find they do not know what "normal" is, having never experienced normal family life growing up.

Without support and help in understanding and coping, many family members may develop substance abuse problems of their own, thus perpetuating the dysfunctional cycle. Treatment and support groups are available to address the issues of family members. The client and family also need information about support groups, their purpose, and their location in the community.

PROMOTING COPING SKILLS

The nurse can encourage the client to identify problem areas in his or her life and explore the ways that substance use may have intensified those problems. The client should not believe that all of life's problems will disappear with sobriety; rather, he or she will be able to think about the problems clearly. The nurse may need to redirect the client's attention to his or her own behavior and how it influenced his or her problems. The nurse should not allow the client to focus on external events or other people without discussing his or her role in the problem.

Nurse: *"Can you describe some of the problems you've been having?"*
Client: *"My wife is always nagging—nothing is ever good enough—so we don't get along very well."*
Nurse: *"How do you communicate with your wife?"*
Client: *"I can't talk to her about anything; she won't listen."*
Nurse: *"Are you saying that you don't talk to her very much?"*

It may be helpful to role-play situations that the client has found difficult in the past. This is also an opportunity to help the client learn to solve problems or discuss situations with others in a calm and more effective manner. In the group setting in treatment, it is helpful to encourage clients to give and receive feedback about how others perceive their interaction or ability to listen.

The nurse can also help the client find ways to relieve stress or anxiety that do not involve substance use. Relaxation, exercise, listening to music, or engaging in activities may be effective. The client may also need to develop new social activities or leisure pursuits if most of his or her friends or habits of socializing involved the use of substances.

The nurse can help the client focus on the present, not what has happened in the past. It is not helpful for the client to dwell on the problems and regrets of the past. Rather, the client needs to focus on what he or she can do now regarding his or her behavior or relationships. The client may need support from the nurse to view life and sobriety in feasible terms—taking it one day at a time. Instead of feeling overwhelmed by thinking, "How can I avoid substances for the rest of my life?" the client can be encouraged to set attainable goals, such as, "What can I do today to stay sober?" The client needs to believe that he or she can succeed.

> ▶ **NURSING INTERVENTIONS FOR CLIENTS WITH SUBSTANCE ABUSE**
>
> • Health teaching for the client and family
> • Dispel myths surrounding substance abuse
> • Decrease codependent behaviors among family members
> • Make appropriate referrals for family members
> • Promote coping skills
> • Role-play potentially difficult situations
> • Focus on the here-and-now with clients
> • Set realistic goals, such as staying sober today

Evaluation

The effectiveness of substance abuse treatment is based heavily on the client's abstinence from substances. In addition, successful treatment should result in more stable role performance, improved interpersonal relationships, and increased satisfaction with quality of life.

COMMUNITY-BASED CARE

Many people receiving treatment for substance abuse do so in community-based settings, such as outpatient treatment, free-standing substance abuse treatment facilities, and recovery programs such as AA and Rational Recovery. Follow-up or aftercare for clients in the community is based on the client's preferences or the programs available in the local community. Some clients remain active in self-help groups. Others may attend aftercare program sessions sponsored by the agency where they completed treatment. Still others may seek individual or family counseling. In addition to formal aftercare, the nurse may also encounter recovering clients in a clinic setting or a physician's office.

SUBSTANCE ABUSE IN HEALTH PROFESSIONALS

Physicians, dentists, and nurses have far higher rates of dependence on controlled substances, such as opioids, stimulants, and sedatives, than other professionals of comparable educational achievement such as lawyers. One reason is thought to be the ease of obtaining controlled substances (Jaffe, 2000c). Health care professionals also have higher rates of alcoholism than the general population.

The issue of reporting colleagues with suspected substance abuse is an important and extremely sensitive one. It is difficult for colleagues and supervisors to report their peers for suspected abuse. Nurses may hesitate to report suspected behaviors for several reasons: they have difficulty believing that a trained health care professional would engage in abuse, they may feel guilty or fear falsely accusing someone, or they may simply want to avoid conflict. However, substance abuse by health professionals is very serious because it can endanger clients. Nurses have an ethical responsibility to report suspicious behavior to a supervisor, and in some states a legal obligation as defined in the state's nurse practice act. Nurses should not try to handle such situations alone by warning the coworker; this often just allows the coworker to continue to abuse the substance without suffering any repercussions.

General warning signs of abuse include poor work performance, frequent absenteeism, unusual behavior, slurred speech, and isolation from peers. More specific behaviors that might indicate substance abuse include:

• Incorrect drug counts
• Excessive amounts of controlled substances that are listed as wasted or contaminated
• Reports by clients of ineffective pain relief from medications, especially if relief had been adequate previously
• Damaged or torn packaging on controlled substances
• Increased reports of "pharmacy error"
• Volunteering consistently to obtain controlled substances from pharmacy
• Unexplained absences from the unit
• Trips to the bathroom after contact with controlled substances
• Coming to work early or staying late consistently for no apparent reason.

Nurses can become involved in substance abuse just as any other person might. Nurses with abuse problems deserve the opportunity for treatment and recovery as well. Reporting suspected substance abuse can be the crucial first step toward a nurse getting the help he or she needs.

➤ KEY POINTS

• Substance use and substance-related disorders can involve the use of alcohol, stimulants, cannabis, opioids, hallucinogens, inhalants, sedatives, hypnotics, and anxiolytics, caffeine, and nicotine.
• Substance use and dependence includes a major impairment in the user's social and

(text continues on page 471)

INTERNET RESOURCES

Resource	Internet Address
▶ Al-Anon/Alateen	http://www.al-anon.org/
▶ Alcoholics Anonymous	http://www.alcoholics-anonymous.org/
▶ Alcoholics Anonymous meetings database	http://www.easydoesit.org/
▶ Center for Substance Abuse Treatment	http://www.samhsa.gov/csat/csat.html
▶ Narcotics & Substance Abuse– U.S. Information Service	http://www.usia.gov/topical/global/drugs/subab.html
▶ Narcotics Anonymous	http://www.na.org/index.html
▶ National Council on Alcoholism and Drug Dependence	http://www.ncadd.org/
▶ National Institute of Mental Health	http://nimh.nih.gov/
▶ National Institute on Alcohol Abuse and Alcoholism	http://www.niaa.nih.gov/
▶ Rational Recovery	http://www.rational.org/recovery
▶ Women for Sobriety	http://www.womenforsobriety.org/

NURSING CARE PLAN FOR A CLIENT WITH ALCOHOL DETOXIFICATION

Nursing Diagnosis

▶ **Altered Health Maintenance** (6.4.2)
Inability to identify, manage, or seek out help to maintain health

ASSESSMENT DATA

- Physical symptoms (impaired nutrition, fluid and electrolyte imbalance, gastrointestinal disturbances, liver impairment)
- Physical exhaustion

EXPECTED OUTCOMES

The client will:
- Establish nutritious eating patterns
- Establish a balance of rest, sleep, and activity
- Maintain personal hygiene and grooming

continued on page 470

continued from page 469

- Sleep disturbances
- Dependence on alcohol

- Agree to participate in a treatment program
- Identify needed health resources
- Follow through with discharge plans regarding physical health, counseling, and legal problems, as indicated

IMPLEMENTATION

Nursing Interventions	**Rationale**
Monitor the client's health status based on predetermined parameters or rating scale. Administer medications as ordered or as indicated by alcohol withdrawal protocol. Observe the client for any behavioral changes as well. Alert the physician to any changes observed or when assessments exceed established parameters.	The client's blood pressure, pulse, and the presence or absence of tongue tremors are the most reliable data to determine the client's need for medication. Use of predetermined parameters or a rating scale ensures consistency of assessments and a reliable data base on which to evaluate the client's progress accurately.
Complete the physical assessment of the client; ask what and how much the client usually drinks, as well as the time and amount of his or her last drink of alcohol.	This information can help you anticipate the onset and severity of withdrawal symptoms.
Offer fluids frequently, especially juices and malts. Serve only decaffeinated coffee. Intravenous therapy may be indicated in severe withdrawal.	Caffeine will increase tremors. Malts and juices offer nutrients and fluids to the client.
Monitor the client's fluid and electrolyte balance.	Clients with alcohol abuse problems are at high risk for fluid and electrolyte imbalances.
Provide food or nourishing fluids as soon as the client can tolerate eating; have something available at night. (Bland food usually is tolerated best at first.)	Many clients who use alcohol heavily experience gastritis, anorexia, and so forth. Therefore, bland foods are tolerated most easily. It is important to re-establish nutritional intake as soon as the client tolerates food.
Administer medication to minimize the progression of withdrawal or complications and to facilitate sleep.	The client will be fatigued and needs rest. Also, he or she should be as comfortable as possible.
Encourage the client to bathe, wash his or her hair, and wear clean clothes.	Personal cleanliness will enhance the client's sense of well-being.

continued on page 471

continued from page 470

Assist the client as necessary; it may be necessary to provide complete physical care, depending on the severity of the client's withdrawal.

The level of client independence is determined by the severity of withdrawal symptoms. The client's needs should be met with the greatest degree of independence he or she can attain.

Teach the client that alcoholism is a disease that requires long-term treatment and follow-up. Refer the client to a substance dependence treatment program.

Detoxification deals only with the client's physical withdrawal from alcohol but does not address the primary disease of alcoholism.

Refer the client's family or significant others to Al-Anon, Alateen, or Adult Children of Alcoholics, as indicated.

Alcoholism is an illness that affects all family members and significant others.

Adapted from Schultz, J. M., & Videbeck, S. L. (1998). Lippincott's manual of psychiatric nursing care plans *(5th ed.)*. Philadelphia: Lippincott-Raven.

occupational functioning and includes behavioral and psychological changes.

- Alcohol is the substance abused most often in the United States; cannabis is second.
- Intoxication is the use of a substance that results in maladaptive behavior.
- Withdrawal syndrome is defined as negative psychological and physical reactions that occur when use of the substance ceases or is dramatically decreased.
- Detoxification is the process of safely withdrawing from a substance. Detoxification from alcohol and barbiturates can be life-threatening and requires medical supervision.
- The most significant risk factors for alcoholism are having an alcoholic parent, genetic vulnerability, and growing up in an alcoholic home.
- Routine screening with tools such as the CAGE questionnaire or AUDIT in a wide variety of settings (clinic, physician's office, emergency services) can be used to detect substance use problems.
- After detoxification, treatment of substance use continues in a variety of outpatient or inpatient settings, which are often based on the 12-step philosophy of abstinence, altered lifestyles, and peer support.
- Substance abuse is a family illness, meaning that all members of the family are affected in some way. Family members and close friends need education and support in coping with their feelings toward the abuser. Many support groups are available to family members and close friends.
- Clients who are dually diagnosed with substance use problems and major psychiatric illness do poorly in traditional treatment settings and need specialized attention.
- Nursing interventions for clients being treated for substance abuse include teaching the client and family about substance abuse, dealing with family issues, and helping the client learn more effective coping skills.

Critical Thinking

Questions

1. You discover that another nurse on your hospital unit has taken Valium from a client's medication supply. You confront the nurse and she replies, "I'm under a lot of stress at home. I've never done anything like this before, and I promise it will never happen again." What should you do, and why?
2. In England, medical clinics provide daily doses of drugs such as heroin at no charge to persons who are addicted to decrease illegal drug traffic and lower crime rates. Is this an effective method? Would you advocate trying this in the United States? Why or why not?

- Health care professionals have increased rates of substance use problems, particularly involving opioids, stimulants, and sedatives. Reporting suspected substance abuse in colleagues is an ethical (and sometimes legal) responsibility of all health care professionals.

REFERENCES

Abraham, H. D. (2000). Hallucinogen-related disorders. In B. J. Sadock & V. A. Sadock (Eds.). *Comprehensive textbook of psychiatry,* Vol. 1 (7th ed., pp. 1015–1025). Philadelphia: Lippincott Williams & Wilkins.

Ackerman, R. J. (1987). A new perspective on adult children of alcoholics. *EAP Digest, 2,* 25–29.

American Psychiatric Association. (2000). *DSM-IV-TR: diagnostic and statistical manual of mental disorders-text revision* (4th ed.). Washington DC: American Psychiatric Association.

Beattie, M. (1987). *Codependent no more: how to stop controlling others and start caring for yourself.* New York: Harper/Hazelden.

Bohn, M. J., Babor, T., F., & Kranzler, H. R. (1995). The alcohol use disorder identification test (AUDIT): Validation of a screening instrument for use in medical settings. *Journal of Studies on Alcohol,* 421–423.

Ciraulo, D. A., & Sarid-Segal, O. (2000). Sedative-, hypnotic- or anxiolytic-related abuse. In B. J. Sadock & V. A. Sadock (Eds.). *Comprehensive textbook of psychiatry,* Vol. 1, (7th ed., pp. 1071–1085). Philadelphia: Lippincott Williams & Wilkins.

Crowley, T. J. (2000). Inhalant-related disorders. In B. J. Sadock & V. A. Sadock (Eds.). *Comprehensive textbook of psychiatry,* Vol. 1 (7th ed., pp. 1035–1033). Philadelphia: Lippincott Williams & Wilkins.

Ewing, J. A. (1984). Detecting alcoholism: The CAGE questionnaire. *JAMA, 252,* 1902–1907.

Finfgeld, D. L. (1997). Resolution of drinking problems without formal treatment. *Perspectives in Psychiatric Care, 33*(3), 14–23.

Freed, P. E., & York, L. N. (1997). Naltrexone: a controversial therapy for alcohol dependence. *Journal of Psychosocial Nursing, 35*(7), 24–28.

Galanter, M., & Kleber, H. D. (Eds.). (1994). *Textbook of substance abuse treatment.* Washington DC: American Psychiatric Association.

Jaffe, J. H. (2000*a*). Amphetamine (or amphetamine-like) related disorders. In B. J. Sadock & V. A. Sadock (Eds.). *Comprehensive textbook of psychiatry,* Vol. 1 (7th ed., pp. 971–982). Philadelphia: Lippincott Williams & Wilkins.

Jaffe, J. H. (2000*b*). Cocaine-related disorders. In B. J. Sadock & V. A. Sadock (Eds.). *Comprehensive textbook of psychiatry,* Vol. 1 (7th ed., pp. 999–1015). Philadelphia: Lippincott Williams & Wilkins.

Jaffe, J. H. (2000*c*). Substance-related disorders: introduction and overview. In B. J. Sadock & V. A. Sadock (Eds.). *Comprehensive textbook of psychiatry,* Vol. 1 (7th ed., pp. 924–952). Philadelphia: Lippincott Williams & Wilkins.

Jaffe, J. H., & Jaffe, A. B. (2000). Opioid-related disorders. In B. J. Sadock & V. A. Sadock (Eds.). *Comprehensive textbook of psychiatry,* Vol. 1 (7th ed., pp. 1038–1169). Philadelphia: Lippincott Williams & Wilkins.

Jerrell, J. M., & Ridgely, M. S. (1995). Evaluating changes in symptoms and functioning of dually diagnosed clients in specialized treatment. *Psychiatric Services, 46*(3), 233–238.

Lehne, R. A. (1998). *Pharmacology for nursing* (3rd ed.). Philadelphia: W. B. Saunders.

Macfadden, W., & Woody, G. E. (2000). Cannabis-related disorders. In B. J. Sadock & V. A. Sadock (Eds.). *Comprehensive textbook of psychiatry,* Vol. 1. (7th ed., pp. 990–999). Philadelphia: Lippincott Williams & Wilkins.

National Institute on Alcohol Abuse and Alcoholism. (2000). *Alcohol and minorities.* Document available: *http://silk.nih.gov/silk/niaaa1/publication/aa23.htm*

Prescott, C. A., & Kendler, K. S. (1999). Genetic and environmental contributions to alcohol abuse and dependence in a population-based sample of male twins. *American Journal of Psychiatry, 156*(1), 34–40.

Schuckit, M. A. (2000). Alcohol-related disorders. In B. J. Sadock & V. A. Sadock (Eds.). *Comprehensive textbook of psychiatry,* Vol. 1 (7th ed., pp. 953–971). Philadelphia: Lippincott Williams & Wilkins.

Schultz, J. M., & Videbeck, S. D. (1998). *Lippincott's manual of psychiatric nursing care plans* (5th ed.). Philadelphia: Lippincott-Raven.

Spratto, G. R., & Woods, A. L. (2000). *PDR nurse's drug handbook.* Montvale, NJ: Medical Economics Co.

Substance Abuse and Mental Health Services Administration. (1997). *National household survey on drug abuse.* Department of Health and Human Services.

Swift, R. M. (1999). Drug therapy for alcohol dependence. *New England Journal of Medicine, 340*(19), 1482–1490.

Tweed, S. H., & Ryff, C. D. (1996). Family climate and parent-child relationships: recollections from a nonclinical sample of adult children of alcoholic fathers. *Research in Nursing & Health, 19*(4), 311–321.

Voth, E. A., & Schwartz, R. H. (1997). Medicinal applications of delta-9-tetrahydrocannabinol and marijuana. *Annals of Internal Medicine, 126*(10), N791–N798.

ADDITIONAL READINGS

Gorman, M. (1997). Substance abuse: when alcoholism hits home. *RN, 97*(7), 68–69.

Markey, B. T., & Stone, J. B. (1997). An alcohol and drug education program for nurses. *AORN, 66*(5), 845–853.

Skinner, H. A. (1982). The drug abuse screening test. *Addictive Behavior, 7,* 363–367.

Zukin, S. R. (2000). Phencyclidine (or phencyclidine-like) related disorders. In B. J. Sadock & V. A. Sadock (Eds.). *Comprehensive textbook of psychiatry,* Vol. 1 (7th ed., pp. 1063–1071). Philadelphia: Lippincott Williams & Wilkins.

Chapter Review

➤ MULTIPLE-CHOICE QUESTIONS

Select the best answer for each of the following questions.

1. Which of the following statements would indicate that teaching about naltrexone (ReVia) had been effective?

   A. "I'll get sick if I use heroin while on this medication."

   B. "This medication will block the effects of any opioid substance I take."

   C. "If I use opioids while taking naltrexone, I'll become extremely ill."

   D. "Using naltrexone may make me dizzy."

2. Clonidine (Catapres) is prescribed for symptoms of opioid withdrawal. Which of the following nursing assessments is essential before giving a dose of this medication?

   A. Assessing the client's blood pressure

   B. Determining when the client last used an opiate

   C. Monitoring the client for tremors

   D. Completing a thorough physical assessment.

3. Which of the following would the nurse recognize as signs of alcohol withdrawal?

   A. Coma, disorientation, and hypervigilance

   B. Tremulousness, sweating, and elevated blood pressure

   C. Increased temperature, lethargy, and hypothermia

   D. Talkativeness, hyperactivity, and blackouts.

4. Which of the following behaviors would indicate stimulant intoxication?

   A. Slurred speech, unsteady gait, impaired concentration

   B. Hyperactivity, talkativeness, euphoria

   C. Relaxed inhibitions, increased appetite, distorted perceptions

   D. Depersonalization, dilated pupils, visual hallucinations.

5. The nurse is caring for a client withdrawing from alcohol. Which of the following assessments would indicate the need to administer diazepam (Valium) for withdrawal symptoms?

   A. Blood pressure 168/106

   B. Pulse 84

   C. Respirations 20

   D. Temperature 99.8°.

➤ TRUE-FALSE QUESTIONS

Identify each of the following statements as T (true) or F (false). Correct any false statements.

_____ 1. Al-Anon is a support group for recovering alcoholics.

_____ 2. When a person intoxicated with alcohol continues to function with no memory of his or her behavior, it is termed a blackout.

3. One of the goals of AA is abstinence from alcohol.

_____

4. Codependence refers to alcoholism in several family members.

_____

5. Cannabis is the most frequently abused illicit drug in the United States.

_____

6. Withdrawal from heroin is not life-threatening.

_____

7. Methadone is a synthetic opioid used to treat alcohol cravings.

_____

8. Dual diagnosis refers to the abuse of two or more substances.

_____

➤ FILL-IN-THE-BLANK QUESTIONS

Give two examples of drugs for each of the following categories.

_____ Stimulants

_____ Opioids

_____ Hallucinogens

_____ Inhalants

➤ SHORT-ANSWER QUESTIONS

1. What are the four questions in the CAGE questionnaire?

2. List four behaviors that might lead the nurse to suspect another health care professional of substance abuse.

3. Explain the concept of tapering medications during detoxification.

➤ **CLINICAL EXAMPLE**

Sharon, age 43, is attending an outpatient treatment program for alcohol abuse. She is divorced, and her two children live with their father. Sharon broke up with her boyfriend of 3 years just last week. She was recently arrested for the second time for driving while intoxicated, which is the reason she is in this treatment program. Sharon tells anyone who will listen that she is "not an alcoholic" but is in this program only to avoid serving time in jail.

1. Identify two nursing diagnoses for Sharon.

2. Write an expected outcome for each of the identified diagnoses.

3. List three interventions for each of the diagnoses.

18

Child and Adolescent Disorders

Learning Objectives

After reading this chapter, the student should be able to:

1. Discuss the characteristics, risk factors, and family dynamics of psychiatric disorders of childhood and adolescence.

2. Describe a developmental assessment for children and adolescents.

3. Apply the nursing process to the care of clients and families with emotional disorders.

4. Provide education to clients, families, teachers, caregivers, and community members for young clients with emotional disorders.

5. Discuss the nurse's role as an advocate for children and adolescents.

6. Evaluate one's own feelings, beliefs, and attitudes about clients with emotional disorders and their parents and caregivers.

Key Terms

attention deficit hyperactivity disorder (ADHD)

autistic disorder

conduct disorder

encopresis

enuresis

limit setting

pervasive developmental disorders

pica

stereotypic movements

therapeutic play

tic

time-out

Tourette's disorder

Psychiatric disorders are not as easily diagnosed in children as in adults. Children often lack the abstract cognitive abilities or verbal skills to describe what is happening. Because children are constantly changing and developing, they have no sense of a stable, normal self that would allow them to discriminate unusual or unwanted symptoms. In addition, behaviors that may be normal for a child of one age may indicate problems for a child of another age. For example, an infant of 10 months might cry and wail when separated from his or her mother, but this is normal for that stage of development. However, if the child is still crying and showing extreme anxiety when separated from his or her mother at 5 years of age, this behavior should be investigated.

Children and adolescents experience some of the same mental health problems as adults, such as depression, bipolar disorder, and anxiety disorders, and are diagnosed with these disorders using the same criteria as for adults. Eating disorders, especially anorexia, usually begin in adolescence and continue into adulthood. Many disorders first seen in infancy, childhood, and adolescence persist into adulthood. Box 18-1 lists the disorders usually first diagnosed in infancy, childhood, or adolescence.

Many children, such as those with learning disorders, communication and motor skills disorders, disorders of eating and feeding, tic disorders and mental retardation, are treated in their homes and communities and make periodic visits to the physician. Children with severe or profound mental retardation may require residential placement or day care services. The disorders most often seen in mental health settings or specialized treatment units include pervasive developmental disorders, attention deficit hyperactivity disorder (ADHD), and disruptive behavior disorders.

This chapter presents an in-depth discussion of ADHD and conduct disorder, with appropriate nursing diagnoses and interventions. Sample nursing care plans for conduct disorder, the most prevalent disruptive behavior disorder, and ADHD are presented.

Box 18-1

➤ DISORDERS FIRST DIAGNOSED IN INFANCY, CHILDHOOD, AND ADOLESCENCE

MENTAL RETARDATION

- Mild
- Moderate
- Severe
- Profound

LEARNING DISORDERS

- Reading disorder
- Mathematics disorder
- Disorder of written expression

MOTOR SKILLS DISORDER

- Developmental coordination disorder

COMMUNICATION DISORDERS

- Expressive language disorder
- Mixed receptive and expressive language disorder
- Phonologic disorder
- Stuttering

PERVASIVE DEVELOPMENTAL DISORDERS

- Autistic disorder
- Rett's disorder
- Childhood disintegrative disorder
- Asperger's disorder

ATTENTION DEFICIT AND DISRUPTIVE BEHAVIOR DISORDERS

- Attention deficit hyperactivity disorder
- Conduct disorder
- Oppositional defiant disorder

FEEDING AND EATING DISORDERS

- Pica
- Rumination disorder
- Feeding disorder of infancy or early childhood

TIC DISORDERS

- Tourette's disorder
- Chronic motor or tic disorder
- Transient tic disorder

ELIMINATION DISORDERS

- Encopresis
- Enuresis

OTHER DISORDERS OF INFANCY, CHILDHOOD, OR ADOLESCENCE

- Separation anxiety disorder
- Selective mutism
- Reactive attachment disorder
- Stereotypic movement disorder

Each category except feeding and eating disorders has an additional diagnosis "Not Otherwise Specified" (NOS) for similar problems that do not meet the criteria for other diagnoses in the category (DSM-IV-TR, 2000). Adapted from DSM-IV-TR (2000).

Less common disorders are also briefly discussed; many of these disorders are not generally treated in inpatient psychiatric units unless they coexist with other disorders.

MENTAL RETARDATION

The essential feature of mental retardation is below-average intellectual functioning (IQ below 70) that is accompanied by significant limitations in adaptive functioning areas, such as communication skills, self-care, home living, social or interpersonal skills, use of community resources, self-direction, academic skills, work, leisure, and health and safety (King et al., 2000). Some persons with mental retardation are passive and dependent, whereas others are aggressive and impulsive. The degree of retardation, based on IQ (mild, IQ 50 to 70; moderate, IQ 35 to 50; severe, IQ 20 to 35; or profound, IQ below 20), has a great impact on the person's ability to function. Causative factors for mental retardation are heredity, such as Tay-Sachs disease or fragile X chromosome syndrome; early alterations of embryonic development, such as trisomy 21 or maternal alcohol intake resulting in fetal alcohol syndrome; pregnancy or perinatal problems, such as fetal malnutrition, hypoxia, infections, and trauma; medical conditions of infancy such as infection or lead poisoning; and environmental influences, such as deprivation of nurturing or stimulation.

LEARNING DISORDERS

Learning disorders are diagnosed when the child's achievement in reading, mathematics, or written expression is below that expected for the child's age, formal education, and level of intelligence. Learning problems interfere with academic achievement and life activities that require reading, math, or writing skills (DSM-IV-TR, 2000). Reading and written expression disorders are usually identified in the first grade; math disorder may go undetected until the child has reached fifth grade. About 5% of children in public schools in the United States are diagnosed with a learning disorder. The school dropout rate for students with learning disorders is 1.5 times higher than the average rate for all students.

Low self-esteem and poor social skills are often seen in children with learning disorders. As adults, some have problems with employment or social adjustment, whereas others have minimal difficulties. Early identification of the problem, effective intervention, and the absence of coexisting problems are associated with better outcomes. Children with learning disorders are assisted with academic achievement through special education classes in public schools.

MOTOR SKILLS DISORDER

The essential feature of developmental coordination disorder is marked impairment in coordination, severe enough to interfere with academic achievement or activities of daily living (DSM-IV-TR, 2000). This diagnosis is not made if the motor coordination problem is part of a general medical condition, such as cerebral palsy or muscular dystrophy. This disorder becomes evident as the child attempts to crawl or walk, or in older children as they try to dress themselves or manipulate toys such as building blocks. Developmental coordination disorder often coexists with communication disorders. The course of motor skills disorder is variable; sometimes lack of coordination persists into adulthood (DSM-IV-TR, 2000).

COMMUNICATION DISORDERS

Communication disorders are diagnosed when the child's communication deficit is severe enough to hinder development, academic achievement, or activities of daily living, including socialization. Expressive language disorder involves an impaired ability to communicate through verbal and sign language. The child has difficulty learning new words and speaking in complete and correct sentences, and the amount of speech is limited. Mixed receptive-expressive language disorder includes the problems of expressive language disorder and difficulties understanding (receiving) words and sentences and determining their meaning. Both of these disorders can be present at birth (developmental), or they may be acquired as a result of neurologic injury or insult to the brain.

Phonologic disorder involves problems with articulation, or forming sounds that are part of speech. Stuttering disorder is a disturbance of the normal fluency and time patterning of speech. Both of these disorders of communication run in families, and they occur more frequently in boys than girls. Speech and language therapists work with children to improve communication skills and teach parents to continue speech therapy activities at home (Johnson & Beitchman, 2000). Communication disorders may be mild to severe, and the resulting difficulties that persist into adulthood are most closely related to the severity of the disorder.

PERVASIVE DEVELOPMENTAL DISORDERS

Pervasive developmental disorders are characterized by pervasive and usually severe impairment of reciprocal social interaction skills, communication deviance, and restricted stereotypical behavioral patterns (Volkmar & Klin, 2000). Included in this category are autistic disorder, Rett's disorder, childhood disintegrative disorder, and Asperger's disorder. Approximately 75% of children with pervasive developmental disorders are mentally retarded (DSM-IV-TR, 2000).

AUTISTIC DISORDER

Autistic disorder, the best known of the pervasive developmental disorders, is more prevalent in boys and is identified no later than age 3 years. The child has little eye contact and makes few facial expressions toward others and does not use gestures to communicate. The child does not relate to peers or parents, lacks spontaneous enjoyment, has apparent absence of mood and emotional affect, and cannot engage in play or make-believe with toys. There is little intelligible speech, and the child engages in stereotyped motor behaviors such as hand-flapping, body-twisting, or head-banging.

Autism was once thought to be rare, but current estimates in the United States suggest there are 58,000 to 115,000 children with autism in the 57.6 million children ages 1 to 15 years (Rapin, 1997). There are no reliable figures on the prevalence of autism among adults.

Autism tends to improve, in some cases substantially, as children start to acquire language and begin to use language to communicate with others. If behavior deteriorates in adolescence, it may reflect the effects of hormonal changes or the difficulty in meeting increasingly complex social demands (Rapin, 1997). Autistic traits persist into adulthood, and most persons with autism remain dependent to some degree on others. The manifestations of autism vary from little speech and poor daily living skills throughout life to adequate social skills that allow the person to function in a relatively independent fashion (Rapin, 1997). Social skills rarely improve enough to permit marriage and child-rearing. Adults with autism may be viewed as merely odd or reclusive, or they may be given a diagnosis of obsessive-compulsive disorder, schizoid personality disorder, or mental retardation.

Until the mid-1970s, children with autism were usually treated in segregated, specialty outpatient, or school programs. Those with more severe behaviors were referred to residential programs. However, since then, most residential programs have been closed, and children are being "mainstreamed" into local school programs whenever possible (Elder, 1994). Short-term inpatient treatment is used when behaviors such as head-banging or tantrums are out of control. When the crisis is over, the child and family are supported by community agencies.

The goals of treatment of children with autism are to reduce behavioral symptoms and to promote learning and development, particularly the acquisition of language skills (Volkmar & Klin, 2000). Comprehensive and individualized treatment, including special education and language therapy, is associated with more favorable outcomes. Pharmacologic treatment with antipsychotics such as haloperidol (Haldol) may be effective for specific target symptoms such as temper tantrums, aggressiveness, self-injury, hyperactivity, and stereotyped behaviors. Other medications such as naltrexone (ReVia), clomipramine (Anafranil), clonidine (Catapres), and stimulants have been used to diminish self-injury and hyperactive and obsessive behaviors with varied but unremarkable results (Volkmar & Klin, 2000).

Rett's Disorder

Rett's disorder is a pervasive developmental disorder characterized by the development of multiple deficits after a period of normal functioning from birth to 5 months. After 5 months, the child loses motor skills and begins showing stereotyped movements instead. There is a loss of interest in the social environment, and severe impairment of expressive and receptive language become evident as the child grows older. This disorder occurs exclusively in girls, is rare, and persists throughout life.

Childhood Disintegrative Disorder

Childhood disintegrative disorder is characterized by marked regression in multiple areas of functioning after a period of at least 2 years of apparently normal growth and development (DSM-IV-TR, 2000). The typical age of onset is 3 to 4 years old. Children have the same social and communication deficits and behavioral patterns seen in autistic disorder. This disorder is rare and occurs slightly more often in boys than girls.

Asperger's Disorder

Asperger's disorder is a pervasive developmental disorder characterized by the same impairments of social interaction and restricted, stereotyped behaviors seen in autistic disorder, but there are no language or cognitive delays. This disorder is rare and occurs more often in boys, and the effects are generally life-long.

ATTENTION DEFICIT HYPERACTIVITY DISORDER

Attention deficit hyperactivity disorder is characterized by inattentiveness, overactivity, and impulsiveness. A common disorder, especially in boys,

ADHD probably accounts for more child mental health referrals than any other single disorder (McCracken, 2000*a*). The essential feature of ADHD is a persistent pattern of inattention and/or hyperactivity and impulsivity that is more common than generally observed in children of the same age. The disorder is most often diagnosed when the child enrolls in preschool or school, although it may be evident starting in infancy in some children.

ADHD affects an estimated 3% to 5% of all school-age children. The ratio of boys to girls ranges from 3 : 1 in nonclinical settings to 9 : 1 in clinical settings (McCracken, 2000*a*). The evaluation of a child for ADHD must be conducted by a qualified specialist, such as a pediatric neurologist or a child psychiatrist, to avoid overdiagnosis of ADHD. Children who are very active or hard to handle in the classroom can be mistakenly diagnosed and treated for ADHD when it does not exist. It is thought that some of these overly active children may suffer from psychosocial stressors in the home, inadequate parenting, or other psychiatric disorders rather than ADHD (Blackman, 1999). Previously, it was believed that children outgrew ADHD some time after puberty, but it is now known that ADHD persists through adolescence and even into adulthood for many people (Wender, 2000).

CLINICAL VIGNETTE: ATTENTION DEFICIT HYPERACTIVITY DISORDER

It is 7 AM and Scott's mother pops her head into 8-year-old Scott's bedroom and sees him playing a hand-held computer game. "Scott, you know the rules: no playing computer games before you are ready for school. Now get dressed and come get some breakfast." Although these rules for a school day have been the routine for the past 7 months of school, still Scott always tests the rules. In about 10 minutes, Scott is still not in the kitchen. His mother checks his room and finds Scott lying on the floor, still in his pajamas, poring over a book on the solar system. Once he gets started with something, it is often difficult to stop him, whether it's talking or something he is doing. Today it is the solar system. He begins to tell her all about the planet Saturn.

"Scott, you need to get dressed first. Your jeans and shirt are over here on the chair." "Mom, after school today, can we go to Toys R Us? There is the coolest Pokemon game that anyone can play. I'd love to try it out." As he is talking, he walks over to the chair and begins to pull his shirt over his head. "Scott, you're putting your shirt over your pajamas. You need to take your pajamas off first," she reminds him.

He laughs at himself. "Oh yeah, oops. Mom, I had the weirdest dream last night. Dad and I were walking along in this strange place. It was sort of like the desert, but rocky terrain, too, and we finally realized we were on this strange planet and there were these alien creatures." "Scott, you need to get dressed first and make your bed, then we can chat at breakfast. I'll be in the kitchen." Ten minutes later, Scott comes bounding into the kitchen, still no socks or shoes on, and his hair is all tousled.

"You forgot your socks, and your hair isn't combed," his mother reminds, him.

"Oh yeah. What's for breakfast?" he says.

"Scott, you need to finish dressing first."

"Well, where are my shoes?"

"By the back door where you left them." This is the special designated place where he is supposed to leave his shoes so he doesn't forget.

Scott starts toward his shoes but spots his younger sister playing with a set of blocks on the floor. He hurries over to her. "Wow, Amy, watch this—I can make these blocks into a huge tower, all the way to the ceiling." "Scott makes a better tower than Amy," he chants as he grabs the blocks and begins to stack them higher and higher. His sister shrieks at this intrusion, but she is used to Scott grabbing things from her. The shriek brings his mother into the room. She notices Scott's feet still do not have socks and shoes.

"Scott, get your socks and shoes on now and leave Amy alone!" He has already backed away from Amy and her blocks and has picked up his set of Pokemon cards and is glancing through them.

"Scott, your socks!" His mother is growing impatient now.

"Where are my socks?" he asks.

"Go to your room and get a clean pair of socks and brush your teeth and hair. Then come eat your breakfast or you'll miss the bus."

"I just want to find this one card, Mom. I've got to check something out."

"No! Now! Go get your socks."

He is still thumbing through the cards. Wearily, his mother directs him toward his room. As he is looking for the socks, he is still chattering away. "Mom, I finished reading the second Harry Potter book last night. Now I've finished all the books in the series so far. Those books are so neat. That lady who writes them sure has a great imagination. Today after school, can we go see if the library has the third book yet? I can't wait to see what happens in the next one!" He finds a pair of socks and bolts off in the direction of the kitchen, grabbing Amy and pinching her cheek as he swirls by her. Amy shrieks again and he begins to chant," Amy's just a baby! Amy's just a baby!"

"Scott, stop it right now and come eat something! You've just got 10 minutes until the bus comes."

Onset and Clinical Course

ADHD is most often identified and diagnosed when the child begins school, although many parents report problems from a much younger age. As infants, children with ADHD are often fussy and temperamental and have poor sleeping patterns. Toddlers may be described as "always on the go" and "into everything," at times dismantling toys and cribs. They dart back and forth, jump and climb on furniture, run through the house, and cannot tolerate sedentary activities, such as listening to a story. At this point in the child's development, it can be difficult for parents to distinguish normal, active behavior from excessive, hyperactive behavior.

By the time the child starts school, the symptoms of ADHD begin to interfere significantly with the child's behavior and performance (Swanson et al., 1999). The child fidgets constantly, is in and out of his or her assigned seat, and makes excessive noise by tapping or playing with pencils or other objects. The child is distracted by normal environmental noises, such as someone coughing. The child cannot listen to directions; he or she interrupts and blurts out the answer before the question is completed and cannot complete tasks. Academic performance suffers because the child makes hurried, careless mistakes in school work, often loses or forgets homework assignments, and fails to follow directions.

Socially, the child may be ostracized by peers or even ridiculed for his or her behavior. It is difficult for the child to form positive peer relationships because the child cannot play cooperatively or take turns and is constantly interrupting others (DSM-IV-TR, 2000). Studies have shown that children with ADHD are perceived by both teachers and peers as more aggressive, more bossy, and less likable (McCracken, 2000a). This perception results from the child's impulsivity, inability to share or take turns, interruptions of others, and failure to listen to and follow directions. Thus, peers and teachers may exclude the child from activities and play, refuse to socialize with the child, or respond to the child in a harsh, punitive, or rejecting manner.

About two thirds of the children diagnosed with ADHD continue to have problems in adolescence. Typical impulsive behaviors in adolescents include cutting class, getting speeding tickets, failing to maintain interpersonal relationships, and adopting risk-taking behaviors such as using drugs or alcohol, sexual promiscuity, fighting, and violating curfew (Ludwikowski & DeValk, 1998). Many adolescents with ADHD have discipline problems in high school that are serious enough to warrant suspension or expulsion (McCracken, 2000a). The secondary complications of ADHD, such as low self-esteem and peer rejection, continue to pose serious problems for the adolescent.

It is estimated that in at least one third of children, symptoms will persist into adulthood (Glod, 1997). In one study, adults who had been treated for hyperactivity 25 years earlier were three to four times more likely than their brothers to experience nervousness, restlessness, depression, lack of friends, and low frustration tolerance (Wender, 2000). Adults in whom ADHD was diagnosed in childhood also have higher rates of impulsivity, alcohol and drug use, trouble with the law, and personality disorder diagnoses.

Etiology

Although there is much research taking place, the definitive causes of ADHD are not known. It is likely that

---

▶ Symptoms of ADHD

Inattentive Behaviors
Misses details
Makes careless mistakes
Difficulty sustaining attention
Doesn't seem to listen
No follow-through on chores or homework
Difficulty with organization
Avoids tasks requiring mental effort
Often loses necessary things
Easily distracted by other stimuli
Often forgetful in daily activities

Hyperactive/Impulsive Behaviors
Fidgets
Often leaves seat, (e.g., during a meal)
Runs or climbs excessively
Can't play quietly
Always on the go; driven
Talks excessively
Blurts out answers
Interrupts
Can't wait for turn
Intrusive with siblings/playmates

Adapted from Ludwikowski, K., & DeValk, M. (1998). ADHD: a neurodevelopmental approach. Journal Child and Adolescent Psychiatric Nursing, 11(1), 17–29.

a combination of factors is responsible, such as environmental toxins, prenatal influences, heredity, and damage to brain structure and functions (McCracken, 2000a). Prenatal exposure to alcohol, tobacco, and lead and severe malnutrition in early childhood increase the likelihood of ADHD (Glod, 1997). Although the relation between ADHD and dietary sugar and vitamins has been studied, results have been inconclusive (McCracken, 2000a; Shealy, 1994).

Brain images of persons with ADHD have suggested decreased metabolism in the frontal lobes of the brain, which are essential for attention, impulse control, organization, and sustained goal-directed activity. Studies have also shown decreased blood perfusion of the frontal cortex in children with ADHD and frontal cortical atrophy in young adults with a history of childhood ADHD. Another study showed decreased glucose utilization in the frontal lobes of parents of children with ADHD who had ADHD themselves (McCracken, 2000a). The evidence is not conclusive, but research in these areas seems promising.

There seems to be a genetic link for ADHD, most likely associated with abnormalities in catecholamine and possibly serotonin metabolism. Having a first-degree relative with ADHD increases the risk of the disorder by four to five times that of the general population (McCracken, 2000a). Despite the strong evidence for a genetic contribution, there are also sporadic cases with no family history of ADHD, furthering the theory that multiple factors contribute to the disorder.

Risk factors for ADHD include a family history of ADHD; male relatives with antisocial personality disorder or alcoholism; female relatives with somatization disorder; lower socioeconomic status; male gender; marital or family discord, including divorce, neglect, abuse, or parental deprivation; low birth weight; and various kinds of brain insult (McCracken, 2000a).

Cultural Considerations

Crijen et al. (1999) conducted a study of 19,647 children from 12 cultures in which parents rated problem behaviors of their children using the Child Behavior Checklist. The total scores for all the categories showed little differences based on culture, but individual category scores varied as much as 10% based on culture. Parents from various cultures have a different threshold for tolerating specific kinds of behavior, and the rates of problems differ among cultures. The authors concluded that an instrument such as the Child Behavior Checklist can be used across cultures to determine the existence of problems (indicated by total score), but the focus of the problems (indicated by individual category scores) would vary according to the culture of the child and parents.

ADHD is known to occur in various cultures. It is more prevalent in Western cultures, but that may be due to different diagnostic practices rather than actual differences in the existence of the disorder (DSM-IV-TR, 2000).

Treatment

No one treatment has been found effective for ADHD, giving rise to many different approaches, such as sugar-controlled diets and megavitamin therapy. Parents need to know that any treatment heralded as the cure for ADHD is probably too good to be true (McCracken, 2000a). ADHD is a chronic disorder, and goals of treatment involve managing symptoms, reducing hyperactivity and impulsivity, and increasing the child's attention so that the child can grow and develop normally. The most effective treatment is a combination of pharmacotherapy and behavioral, psychosocial, and educational interventions (Glod, 1997).

PSYCHOPHARMACOLOGY

Medications are often effective in decreasing hyperactivity and impulsiveness and improving the child's attention, giving the child the ability to participate in school and family life. The most common medication is methylphenidate (Ritalin) (Ludwikowski & DeValk, 1998; McCracken, 2000a). Methylphenidate is effective in 70% to 80% of children with ADHD; it reduces hyperactivity, impulsivity, and mood lability and helps the child pay attention more appropriately (Julien, 1998). Dextroamphetamine (Dexedrine), amphetamine (Adderall), and pemoline (Cylert) are other stimulants used to treat ADHD. The most common side effects of these drugs are insomnia, loss of appetite, and weight loss or failure to gain weight. Because pemoline can cause liver damage, it is the last of these drugs to be prescribed. Table 18-1 lists drugs, dosages, and nursing considerations.

Giving stimulants during daytime hours is usually effective in combating insomnia. Eating a good breakfast with the morning dose of medication and eating substantial, nutritious snacks late in the day and at bedtime will help the child maintain an adequate dietary intake. When stimulant medications are not effective or their side effects are intolerable, the second choice for treatment of ADHD is antidepressants (see Chap. 2).

STRATEGIES FOR HOME AND SCHOOL

Medications do not automatically improve the child's academic performance or ensure that he or she makes friends. Behavioral strategies are needed to help the child master appropriate behaviors, and environmen-

Table 18-1

STIMULANT DRUGS USED TO TREAT ADHD

Drug	Dosage (mg/day)	Nursing Considerations
methylphenidate (Ritalin)	10–60 in 3 or 4 divided doses	Monitor for lowered appetite suppression, or growth delays; give after meals; full drug effect in 2 days
dextroamphetamine (Dexedrine), amphetamine (Adderall)	5–40 in 2 or 3 divided doses	Monitor for insomnia; give after meals to reduce appetite-suppressing effects; full drug effect in 2 days
pemoline (Cylert)	37.5–112.5 in one daily dose	Monitor for elevated liver function tests and appetite supression; may take 2 weeks for full drug effect

Julien, R. M. (1998). *A primer of drug action* (8th ed.). New York: W. H. Freeman & Co.; Lehne, 1998

tal strategies at school and home help the child succeed in those settings. Educating parents and helping them with parenting strategies are crucial components of effective treatment of ADHD. Effective approaches include providing consistent rewards and consequences for behavior, offering consistent praise, using time-out, and giving verbal reprimands. Additional strategies are issuing daily report cards for behavior and using point systems for positive and negative behavior (McCracken, 2000*a*).

In **therapeutic play**, play techniques are used to understand the child's thoughts and feelings and to promote communication. This should not be confused with play therapy, a psychoanalytic technique used by psychiatrists. Dramatic play is acting out an anxiety-producing situation, such as allowing the child to be a doctor, using a stethoscope or other equipment to take care of a patient (a doll). Play techniques to release energy could include pounding pegs, running, or working with modeling clay. Creative play techniques can help children express themselves, for instance by drawing a picture of themselves or their family or peers. These techniques are especially useful when the child is unable or unwilling to express himself or herself verbally.

CONDUCT DISORDER

Conduct disorder is a persistent antisocial behavior of children and adolescents that significantly impairs their ability to function in the social, academic, or occupational areas. Symptoms are clustered in four areas: aggression to people and animals, destruction of property, deceitfulness and theft, and serious violation of rules (Steiner, 2000). Persons with conduct disorder have little empathy for others; they have low self-esteem, poor frustration tolerance, and temper outbursts. Conduct disorder is often associated with early onset of sexual behavior, drinking, smoking, use

CLINICAL VIGNETTE: CONDUCT DISORDER

Tom, age 14, leaves the principal's office after being involved in a physical fight in the hall. He knows his parents will be furious because he is suspended for a week. "It wasn't my fault," he thinks to himself. "What am I supposed to do when someone calls me names?" Tom is angry that he even came to school today; he'd much rather spend time hanging out with his friends and having a few drinks or smoking pot.

On his way home, Tom sees a car parked next to the grocery store, and it is unlocked and running. Tom jumps in, thinking, "This is my lucky day!" He speeds away, but soon he can hear police sirens as a patrol car closes in on him. He is eventually stopped and arrested. As he waits for his parents at the station, he's not sure what to do next. He tells the police officer that the car belongs to a friend and he just borrowed it. He promises never to get into trouble again if the officer will let him go. But the officer has Tom's record, which includes school truancy, underage drinking, suspicion in the disappearance of a neighbor's pet cat, and shoplifting.

When Tom's father arrives, he smacks Tom across the face and says, "You stupid kid! I told you the last time you'd better straighten up. And look at you now! What a sorry excuse for a son!" Tom slumps in his chair with a sullen, defiant look on his face. "Go ahead and hit me! Who cares? I'm not gonna do what you say, so you might as well give up!"

of illegal substances, and other reckless or risky behaviors. This disorder occurs three times more often in boys than girls, and as many as 30% to 50% of these children are diagnosed with antisocial personality disorder as adults.

Onset and Clinical Course

Two subtypes of conduct disorder are based on age of onset. The childhood-onset type involves symptoms that occur before age 10 years, including physical aggression toward others and disturbed peer relationships. These children are more likely to have persistent conduct disorder and to develop antisocial personality disorder as adults. Adolescent-onset type is defined by the absence of any conduct disorder behaviors until after the age of 10 years. These adolescents are less likely to be aggressive, and they have more normal peer relationships. They are less likely to have persistent conduct disorder or antisocial personality disorder as an adult (DSM-IV-TR, 2000).

Conduct disorders can be classified as mild, moderate, or severe (DSM-IV-TR, 2000):

- *Mild:* The person has a few conduct problems that cause relatively minor harm to others, such as lying, truancy, or staying out late without permission.
- *Moderate:* The number of conduct problems increases, as does the amount of harm to others, such as vandalism or theft.
- *Severe:* Many conduct problems are present, and there is considerable harm to others, such as forced sex, cruelty to animals, use of a weapon, burglary, or robbery.

The course of conduct disorder is variable. Persons with the adolescent-onset type and few or milder problems can achieve adequate social relationships and academic or occupational success as adults. Those with the childhood-onset type and more severe problem behaviors are more likely to develop antisocial personality disorder as adults. Only about 40% of persons with conduct disorder go on to develop antisocial personality disorder, but even those who do not may lead troubled lives, difficulty with interpersonal relationships, unhealthy lifestyles, and an inability to support themselves (Steiner, 2000).

Etiology

It is generally accepted that genetic vulnerability, environmental adversity, and factors such as poor coping interact to cause the disorder. Risk factors include poor parenting, low academic achievement, poor peer relationships, and low self-esteem; protective factors include resilience, family support, positive peer relationships, and good health (Steiner, 2000).

There is a genetic risk for conduct disorder, although no specific gene marker has been identified (Steiner, 2000). The disorder is more common in children who have a sibling with conduct disorder or a parent with antisocial personality disorder, substance abuse, mood disorders, schizophrenia, or ADHD (DSM-IV-TR, 2000).

A lack of reactivity of the autonomic nervous system has been found in children with conduct disorder, similar to adults with antisocial personality disorder. This abnormality may cause more aggression in social relationships as a result of a decrease in normal avoidance or social inhibitions. Research into the role of neurotransmitters is a promising area (Steiner, 2000).

Poor family functioning, marital discord, poor parenting, and a family history of substance abuse and psychiatric problems are all associated with the development of conduct disorder. Child abuse is an especially significant risk factor. The specific parenting patterns that are considered ineffective are inconsistent responses by parents to the child's demands, and giving in to demands as the child's behavior escalates. Exposure to violence in the media and in the community is a contributing factor for the child who is at risk in other areas. Socioeconomic disadvantages such as inadequate housing, crowded conditions, and poverty also increase the likelihood of conduct disorder in the at-risk child (Steiner, 2000).

Academic underachievement, learning disabilities, hyperactivity, and problems with attention span are all associated with conduct disorder. Children with conduct disorder have difficulty functioning in social situations. They lack the abilities to respond appropriately to others or to negotiate conflict, and they lose their ability to restrain themselves when emotionally stressed. They are often accepted only by peers who have similar problems (Steiner, 2000).

Cultural Considerations

Concerns have been raised that "difficult" children may be mistakenly labeled as having a conduct disorder. It is important to know the history and circumstances of the client to make an accurate diagnosis. In areas that have high crime rates, aggressive behavior may be protective and may not necessarily indicate a conduct disorder. In immigrants from war-ravaged countries, aggressive behavior may have been a matter of survival, and they should not be diagnosed with a conduct disorder (DSM-IV-TR, 2000).

Treatment

A wide variety of treatments have been used for conduct disorder with only modest effectiveness. Early

> ### SYMPTOMS OF CONDUCT DISORDER

Aggression to people and animals
Bullies, threatens, or intimidates others
Physical fights
Use of weapons
Forced sexual activity
Cruelty to people or animals
Destruction of property
Fire setting
Vandalism
Deliberate property destruction
Deceitfulness and theft
Lying
Shoplifting
Breaking into house, building, or car
Cons other to avoid responsibility
Serious violation of rules
Stays out overnight without parental consent
Runs away from home overnight
Truancy from school

attempts to improve academic performance and increase the child's ability to comply with demands from authority figures are included. Family therapy is considered essential for children in this age group (Steiner, 2000).

Adolescents rely less on their parents and more on peers, so treatment for this age group includes individual therapy. Many clients in this age group have some involvement with the legal system as a result of criminal behavior, and they may have restrictions on their freedom as a result. Use of alcohol and other drugs plays a more significant role for this age group and must be addressed in any treatment plan. The most promising treatment approach includes keeping the client in his or her environment, with family and individual therapy. Conflict resolution, anger management, and teaching of social skills are frequently included in the treatment plan.

Medications alone have little effect but may be used in conjunction with treatment for specific symptoms. For example, the client who presents a clear danger to others may be prescribed an antipsychotic medication, or a client with a labile mood may benefit from lithium or another mood stabilizer, such as carbamazepine (Tegretol) or valproic acid (Depakote) (Steiner, 2000).

OPPOSITIONAL DEFIANT DISORDER

Oppositional defiant disorder consists of an enduring pattern of uncooperative, defiant, and hostile behavior toward authority figures that does not involve major antisocial violations. A certain level of oppositional behavior is common in children and adolescents; indeed, it is almost expected at some developmental phases, such as 2 to 3 years of age and in early adolescence. Table 18-2 contrasts acceptable characteristics with abnormal behavior in adolescents. Op-

intervention is more effective, and prevention is more effective than treatment. Dramatic interventions such as "boot camp" or incarceration have not proven effective and may even worsen the situation (Steiner, 2000). Treatment must be geared toward the client's developmental age; no one type of treatment is suitable for all ages. Preschool programs such as Head Start result in lower rates of delinquent behavior and conduct disorder through use of parental education about normal growth and development, stimulation for the child, and support of parents during crises.

For school-age children with conduct disorder, the child, the family, and the school environment are the focus of treatment. Parenting education, social skills training to improve peer relationships, and

Table 18-2

ACCEPTABLE CHARACTERISTICS AND ABNORMAL BEHAVIOR IN ADOLESCENCE

Acceptable	Abnormal
Occasional psychosomatic complaints	Fears, anxiety, and guilt about sex, health, education
Inconsistent and unpredictable behavior	Defiant, negative, or depressed behavior
Eagerness for peer approval	Frequent hypochondriacal complaints
Competitive in play	Learning irregular or deficient
Erratic work–leisure patterns	Poor personal relationships with peers
Critical of self and others	Inability to postpone gratification
Highly ambivalent toward parents	Unwillingness to assume greater autonomy
Anxiety about lost parental nurturing	Acts of delinquency, ritualism, obsessions
Verbal aggression to parents	Sexual aberrations
Strong moral and ethical perceptions	Inability to work or socialize

Adapted from Cotton, N. S. (2000). Normal adolescence. In B. J. Sadoch & V. A. Sadoch (Eds.). *Comprehensive textbook of psychiatry* (7th ed., pp. 2550–2557). Philadelphia: Lippincott Williams & Wilkins.

positional defiant disorder is diagnosed only when the behaviors are more frequent and intense than in unaffected peers and when the behaviors cause dysfunction in social, academic, or work situations (Steiner, 2000). This disorder is diagnosed in about 5% of the population and occurs equally among male and female adolescents. Most authorities believe that genes, temperament, and adverse social conditions interact to create oppositional defiant disorder. Twenty-five percent of people with this disorder go on to develop a conduct disorder, and 10% are diagnosed with antisocial personality disorder as adults (Steiner, 2000).

FEEDING AND EATING DISORDERS OF INFANCY OR EARLY CHILDHOOD

The disorders of eating and feeding included in this category are persistent in nature and are not explained by underlying medical conditions.

Pica

Pica is the persistent ingestion of nonnutritive substances, such as paint, hair, cloth, leaves, sand, clay, or soil. Pica is commonly seen in mentally retarded children and occasionally in pregnant women. It comes to the attention of clinicians only if there is a medical complication that occurs, such as a bowel obstruction, infection, or a toxic condition such as lead poisoning. In most instances, the behavior lasts for several months and then remits.

Rumination Disorder

Rumination disorder is the repeated regurgitation and rechewing of food. Partially digested food is brought up into the mouth and usually rechewed and reswallowed. The regurgitation does not involve nausea, vomiting, or any medical condition (DSM-IV-TR, 2000). This disorder is relatively uncommon and occurs more often in boys; it results in malnutrition, weight loss, and even death in about 25% of affected infants. In infants, the disorder frequently remits spontaneously, but in severe cases it may continue.

Feeding Disorder

Feeding disorder of infancy or early childhood is characterized by persistent failure to eat adequately, resulting in a significant weight loss or failure to gain weight. Feeding disorder is equally common in boys and girls and occurs most often during the first year of life. It is estimated that 5% of all pediatric hospital admissions are for failure to gain weight, and up to half of those admissions reflect a feeding disorder with no predisposing medical condition. In severe cases malnutrition and death can result, but most children have improved growth after a variable period of time (DSM-IV-TR, 2000).

TIC DISORDERS

A **tic** is a sudden, rapid, recurrent, nonrhythmic, stereotyped motor movement or vocalization (DSM-IV-TR, 2000). Tics can be suppressed for a period of time, but not indefinitely. Tics are exacerbated by stress and diminished during sleep and when the person is engaged in an absorbing activity. Common simple motor tics include blinking, jerking the neck, shrugging the shoulders, grimacing, and coughing. Common simple vocal tics include clearing the throat, grunting, sniffing, snorting, and barking. Complex motor tics include facial gestures, jumping, or touching or smelling an object. Complex vocal tics include repeating words or phrases out of context, coprolalia (use of socially unacceptable words, frequently obscene), palilalia (repeating one's own sounds or words), and echolalia (repeating the last-heard sound word or phrase) (DSM-IV-TR, 2000).

Tic disorders tend to run in families. Abnormal transmission of the neurotransmitter dopamine is thought to play a part in tic disorders (McCracken, 2000b). Tic disorders are frequently treated with risperidone (Risperdal) or olanzapine (Zyprexa), both atypical antipsychotics. It is important for clients with tic disorders to get plenty of rest and manage stress, because stress and fatigue increase the frequency of symptoms.

Tourette's Disorder

Tourette's disorder involves multiple motor tics and one or more vocal tics. The tics occur many times a day for a period of more than 1 year. The complexity and severity of the tics change over time, and the person experiences almost all the possible tics described above during his or her lifetime. The person has significant impairment in academic, social, or occupational areas and feels ashamed and self-conscious. This rare disorder (4 or 5 in 10,000) is more common in boys and is usually identified by age 7 years. Some people have lifelong problems, but others have no symptoms after early adulthood (DSM-IV-TR, 2000).

Chronic Motor or Tic Disorder

Chronic motor or vocal tic is different from Tourette's disorder in that only motor or vocal tics are seen, but not both types. Transient tic disorder may involve single or multiple vocal or motor tics, but for no longer than 12 months.

ELIMINATION DISORDERS

Encopresis is the repeated passage of feces into inappropriate places, such as clothing or the floor, by a child who is at least 4 years old, either chronologically or developmentally. It is often involuntary, but it can be intentional. Involuntary encopresis is usually associated with constipation that occurs for psychological, not medical, reasons. Intentional encopresis is often associated with oppositional defiant disorder or conduct disorder.

Enuresis is the repeated voiding of urine during the day or at night into clothing or bed by a child at least 5 years old, either chronologically or developmentally. Most often enuresis is involuntary, but when it is intentional, it is associated with a disruptive behavior disorder. Seventy-five percent of children with enuresis have a first-degree relative who had the disorder. Most children with enuresis do not have a coexisting mental disorder.

Both encopresis and enuresis are more common in boys, with 1% of all 5-year-olds having encopresis and 5% of all 5-year-olds having enuresis. Encopresis can persist with intermittent exacerbations for years, but it is rarely chronic. Most children with enuresis are continent by adolescence, with only 1% of all cases persisting into adulthood.

The amount of impairment associated with elimination disorders depends on the limitations on the child's social activities, the effects on self-esteem, the degree of social ostracism by peers, and the anger, punishment, and rejection on the part of parents or caregivers (DSM-IV-TR, 2000).

Enuresis can be effectively treated with imipramine (Tofranil), an antidepressant with a side effect of urinary retention. Both elimination disorders respond to behavioral approaches, such as a pad with a warning bell for enuresis, and to positive reinforcement for continence. For children with a disruptive behavior disorder, psychological treatment of that disorder may result in improvement in the elimination disorder (Mikkelsen, 2000).

OTHER DISORDERS OF INFANCY, CHILDHOOD, OR ADOLESCENCE

Separation Anxiety Disorder

Separation anxiety disorder is characterized by excessive anxiety about separation from the home or from those to whom the child is attached, with the anxiety exceeding what would be expected for the child's developmental level (DSM-IV-TR, 2000). When separated from attachment figures, the child insists on knowing their whereabouts and may need to make frequent contact with them, such as phone calls. These children are miserable when away from home and may fear never seeing their home or loved ones again. Children with separation anxiety often follow the parent like a shadow, will not be in a room alone, and have trouble going to bed at night unless someone stays with them. The fear of separation may lead to avoidance behaviors, such as refusal to attend school or go on errands. Separation anxiety disorder is often accompanied by nightmares and multiple physical complaints such as headaches, nausea, vomiting, and dizziness.

Separation anxiety disorders are thought to result from an interaction between temperament and parenting behaviors. Inherited temperament traits, such as passivity, avoidance, fearfulness, or shyness in novel situations, coupled with parenting behaviors that encourage avoidance as a way to deal with strange or unknown situations are thought to result in anxiety in the child (Sylvester, 2000).

Depending on the severity of the disorder, children may have academic difficulties and social withdrawal if their avoidance behavior keeps them from school or relationships with others. Children may be described as demanding, intrusive, and in need of constant attention, or they may be compliant and eager to please. As adults, they may be slow to leave the family home, they may be overly concerned about and protective of their own spouses and children, and they may continue to have marked discomfort when separated from home or family. Parent education and family therapy are essential components of treatment, and 80% of children experience remission at 4-year follow-up (Sylvester, 2000).

Selective Mutism

Selective mutism is characterized by persistent failure to speak in social situations where speaking is expected, such as school (DSM-IV-TR, 2000). Children may communicate by gestures, nodding or shaking the head, or occasionally one-syllable vocalizations in a voice different than their natural voice. These children are often excessively shy, socially withdrawn or isolated, and clinging, and they may have temper tantrums. Selective mutism is rare and slightly more common in girls. It usually lasts only a few months but may persist for years.

Reactive Attachment Disorder

Reactive attachment disorder involves a markedly disturbed and developmentally inappropriate social relatedness that occurs in most situations. This disorder usually begins before age 5 years and is associated with grossly pathogenic care, such as parental neglect, abuse, or failure to meet the child's basic physical or emotional needs. Repeated changes in the child's primary caregiver, such as multiple foster care placements, can also prevent the formation of stable attachments (DSM-IV-TR, 2000). The disturbed social relatedness may be evidenced by the child's failure to initiate or respond to social interaction (inhibited type) or indiscriminate sociability or lack of selectivity in the choice of attachment figures (disinhibited type). In the first type, the child will not cuddle or desire to be close to anyone; in the second type, the child's response is the same to a stranger or a parent.

Initially, treatment focuses on the child's safety, including removal of the child from the home if neglect or abuse is found. Individual and family therapy (either with parents or foster caregivers) is the most effective treatment. With early identification and effective intervention, remission or considerable improvements can be attained. Otherwise, the disorder follows a continuous course, with relationship problems persisting into adulthood.

Stereotypic Movement Disorder

Stereotypic movement disorder is associated with many genetic, metabolic, and neurologic disorders and often occurs with mental retardation, but the precise cause is unknown. It involves repetitive motor behavior that is nonfunctional and either interferes with normal activities or results in self-injury that requires medical treatment (DSM-IV-TR, 2000). The **stereotypic movements** may include waving, rocking, twirling objects, biting fingernails, banging the head, biting or hitting oneself, or picking at the skin or body orifices. Generally speaking, the more severe the retardation, the higher the risk for self-injury behaviors. Stereotypic movement behaviors are relatively stable over time but may diminish with age (Luby, 2000).

No specific treatment has been shown to be effective. Clomipramine (Anafranil) and desipramine (Norpramin) are effective in treating severe nail-biting, and haloperidol (Haldol) and chlorpromazine (Thorazine) have been effective for stereotypic movement disorder associated with mental retardation and autistic disorder.

APPLICATION OF THE NURSING PROCESS: ADHD

Assessment

During the assessment phase, the nurse gathers information from the child's parents, day care providers (if any), and teachers, as well as through direct observation. Assessing the child in a group of peers is likely to yield useful information, because the child's behavior may be subdued or different in a focused one-to-one interaction with the nurse. It is often help-

ful to use a checklist when talking with parents to help focus their input on the target symptoms or behaviors their child exhibits.

HISTORY

The parents may report that the child was fussy and had problems as an infant, or the hyperactive behavior may have gone unnoticed until the child was a toddler or entered day care or school. The child probably has difficulties in all major life areas, such as school or play, and displays overactive or even dangerous behavior at home. Often parents say the child is "out of control," and they feel unable to deal with the child's behavior. Parents may report many attempts to discipline the child or change his or her behavior, all largely unsuccessful.

GENERAL APPEARANCE AND MOTOR BEHAVIOR

The child cannot sit still in a chair, and squirms and wiggles while trying to do so. The child may dart around the room from one thing to another with little or no apparent purpose. The child's ability to speak is unimpaired, but he or she cannot carry on a conversation; he or she interrupts, blurts out answers before the question is finished, and fails to pay attention to what has been said. The child's conversation may jump abruptly from one thing to another. The child may appear immature or may lag behind in developmental milestones.

MOOD AND AFFECT

The child's mood may be labile, even to the point of verbal outbursts or temper tantrums. Anxiety, frustration, and agitation are common. The child appears to be driven to keep moving or talking and appears to have little control over either one. Attempts to focus the child's attention or redirect the child back to a topic may evoke resistance and anger.

THOUGHT PROCESS AND CONTENT

There are generally no impairments in this area, although it can be difficult to assess depending on the child's level of activity and age or developmental stage.

SENSORIUM AND INTELLECTUAL PROCESSES

The child is alert and oriented, and there are no sensory or perceptual alterations such as hallucinations. The child's ability to pay attention or concentrate is markedly impaired. The child's attention span may be as little as 2 or 3 seconds with severe

ADHD, or 2 or 3 minutes in milder forms of the disorder. It may be difficult to assess the child's memory; he or she frequently answers, "I don't know" because he or she cannot pay attention to the question or cannot stop the mind from racing. The child with ADHD is very distractible and is rarely able to complete tasks.

JUDGMENT AND INSIGHT

Children with ADHD usually exhibit poor judgment and often do not think before acting. They may fail to perceive harm or danger and engage in impulsive acts, such as running into the street or jumping off high objects. Although it is difficult to assess judgment and insight in young children, children with ADHD display more lack of judgment when compared with those of the same age. Most young children with ADHD are totally unaware that their behavior is different from that of others and cannot perceive how it harms others. Older children might report, "No one at school likes me," but they cannot relate the lack of friends to their own behavior.

SELF-CONCEPT

Again, this may be difficult to assess in a very young child, but generally the self-esteem of children with ADHD is low. Because they are not successful at school, may not develop many friends, and have trouble getting along at home, they generally feel out of place and bad about themselves. The negative reactions their behavior evokes from others often cause them to see themselves as bad or stupid.

ROLES AND RELATIONSHIPS

The child is usually unsuccessful at school, both academically and socially. The child is often disruptive and intrusive at home, causing friction with siblings and parents. Until the child is diagnosed and treated, parents often believe the child is willful and stubborn and purposefully misbehaves. Generally, measures to discipline the child have limited success; in some cases, the child becomes physically out of control, even hitting parents or destroying family possessions. Parents find themselves chronically exhausted both mentally and physically. Teachers often feel the same frustration as parents, and day care providers or babysitters may refuse to care for the child with ADHD, adding to the child's rejection.

PHYSIOLOGIC AND SELF-CARE CONSIDERATIONS

Children with ADHD may be thin if they do not take time to eat properly or if they cannot sit through a meal. Trouble settling down for bed and difficulty sleeping are problems as well. If the child engages in reckless or risk-taking behaviors, there may also be a history of physical injuries.

Data Analysis and Planning

Nursing diagnoses commonly used when working with children with ADHD include:
- Risk for Injury
- Altered Role Performance
- Impaired Social Interaction
- Ineffective Family Coping.

Outcome Identification

Treatment outcomes for clients with ADHD may include:
1. The client will be free of injury.
2. The client will not violate the boundaries of others.
3. The client will demonstrate age-appropriate social skills.
4. The client will complete tasks.
5. The client will follow directions.

Intervention

The interventions described in this section can be adapted to a variety of settings and can be used by nurses and other health professionals, teachers, and parents or caregivers.

▶ INTERVENTIONS FOR **ADHD**

- Ensuring the child's safety and that of others
  Stop unsafe behavior.
  Provide close supervision.
  Give clear directions about acceptable and unacceptable behavior.
- Improved role performance
  Give positive feedback for meeting expectations.
  Environmental management (e.g., a quiet place free of distractions for task completion)
- Simplifying instructions/directions
  Get child's full attention.
  Break complex tasks into small steps.
  Allow breaks.
- Structured daily routine
  Establish a daily schedule.
  Minimize changes.
- Client/family education and support
  Listen to parent's feelings and frustrations.

ENSURING SAFETY

The child's safety and the safety of others is always a priority. If the child is engaged in a potentially dangerous activity, the first step is to stop the behavior. This may require physical intervention if the child is running into the street or attempting to jump from a high place. Attempting to talk to or reason with a child engaged in a dangerous activity is unlikely to be successful, because his or her ability to pay attention and listen is limited. When the incident is over and the child is safe, the adult should talk to the child directly about the expectations for safe behavior. Close supervision may be required for a time to ensure compliance and avoid injury.

The explanation should be short and clear, and the adult should not use a punitive or belittling tone of voice. The adult should not assume that the child knows what is acceptable behavior, but instead should state expectations in clear terms. For example, if the child was jumping down a flight of stairs, the adult might say, *"It is unsafe to jump down stairs. From now on, you are to walk down the stairs, one at a time."* If the child crowded ahead of others, the adult would walk the child back to the proper place in line and say, *"It is not OK to crowd ahead of others. Take your place at the end of the line."*

It may also be necessary to supervise the child closely while he or she is playing to prevent physically intrusive behavior. Again, it is often necessary to act first to stop the harmful behavior by separating the child from the friend, such as stepping between them or physically removing the child. Afterward, the adult should explain clearly what is expected behavior and what is unacceptable behavior. For example, the adult might say, *"It is not OK to grab other people. When you are playing with others, you must ask for the toy."*

IMPROVED ROLE PERFORMANCE

It is extremely important to give the child specific, positive feedback when he or she meets the stated expectations. This reinforces the desired behavior and gives the child a sense of accomplishment. For example, the adult might say, *"You walked down the stairs in a safe way"* or *"You did a good job of asking to play with the guitar, and waited until it was your turn to play with it."*

Managing the environment helps the child improve his or her ability to listen, pay attention, and complete tasks. A quiet place with minimal noise and distraction is desirable. At school, this may be a seat at the front of the room, directly facing the teacher and away from the distraction of a window or the door. At home, the child should have a quiet area for homework that is away from the television or radio (Shealy, 1994).

SIMPLIFYING INSTRUCTIONS

Before beginning any tasks, it is important to gain the child's full attention. It is helpful to face the child, on his or her level, using good eye contact. The adult should tell the child what needs to be done, breaking the task into smaller steps if necessary. For example, if the child has 25 math problems to do, it may help to give him or her 5 problems at a time, then 5 more when those are completed, and so on. This approach keeps the child from being overwhelmed and provides the opportunity for positive feedback for each set of problems he or she completes. It is also important to allow breaks or opportunities to move around when performing sedentary tasks.

The same approach can be used for tasks such as cleaning or picking up toys. Initially, the child needs supervision, or at least the presence of the adult. The child can be directed to do one portion of the task at a time; with time, the adult can give only occasional reminders, and then allow the child to complete the task independently. Again, rather than giving a general direction ("Please clean your room"), it helps to provide specific, step-by-step directions. The adult could say, *"Put your dirty clothes in the hamper."* After this step is completed, the adult gives another direction: *"Now make the bed."* Specific tasks are assigned until the overall chore is completed.

STRUCTURED DAILY ROUTINE

Having a structured daily routine is helpful. Getting up, dressing, doing homework, playing, going to bed, and so forth are accomplished much more readily if there is a routine time for these daily activities. Children with ADHD do not readily adjust to changes and are less likely to meet expectations if the times for activities are arbitrary or differ from day to day.

CLIENT AND FAMILY EDUCATION AND SUPPORT

It is important to include parents in planning and providing care for the child with ADHD. The nurse can teach the parents the approaches described above for use at home. Parents feel empowered and relieved to have specific strategies that can help both them and their child be more successful.

The nurse must listen to parents' feelings and frustrations. They may feel frustrated, angry, or guilty and may blame themselves or the school system for their child's problems. Parents need to hear that

> ▶ CLIENT/FAMILY TEACHING FOR ADHD
>
> Include parents in planning and providing care.
> Refer parents to support groups.
> Focus on child's strengths as well as problems.
> Teach accurate administration of medication and
>   possible side effects.
> Inform parents that child is eligible for special
>   school services.

Box 18-2

> ➤ READING LIST FOR PARENTS OF CHILDREN
>   WITH ADHD
>
> Edward M. Hallowell, M.D., & John J. Ratey, M.D.
>   *Driven to distraction: Recognizing and coping*
>   *with attention deficit disorder from childhood*
>   *through adulthood.* New York: Touchstone—
>   Simon & Schuster, 1994.
> Edward M. Hallowell, M.D., & John J. Ratey, M.D.
>   *Answers to distraction.* New York: Pantheon
>   Books, Division of Random House, Inc., 1994.
> Lynn Weiss, PhD. *A.D.D. and Creativity.* Dallas:
>   Taylor Publishing Co. 1997.
> Jeffrey Freed, M.A.T., and Laurie Parsons. *Right-*
>   *brained children in a left-brained world:*
>   *Unlocking the potential of your ADD child.*
>   New York: Simon & Schuster, 1997.
> Mary Sheedy Kurcinka. *Raising your spirited child:*
>   *A guide for parents whose child is more intense,*
>   *sensitive, perceptive, persistent, energetic.* New
>   York: Harper Perennial, division of Harper Collins
>   Publishers, 1991.

neither they nor their child are at fault, and that there are techniques and school programs designed to help these children. Children with ADHD qualify for special school services under the Individuals with Disabilities Education Act (IDEA).

Because raising a child with ADHD can be frustrating and exhausting, it often helps for parents to attend support groups to obtain information and support from other parents with the same problems. Parents must be taught strategies to help their child improve his or her social and academic abilities, but they must also be encouraged to help rebuild their child's self-esteem. Most of these children have low self-esteem because they have been labeled as having behavior problems and have been corrected continually by parents and teachers for not listening, not paying attention, and misbehaving. Parents must try to encourage the child and recognize the child's strengths, giving positive comments as much as possible. One technique to help parents achieve a good balance is to ask them to count the numbers of times they praise or criticize their child each day or for several days. Box 18-2 lists books the nurse can recommend to parents of a child with ADHD.

Although medication can help reduce hyperactivity and inattention and allow the child to focus and learn during school, it is by no means a cure-all for the child's problems. The child needs strategies and practice to improve social skills and academic performance. Because these children are often not diagnosed until the second or third grade, they may have missed much of the basic learning for reading and math. Parents should know that it will take time for them to catch up to other children of the same age (Ludwikowski & DeValk, 1998).

Evaluation

Parents and teachers are likely to notice positive outcomes of treatment before the child does. Medications are often effective in decreasing hyperactivity and impulsivity and improving attention relatively quickly, if the child responds to them. Improved sociability, peer relationships, and academic achievement happen more slowly and gradually but are possible with effective treatment.

APPLICATION OF THE NURSING PROCESS: CONDUCT DISORDER

Assessment

HISTORY

The child with a conduct disorder has a history of disturbed relationships with peers, aggression toward people or animals, destruction of property, deceitfulness or theft, and serious violation of rules such as truancy, running away from home, and staying out all night without permission. The behaviors and problems may be mild to severe.

GENERAL APPEARANCE AND MOTOR BEHAVIOR

The client's appearance, speech, and motor behavior are typically normal for his or her age group but may be somewhat extreme (in terms of body piercings, tattoos, hairstyle, and clothing). The client often slouches in the chair and is sullen and unwilling to be interviewed. He or she may use profanity, call the nurse or physician names, and make disparaging remarks about parents, teachers, police, and other authority figures.

MOOD AND AFFECT

The client may be quiet and reluctant to talk or may be openly hostile or angry. The client's attitude is likely to be disrespectful toward parents, the nurse, or anyone perceived to be in a position of authority. Irritability, frustration, and temper outbursts are common. The client may be unwilling to answer questions or cooperate with the interview, believing that he or she does not need help or treatment. If the client has legal problems, he or she may express superficial feelings of guilt or remorse, but it is unlikely that these emotions are sincere.

THOUGHT PROCESS AND CONTENT

The client's thought processes are usually intact— that is, he or she has the capacity for logical, rational thinking. However, the client often perceives the world to be aggressive and threatening and responds in the same manner. The client may be preoccupied with looking out for himself or herself, behaving as though everyone is "out to get me." Thoughts or fantasies about death or violence are common.

SENSORIUM AND INTELLECTUAL PROCESSES

The client is alert and oriented, memory is intact, and there are no sensory-perceptual alterations. Intellectual capacity is not impaired, but typically the client has poor grades due to academic underachievement, behavioral problems in school, or failure to attend class, complete assignments, and so forth.

JUDGMENT AND INSIGHT

Judgment and insight are limited even when the client's developmental stage is taken into consideration. The client consistently breaks rules with no regard for the consequences. Thrill-seeking or risky behavior is common, such as the use of drugs or alcohol, reckless driving, sexual activity, and illegal activities such as theft. The client lacks insight, usually blaming others or society for his or her problems; the client rarely believes that his or her behavior is the cause of difficulties.

SELF-CONCEPT

Although clients generally try to appear tough, their self-esteem is low. They do not value themselves as persons any more than they value other people. Their identity is related to the types of behavior they display, such as being cool if they have had many sexual encounters or important if they have stolen expensive merchandise or been expelled from school.

ROLES AND RELATIONSHIPS

Relationships with others, especially those in authority, are disrupted and may even be violent. This includes parents, teachers, police, and most other adults they encounter. Verbal and physical aggression are common. Siblings may be a target for the client's ridicule or aggression. Relationships with peers are limited to others displaying the same behavior as the client; peers at school are seen as dumb or afraid if they follow rules. The client is usually getting poor grades in school or has been expelled or dropped out. It is unlikely that the client has a job (if old enough), since he or she would prefer to steal what is needed. The client's idea of fulfilling roles is being tough, breaking rules, and taking advantage of others.

PHYSIOLOGIC AND SELF-CARE CONSIDERATIONS

Clients are often at risk for unplanned pregnancy and sexually transmitted diseases due to their early and frequent sexual behavior. The use of drugs and alcohol is an additional risk to health. Clients with conduct disorders are involved in physical aggression and violence, including the use of weapons; this results in more injuries and deaths than others of the same age.

Data Analysis and Planning

Nursing diagnoses commonly used for clients with conduct disorders include:
- Risk for Violence
- Noncompliance
- Ineffective Individual Coping
- Impaired Social Interaction
- Self-Esteem Disturbance.

Outcome Identification

Treatment outcomes for clients with conduct disorders may include:
1. The client will not hurt others or damage property.
2. The client will participate in treatment.
3. The client will learn effective problem-solving and coping skills.
4. The client will interact with others using age-appropriate and acceptable behaviors.
5. The client will verbalize positive statements about self that are age-appropriate.

> ## ▶ INTERVENTIONS FOR CONDUCT DISORDER
>
> - Decreasing violence and increasing compliance with treatment
>   - Protect others from client's aggression and manipulation.
>   - Set limits for unacceptable behavior.
>   - Provide consistency with client's treatment plan.
>   - Use behavioral contracts.
>   - Institute time-out.
>   - Provide a routine schedule of daily activities.
> - Improving coping skills and self-esteem
>   - Show acceptance of the person, not necessarily the behavior.
>   - Encourage the client to keep a diary.
>   - Teach and practice problem-solving skills.
> - Promoting social interaction
>   - Teach age-appropriate social skills.
>   - Role-model and practice social skills.
>   - Provide positive feedback for acceptable behavior.
> - Client and family education

Intervention

DECREASING VIOLENCE AND INCREASING COMPLIANCE WITH TREATMENT

Others must be protected from manipulation or aggressive behavior by the client. Setting limits on unacceptable behavior must be instituted at the beginning of treatment. **Limit setting** involves three steps: informing the client of the rule or limit, explaining the consequences if the limit is exceeded, and a statement of expected behavior. Providing consistent enforcement of the limit with no exceptions by all members of the health team, including parents, is essential. For example, the nurse might say, *"It is unacceptable to hit another person. If you are angry, tell a staff person about your anger. If you hit someone, you will be restricted from recreation time for 24 hours."*

For limit setting to be effective, the consequences must have meaning for the client—that is, the client needs to value or desire recreation time (in this example). If the client wanted to be alone in his or her room, then this would not be an effective consequence.

A behavioral contract outlining expected behaviors, limits, and rewards can be negotiated with the client to increase treatment compliance. The client can refer to the written agreement to keep expectations in mind, and staff can refer to the agreement should the client try to change any of the terms. A contract can help staff avoid power struggles over the client's requests for special favors or attempts to alter treatment goals or expectations of behavior.

Whether there is a written contract or a treatment plan, the staff must be consistent with the client. He or she will make attempts to bend or break the rules, blame others for his or her noncompliance, or make excuses for his or her behavior. Consistency in following the treatment plan is essential to decrease manipulation.

Time-out is retreat to a neutral place so the client can regain his or her self-control. It is not a punishment. When the client's behavior begins to escalate, such as yelling at or threatening someone, aggression or acting out may be avoided if the client can take a time-out. Staff may need to institute a time-out for the client if he or she is unwilling or unable to do so. Eventually, the goal is for the client to recognize signs of increasing agitation and take a self-instituted time-out as a means of controlling emotions and outbursts. The nurse should discuss the events with the client after the time-out period. Discussing such events can help the client to recognize situations that trigger his or her emotional responses and to learn more effective ways of dealing with similar situations in the future. Providing positive feedback for successful efforts at avoiding aggression helps to reinforce new behaviors for the client.

It helps for the client to have a schedule of daily activities, including hygiene, school, homework, leisure time, and so forth. The client is more likely to establish positive habits if he or she has routine expectations about tasks and responsibilities. The client is more likely to follow a daily routine if he or she has input concerning the schedule.

IMPROVING COPING SKILLS AND SELF-ESTEEM

The nurse must show the client that he or she is accepted as a worthwhile person, even if his or her behavior is unacceptable. This means the nurse must be matter-of-fact about setting limits and must not make judgmental statements about the client, focusing only on the behavior. For example, if the client broke a chair during an angry outburst, the nurse would say, *"John, breaking chairs is unacceptable behavior. You need to let staff know you're upset so you can talk about it instead of acting out."* The nurse must avoid saying things like, *"What's the matter with you? Don't you know any better?"* Comments such as these are personal and do not focus on the specific behavior; they reinforce the client's self-image as a "bad person."

Clients with a conduct disorder often have a tough exterior and are unable or reluctant to discuss feelings and emotions. Keeping a diary may help them identify and express their feelings. The nurse can discuss these feelings with clients and explore better, safer ways to express feelings than through aggression or acting out.

The client may also need to learn how to solve problems effectively. Problem-solving involves identifying the problem, exploring all possible solutions, choosing and implementing one of the alternatives, and evaluating the results. The nurse can help the client work on actual problems using this process. The client's skill at solving problems is likely to improve with practice.

PROMOTING SOCIAL INTERACTION

The client with conduct disorder may not have age-appropriate social skills, so teaching social skills is important. The nurse can role-model these skills and help the client practice appropriate social interaction. The nurse should identify what is not appropriate, such as profanity and name-calling, and also what *is* appropriate. The client may have little experience discussing the news, current events, sports, or other topics of interest. As the client begins to develop social skills, the nurse can include other peers in these discussions. Positive feedback is essential to let the client know he or she is meeting expectations.

CLIENT AND FAMILY EDUCATION

The client's parents may also need help learning social skills, solving problems, and behaving appropriately. Often parents have problems of their own, and they have had difficulties with the client for a long time before treatment was instituted. Old patterns of parenting, such as yelling, hitting, or simply ignoring the client's behavior, need to be replaced with more effective strategies. The nurse can teach parents about age-appropriate activities and expectations for the client, such as reasonable curfew, household responsibilities, and acceptable behavior at home. The parents may need to learn effective limit setting with appropriate consequences. Parents often need to learn to communicate their feelings and expectations in a clear and direct manner to the client. Some parents may need to let the client experience the consequences of his or her behavior rather than rescuing the client. For example, if the client gets a speeding ticket, the parents should not pay the fine for him or her. If the client causes a disturbance in school and receives detention, the parents can support the teacher's actions instead of blaming the teacher or school for the situation.

Evaluation

Treatment is considered effective if the client stops behaving in an aggressive or illegal way, attends school, and follows reasonable rules and expectations at home. The client will not become a model child in a short period of time; instead, he or she may make modest progress with some setbacks over time.

Community-Based Care

Clients with conduct disorders are seen in acute care settings only when their behavior is more severe, and for short periods of stabilization. Much of the long-term work takes place at school and home or another community setting. Some clients are placed outside their parents' home for short or long periods. Group homes, halfway houses, and residential treatment settings are designed to provide a safe, structured environment and adequate supervision if that cannot be provided in the client's home. Clients with legal issues may be placed in detention facilities, jails, or jail-diversion programs. Chapter 4 discusses treatment settings and programs.

SELF-AWARENESS ISSUES

Working with children and adolescents can be both rewarding and difficult. Many disorders of childhood place severe limitations on the child's ability, as in severe forms of developmental disorders. It may be difficult for the nurse to remain positive with the child and parents when the prognosis for improvement may not be good. Even in overwhelming and depressing situations, the nurse has an opportunity to have a positive impact on children and adolescents, who are still in crucial phases of development. The nurse can often help them develop coping mechanisms that can help them throughout adulthood.

Working with parents is a crucial part of dealing with children with these disorders. Parents often have the most influence on how these children learn to cope with their disorders. The nurse's beliefs and values about raising children affect how he or she deals with children and parents. The nurse must not be overly critical about how parents handle their children's problems until the situation is fully understood: caring for a child as a nurse is very different than being

(text continues on page 500)

> ### CLIENT/FAMILY TEACHING FOR CONDUCT DISORDER
> Teach parents social and problem-solving skills when needed.
> Encourage parents to seek treatment for their own problems.
> Help parents identify age-appropriate activities and expectations.
> Assist parents with direct, clear communication.
> Help parents avoid "rescuing" the client.

INTERNET RESOURCES

Resource	Internet Address
▶ American Academy of Child and Adolescent Psychiatry	http://www.aacap.org/
▶ Autism Society of America	http://www.autism-society.org
▶ National Tourette Syndrome Association, Inc.	http://tsa.mgh.harvard.edu
▶ ADHD	http://www.mediconsult.com/add/
▶ Children and Adults with Attention Deficit Disorders (CHADD)	http://www.chadd.org/

NURSING CARE PLAN   FOR A CLIENT WITH CONDUCT DISORDER

Nursing Diagnosis

➤ **Ineffective Individual Coping** (5.1.1.1)
A person's impairment of adaptive behaviors and problem-solving abilities in meeting life's demands and roles

ASSESSMENT DATA

- Few or no meaningful peer relationships
- Inability to empathize with others
- Inability to give and receive affection
- Low self-esteem, masked by "tough" act

EXPECTED OUTCOMES

The client will:
- Engage in social interaction
- Verbalize feelings
- Learn problem-solving skills
- Demonstrate development of relationships with peers
- Verbalize real feelings of self-worth
- Perform at a satisfactory academic level

IMPLEMENTATION

Nursing Interventions

Encourage the client to openly discuss his or her thoughts and feelings.

Nursing Interventions

Verbalizing feelings is an initial step toward dealing with them in an appropriate manner.

continued on page 497

continued from page 496

Give positive feedback for appropriate discussions.	Positive feedback increases the likelihood of continued performance.
Tell the client that he or she is accepted as a person, although his or her particular behavior may not be acceptable.	Clients with conduct disorders frequently experience rejection. The client needs support to increase self-esteem, while understanding that behavioral changes are necessary.
Give the client positive attention when his or her behavior is not problematic.	The client may have been receiving the majority of attention from others when he or she was engaged in problematic behavior, a pattern that needs to change.
Teach the client about limit setting and the need for these limits. Include time for discussion.	The client may have no knowledge of the concept of limits and how limits can benefit him or her. The client has an opportunity to ask questions when manipulation is not needed. This allows the client to hear about the relationship between aberrant behavior and consequences.
Teach the client a simple problem-solving process as an alternative to acting out (identify the problem, consider alternatives, select and implement an alternative, evaluate the effectiveness of the solution).	The client may not know how to solve problems constructively or may not have seen this behavior modeled in the home.
Help the client practice the problem-solving process with situations on the unit, then situations the client may face at home, school, and so forth.	The client's ability and skill will increase with practice. He or she will experience success with practice.
Role-model appropriate conversation and social skills for the client.	This allows the client to see what is expected in a nonthreatening situation.
Practice social skills with the client on a one-to-one basis.	As the client gains comfort with the skills through practice, he or she will increase their use.
Gradually introduce other clients into the interactions and discussions.	Success with others is more likely to occur once the client has been successful with the staff.
Assist the client to focus on age- and situation-appropriate topics.	Peer relationships are enhanced when the client is able to interact as other adolescents do.
Encourage the client to give and receive feedback with others in his or her age group.	Peer feedback can be influential in shaping the behavior of an adolescent.
Promote expression of feelings among clients in supervised group situations.	Adolescents are reluctant to be vulnerable to peers, and they may need encouragement to be open and honest with their feelings.

Adapted from Schultz, J. M. & Videbeck, S. L. (1998). Lippincott's manual of psychiatric nursing care plans *(5th ed.). Philadelphia: Lippincott-Raven.*

NURSING CARE PLAN   FOR A CLIENT WITH ADHD

Nursing Diagnosis

➤ **Impaired Social Interaction** (3.1.1)
The state in which an individual participates in an insufficient or excessive quantity or ineffective quality of social exchange

ASSESSMENT DATA

- Short attention span
- High level of distractibility
- Labile moods
- Low frustration tolerance
- Inability to complete tasks
- Inability to sit still or fidgeting
- Excessive talking
- Inability to follow directions

EXPECTED OUTCOMES

The client will:
- Successfully complete tasks or assignments with assistance
- Demonstrate acceptable social skills while interacting with staff or family member
- Participate successfully in the educational setting
- Demonstrate the ability to complete single tasks independently
- Demonstrate the ability to complete tasks with reminders
- Verbalize positive statements about himself or herself
- Demonstrate successful interactions with family members

IMPLEMENTATION

Nursing Interventions

Identify the factors that aggravate and alleviate the client's performance.

Provide an environment as free of distractions as possible. Institute interventions on a one-to-one basis. Gradually increase the amount of environmental stimuli.

Engage the client's attention before giving instructions (that is, call the client's name and establish eye contact).

Nursing Interventions

The external stimuli that exacerbate the client's problems can be identified and minimized. Likewise, any that positively influence the client can be effectively used.

The client's ability to deal with external stimulation is impaired.

The client must hear instructions as a first step toward compliance.

continued on page 499

continued from page 498

Give instructions slowly, using simple language and concrete directions.	The client's ability to comprehend instructions (especially if they are complex or abstract) is impaired.
Ask the client to repeat instructions before beginning tasks.	Repetition demonstrates that the client has accurately received the information.
Separate complex tasks into small steps.	The likelihood of success is enhanced with less complicated components of a task.
Provide positive feedback for completion of each step.	The client's opportunity for successful experiences is increased by treating each step as an opportunity for success.
Allow breaks, during which the client can move around.	The client's restless energy can be given an acceptable outlet, so he or she can attend to future tasks more effectively.
State expectations for task completion clearly.	The client must understand the request before he or she can attempt task completion.
Initially, assist the client to complete tasks.	If the client is unable to complete a task independently, having assistance will allow success and will demonstrate how to complete the task.
Progress to prompting or reminding the client to perform tasks or assignments.	The amount of intervention gradually is decreased to increase client independence as the client's abilities increase.
Give the client positive feedback for performing behaviors that come close to task achievement.	This approach, called *shaping,* is a behavioral procedure in which successive approximations of a desired behavior are positively reinforced. It allows rewards to occur as the client gradually masters the actual expectation.
Gradually decrease reminders.	Client independence is prompted as staff participation is decreased.
Assist the client to verbalize by asking sequencing questions to keep on the topic ("Then what happens?" and "What happens next?").	Sequencing questions provide a structure for discussions to increase logical thought and decrease tangentiality.
Teach the client's family or caregivers to use the same procedures for the client's tasks and interactions at home.	Successful interventions can be instituted by the client's family or caregivers by using this process. This will promote consistency and enhance the client's chances for success.

continued on page 500

continued from page 499

Explain and demonstrate "positive parenting" techniques to family or caregivers such as: *Time-in* for good behavior, or being vigilant in identifying the child's first bid for attention, and responding positively to that behavior; *Special time,* or guaranteed time a parent or surrogate spends daily with the child with no interruptions and no discussion of problem-related topics; *Ignoring minor transgressions* by immediate withdrawal of eye contact or physical contact and cessation of discussion with the child to avoid secondary gains.

It is important for parents or caregivers to engage in techniques that will maintain their loving relationship with the child while promoting, or at least not interfering with, therapeutic goals. Children need to have a sense of being lovable to their significant others that is not crucial to the nurse–client therapeutic relationship.

responsible around the clock. Parents are often making their best efforts, given their own skills and problems. Given the opportunity, resources, support, and education, many parents can improve their parenting.

Helpful Hints for Working With Children and Adolescents and Their Parents

- Remember to focus on the client's and parent's strengths and assets, not just their problems.
- Support parents' efforts to remain hopeful while dealing with the reality of their child's situation.
- Ask parents how they are doing. Offer to answer questions, and provide support or make referrals to meet their needs as well as those of the client.

➤ KEY POINTS

- Psychiatric disorders are more difficult to diagnose in children than adults because their basic development is not completed and they may lack the ability to recognize or describe what they are experiencing.
- Children and adolescents can experience some of the same mental health problems seen in the adult population, such as depression, bipolar disorder, and anxiety.
- The disorders of childhood and adolescence most often encountered in mental health settings include pervasive developmental disorders, attention deficit hyperactivity disorder, and disruptive behavior disorders.
- Pervasive developmental disorders are characterized by severe impairment of reciprocal

social interaction skills, communication deviance, and restricted stereotyped behavioral patterns.

- The child with autism, the best known of the pervasive developmental disorders, seems detached, with little eye contact and few facial expressions toward others. He or she does not relate to peers or parents, lacks spontaneous enjoyment, and cannot engage in play or make-believe with toys.
- Autism is often treated with behavioral approaches. Months or years of treatment may be needed before positive outcomes appear.
- Mental retardation involves below-average intellectual functioning (IQ below 70) and is accompanied by significant limitations in adaptive functioning such as communication, self-care, self-direction, academic achievement, work, and health and safety. The degree of impairment is directly related to the IQ.

Critical Thinking

Questions

1. In an effort to protect the fetus from neurologic damage, many states are attempting to enact legislation providing penalties for pregnant women who drink heavily or use drugs. What is your position on this issue? What, if anything, should be done? Why do you believe the way you do?
2. What values or beliefs about child-rearing and families do you have as a result of your own experiences growing up? Have these values and beliefs changed over time? If so, how?

- Learning disorders include categories for substandard achievement in reading, mathematics, and written expression. They are treated through special education in schools.
- Communication disorders may be expressive or receptive and expressive. They primarily involve articulation or stuttering and are treated by speech and language therapists.
- The essential feature of attention deficit hyperactivity disorder is a persistent pattern of inattention and/or hyperactivity and impulsivity. ADHD, the most common disorder of childhood, results in poor academic performance, strained family relations, and rejection by peers.
- Interventions for ADHD include a combination of medication, behavioral interventions, and parental education. Often special educational assistance is needed to help with academic achievement.
- Conduct disorder, the most common disruptive behavior disorder, is characterized by aggression to people and animals, destruction of property, deceitfulness and theft, and serious violation of rules.
- Interventions for conduct disorder include decreasing violent behavior, increasing compliance, improving coping skills and self-esteem, promoting social interaction, and educating and supporting parents.
- Feeding and eating disorders of infancy and childhood include pica, rumination, and feeding disorders of infancy or early childhood. Pica and rumination often improve with time, and most cases of feeding disorders can be successfully treated.
- Tic disorders involve various combinations of involuntary vocal and/or motor tics. Tourette's disorder is most common. Tic disorders are usually treated successfully with atypical antipsychotic medications.
- Elimination disorders cause impairment for the child based on the response of parents, the level of self-esteem, and the degree of ostracism by peers.

REFERENCES

American Psychiatric Association. (2000). *DSM-IV-TR: diagnostic and statistical manual of mental disorders-text revision* (4th ed.). Washington DC: American Psychiatric Association.

Blackman, J. A. (1999). Attention-deficit/hyperactivity disorder in preschoolers: does it exist and should we treat it? *Pediatric Clinics of North America, 46*(5), 1011–1045.

Cotton, N. S. (2000). Normal adolescence. In B. J. Sadock & V. A. Sadock (Eds.). *Comprehensive textbook of psychiatry* (7th ed., pp. 2550–2557). Philadelphia: Lippincott Williams & Wilkins.

Crijen, A. A. M., Achenbach, T. M., & Verhulst, F. C. (1999). Problems reported by parents of children in multiple cultures: the child behavior checklist syndrome constructs. *American Journal of Psychiatry, 156*(4), 569–574.

Elder, J. H. (1994). Beliefs held by parents of autistic children. *Journal of Child and Adolescent Psychiatric Nursing, 7*(1), 9–16.

Glod, C. A. (1997). Attention deficit hyperactivity disorder throughout the lifespan: diagnosis, etiology, and treatment. *Journal of the American Psychiatric Nurses Association, 3*(3), 89–92.

Johnson, C. J., & Beitchman, J. T. (2000). Communication disorders. In B. J. Sadock & V. A. Sadock (Eds.). *Comprehensive textbook of psychiatry* (7th ed., pp. 2634–2650). Philadelphia: Lippincott Williams & Wilkins.

Julien, R. M. (1998). *A primer of drug action: a concise, nontechnical guide to the actions, uses, and side effects of psychoactive drugs* (8th ed.). New York: W. H. Freeman & Co.

King, B. H., Hodapp, R. M., & Dykens, E. M. (2000). Mental retardation. In B. J. Sadock & V. A. Sadock (Eds.). *Comprehensive textbook of psychiatry* (7th ed., pp. 2587–2613). Philadelphia: Lippincott Williams & Wilkins.

Lehne, R. A. (1998). *Pharmacology for nursing* (3rd ed.). Philadelphia: W.B. Saunders.

Luby, J. L. (2000). Stereotypic movement disorder of infancy and disorders of infancy and childhood not otherwise specified. In B. J. Sadock & V. A. Sadock (Eds.). *Comprehensive textbook of psychiatry* (7th ed., pp. 2735–2739). Philadelphia: Lippincott Williams & Wilkins.

Ludwikowski, K., & DeValk, M. (1998). Attention deficit/hyperactivity disorder: a neurodevelopmental approach. *Journal of Child and Adolescent Psychiatric Nursing, 11*(1), 17–29.

McCracken, J. T. (2000a). Attention deficit disorders. In B. J. Sadock & V. A. Sadock (Eds.). *Comprehensive textbook of psychiatry* (7th ed., pp. 2679–2687). Philadelphia: Lippincott Williams & Wilkins.

McCracken, J. T. (2000b). Tic disorders. In B. J. Sadock & V. A. Sadock (Eds.). *Comprehensive textbook of psychiatry* (7th ed., pp. 2711–2719). Philadelphia: Lippincott Williams & Wilkins.

Mikkelsen, E. J. (2000). Elimination disorders. In B. J. Sadock & V. A. Sadock (Eds.). *Comprehensive textbook of psychiatry* (7th ed., pp. 2720–2728). Philadelphia: Lippincott Williams & Wilkins.

Rapin, I. (1997). Autism. *New England Journal of Medicine, 337*(2), 97–104.

Shealy, A. H. (1994). Attention-deficit hyperactivity disorder: etiology, diagnosis, and management. *Journal of Child and Adolescent Psychiatric Nursing, 7*(2), 24–36.

Steiner, H. (2000). Disruptive behavior disorders. In B. J. Sadock & V. A. Sadock (Eds.). *Comprehensive textbook of psychiatry* (7th ed., pp. 2770–2777). Philadelphia: Lippincott Williams & Wilkins.

Swanson, J., Lerner, M., March, J., & Greshem, F. M. (1999). Assessment and intervention for attention-deficit/hyperactivity disorder in the schools: lessons from the MTA study. *Pediatric Clinics of North America, 46*(5), 993–1009.

Sylvester, C. (2000). Separation anxiety disorder and other anxiety disorders. In B. J. Sadock & V. A. Sadock (Eds.). *Comprehensive textbook of psychiatry* (7th ed., pp. 2659–2678). Philadelphia: Lippincott Williams & Wilkins.

Volkmar, F. R., & Klin, A. (2000). Pervasive developmental disorders. In B. J. Sadock & V. A. Sadock (Eds.). *Comprehensive textbook of psychiatry* (7th ed., pp. 2659–2678). Philadelphia: Lippincott Williams & Wilkins.

Wender, P. H. (2000). Adult manifestations of attention deficit/hyperactivity disorder. In B. J. Sadock & V. A. Sadock (Eds.). *Comprehensive textbook of psychiatry* (7th ed., pp. 2688–2692). Philadelphia: Lippincott Williams & Wilkins.

ADDITIONAL READINGS

Baker, C. (1999). Innovative new program: from chaos to order: a nursing-based psychoeducation program for parents of children with attention deficit-hyperactivity

disorder. *Canadian Journal of Nursing Research, 31*(2), 71–75.

Concouvanis, J. (1997). Behavioral intervention for children with autism. *Journal of Child and Adolescent Psychiatric Nursing, 10*(1), 37–44.

Gordon, M. F. (2000). Normal child development. In B. J. Sadock & V. A. Sadock (Eds.). *Comprehensive textbook of psychiatry* (7th ed., pp. 2534–2557). Philadelphia: Lippincott Williams & Wilkins.

Kendall, J. (1997). The use of qualitative methods in the study of wellness in children with attention deficit hyperactivity disorder. *Journal of Child and Adolescent Psychiatric Nursing, 10*(4), 27–38.

Parker, J. G. (1995). Chemical restraints and children: autonomy or veracity? *Perspectives in Psychiatric Care, 31*(2), 25–29.

Pataki, C. S. (2000). Child psychiatry: introduction and overview. In B. J. Sadock & V. A. Sadock (Eds.). *Comprehensive textbook of psychiatry* (7th ed., pp. 2532–2534). Philadelphia: Lippincott Williams & Wilkins.

Puskar, K. R., Lamb, J., & Tusaie-Mumford, K. (1997). Teaching kids to cope: a preventive mental health nursing strategy for adolescents. *Journal of Child and Adolescent Psychiatric Nursing, 10*(3), 18–28.

Chapter Review

> ## MULTIPLE-CHOICE QUESTIONS

Select the best answer for each of the following questions.

1. A child is taking pemoline (Cylert) for ADHD. The nurse must be aware of which of the following side effects?

   A. Decreased thyroid-stimulating hormone

   B. Decreased red blood cell count

   C. Elevated white blood cell count

   D. Elevated liver function tests.

2. Teaching for methylphenidate (Ritalin) should include which of the following?

   A. Give the medication after meals.

   B. Give the medication when the child becomes overactive.

   C. Increase the child's fluid intake when taking the medication.

   D. Take the child's temperature daily.

3. The nurse would expect to see all of the following symptoms in a child with ADHD except:

   A. Easily distracted and forgetful

   B. Excessive running, climbing, and fidgeting

   C. Moody, sullen, and pouting behavior

   D. Interrupts others and can't take turns.

4. Which of the following is a characteristic of normal adolescent behavior?

   A. Critical of self and others

   B. Defiant, negative, and depressed behavior

   C. Frequent hypochondriacal complaints

   D. Unwillingness to assume greater autonomy.

5. Which of the following is used to treat enuresis?

   A. Imipramine (Tofranil)

   B. Methylphenidate (Ritalin)

   C. Olanzapine (Zyprexa)

   D. Risperidone (Risperdal).

> ## TRUE-FALSE QUESTIONS

Identify each of the following statements as T (true) or F (false). Correct any false statements.

_____ 1. Oppositional defiant disorder is the most common type of disruptive behavior disorder.

_____

_____ 2. Encopresis is the repeated passage of feces in inappropriate places.

_____ 3. Enuresis is usually a sign of underlying psychiatric pathology.

_____

_____ 4. Forty percent of clients with conduct disorders develop antisocial personality disorder as adults.

_____

_____ 5. A tic is usually a sign of an anxiety disorder.

_____

_____ 6. Having a child draw a picture of his or her family is an example of creative play therapy.

_____

_____ 7. Examples of stereotypic movements include nail-biting, rocking, and head-banging.

_____

_____ 8. Children with the disinhibited type of reactive attachment disorder would be expected to reject contact with anyone who approaches them.

_____

➤ FILL-IN-THE-BLANK QUESTIONS

Identify the disorder associated with the following behaviors.

_____ Ingestion of paint, clay, sand, or soil

_____ Repeated regurgitation and rechewing of food

_____ Disturbed and developmentally inappropriate social relatedness

_____ Persistent failure to speak in specific social situations

➤ SHORT-ANSWER QUESTIONS

1. Define the steps in limit setting.

2. Explain the therapeutic use of time-out.

Dixie, age 7, has been brought by her parents to the mental health center because she has been very rough with her 18-month-old brother, cannot sit still at school or at meals, and is beginning to fall behind academically in the first grade. Her parents report that they have "tried everything," but Dixie will not listen to them. She cannot follow directions, pick up toys, or get ready for school on time.

After a thorough examination of Dixie and a lengthy interview with the parents, the psychiatrist diagnoses attention deficit hyperactivity disorder and prescribes methylphenidate (Ritalin), 10 mg in the morning, 5 mg at noon, and 5 mg in the afternoon. The nurse meets with the parents to provide teaching and answer questions before they go home.

1. What teaching will the nurse include about methylphenidate?

2. What information should the nurse provide about attention deficit hyperactivity disorder?

3. What suggestions for managing the home environment might be helpful for the parents?

4. What referrals can the nurse can make for Dixie and her parents?

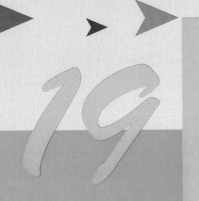

19

Somatoform Disorders

Key Terms

conversion disorder

emotion-focused coping strategies

factitious disorders

hypochondriasis

hysteria

internalization

la belle indifference

malingering

Munchausen's syndrome

Munchausen's by proxy

primary gain

problem-focused coping strategies

psychosomatic

secondary gain

somatization

somatoform disorders

The term **hysteria** refers to multiple physical complaints with no organic basis, usually described in a dramatic fashion. The concept of hysteria probably originated in Egypt and is about 4000 years old. In the Middle Ages, hysteria was associated with witchcraft, demons, and sorcerers. People with hysteria, usually women, were considered to be evil or possessed by evil spirits (Goodwin & Guze, 1989).

In the early 1800s, the medical field began to consider the various social and psychological factors that influence illness. The term **psychosomatic** began to be used to convey the connection between the mind (*psyche*) and the body (*soma*) in states of health and illness. Paul Briquet and Jean Martin Charcot, both French physicians, identified hysteria as a disorder of the nervous system. Sigmund Freud, working with Charcot, observed that patients with hysteria improved with hypnosis and experienced relief from their physical symptoms when memories were recalled and emotions were expressed. This led Freud to propose that unexpressed emotions can be converted into physical symptoms (Guggenheim, 2000).

Somatization is defined as the transference of mental experiences and states into bodily symptoms. **Somatoform disorders** can be characterized as the presence of physical symptoms that suggest a medical condition without a demonstrable organic basis to account for the symptoms fully. There are three central features of somatoform disorders:

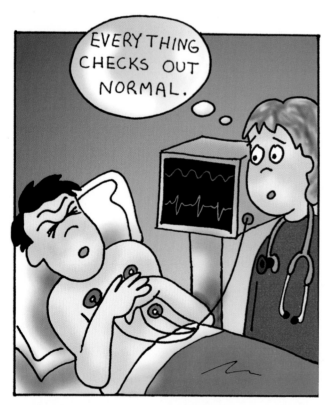

Somatoform disorders

- Physical complaints that suggest major medical illness but have no demonstrable organic basis
- Psychological factors and conflicts that seem important in initiating, exacerbating, and maintaining the symptoms
- Symptoms or magnified health concerns that are not under the patient's conscious control (Guggenheim, 2000).

Clients are convinced that they harbor serious physical problems despite negative diagnostic tests. They actually experience these physical symptoms as well as the accompanying pain and distress and functional limitations induced by them. Their physical symptoms are not willfully controlled. Their illnesses are viewed as psychiatric in nature, although many do not seek help from mental health professionals. Unfortunately, many in the health care community who do not understand the nature of this disorder may not understand or be sympathetic to these clients' complaints (Bartol & Eakes, 1995). Nurses must remember that these clients really do experience the symptoms they describe and cannot voluntarily control them.

There are five specific somatoform disorders:

- **Somatization disorder** is characterized by multiple physical symptoms. It begins by age 30, extends over a period of years, and is characterized by a combination of pain and gastrointestinal, sexual, and pseudo-neurologic symptoms.
- **Conversion disorder**, sometimes called conversion reaction, involves unexplained, usually sudden, deficits in sensory or motor function, such as blindness or paralysis, that suggest a neurologic disorder but are associated with psychological factors. An attitude of **la belle indifference,** a seeming lack of concern or distress, is a key feature.
- **Pain disorder** has the primary physical symptom of pain. The pain is generally unrelieved by analgesics and is greatly affected by psychological factors in terms of onset, severity, exacerbation, and maintenance.
- **Hypochondriasis** is the preoccupation with the fear that one has or will get a serious disease. It is thought these clients misinterpret bodily sensations or functions.
- **Body dysmorphic disorder** is the preoccupation with an imagined or exaggerated defect in physical appearance.

Somatization disorder, conversion disorder, and pain disorder are more common in women than men; hypochondriasis and body dysmorphic disorder are distributed equally by gender. Somatization disorder exists in 0.2% to 2% of the general population, con-

SYMPTOMS OF SOMATIZATION DISORDER

Pain symptoms: complaints of headache; pain in the abdomen, head, joints, back, chest, rectum; pain during urination, menstruation, or sexual intercourse

Gastrointestinal symptoms: nausea, bloating, vomiting (other than during pregnancy), diarrhea, or intolerance of several foods

Sexual symptoms: sexual indifference, erectile or ejaculatory dysfunction, irregular menses, excessive menstrual bleeding, vomiting throughout pregnancy

Pseudoneurologic symptoms: conversion symptoms such as impaired coordination or balance, paralysis or localized weakness, difficulty swallowing or lump in throat, aphonia, urinary retention, hallucinations, loss of touch or pain sensation, double vision, blindness, deafness, seizures; dissociative symptoms such as amnesia; or loss of consciousness other than fainting

---

Adapted from American Psychiatric Association. (2000). DSM-IV-TR: diagnostic and statistical manual of mental disorders-text revision (4th ed.). Washington, DC: APA.

version disorder occurs in less than 1% of the population, and no statistics are available for body dysmorphic disorder. Hypochondriasis is estimated to occur in 4% to 9% of persons seen in a general medical practice. Pain disorder is commonly seen in a medical practice, with 10% to 15% of persons in the United States reporting work disability related to back pain alone (DSM-IV-TR, 2000).

ONSET AND CLINICAL COURSE

Clients with somatization disorder and body dysmorphic disorder often experience symptoms in adolescence, although these diagnoses may not be made until early adulthood (about age 25). Conversion disorder usually occurs between the ages of 10 and 35 years. Pain disorder and hypochondriasis can occur at any age (DSM-IV-TR, 2000).

All the somatoform disorders are either chronic or recurrent in nature, lasting for decades for many people. Clients with somatization disorder and conversion disorder are most likely encountered in the mental health setting after they have exhausted efforts at a diagnosis for a medical condition. Persons with hypochondriasis, pain disorder, and body dysmorphic disorder are not likely to be treated in mental health settings unless there is a comorbid condition. Persons with somatoform disorders tend to go from one physician or clinic to another, or may see multiple providers at one time in an effort to obtain relief of symptoms. These clients tend to be pessimistic about the medical establishment, often believing their disease could be diagnosed if providers were more competent.

RELATED DISORDERS

Somatoform disorders need to be distinguished from other body-related mental disorders such as malingering and factitious disorders, in which the client feigns or intentionally produces symptoms for some purpose or gain and has willful control over those symptoms. The difference is that clients with somatoform disorders have no willful control over their physical symptoms.

Malingering is the intentional production of false or grossly exaggerated physical or psychological

CLINICAL VIGNETTE: CONVERSION DISORDER

Matthew, 13, has just been transferred from a medical unit to the adolescent psychiatric unit. He had been on the medical unit for 3 days, undergoing extensive tests to determine the cause of a sudden onset of blindness. No organic pathology was discovered, and Matthew was diagnosed with a conversion disorder.

As the nurse is interviewing Matthew, she notices that he is calm and speaks of his inability to see in a matter-of-fact manner, demonstrating no distress at his blindness. Matthew seems to have the usual interests of a 13-year-old, describing his activities at school and with his friends. However, the nurse finds that Matthew has little to say about his parents, his younger brother, or activities at home.

Later, the nurse has a chance to talk with Matthew's mother when she comes to the unit after work. Soon, Matthew's mother is crying, telling the nurse that her husband has a drinking problem and has been increasingly violent at home. Two days before Matthew's symptoms developed, Matthew witnessed one of his father's rages, which included breaking furniture and hitting his wife. When Matthew tried to help his mother, his father called him spineless and worthless and told him to go to the basement and stay there. The nurse understands that the violence Matthew has witnessed and his inability to change the situation may be the triggering event for his conversion disorder.

symptoms, motivated by external incentives such as avoiding work, evading criminal prosecution, obtaining financial compensation, or obtaining drugs. Persons who malinger have no real physical symptoms or grossly exaggerate relatively minor symptoms. Their purpose in doing so is some type of external incentive or outcome viewed as important to the person that is a direct result of the illness. Examples include no longer having to work, getting a large financial settlement based on reported injuries, or avoiding unpleasant consequences, such as jail. Persons who malinger can stop the physical symptoms as soon as they have gained what they wanted.

Factitious disorder occurs when physical or psychological symptoms are intentionally produced or feigned to gain attention. The sole purpose is to draw others' attention to themselves because of their "sickness." They may even inflict injury to themselves to receive attention. Factitious disorder is known by the common term **Munchausen's syndrome.** A variation of factitious disorder called **Munchausen's by proxy** occurs when the person inflicts illness or injury on someone else to gain the attention of emergency medical personnel or to be a "hero" for saving the victim. An example of Munchausen's by proxy would be a nurse giving excess intravenous potassium to a client and then "saving his life" by performing CPR. Although factitious disorders are not common, they occur most often in people who are in or familiar with medical professions, such as nurses, physicians, medical technicians, or hospital volunteers (Kent et al., 1995). Persons who injure clients or their children are generally arrested and prosecuted in the legal system.

ETIOLOGY

Psychosocial Theories

Psychosocial theorists believe that persons with somatoform disorders keep feelings of stress, anxiety, or frustration inside themselves rather than expressing them outwardly. This is called **internalization**. These internalized feelings and stress are expressed through physical symptoms rather than emotions; this is called **somatization**. Both internalization and somatization are unconscious defense mechanisms. The person is not consciously aware of the process, nor does he or she have voluntary control over these mechanisms.

Persons with somatoform disorders do not readily express their feelings and emotions verbally and directly and have tremendous difficulty dealing with interpersonal conflict. When placed in situations involving conflict with others, or under emotionally stressful circumstances, their physical symptoms appear to grow worse. The worsening of physical symptoms helps the person meet psychological needs for security, attention, and affection through primary and secondary gain (Guggenheim, 2000). **Primary gains** are the direct external benefits gained by the person by being sick, such as relief of anxiety, conflict, or distress. **Secondary gains** are the internal or personal benefits gained by the special attention and concern received from others because one is sick (e.g., attention from family members, comfort measures such as bringing tea or giving a back rub).

Somatization is most often associated with women, as evidenced by the old term *hysteria* (Greek for "wandering uterus"). Unexplained female pains were thought to be caused by the migration of the uterus throughout the woman's body. Psychosocial theorists believe this may be related to a variety of reasons:

- Boys in the United States are taught to be stoic and "take it like a man," causing them to offer fewer physical complaints as adults.
- Women seek medical treatment more often than men, and it is more socially acceptable for them to do so.
- Childhood sexual abuse, which is related to somatization, happens more frequently to girls.
- Women are more often treated for psychiatric disorders that have a strong somatic component, such as depression (Wool & Barsky, 1994).

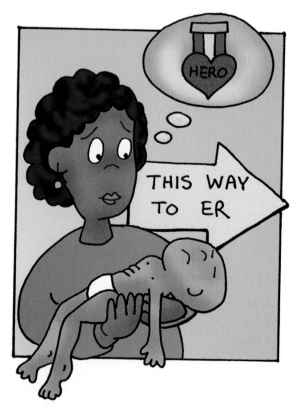

Factitious disorder

Biologic Theories

Research has shown differences in the way these clients regulate and interpret stimuli. Persons with somatoform disorders cannot sort relevant from irrelevant stimuli and respond equally to both types. In other words, the person may experience a normal body sensation such as peristalsis and attach a pathologic rather than a normal meaning to it (Guggenheim, 2000). Too little inhibition of sensory input causes an amplified awareness of physical symptoms, as well as an exaggerated response to bodily sensations. For example, minor discomfort, such as muscle tightness, becomes amplified because of the concern and attention given to the tightness by the person. This amplified sensory awareness causes the person to experience somatic sensations as more intense, noxious, and disturbing (Barsky et al., 1988).

Somatization disorder is found in 10% to 20% of female first-degree relatives of persons with somatization disorder. Conversion symptoms are found more often in relatives of persons with conversion disorder. First-degree relatives of persons with pain disorder are more likely to have depressive disorders, alcohol dependence, and chronic pain (DSM-IV-TR, 2000).

CULTURAL CONSIDERATIONS

The type and frequency of somatic symptoms and their meaning may vary across cultures. Pseudoneurologic symptoms of somatization disorder in Africa and South Asia include burning hands and feet, or the nondelusional sensation of worms in the head or ants under the skin. Symptoms related to male reproduction are more common in some countries or cultures— for example, in India men often have a hypochondriacal concern about loss of semen, called *dhat*. Somatization disorder is rare in men in the United States but is more common in Greece and Puerto Rico.

There are many culture-bound syndromes that have corresponding somatic symptoms that are not explained by a medical condition (Table 19-1). *Koro* occurs in Southeast Asia and may be related to body dysmorphic disorder. It is characterized by the belief that the penis is shrinking and will disappear into the abdomen, causing the man to die. Falling-out episodes, found in the southern United States and the Caribbean islands, are characterized by a sudden collapse during which the person cannot see or move. *Hwa-byung* is a Korean folk syndrome attributed to the suppression of anger and includes insomnia, fatigue, panic, indigestion, and generalized aches and pains. *Sangue dormido* ("sleeping blood") occurs among Portuguese Cape Verde Islanders who report pain, numbness, tremors, paralysis, seizures, blindness, heart attack, and miscarriages. *Shenjing shuariuo* occurs in China and includes physical and mental fatigue, dizziness, headache, pain, sleep disturbance, memory loss, gastrointestinal problems, and sexual dysfunction (Mezzich et al, 2000).

TREATMENT

Treatment is focused on managing symptoms and improving the quality of life. The health care provider must show empathy and sensitivity to the client's physical complaints. Building a trusting relationship with the client will help keep the client with one care provider. Depression may accompany or result from somatoform disorders for many persons; therefore, antidepressants have been helpful in some cases. The selective serotonin reuptake inhibitors, such as

Table 19-1

CULTURE-BOUND SYNDROMES

Syndrome	Culture	Characteristics
Dhat	India	Hypochondriacal concern about semen loss
Koro	Southeast Asia	Belief that penis is shrinking and will disappear into abdomen, resulting in death
Falling-out episodes	Southern United States, Caribbean islands	Sudden collapse; person cannot see or move
Hwa-byung	Korea	Suppressed anger causes insomnia, fatigue, panic, indigestion, and generalized aches and pains
Sangue dormido ("sleeping blood")	Portuguese Cape Verde Islands	Pain, numbness, tremors, paralysis, seizures, blindness, heart attack, miscarriage
Shenjing shuariuo	China	Physical and mental fatigue, dizziness, headache, pain, sleep disturbance, memory loss, GI problems, sexual dysfunction

Adapted from Mezzich, J. E., Lin, K., & Hughes, C. C. (2000). Acute and transient psychotic disorders and culture-bound syndromes. In B. J. Sadock & V. A. Sadock (Eds.). *Comprehensive textbook of psychiatry*, Vol. 1. (7th ed., pp. 1264–1276). Philadelphia: Lippincott Williams & Wilkins. © American Psychiatric Association. Reprinted with permission.

fluoxetine (Prozac), sertraline (Zoloft), and paroxetine (Paxil), are most commonly used (Table 19-2).

For clients with pain disorder, referral to a chronic pain clinic may be useful. Pain clinics help clients learn methods of pain management such as visual imaging and relaxation and help improve the client's functional abilities through physical therapy, which maintains and builds muscle tone. Narcotic analgesics are avoided because of the risk of dependence or abuse, and nonsteroidal anti-inflammatory agents are used to help reduce the pain.

Involvement in therapy groups is also beneficial for some people with somatoform disorders. Studies of clients with somatization disorder who participated in a structured cognitive-behavioral group showed evidence of improved physical and emotional health 1 year afterward (Guggenheim, 2000). The overall goals of the group were offering peer support, sharing methods of coping, and perceiving and expressing emotions.

In terms of prognosis, somatoform disorders tend to be chronic or recurrent. Conversion disorder often remits in a few weeks with treatment but recurs in 25% of clients. Somatization disorder, hypochondriasis, and pain disorder often last for many years, and clients report being in poor health. Persons with body dysmorphic disorder may be preoccupied with the same or a different perceived body flaw throughout their lives (DSM-IV-TR, 2000).

APPLICATION OF THE NURSING PROCESS

The underlying mechanism of somatization is consistent for clients with somatoform disorders of all types. In this section, application of the nursing process will be discussed for clients with somatization; differences among the disorders are highlighted in the appropriate places.

Assessment

The client's physical health status must be thoroughly investigated to ensure there is no underlying pathology requiring treatment. Box 19-1 contains a screening test for symptoms of somatization disorder that may be useful. Once a client has been diagnosed with a somatoform disorder, it is important not to dismiss all future complaints, because the client could at any time develop a physical condition that would require medical attention.

HISTORY

The client usually provides a lengthy and detailed account of previous physical problems, numerous diagnostic tests, and perhaps even a number of surgical procedures. It is likely that the client has seen multiple health care providers over a period of years. The client may express dismay or anger at the medical community, with comments such as, "They just can't find out what's wrong with me" or "They're all incompetent, and they're trying to tell me I'm crazy!" The exception may be the client with a conversion disorder who shows little emotion when describing physical limitations or lack of a medical diagnosis.

GENERAL APPEARANCE AND MOTOR BEHAVIOR

The overall appearance is usually not remarkable. Often, the client may walk slowly or with an unusual gait due to the pain or disability caused by the symptoms. The client may exhibit a facial expression of discomfort or physical distress. In many cases, the client will brighten and look much better as the assessment interview begins because the client has the nurse's undivided attention. The client with somatization disorder usually describes his or her complaints in colorful, exaggerated terms but often lacks specific information.

Table 19-2

Antidepressants Used to Treat Somatoform Disorders

Drug	Usual dose (mg/day)	Nursing Considerations
fluoxetine (Prozac)	20–60	Monitor for rash, hives, insomnia, headache, anxiety, drowsiness, nausea, loss of appetite; avoid alcohol
paroxetine (Paxil)	20–60	Monitor for nausea, loss of appetite, dizziness, dry mouth, somnolence or insomnia, sweating, sexual dysfunction; avoid alcohol
sertraline (Zoloft)	50–200	Monitor for nausea, loss of appetite, diarrhea, headache, insomnia, sexual dysfunction; avoid alcohol

Adapted from Spratto, G. R., & Woods, A. L. (2000). *PDR nurse's drug handbook.* Montvale, NJ: Medical Economics Co.

Box 19-1

➤ ASSESSMENT QUESTIONS FOR SYMPTOMS IN SCREENING TEST FOR SOMATIZATION DISORDER

1. Have you ever had trouble breathing?
2. Have you ever had trouble with menstrual cramps?
3. Have you ever had burning sensations in your sexual organs, mouth, or rectum?
4. Have you ever had difficulties swallowing or had an uncomfortable lump in your throat that stayed for at least an hour?
5. Have you ever found that you could not remember what you had been doing for hours or days at a time? If yes, did this happen even though you had not been drinking or using drugs?
6. Have you ever had trouble with frequent vomiting?
7. Have you ever had frequent pain in your fingers or toes?

Adapted from Othmer, E., & DeSouza, C. (1983). A screening test for somatization disorder (hysteria). American Journal of Psychiatry, 142*(10), 1146–1149.* © American Psychiatric Association. Reprinted with permission.

MOOD AND AFFECT

The client's mood is often labile, shifting from depressed and sad when describing physical problems to looking bright and excited when talking about how he or she had to go to the hospital in the middle of the night by ambulance. Emotions are often exaggerated, as are the client's reports of physical symptoms. The client may describe a series of personal crises related to his or her physical health, appearing pleased about these situations rather than distressed. The client with conversion disorder displays an unexpected lack of distress.

THOUGHT PROCESS AND CONTENT

Clients who somatize do not experience disordered thought processes. The content of their thinking is primarily about physical concerns, often exaggerated; for example, when they have a simple cold, they may be convinced it is pneumonia. They may even talk about dying and what music they want played at their funeral.

The client is unlikely to be able to think about or respond to questions about emotional feelings. Questions about how the client feels will be answered in terms of physical health or sensations. For example, the nurse may ask, "How did you feel about having to quit your job?" The client might respond "Well, I thought I'd feel better with the extra rest, but my back pain was just as bad as ever."

Clients with hypochondriasis focus on the fear of serious illness rather than the existence of illness seen in clients with other somatoform disorders. They are just as preoccupied with physical concerns as other somatizing clients and are likewise very limited in their abilities to identify emotional feelings or interpersonal issues.

SENSORIUM AND INTELLECTUAL PROCESSES

Clients are alert and oriented. Intellectual functions are unimpaired.

JUDGMENT AND INSIGHT

Clients' judgment may be affected by their exaggerated responses to their physical health. They have little or no insight into their behavior. They are firmly convinced that their problem is entirely physical and often believe that others don't understand.

SELF-CONCEPT

Clients are focused only on the physical part of themselves. They are unlikely to think about personal characteristics or strengths and are uncomfortable when asked to do so. Clients who somatize have low self-esteem and seem to deal with this by a total focus on physical concerns. They lack confidence, have little success in work situations, and have difficulty managing daily life issues, which they relate solely to their physical status.

ROLES AND RELATIONSHIPS

The client is not likely to be employed, although there may be a past work history. Jobs are often lost due to excessive absenteeism or inability to perform the work; the client may have quit working voluntarily due to poor physical health. The client has difficulty fulfilling family roles, being consumed with seeking medical care. It is likely that the client has few friends and spends little time in social activities. He or she may decline to see friends or go out socially for fear that he or she would become desperately ill away from home. Most of the client's socialization takes place with members of the health care community.

The client may report a lack of family support and understanding. Family members may tire of the client's ceaseless complaints and the client's refusal to accept the absence of a medical diagnosis. The client's illnesses and physical conditions often interfere with planned family events, such going on vacations or attending family gatherings. Home life is often chaotic and unpredictable.

PHYSIOLOGIC AND SELF-CARE CONCERNS

In addition to the multitude of physical complaints, there are often legitimate needs in terms of the client's health practices. Clients who somatize often have sleep pattern disturbances, lack basic nutrition, and get no exercise. In addition, they may be taking multiple prescriptions for pain or other complaints. If the client has been using anxiolytics or medications for pain, the possibility of withdrawal needs to be considered (see Chap. 17).

Data Analysis and Planning

Nursing diagnoses commonly used when working with clients who somatize include:

- Ineffective Individual Coping
- Ineffective Denial
- Impaired Social Interaction
- Anxiety
- Sleep Pattern Disturbance
- Fatigue
- Pain.

The client with conversion disorder may be at risk for disuse syndrome from having pseudoneurologic paralysis symptoms. In other words, if the client does not use a limb for a long time, the muscles may be weakened or atrophied from lack of use.

Outcome Identification

Treatment outcomes for clients with a somatoform disorder may include:

1. The client will identify the relationship between stress and physical symptoms.
2. The client will verbally express emotional feelings.
3. The client will follow an established daily routine.
4. The client will demonstrate alternative ways to deal with stress, anxiety, and other feelings.
5. The client will demonstrate healthier behaviors regarding rest, activity, and nutritional intake.

Intervention

HEALTH TEACHING

The nurse must help the client establish a daily routine that includes improved health behaviors. Adequate nutritional intake, improved sleep patterns, and a realistic balance of activity and rest are all areas with which the client may need assistance. The nurse should expect resistance from the client, with protests that he or she does not feel well enough to do these things. The challenge for the nurse is to validate the client's feelings while encouraging him or her to participate in the activities.

Nurse: *"Let's take a walk outside for some fresh air."* (encouraging collaboration)

Client: *"I wish I could, but I feel so terrible, I just can't do it."*

Nurse: *"I know this is difficult, but some exercise is essential. It will be a short walk."* (validation, encouraging collaboration)

A similar approach can be used to gain the client's participation in eating more nutritious foods, getting up and dressed at a certain time every morning, and setting a regular bedtime. The nurse can also explain that inactivity and poor eating habits perpetuate the client's discomfort, and that often it is necessary to engage in behaviors even when one doesn't feel like doing it.

Client: *"I just can't eat anything. I have no appetite."*

Nurse: *"I know you don't feel well, but it is important to begin eating."* (validation, encouraging collaboration)

Client: *"I promise I'll eat just as soon as I'm hungry."*

Nurse: *"Actually, if you begin to eat a few bites, you'll begin to feel better, and your appetite may improve."* (encouraging collaboration)

> ### ▶ CLIENT AND FAMILY TEACHING
>
> - Establish daily health routine including adequate rest, exercise, and nutrition.
> - Teach about relationship of stress and physical symptoms and mind/body relationship.
> - Educate about proper nutrition, rest, and exercise.
> - Educate client in relaxation techniques: progressive relaxation, deep breathing, guided imagery, and distraction such as music or other activities.
> - Educate client by role-playing social situations and interactions.
> - Encourage family to provide attention and encouragement when client has fewer complaints.
> - Encourage family to decrease special attention when client is in "sick" role.

The client should not be stripped of his or her somatizing defenses until adequate assessment data are collected and other coping mechanisms are learned. The nurse should not attempt to confront the client about somatic symptoms or attempt to tell him or her that these symptoms are not "real." They are very real to the client, and the client actually does experience the symptoms and associated distress.

EXPRESSION OF EMOTIONS

Teaching about the relationship between stress and physical symptoms is a useful way to help the client to begin to see the mind–body relationship. The client may keep a detailed journal of his or her physical symptoms. The nurse might ask the client to describe the situation at the time, such as whether the client was alone or with others, whether any disagreements were occurring, and so forth. This may help the client see when the physical symptoms seemed worse or better, and what other factors may have affected that perception.

It may be necessary to limit the amount of time the client can focus on physical complaints alone. Encouraging the client to focus on emotional feelings is important, although this can be difficult for the client. The nurse should provide attention and positive feedback for the client's efforts to identify and discuss feelings.

It may help for the nurse to explain to the family about primary and secondary gains. For example, if the family can provide attention to the client when he or she is feeling better or fulfilling responsibilities, the client is more likely to continue doing so. If the family members have lavished attention on the client when he or she has more physical complaints, they can be encouraged to stop reinforcing the client's sick role.

COPING STRATEGIES

Two categories of coping strategies are important for the client to learn and practice: **emotion-focused coping strategies**, which help the client relax and reduce feelings of stress, and **problem-focused coping strategies**, which help resolve or change the client's behavior or situation or manage life stressors. Emotion-focused strategies include progressive relaxation, deep breathing, guided imagery, and distractions such as music or other activities. There are many approaches to stress relief that the client can try. The nurse should help the client learn and practice these techniques, emphasizing that their effectiveness usually improves with routine use. The client must not expect such techniques to eliminate his or her pain or physical symptoms; rather, the focus is helping the client manage or diminish the intensity of the symptoms.

Problem-focused coping strategies include learning problem-solving methods, applying the process to identified problems, and role-playing interactions with others. For example, the client may complain that no one comes to visit or he or she has no friends. The nurse can help the client plan social contact with others, role-play what to talk about (other than the client's complaints), and improve the client's confidence in making relationships. The nurse can also help the client to identify life situations that are stressful to him or her and plan strategies to deal with these situations. For example, if the client finds it difficult to accomplish daily household tasks, the nurse can help him or her to plan a schedule of tasks, followed by something fun the client may enjoy.

Evaluation

Somatoform disorders are chronic or recurrent, so changes are likely to occur slowly. If treatment is effective, the client should make fewer visits to physicians with physical complaints, use less medication and more positive coping techniques, and increase his or her functional abilities. Improved family and social relationships are also a positive outcome that may follow improvements in the client's coping abilities.

▶ **INTERVENTIONS FOR SOMATOFORM DISORDERS**

- Health teaching
    Establish a daily routine.
    Promote adequate nutrition and sleep.
- Expression of emotional feelings
    Recognize relationship between stress/coping and physical symptoms.
    Keep a journal.
    Limit time spent on physical complaints.
    Limit primary and secondary gains.
- Coping strategies
    Emotion-focused coping strategies such as relaxation techniques, deep breathing, guided imagery, and distraction
    Problem-focused coping strategies such as problem-solving strategies and role-playing

---

Box 19-2

➤ **CLINICAL NURSE ALERT**

Just because a client has been diagnosed with a somatoform disorder, do not automatically dismiss all future complaints. They should be completely assessed because the client could at any time develop a physical condition that would require medical attention.

COMMUNITY-BASED CARE

Clients with somatoform disorders are often encountered in clinics, physicians' offices, or settings other than mental health. Building a trusting relationship with the client, providing empathy and support, and being sensitive to rather than dismissive of the client's complaints are skills the nurse can use in any setting where clients are seeking assistance. Making appropriate referrals, such as a pain clinic for clients with pain disorder, or providing information about support groups in the community may be helpful to the client. Encouraging clients to find pleasurable activities or hobbies may help meet their needs for attention and security, thus diminishing the psychological needs for somatic symptoms.

SELF-AWARENESS ISSUES

Clients who cope through physical symptoms can be frustrating for the nurse. Initially, they are unwilling to consider that anything other than major physical illness is the root of all their problems. When health professionals tell clients there is no physical illness present and they are referred to a mental health professional, their response is often one of anger. They may express anger directly or passively at the medical community and be highly critical of the inadequate care they believe they have received. The nurse must not respond with anger to such outbursts or criticism.

The client's progress is slow and painstaking, if there is any at all. The client coping with somatization has been doing so for years. Changes do not occur rapidly or drastically in a few days or weeks. The nurse may feel frustrated because after giving the client his or her best efforts, the client returns time after time with the same focus on physical symptoms. The nurse should be realistic about the small successes that can be achieved in any given period of time. To enhance the ongoing relationship, the nurse must be able to accept the client and his or her continued complaints and criticisms while remaining nonjudgmental.

Helpful Hints for Working With Clients With Somatoform Disorders

- Carefully assess the client's physical complaints. Even when a client has a history of a somatoform disorder, physical complaints must not be dismissed or assumed to be psychological in nature. The client may actually have a medical condition.
- Validate the client's feelings while trying to engage him or her in treatment, such as "I know you're not feeling well, but it is important to get some exercise each day."
- Remember that the somatic complaints are not under the client's voluntary control. The

(*text continues on page 521*)

INTERNET RESOURCES

Resource	Internet Address
▸ **Differential diagnosis of somatoform disorders**	http://202.30.011/~lmk/somatoform.htm
▸ **Hypochondria and Munchausen syndrome**	http://www.seanet.com/~tzhre/hypochon.htm
▸ **Body dysmorphic disorder**	http://www.sfwed.org/bdd.htm
▸ **Conversion disorder**	http://www.emedicine.com/emerg/topic112.htm
▸ **Somatoform disorders: Life Wellness Education Center**	http://www.lifewell.com/educenter/295.cfm
▸ **Psychosomatics**	http://www.appi.org/psytoc.html
▸ **Journal of Psychosomatic Research**	http://www.elsevier.n1/inca/publications/store/5/2/5/4/7/4/525474.pub.shtml

NURSING CARE PLAN FOR A CLIENT WITH HYPOCHONDRIASIS

Nursing Diagnosis

> **Ineffective Individual Coping** (5.1.1.1)
Impairment of adaptive behaviors and problem-solving abilities of a person in meeting life's demands and roles

ASSESSMENT DATA

- Denial of emotional problems
- Difficulty identifying and expressing feelings
- Lack of insight
- Self-preoccupation, especially with physical functioning
- Fears of or rumination on disease
- Numerous somatic complaints (may involve many different organs or systems)
- Sensory complaints (pain, loss of taste sensation, olfactory complaints)
- Reluctance or refusal to participate in psychiatric treatment program or activities
- Limited gratification from interpersonal relationships
- Lack of emotional support system
- Anxiety
- Secondary gains (attention, evasion of responsibilities) received for physical problems
- History of repeated visits to physicians or hospital admissions
- History of repeated medical evaluations with no findings of abnormalities

EXPECTED OUTCOMES

The client will:
- Decrease the number and frequency of physical complaints
- Demonstrate compliance with medical therapy and medications
- Demonstrate adequate energy, food and fluid intake
- Identify life stresses and anxieties
- Identify the relationship between stress and physical symptoms
- Express feelings verbally
- Identify alternative ways to deal with stress, anxiety, or other feelings
- Eliminate overuse of medications or physical treatments
- Decrease physical attention-seeking complaints
- Demonstrate alternative ways to deal with stress, anxiety, or other feelings
- Verbalize increased insight into the dynamics of hypochondriacal behavior, including secondary gains
- Verbalize an understanding of therapeutic regimens and medications, if any

IMPLEMENTATION

Nursing Interventions

The initial nursing assessment should include a complete physical assessment, a history of previous complaints and treatment, and a consideration of each current complaint.

Rationale

The nursing assessment provides a baseline from which to begin planning care.

continued on page 518

continued from page 517

Each time the client voices a new complaint (or claims injury), the client should be referred to the medical staff for assessment (and treatment if appropriate).

It is unsafe to assume that all physical complaints are hypochondriacal—the client could really be ill or injured. The client may attempt to establish the legitimacy of complaints by being genuinely injured or ill.

Minimize the amount of time and attention given to complaints. When the client makes a complaint, refer him or her to the medical staff (if it is a new complaint) or follow the team treatment plan; then tell the client you will discuss something else but not bodily complaints. Tell the client that you are interested in the client as a person, not just in his or her physical complaints. If the complaint is not acute, ask the client to save the complaint until a regular appointment with the medical staff.

If physical complaints are unsuccessful in gaining attention, they should decrease in frequency over time.

Withdraw your attention if the client insists on making complaints the sole topic of conversation. Tell the client your reason for withdrawal and that you desire to discuss other topics or will interact at a later time.

It is important to make clear to the client that attention is withdrawn from physical complaints, not from the client as a person.

Allow the client a specific time limit (like 5 minutes per hour) to discuss physical complaints with one person. The remaining staff will discuss only other issues with the client.

Because physical complaints have been the client's primary coping strategy, it is less threatening to the client if you limit this behavior initially rather than forbid it. The client's hypochondriacal behavior may abruptly worsen if he or she is denied this coping mechanism before new skills can be developed.

Do not argue with the client about his or her somatic complaints. Acknowledge the complaint as the client's feeling or perception and then follow the previous approaches.

Arguing with the client still constitutes attention, even though it is negative. The client is able to avoid discussing feelings.

Encourage the client to discuss his or her feelings about the fears rather than the fears themselves.

The focus is on feelings of fear, not fear of physical problems.

Explore the client's feelings of lack of control over stress and life events.

The client may have helpless feelings but may not recognize this independently.

Initially, carefully assess the client's self-image, social patterns, and ways of dealing with anger, stress, and so forth.

This assessment provides a knowledge base regarding hypochondriacal behaviors.

continued on page 519

continued from page 518

Talk with the client about sources of satisfaction and dissatisfaction in his or her daily life, family and other significant relationships, employment, and so forth.

Open-ended discussion usually is nonthreatening and helps the client begin self-assessment.

After some discussion of the above and the continued strengthening of your trust relationship, talk more directly with the client, and encourage the client to talk more openly about specific stresses, recent and ongoing. What does the client perceive as stressful?

The client's perception of stressors usually is more significant than others' perception of those stressors. The client will operate on the basis of what he or she believes.

If the client is using denial as a defense mechanism, the discussion of stresses may need to be less direct. Point out apparent, probable, or possible stresses to the client (in a nonthreatening way) and ask the client for feedback.

If the client is in denial, more direct approaches may produce anger or hostility and threaten the trust relationship.

Gradually, help the client identify possible connections between stress and anxiety and the occurrence or exacerbation of physical symptoms. Points you might help the client assess are: What makes the client more or less comfortable? What is the client doing or what is going on around the client when he or she feels more or less comfortable or is experiencing symptoms?

The client can begin to see the relatedness of stress and physical problems at his or her own pace. Self-realization will be more acceptable to the client, as opposed to the nurse telling the client the problem.

Encourage the client to keep a diary of events or situations, stresses, and occurrence of symptoms. This diary can then be used to identify relationships between stresses and symptoms.

Reflecting on written items may be more accurate and less threatening to the client.

Encourage the client to ventilate feelings by talking or crying, through physical activities, and so forth.

The client may have difficulty identifying and expressing feelings directly. Your encouragement and support may help him or her develop these skills.

Teach the client and his or her family or significant others about the dynamics of hypochondriacal behavior and the treatment plan, including plans after discharge.

The client and his or her family or significant others may have little or no knowledge of stress, interpersonal dynamics, hypochondriacal behavior, and so on. Knowledge of the treatment plan will promote long-term behavior change.

Talk with the client and his or her significant others about the concept of secondary gains, and together develop a plan to reduce those gains. Identify the needs the client is attempting to meet with secondary gains (such as attention or escape from perceived responsibilities or from stress).

Maintaining limits to reduce secondary gain requires everyone's participation to be successful. The client's family and significant others must be aware of the client's needs if they want to be effective in helping to meet those needs.

continued on page 520

continued from page 519

Help the client plan to meet his or her needs in more direct ways. (Show the client that attention and support are available when he or she is not exhibiting symptoms or complaints and when he or she deals with responsibilities directly or asserts himself or herself in the face of stress or discomfort.)

Positive feedback and support for healthier behavior tends to make that behavior recur more frequently. The client's family and significant others also must use positive reinforcement.

Reduce the benefits of illness as much as possible. Do not allow the client to avoid responsibilities by voicing somatic discomfort; do not excuse the client from activities or allow special privileges, such as staying in bed or dressing in night clothes.

If physical problems do not get the client what he or she wants, the client is less likely to cope in that manner.

Observe and record the circumstances surrounding the occurrence or exacerbation of complaints; talk about your observations with the client.

Alerting the client to situations surrounding the complaint helps him or her see the relatedness of stress and physical symptoms.

Help the client identify and use nonchemical methods of pain relief, such as relaxation techniques.

Learning nonchemical pain relief techniques will shift the focus of coping away from physical means and increase the client's sense of control.

Teach the client more healthful daily living habits with regard to diet, sleep, comfort measures, stress management techniques, daily fluid intake, daily exercise, decreased stimuli, rest, possible connection between caffeine and anxiety symptoms, and so forth.

Optimal physical wellness is especially important with clients using physical symptoms as a coping strategy.

Encourage the client to identify and express feelings directly in interpersonal relationships or stressful situations, especially feelings with which the client is uncomfortable (such as anger or resentment).

Direct expression of feelings will minimize the need to use physical symptoms to express them.

Notice the client's interactions with others (other clients, staff members, visitors, significant others, yourself), and give positive feedback for self-assertion and the direct expression of feelings, especially anger, resentment, and other so-called negative emotions.

The client can gain confidence in dealing with stress. The client needs to know that appropriate expressions of anger or other negative emotions are acceptable and that he or she can feel better physically as a result of these expressions.

Adapted from Schultz, J. M. & Videbeck, S. L. (1998). Lippincott's manual of psychiatric nursing care plans *(5th ed.). Philadelphia: Lippincott-Raven.*

client will have fewer somatic complaints when he or she improves his or her coping skills and interpersonal relationships.

➤ KEY POINTS

- Somatization means transforming mental experiences and states into bodily symptoms.
- The three central features of somatoform disorders are physical complaints that suggest major medical illness but have no demonstrable organic basis; psychological factors and conflicts that seem important in initiating, exacerbating, and maintaining the symptoms; and symptoms or magnified health concerns that are not under the patient's conscious control.
- Somatoform disorders include somatization disorder, conversion disorder, hypochondriasis, pain disorder, and body dysmorphic disorder
- Malingering means feigning physical symptoms for some external gain, such as avoiding work.
- Factitious disorders are characterized by physical symptoms that are feigned or inflicted for the sole purpose of drawing attention to oneself and gaining the emotional benefits of assuming the sick role.

- Internalization and somatization are the chief defense mechanisms seen in somatoform disorders.
- Clients with somatization disorder and conversion reactions may eventually be treated in mental health settings. Clients with other somatoform disorders are typically seen in medical settings.
- Clients who cope with stress through somatizing are reluctant or unable to identify emotional feelings and interpersonal issues and have few coping abilities unrelated to physical symptoms.
- Nursing interventions that may be effective with clients who somatize involve health teaching, identifying emotional feelings and stress, and learning alternative coping strategies.
- Coping strategies that are helpful to clients with somatoform disorders include relaxation techniques such as guided imagery, deep breathing, or distraction such as music, and problem-solving strategies such as identifying stressful situations and new methods of managing them and role-playing social interactions.
- Clients with somatization disorder actually experience symptoms and the associated discomfort and pain. The nurse should never try to confront the client about the origin of these symptoms until the client has learned other coping strategies.
- Somatoform disorders are chronic or recurrent, so progress toward treatment outcomes can be slow and difficult.
- Nurses caring for clients with somatoform disorders must show patience and understanding toward them as they struggle through years of recurrent somatic complaints and attempts to learn new emotion- and problem-focused coping strategies.

Critical Thinking

Questions

1. When a client has somatoform pain disorder, powerful analgesics such as narcotics are generally contraindicated, even though the client is suffering unremitting pain. How might the nurse feel when working with this client? How does the nurse respond when the client says, "You know I'm in pain! Why won't you do anything? Why do you let me suffer?"
2. Should there be limits on expensive medical tests and procedures for clients with somatoform disorder? Who should decide when health care benefits are limited?
3. A mother is found to have caused a medical crisis by giving her 6-year-old child a medication to which the child has a known severe allergy. The mother is diagnosed as having Munchausen's by proxy. Should she be treated in the mental health setting? Charged with a criminal act? Why?

REFERENCES

American Psychiatric Association. (2000). *DSM-IV-TR: diagnostic and statistical manual of mental disorders-text revision* (4th ed.). Washington, DC: American Psychiatric Association.

Barsky, A. J., Goodson, J. D., Lane, R. S., & Cleary, P. D. (1988). The amplification of somatic symptoms. *Psychosomatic Medicine, 50*, 510–518.

Bartol, G. M., & Eakes, G. G. (1995). A study of the meanings assigned to the term psychosomatic among health professionals. *Perspectives in Psychiatric Care, 31*(1), 24–29.

Goodwin, D. W., & Guze, S. B. (1989). *Psychiatric diagnosis* (4th ed.). New York: Oxford University Press.

Guggenheim, F. G. (2000). In B. J. Sadock & V. A. Sadock (Eds.). *Comprehensive textbook of psychiatry,* vol. 1. (7th ed., pp. 1504–1532). Philadelphia: Lippincott Williams & Wilkins.

Kent, D., Tomasson, K., & Coryell, W. (1995). Course and outcome of conversion and somatization disorders. *Psychosomatics, 36*(2), 138–144.

Mezzich, J. E., Lin, K., & Hughes, C. C. (2000). Acute and transient psychotic disorders and culture-bound syndromes. In B. J. Sadock & V. A. Sadock (Eds.). *Comprehensive textbook of psychiatry*, Vol. 1. (7th ed., pp. 1264–1276). Philadelphia: Lippincott Williams & Wilkins.

Othmer, E., & DeSouza, C. (1985). A screening test for somatization disorder (hysteria). *American Journal of Psychiatry, 142*(10), 1146–1149.

Schultz, J. M., and Videbeck, S. D. (1998). *Lippincott's manual of psychiatric nursing care plans* (5th ed.). Philadelphia: Lippincott-Raven.

Spratto, G. R., & Woods, A. L. (2000). *PDR nurse's drug handbook.* Montvale, NJ: Medical Economics Co.

Wool, C., & Barsky, A. (1994). Do women somatize more than men? *Psychosomatics, 35*(5), 445–452.

ADDITIONAL READINGS

Langford, L. (1992). Nursing people with psychosomatic illness. *Nursing Standard, 7*(8), 35–37.

Leibbrand, R., Hiller, W., & Fichter, M. M. (1999). Effect of comorbid anxiety, depressive, and personality disorders on treatment outcomes of somatoform disorders. *Comprehensive Psychiatry, 40*(3), 203–209.

Lenze, E. J., Miller, A. R., Munir, Z. R., Pornnoppadol, C., & North, C. (1999). Psychiatric symptoms endorsed by somatization disorder patients in a psychiatric clinic. *Annals of Clinical Psychiatry, 11*(2), 73–79.

Roberts, S. J. (1994). Somatization in primary care: the common presentation of psychosocial problems through physical complaints. *Nurse Practitioner, 19*(5), 47–56.

Russo, J., Katon, W. J., Sullivan, M., Clark, M., & Buchwald, D. (1994). Severity of somatization and its relationship to psychiatric disorders and personality. *Psychosomatics, 35*(6), 546–555.

Tyrer, P., Seivewright, N., & Sievewright, H. (1999). Long- term outcome of hypochondriacal personality disorder. Journal of Psychosomatic Research, 46(2), 177–185.

Chapter Review

➤ **MULTIPLE-CHOICE QUESTIONS**

Select the best answer for each of the following questions.

1. The nurse is caring for a client with a conversion disorder. Which of the following assessments will the nurse expect to see?

    A. Extreme distress over the physical symptom

    B. Indifference about the physical symptom

    C. Labile mood

    D. Multiple physical complaints.

2. Which of the following statements would indicate that teaching about somatization disorder has been effective?

    A. "The doctor believes I am faking my symptoms."

    B. "If I try harder to control my symptoms, I will feel better."

    C. "I will feel better when I begin handling stress more effectively."

    D. "Nothing will help me feel better physically."

3. Paroxetine (Paxil) has been prescribed for a client with a somatoform disorder. The nurse instructs the client to watch for which of the following side effects?

    A. Constipation

    B. Increased appetite

    C. Increased flatulence

    D. Nausea.

4. Emotion-focused coping strategies are designed to accomplish which of the following outcomes?

    A. Helping the client to manage difficult situations more effectively

    B. Helping the client to manage the intensity of symptoms

    C. Teaching the client the relationship between stress and physical symptoms

    D. Relieving the client's physical symptoms.

5. Which of the following is true about clients with hypochondriasis?

    A. They may interpret normal body sensations as signs of disease.

    B. They often exaggerate or fabricate physical symptoms for attention.

    C. They do not show signs of distress about their physical symptoms.

    D. All of the above are true statements.

➤ **TRUE-FALSE QUESTIONS**

Identify each of the following statements as T (True) or F (False). Correct any false statements.

_____ 1. Clients with hypochondriasis are usually reassured by medical tests that show no presence of disease.

_____ 2. Conversion disorders rarely occur before the age of 25 years.

_____ 3. Clients with a somatization disorder often believe their medical care has been inadequate.

_____

_____ 4. Malingering involves feigning or exaggerating physical symptoms.

_____

_____ 5. Learning relaxation exercises is an example of an emotion-focused coping strategy.

_____

_____ 6. Narcotics are the only effective method of treating pain disorder.

_____

_____ 7. Clients with somatoform disorders are thought to have deficits in processing sensory stimuli.

_____

_____ 8. All somatoform disorders are more common in women than in men.

_____

➤ **FILL-IN-THE-BLANK QUESTIONS**

Identify the type of somatoform disorder that is described by each of the following statements.

_____ Preoccupation with an imagined or exaggerated body defect

_____ Multiple physical symptoms including pain and gastro-intestinal, sexual, and pseudoneurologic symptoms

_____ Sudden, unexplained deficits in sensory or motor function

_____ Pain that is unrelieved by analgesics and is greatly affected by psychological factors

_____ Preoccupation with the fear of having or acquiring a serious illness.

➤ **SHORT-ANSWER QUESTIONS**

Define each of the following and provide an example.

Primary gain

Secondary gain

La belle indifference.

Mary Jones, 34, was referred to a chronic pain clinic with a diagnosis of pain disorder. She has been unable to work for 7 months due to back pain. Mary has seen several doctors, has had an MRI, and has tried a variety of anti-inflammatory medications. She tells the nurse that she is at the clinic as a last resort because none of her doctors will "do anything" for her. Mary's gait is slow, her posture is stiff, and she grimaces frequently while trying to sit in a chair. She reports being unable to drive a car, play with her children, do housework, or enjoy any of her previous leisure activities.

1. Identify three nursing diagnoses that would be pertinent for Mary's plan of care.

2. Identify two expected outcomes for Mary's plan of care.

3. Describe five interventions the nurse might implement to achieve the outcomes.

4. What other disciplines might make a contribution to Mary's care at the clinic?

5. Identify any community referrals the nurse might make for Mary.

20

Eating Disorders

Learning Objectives

After reading this chapter, the student should be able to:

1. Compare and contrast the symptoms of anorexia nervosa and bulimia nervosa.
2. Discuss various etiologic theories for eating disorders.
3. Identify effective treatment for clients with eating disorders.
4. Apply the nursing process to the care of clients with eating disorders.
5. Provide teaching to clients, families, and community members to increase knowledge and understanding of eating disorders.
6. Evaluate one's own feelings, beliefs, and attitudes about clients with eating disorders.

Key Terms

anorexia nervosa

binge eating

body image

body image disturbance

bulimia nervosa

enmeshment

purging

satiety

self-monitoring

separation-individuation

Although we think of eating disorders as relatively new, documentation from the Middle Ages indicates willful dieting leading to self-starvation in female saints, who fasted to achieve purity. In the late 1800s, doctors in England and France described young women who apparently used self-starvation to avoid obesity. However, it was not until the 1960s that anorexia nervosa was established as a mental disorder. Bulimia nervosa was first described as a distinct syndrome in 1979 (Halmi, 2000).

Eating disorders can be viewed on a continuum with the anorexic person eating too little or starving herself, the bulimic person eating in a chaotic way, and the obese person eating too much (White, 1991). There is much overlap among the eating disorders: 30% to 35% of normal-weight people with bulimia have a history of anorexia nervosa and low body weight, and about 50% of people with anorexia nervosa exhibit bulimic behavior (Kaye, Klump, Frank & Strober, 2000). The distinguishing features of anorexia include an earlier age of onset and below-normal body weight; the person fails to recognize the eating behavior as a problem. The client with bulimia has a later age of onset and near-normal body weight and is ashamed and embarrassed by the eating behavior.

More than 90% of cases of anorexia nervosa and bulimia occur in females (DSM-IV-TR, 2000). The prevalence of both eating disorders is estimated to be 1% to 3% of the general population in the United States (Halmi, 2000). This chapter focuses on anorexia nervosa and bulimia nervosa, the two most common eating disorders encountered in the mental health setting. Strategies for early identification and prevention of these disorders are also discussed.

ANOREXIA NERVOSA

Anorexia nervosa is a life-threatening eating disorder characterized by the client's refusal or inability to maintain a minimally normal body weight, intense fear of gaining weight or becoming fat, a significantly disturbed perception of the shape or size of the body, and a steadfast inability or refusal to acknowledge the seriousness of the problem or even that there is a problem (DSM-IV-TR, 2000). Clients with anorexia have a body weight that is 85% less than the weight expected for their age and height, have experienced amenorrhea for at least three consecutive cycles, and have a preoccupation with food and food-related activities.

Clients with anorexia nervosa can be classified into two subgroups, depending on how they control their weight. Clients with the restricting subtype lose weight primarily through dieting, fasting, or excessive exercise. Those with the binge eating and purging subtype engage regularly in binge eating, followed by purging. Some clients with anorexia do not binge but still engage in purging behaviors after ingesting small amounts of food. **Binge eating** means consuming a large amount of food in a discrete period of time, usually 2 hours or less. The amount of food eaten is far greater than most people eat at one time. **Purging** means the compensatory behaviors designed to eliminate food by means of self-induced vomiting or misuse of laxatives, enemas, and diuretics.

Clients with anorexia become totally absorbed in their quest for weight loss and thinness. The term "anorexia" is actually a misnomer: these clients do not lose their appetites but actually experience hunger. They ignore their feelings of hunger and signs of physical weakness and fatigue, often believing that if they eat anything, they will not be able to stop eating and will become fat. Clients with anorexia often become preoccupied with food-related activities such as preparing food, collecting recipes or cookbooks, counting calories, cooking fat-free meals, or cooking family meals. Clients also may engage in unusual or ritualistic food behaviors, such as refusing to eat in the presence of others, cutting food into minute pieces, or

---

▶ SYMPTOMS OF ANOREXIA NERVOSA

Fear of gaining weight or becoming fat, even when severely underweight
Body image disturbance
Amenorrhea
Depressive symptoms such as depressed mood, social withdrawal, irritability, and insomnia
Preoccupation with thoughts of food
Feelings of ineffectiveness
Inflexible thinking
Strong need to control environment
Limited spontaneity and overly restrained emotional expression

Complaints of constipation and abdominal pain
Cold intolerance
Lethargy
Emaciation
Hypotension, hypothermia, and bradycardia
Hypertrophy of salivary glands
Elevated BUN (blood urea nitrogen)
Electrolyte imbalances
Leukopenia and mild anemia
Elevated liver function studies

not allowing the food they eat to touch their lips. These ritualistic behaviors increase their sense of control. Excessive exercise is common; it may occupy several hours a day.

Onset and Clinical Course

Anorexia nervosa typically begins between the ages of 14 to 18 years. In the early stages, the client often denies having anxiety regarding her appearance and denies that she has a negative body image. She is very pleased with her ability to control her weight and may express this. When she initially comes for treatment, she may be unable to identify or explain her emotions regarding events in her life, such as school or relationships with family or friends. A profound sense of emptiness is not uncommon.

As the illness progresses, depression and lability in mood become more apparent. As the client's dieting and compulsive behaviors increase, she isolates herself from others. This social isolation can lead to a basic mistrust of others and even paranoia. The client may believe that her peers are jealous of her weight loss and may see family and health care professionals as trying to make her "fat and ugly."

In a long-term outcome study of clients with anorexia nervosa, Zipfel et al. (2000) found that after 21 years, 50% had recovered fully, 25% had intermediate outcomes, 10% still met all the criteria for anorexia nervosa, and 15% had died of causes related to anorexia. Clients with the lowest body weights and a longer duration of illness tend to relapse more often and have poorer outcomes (Herzog et al., 1999). Clients who abuse laxatives are at a greater risk for medical complications (Turner et al., 2000). Table 20-1 lists common medical complications of eating disorders.

BULIMIA NERVOSA

Bulimia nervosa, often simply called bulimia, is an eating disorder characterized by recurrent episodes (at least twice a week for 3 months) of binge eating followed by inappropriate compensatory behaviors to avoid weight gain, such as purging (self-induced vomiting or use of laxatives, diuretics, enemas, or emetics), fasting, or excessive exercise (DSM-IV-TR, 2000). The amount of food consumed during a binge episode is much larger than a person would normally eat, and binge eating is often done secretly. Between binges, the client may eat low-calorie food or have periods of fasting. Bingeing or purging episodes are often precipitated by strong emotions and followed by guilt, remorse, shame, or self-contempt.

Clients with bulimia are usually in the normal weight range, but they may be overweight or underweight. Tooth enamel is lost because of recurrent vomiting, and there is an increased incidence of dental caries and ragged or chipped teeth. Dentists are often the first health care professionals to identify bulimia nervosa.

Onset and Clinical Course

Bulimia nervosa usually begins in late adolescence or early adulthood; 18 or 19 is the typical age of onset. Binge eating frequently begins during or after an episode of dieting. Between bingeing and purging episodes, the person may eat restrictively, choosing salads and other low-calorie foods. This restrictive eating effectively sets the person up for the next episode of bingeing and purging, and the cycle continues.

Clients with bulimia are aware that their eating behavior is pathologic and go to great lengths to hide it from others. They may store food in their cars, desks, or secret locations around the house. They may drive

---

CLINICAL VIGNETTE: ANOREXIA NERVOSA

Maggie is a 15-year-old girl, 5'7", and weighs 92 pounds. Though it is August, she is wearing sweatpants and three layers of shirts. Her hair is dry, brittle, and uncombed, and she wears no makeup. Maggie's family physician has referred her to the eating disorders unit because she has lost 20 pounds in the last 4 months and her menstrual periods have ceased. She also is lethargic and weak, yet has trouble sleeping. Maggie is an avid ballet student, and believes she still needs to lose more weight to achieve the figure she wants. Her ballet instructor has expressed concern to Maggie's parents about her appearance and fatigue.

Maggie's family reports that she has gone from being an A and B student to barely passing in school. She spends much of her time isolated in her room and is often exercising for long hours, even in the middle of the night. Maggie seldom goes out with friends, and they have stopped calling her on the phone. The nurse interviews Maggie, but gains little information as she is reluctant to discuss her eating. Maggie does say she is too fat, has no interest in gaining weight, and she does not understand why her parents are forcing her to come to "this place where all they want to do is fatten you up and keep you ugly."

Table 20-1

MEDICAL COMPLICATIONS OF EATING DISORDERS

Body System	Symptoms
RELATED TO WEIGHT LOSS	
Musculoskeletal	Loss of muscle mass, loss of fat, osteoporosis, and pathologic fractures
Metabolic	Hypothyroidism (symptoms include lack of energy, weakness, intolerance to cold, and bradycardia) hypoglycemia, and decreased insulin sensitivity
Cardiac	Bradycardia, hypotension, loss of cardiac muscle, small heart, cardiac arrhythmias (including atrial and ventricular premature contractions, prolonged QT interval, ventricular tachycardia), and sudden death
Gastrointestinal	Delayed gastric emptying, bloating, constipation, abdominal pain, gas, and diarrhea
Reproductive	Amenorrhea and low levels of luteinizing and follicle-stimulating hormones
Dermatologic	Dry, cracking skin due to dehydration, lanugo (ie, fine, baby-like hair over body), edema, and acrocyanosis (ie, blue hands and feet)
Hematologic	Leukopenia, anemia, thrombocytopenia, hypercholesterolemia, and hypercarotenemia
Neuropsychiatric	Abnormal taste sensation, apathetic depression, mild organic mental symptoms, and sleep disturbances
RELATED TO PURGING (VOMITING AND LAXATIVE ABUSE)	
Metabolic	Electrolyte abnormalities, particularly hypokalemia, hypochloremic alkalosis, hypomagnesemia, and elevated blood urea nitrogen (BUN)
Gastrointestinal	Salivary gland and pancreas inflammation and enlargement with an increase in serum amylase, esophageal and gastric erosion or rupture, dysfunctional bowel, and superior mesenteric artery syndrome
Dental	Erosion of dental enamel (perimyolysis), particularly front teeth
Neuropsychiatric	Seizures (related to large fluid shifts and electrolyte disturbances), mild neuropathies, fatigue, weakness, and mild organic mental symptoms

Adapted from Halmi, K. A. (2000). Eating disorders. In B. J. Sadock & V. A. Sadock (Eds.). *Comprehensive textbook of psychiatry*, Vol. 2, (7th ed., pp. 1663–1676). Philadelphia: Lippincott Williams & Wilkins.

▶ SYMPTOMS OF BULIMIA NERVOSA

- Recurrent episodes of binge eating
- Compensatory behavior such as self-induced vomiting, misuse of laxatives, diuretics, enema or other medications, or excessive exercise
- Self-evaluation overly influenced by body shape and weight
- Usually within normal weight range, possible underweight or overweight
- Restriction of total calorie consumption between binges, selecting low-calorie foods while avoiding foods perceived to be fattening or likely to trigger a binge
- Depressive and anxiety symptoms
- Possible substance use involving alcohol or stimulants
- Loss of dental enamel
- Chipped, ragged, or moth-eaten appearance of teeth
- Increased dental caries
- Menstrual irregularities
- Dependence on laxatives
- Esophageal tears
- Fluid and electrolyte abnormalities
- Metabolic alkalosis (from vomiting) or metabolic acidosis (from diarrhea)
- Mildly elevated serum amylase levels

from one fast-food restaurant to another, ordering a normal amount of food at each one but stopping at six places in an hour or two. This type of eating pattern may exist for years until family or friends discover the client's behavior, or medical complications develop for which she seeks treatment.

About 50% of bulimic clients recover fully, 20% continue to meet all the criteria for the disease, and 30% have episodic bouts of bulimia. One third of fully recovered clients have a relapse. Clients with a comorbid personality disorder tend to have poorer outcomes than those without a personality disorder. The death rate for bulimia is estimated to be 0% to 3% (Halmi, 2000).

RELATED DISORDERS

Eating disorders that are usually first diagnosed in infancy and childhood include rumination disorder, pica, and feeding disorder (see Chap. 18). Family dysfunction and parent–child conflicts may be seen in these families (Patel et al., 1998).

Binge eating disorder is listed as a research category in DSM-IV-TR, 2000; it is undergoing study to determine whether it will be classified as a mental disorder in the future. The essential features are re-

CLINICAL VIGNETTE: BULIMIA NERVOSA

Susan is driving home from the grocery store, eating from the grocery bags as she drives. In the 15-minute trip, she has already consumed a package of cookies, a large bag of potato chips, and a pound of ham from the deli. She thinks "I have to hurry, I'll be home soon. No one can see me like this!" She knew when she bought these food items that she would never get home with them.

Susan hurriedly drops the groceries on the kitchen counter and races for the bathroom. Tears are streaming down her face as she vomits to get rid of what she has just eaten. She feels guilty and ashamed, and does not understand why she cannot stop her behavior. If only she did not eat those things. She thinks, "I'm 30 years old, married, with two beautiful daughters, and a successful interior design consultant. What would my clients say if they could see me now? If my husband and daughters saw me, they would be disgusted." As Susan leaves the bathroom to put away the remainder of the groceries, she promises herself to stay away from all those bad foods. If she just does not eat them, this won't happen. This is a promise she has made many times before.

current episodes of binge eating without the regular use of inappropriate compensatory behaviors seen in bulimia, guilt and shame about eating behaviors, and psychological distress. Clients are more likely to be overweight or obese, were overweight as children, and were more likely to be teased about their weight at an early age. Thirty-five percent reported that binge eating preceded dieting; 65% reported dieting before the onset of binge eating (Grilo & Masheb, 2000).

Comorbid psychiatric disorders are common in patients with anorexia nervosa and bulimia nervosa. Clients with anorexia nervosa have a high rate of major depression (68%), anxiety disorders (65%), obsessive-compulsive disorder (26%), and social phobia (34%). Personality disorders also are prevalent: 25% of clients with the restricting type of anorexia have cluster C anxious personality traits, and 40% of clients with the binge and purge type of anorexia have cluster B impulsive personality traits. Clients with bulimia have comorbid psychiatric diagnoses of major depressive disorder (36% to 70%), substance abuse (18% to 32%), and personality disorders (28% to 77%), primarily cluster B impulsive personality traits (Halmi, 2000).

Eating disorders are often linked to a past history of sexual abuse. Wiederman (1996) found that a history of sexual abuse in women with anorexia nervosa or bulimia was a factor contributing to problems with intimacy, sexual attractiveness, and low levels of interest in sexual activity. Matsunaga et al. (1999) studied women recovering from bulimia and found that women with a history of physical or sexual abuse had higher rates of borderline personality disorder and posttraumatic stress disorder and more severe core eating disorder symptoms such as a drive for thinness, body dissatisfaction, and ineffectiveness. However, whether sexual abuse has a cause-and-effect relationship to the development of eating disorders remains unclear.

ETIOLOGY

A specific cause for eating disorders is unknown. Initially, dieting is the stimulus that leads to the development of the serious eating disorders. Biologic vulnerability, development problems, and family and social influences can turn the dieting behavior into an eating disorder (Table 20-2). Psychological and physiologic reinforcement of the maladaptive eating behavior sustains the cycle (Halmi, 2000).

Biologic Factors

Studies of anorexia nervosa and bulimia nervosa have shown that these disorders tend to run in families. Thus, a genetic vulnerability may exist that is triggered by inappropriate dieting or emotional stress. This genetic vulnerability might be due to a particular personality type or a general susceptibility to psychiatric disorders, or it may directly involve a dysfunction of the hypothalamus (Halmi, 2000). A family history of mood or anxiety disorders or obsessive-compulsive disorders places a person at risk for developing an eating disorder. Wade et al. (2000) attributed 58% of cases of anorexia nervosa to heritability but could not totally discount the effect of a shared environment.

Many of the symptoms of eating disorders may be produced by disruptions of the nuclei of the hypothalamus. Two sets of nuclei are particularly important in many aspects of hunger and **satiety** (satisfaction of appetite): the lateral hypothalamus and the ventromedial hypothalamus. Deficits in the lateral hypothalamus result in decreased eating and decreased responses to sensory stimuli, which are important to eating. Disruption of the ventromedial hypothalamus leads to excessive eating, weight gain, and decreased responsiveness to the satiety effects of glucose, which are behaviors seen in bulimia.

Table 20-2

RISK FACTORS FOR EATING DISORDERS

Disorder	Biologic Risk Factors	Developmental Risk Factors	Family Risk Factors	Sociocultural Risk Factors
Anorexia nervosa	Obesity; dieting at an early age	Issues of developing autonomy and having control over one's self and environment; developing a unique identity; dissatisfaction with body image	Family is rigid about values and rules; overprotective; unable to deal with conflict	Cultural ideal of being thin; media focus on beauty, thinness, fitness; preoccupation with achieving the ideal body
Bulimia nervosa	Obesity; early dieting; possible serotonin and norepinephrine disturbances	Separation–individuation issues; physical or emotional separation is stressful; dissatisfaction with body image	Family is chaotic, with loose boundaries; achievement oriented; perceived as less caring; parental concerns about weight	Same as above; weight-related teasing

Adapted from Stice, E., Akutagawa, D., Guggar, A., & Agras, W. S. (2000). Negative effect moderates the relation between dieting and binge eating. *International Journal of Eating Disorders, 27*(2), 218–229).

Many neurochemical changes occur with eating disorders, but it is difficult to tell whether these cause eating disorders or are a result of anorexia and bulimia because of the starvation, bingeing, and purging. For example, norepinephrine levels rise in normal people in response to eating, allowing nutrients to be metabolized and used by the body. However, norepinephrine levels do not rise to normal levels during periods of starvation, because there are few nutrients to metabolize. Therefore, low norepinephrine levels are seen in clients during periods of restricted food intake. Also, low epinephrine levels are related to the decreased heart rate and blood pressure seen in clients with anorexia.

Higher levels of the neurotransmitter serotonin and its precursor tryptophan have been linked to increased satiety, the body's signal that indicates we have had enough to eat. Low levels of serotonin, as well as lowered platelet levels of monoamine oxidase, have been found in clients with bulimia and clients with the binge and purge subtype of anorexia nervosa (Carrasco et al., 2000); this may explain bingeing behavior. The positive response of some clients with bulimia to treatment with selective serotonin reuptake inhibitor antidepressants supports the idea that serotonin levels at the synapse may be low in these clients.

Developmental Factors

ANOREXIA NERVOSA

The onset of anorexia nervosa usually occurs during adolescence or young adulthood, and it is believed that some of the causes are related to developmental issues in this stage of life. The struggle to develop autonomy and the establishment of a unique identity are two essential tasks.

The developmental task of autonomy, or exerting control over oneself and the environment, may be difficult in families that are overprotective or where **enmeshment** (lack of clear role boundaries) exists. The adolescent's efforts to gain independence are not supported, and she may feel as though she has little or no control in her life. She begins to control her eating by severe dieting and thus gain control over her weight. Losing weight becomes reinforcing: by continuing to lose weight, she is in control of some aspect of her life.

Serpell et al. (1999) studied girls with anorexia nervosa to determine positive or reinforcing aspects of the disorder. Two main themes were discovered: conforming to a strict diet and fitting into smaller clothes (slim cultural ideal), and feelings of power, control, and even superiority over others by losing weight.

The need to develop a unique identity, or a sense of who one is as a person, is another essential task of adolescence. This coincides with the onset of puberty, bringing with it many emotional and physiologic changes. Self-doubt and confusion can result if the adolescent does not measure up to who she wants to be.

Advertisements, magazines, and movies that feature thin models reinforce the cultural belief that slimness is attractive. Excessive dieting and weight loss may be the way the adolescent chooses to achieve this ideal. **Body image** is how a person perceives his or her body, a mental image of oneself. For most people, body image is consistent with how others view them. However, for persons with anorexia nervosa, their body image differs greatly from the perception of others. They perceive themselves as fat, unattractive, and undesirable, even when they are severely underweight and malnourished. **Body image disturbance** occurs when there is an extreme discrepancy between one's body image and the perceptions of others and extreme dissatisfaction with one's body image (Gardner et al., 1999).

BULIMIA NERVOSA

A normal part of development in later adolescence or early adulthood is the physical and emotional separation of the child from the nuclear family, known as **separation-individuation**. This often coincides with going to college, getting a job, or moving into an apartment. When this separation from the family is difficult, anxiety can develop. Binge eating can be a way to deal with the anxiety, and purging behaviors are used as a way to get rid of the food to avoid becoming fat (White, 1993). In clients with bulimia nervosa, body dissatisfaction also exists as well as the belief that one is fat, unattractive, and undesirable.

Family Influences

The family structure of the client with anorexia nervosa is often rigid in terms of values and rules, and

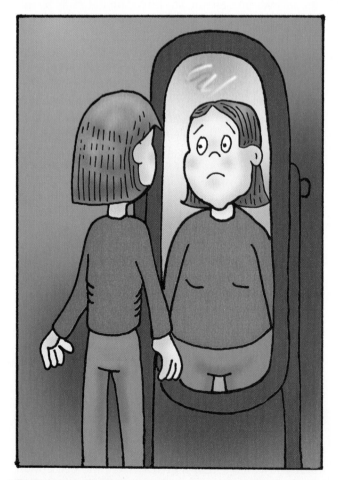

Body image disturbance

parents are often overprotective of the child. This rigidity and overprotection may stifle the adolescent's attempts to become autonomous and develop her own identity. The family tends to avoid conflict and prefers to present a united front of harmony, both to themselves and outsiders. This inability to experience conflict and negotiate solutions puts additional pressure on the adolescent. Resorting to dieting and weight control can be a response to such situations in the family (White, 1993).

Families of clients with bulimia are chaotic, lack clear boundaries between members, and are achievement-oriented (White, 1993). The client may have difficulty identifying her appropriate role, may have trouble separating from the family, and may believe she is judged by her "success." Soothing herself with certain foods becomes a way of dealing with the family pressures and the resulting anxiety and unhappiness. Bingeing to find comfort is followed by guilt and shame at the lack of control, so purging behaviors become necessary to deal with the guilt and get rid of the unwanted food. Even when the client gets older, marries, and has a family of her own, she strives to please others and maintain harmony and continues to deal with her feelings in food-related ways.

Sociocultural Factors

In the United States and other Western countries, the media fuels the image of the "ideal woman" as thin. Beauty, desirability, and ultimately happiness are equated with being very thin, perfectly toned, and physically fit. Actresses and models often are idealized by adolescents as having the perfect "look" or body, even though many of them are underweight or use special effects to appear thinner than they are. Books, magazines, dietary supplements, exercise equipment, plastic surgery advertisements, and weight loss programs abound; the dieting industry is a billion-dollar business. Being overweight is considered a sign of laziness, lack of self-control, or indifference; pursuing the "perfect" body is equated with beauty, desirability, success, and will power. Thus, many women speak of being "good" when they stick to their diet and "bad" when they eat desserts or snacks.

Pressure from others may also contribute to the development of eating disorders. Picard (1999) noted that pressure from coaches, parents, and peers and the emphasis placed on body form in certain sports can promote eating disorders in athletes. Parental concern over a girl's weight and teasing from parents or peers about her weight reinforces a girl's body dissatisfaction and her need to diet or control eating in some way.

CULTURAL CONSIDERATIONS

Both anorexia and bulimia nervosa appear to be far more prevalent in industrialized societies, where there is abundant food and where beauty is linked to being thin (Patel et al., 1998). Eating disorders are most common in the United States, Canada, Europe, Australia, Japan, New Zealand, and South Africa. Immigrants from cultures in which eating disorders are rare may develop eating disorders as they assimilate the thin-body ideal (DSM-IV, 1994). Eating disorders appear to be equally common among Hispanic and white women and less common among African American and Asian women (Halmi, 2000). Minority women who are younger, better educated, and more closely identified with white, middle-class values are at greater risk for developing an eating disorder.

Dieting is becoming a fad in countries such as China (Patel et al., 1998). With today's technology, the entire world is exposed to the Western ideal equating thinness with beauty and desirability. As this ideal becomes widespread in non-Western cultures, it is likely there will be an increase in anorexia and bulimia as well.

TREATMENT
Anorexia Nervosa

Clients with anorexia nervosa can be very difficult to treat because they are often resistant to treatment and appear uninterested in treatment because of their denial that problems exist. Treatment settings include inpatient specialty eating disorder units, partial hospitalization or day treatment programs, and outpatient therapy. The choice of setting depends on the severity of the illness, such as weight, physical symptoms, duration of bingeing and purging, drive for thinness, body dissatisfaction, and the existence of comorbid psychiatric conditions (White & Litovitz, 1998). Major life-threatening complications that indicate the need for hospital admission include severe fluid, electrolyte, and metabolic imbalances, cardiovascular complications, severe weight loss and its consequences (Patel et al., 1998), and the risk of suicide. Outpatient therapy has the best success with clients who have been ill for less than 6 months, are not bingeing and purging, and have parents who are likely to participate effectively in family therapy (Halmi, 2000).

MEDICAL MANAGEMENT

Medical management focuses on weight restoration, nutritional rehabilitation, rehydration, and correction of electrolyte imbalances. The client is given nutritionally balanced meals and snacks, gradually increasing caloric intake to a normal level for her size, age, and activity. Clients who are severely malnourished may require total parenteral nutrition, tube feedings, or hyperalimentation to provide adequate nutritional intake. Generally, the client's access to a bathroom is supervised to prevent purging as the client begins to eat more food. Weight gain and adequate food intake are most often the criteria for determining the effectiveness of treatment.

PSYCHOPHARMACOLOGY

Several classes of drugs have been studied, but few have shown clinical success. Amitriptyline (Elavil) and the antihistamine cyproheptadine (Periactin) in high doses (up to 28 mg/day) can promote weight gain in inpatients with anorexia nervosa (Halmi, 2000; Peterson & Mitchell, 1999). Fluoxetine (Prozac) has shown some effectiveness in preventing relapse in clients whose weight has been partially or completely restored (Peterson & Mitchell, 1999). Close monitoring is needed, because weight loss can be a side effect of fluoxetine.

PSYCHOTHERAPY

Family therapy may be beneficial for families of clients younger than 18 years of age. Families who demonstrate enmeshment, unclear boundaries between members, and difficulty handling emotions and conflict can begin to resolve these issues and improve communication in the family. Family therapy also is useful to help family members to be effective participants in the client's treatment. Studies have shown that dysfunctional families may take as long as 2 years to demonstrate improvement in functioning (Gowers & North, 1999; North et al., 1997).

Individual therapy for the client with anorexia nervosa may be indicated in some circumstances, such as if the family cannot participate in family therapy, if the client is older or separated from the nuclear family, or if the client has individual issues requiring psychotherapy. McIntosh et al. (2000) reported that interpersonal functioning can be improved and symptoms decreased with therapy that focuses on grief issues, interpersonal disputes, interpersonal deficits, and role transitions.

Bulimia Nervosa

Most clients with bulimia are treated on an outpatient basis. Hospital admission would be indicated if bingeing and purging behaviors were out of control and the client's medical status was compromised. Most clients with bulimia have near-normal weight, reducing the concern about severe malnutrition (which is a factor in clients with anorexia nervosa).

COGNITIVE-BEHAVIORAL THERAPY

Cognitive-behavioral therapy has been found to be the most effective treatment for bulimia (Halmi, 2000). This outpatient approach often uses a detailed manual to guide treatment. Strategies designed to change the client's thinking (cognition) and actions (behavior) about food focus on interrupting the cycle of dieting, bingeing, and purging and altering the client's dysfunctional thoughts and beliefs about food, weight, body image, and overall self-concept (Halmi, 2000). Combining cognitive-behavioral therapy with psychoeducation using both individual and group formats has been effective in terms of outcomes, cost, and client satisfaction (White, 1999). Agras et al. (2000) found that cognitive-behavioral therapy produced more rapid improvement for clients with bulimia than did interpersonal psychotherapy.

PSYCHOPHARMACOLOGY

Since the 1980s, several controlled studies have been conducted to evaluate the effectiveness of antidepressant medication to treat bulimia. Drugs such as desipramine (Norpramin), imipramine (Tofranil), amitriptyline (Elavil), nortriptyline (Pamelor), phenelzine (Nardil), and fluoxetine (Prozac) were prescribed in the same dosages used to treat depression (see Chap. 2). In all the studies, the antidepressants were more effective than placebos in reducing binge eating. The medication also improved mood and reduced preoccupation with shape and weight (Halmi, 2000; Peterson & Mitchell, 1999). However, only 22% to 25% of the clients were completely abstinent from binge eating and purging by the end of treatment (Agras, 1997; Halmi, 2000).

APPLICATION OF THE NURSING PROCESS

Although there are differences between clients with anorexia and bulimia, there are many similarities in assessing, planning, implementing, and evaluating nursing care for these clients. For that reason, this section will address both eating disorders, highlighting the differences between anorexia and bulimia where they exist.

Assessment

Several specialized tests have been developed for eating disorders. An assessment tool such as the Eating Attitudes Test is often used in studies of anorexia and bulimia. This test can also be used at the end of treatment to evaluate outcomes because it is sensitive to clinical changes.

HISTORY

Before the development of anorexia nervosa, clients are often described as perfectionists with above-average intelligence and as being achievement-oriented, dependable, eager to please, and seeking approval. Parents describe the client as being "good, causing us no trouble" until the onset of anorexia. Likewise, clients with bulimia are often focused on pleasing others and avoiding conflict. However, clients with bulimia often have a history of impulsive behavior such as substance abuse and shoplifting, as well as anxiety, depression, and personality disorders (Schultz & Videbeck, 1998).

GENERAL APPEARANCE AND MOTOR BEHAVIOR

The client with anorexia appears slow, lethargic, and fatigued; she may be emaciated, depending on the amount of weight loss. She may be slow to respond to questions and have difficulty deciding what to say. She is often reluctant to answer questions fully, not wanting to acknowledge that a problem exists. She often wears loose-fitting clothes in layers, regardless of the weather, both to hide her weight loss and to keep warm (clients with anorexia are generally cold). Eye contact may be limited, and the client may turn away from the nurse, indicating her unwillingness to discuss her problems or enter treatment.

The client with bulimia may be underweight or overweight but is generally close to the expected body weight for her age and size. The general appearance of the client is not unusual, and she appears open and willing to talk.

MOOD AND AFFECT

Clients with eating disorders have labile moods, usually corresponding to their eating or dieting behaviors. Avoiding "bad" or fattening foods gives them a sense of power and control over their bodies, whereas eating, bingeing, or purging leads to anxiety, depression, and feeling out of control. Clients often appear sad, anxious, and worried. Clients with anorexia seldom smile, laugh, or enjoy any attempts at humor; they are somber and serious most of the time.

In contrast, the client with bulimia is initially pleasant and cheerful, as though nothing is wrong. The pleasant façade usually disappears when the client begins describing binge eating and purging behaviors, and the client may express intense emotions of guilt, shame, and embarrassment.

It is important to ask clients with eating disorders about thoughts of self-harm or suicide. It is not uncommon for clients with eating disorders to engage in self-mutilating behaviors such as cutting.

▸ EATING ATTITUDES TEST

Please place an (X) under the column that applies best to each of the numbered statements. All of the results will be strictly confidential. Most of the questions relate to food or eating, although other types of questions have been included. Please answer each question carefully. Thank you.

	Always	Very Often	Often	Sometimes	Rarely	Never
1. Like eating with other people.						X
2. Prepare foods for others but do not eat what I cook.	X					
3. Become anxious prior to eating.	X					
4. Am terrified about being overweight.	X					
5. Avoid eating when I am hungry.	X					
6. Find myself preoccupied with food.	X					
7. Have gone on eating binges where I feel that I may not be able to stop.	X					
8. Cut food into small pieces.	X					
9. Aware of the calorie content of foods that I eat.	X					
10. Particularly avoid foods with a high carbohydrate content (eg, bread, potatoes, rice, etc.).	X					
11. Feel bloated after meals.	X					
12. Feel that others would prefer I ate more.	X					
13. Vomit after I have eaten.	X					
14. Feel extremely guilty after eating.	X					
15. Am preoccupied with a desire to be thinner.	X					
16. Exercise strenuously to burn off calories.	X					
17. Weigh myself several times a day.	X					
18. Like my clothes to fit tightly.						X
19. Enjoy eating meat.						X
20. Wake up early in the morning.	X					
21. Eat the same foods day after day.	X					
22. Think about burning up calories when I exercise.	X					
23. Have regular menstrual periods.						X
24. Other people think I am too thin.	X					
25. Am preoccupied with the thought of having fat on my body.	X					
26. Take longer than others to eat.	X					
27. Enjoy eating at restaurants.						X
28. Take laxatives.	X					
29. Avoid foods with sugar in them.	X					
30. Eat diet foods.	X					
31. Feel that food controls my life.	X					
32. Display self-control around food.	X					
33. Feel that others pressure me to eat.	X					
34. Give too much time and thought to food.	X					
35. Suffer from constipation.		X				
36. Feel uncomfortable after eating sweets.	X					
37. Engage in dieting behavior.	X					
38. Like my stomach to be empty.	X					
39. Enjoy trying new rich foods.						X
40. Have impulse to vomit after meals.	X					

Scoring: The patient is given the questionnaire without the X's, just blank. 3 points are assigned to endorsements that coincide with the X's; the adjacent alternatives are weighted as 2 points and 1 point, respectively. A total score of over 30 indicates significant concerns with eating behavior.

Concern about self-harm and suicidal behavior is increased in clients with a history of sexual abuse (see Chaps. 11 and 14).

THOUGHT PROCESSES AND CONTENT

Clients with eating disorders spend most of the time thinking about dieting, food, and food-related behavior. They are preoccupied with food and their attempts to avoid eating or eating "bad" or the "wrong" foods. Clients cannot think about themselves without thinking about weight and food. The body image disturbance can be almost delusional: even if they are severely underweight, they can point to areas on their buttocks or thighs that are "still fat," fueling their need to continue dieting. Clients with anorexia who are severely underweight may have paranoid ideas about their family and health care professionals, believing that they are their "enemies" who are trying to make them fat by getting them to eat.

SENSORIUM AND INTELLECTUAL PROCESSES

Generally, clients with eating disorders are alert and oriented, and intellectual functions are intact. The exception is clients with anorexia who are severely malnourished and showing signs of starvation such as mild confusion, slowed mental processes, and difficulty with concentration and attention.

JUDGMENT AND INSIGHT

The client with anorexia has very limited insight and poor judgment about her health status. She does not believe she has a problem but believes that other people are trying to interfere with her ability to lose weight and achieve the body image she desires. Factual information about her failing health status is not enough to convince her that problems truly exist. The client with anorexia continues to restrict her food intake or engage in purging behaviors despite the negative effect on her health.

In contrast, the client with bulimia is ashamed of the binge eating and purging behaviors. She recognizes these behaviors as abnormal and goes to great lengths to hide them from others. She feels out of control and unable to change these behaviors, even though she recognizes them as pathologic.

SELF-CONCEPT

Low self-esteem is prominent in clients with eating disorders. They see themselves only in terms of their ability to control their food intake and weight. They tend to judge themselves harshly and see themselves as "bad" if they eat certain foods or fail to lose weight. Other personal characteristics or achievements are overlooked or ignored as not being as important as thinness. Clients often perceive themselves as helpless, powerless, and ineffective. This feeling of lack of control over themselves and their environment only strengthens their desire to control their intake and weight.

ROLES AND RELATIONSHIPS

An eating disorder interferes with the client's ability to fulfill roles and have satisfying relationships with others. The client with anorexia may begin to have failing grades in school, in sharp contrast to her previously successful academic performance. She withdraws from peers and pays little attention to friendships. She believes that others will not understand or fears that she will begin out-of-control eating in the presence of others.

The client with bulimia feels a great deal of shame about her binge eating and purging behaviors. This causes her to lead a secret life, sneaking behind the backs of her friends and family to binge and purge in privacy. The amount of time spent buying and eating food and then purging can interfere with role performance both at home and at work.

PHYSIOLOGIC AND SELF-CARE CONSIDERATIONS

The health status of the client with an eating disorder is directly related to the severity of self-starvation and the purging behaviors in which she engages, or both (see Table 20-1). In addition, the client may engage in excessive exercise, almost to the point of exhaustion, in an effort to control her weight. Many clients have sleep disturbances such as insomnia, reduced sleep time, and early-morning wakening. Clients who engage in frequent vomiting have many dental problems such as loss of tooth enamel, chipped and ragged teeth, and dental caries. Frequent vomiting may also result in sores in the mouth. Complete medical and dental examinations are essential.

Data Analysis

Nursing diagnoses for clients with eating disorders include:
- Altered Nutrition: Less Than/More Than Body Requirements
- Ineffective Individual Coping
- Body Image Disturbance.

Other nursing diagnoses may be pertinent, such as fluid volume deficit, constipation, fatigue, and activity intolerance.

Outcome Identification

For the client who is severely malnourished, her medical condition must be stabilized before psychiatric treatment can begin. Medical stabilization may include parenteral fluids, total parenteral nutrition, and cardiac monitoring.

Examples of expected outcomes for clients with eating disorders include:

1. The client will establish adequate nutritional eating patterns.
2. The client will eliminate use of compensatory behaviors such as excessive exercise and use of laxatives and diuretics.
3. The client will demonstrate non–food-related coping mechanisms.
4. The client will verbalize feelings of guilt, anger, anxiety, or an excessive need for control.
5. The client will verbalize acceptance of body image with stable body weight.

Interventions

ESTABLISHING NUTRITIONAL EATING PATTERNS

Typically, treatment in an inpatient setting is for clients with anorexia nervosa who are severely malnourished, and clients with bulimia whose binge eating and purging behaviors are out of control. A primary role of the nurse is to implement and supervise the regimen for nutritional rehabilitation. Total parenteral nutrition or enteral feedings may be prescribed initially when the client's health status is severely compromised.

When the client can eat, a diet of 1,200 to 1,500 calories per day is ordered, with gradual increases in calories until the client is ingesting adequate amounts for her height, level of activity, and growth needs. Typically, the allotted calories are divided into three meals and three snacks. A liquid protein supplement is given to replace any food not eaten to ensure that the total number of prescribed calories is consumed. The nurse is responsible for monitoring the client's meals and snacks and often will sit with the client while she eats, at a table away from other clients initially. Depending on the treatment program, diet beverages and food substitutions may be prohibited, and a specified amount of time may be set for consuming each meal or snack. The client also may be discouraged from performing food rituals such as cutting food into tiny pieces or mixing food in unusual combinations. The nurse must be alert for any attempts by the client to hide or discard food.

After each meal or snack, the client may be required to remain in view of staff for 1 to 2 hours to ensure she does not empty her stomach by vomiting. Some treatment programs limit the client's access to the bathroom without supervision, particularly after meals, to discourage vomiting. As the client begins to gain weight, these restrictions are lessened gradually as the client becomes more independent in her eating behavior.

> ▶ **INTERVENTIONS FOR CLIENTS WITH EATING DISORDERS**
>
> - **Establishing nutritional eating patterns**
>   Sit with the client during meals and snacks
>   Offer liquid protein supplement if unable to complete meal
>   Adhere to treatment program guidelines regarding restrictions
>   Observe client following meals and snacks for 1 to 2 hours
>   Weigh client daily in uniform clothing
>   Be alert for attempts to hide or discard food or inflate weight
> - **Helping the client identify emotions and develop non–food-related coping strategies**
>   Ask the client to identify feelings
>   Self-monitoring using a journal
>   Relaxation techniques
>   Distraction
>   Assist client to change stereotypical beliefs
> - **Helping the client deal with body image issues**
>   Recognize benefits of a more near-normal weight
>   Assist to view self in ways not related to body image
>   Identify personal strengths, interests, talents
> - **Providing client and family education** (See Client and Family Teaching)

In most treatment programs, the client is weighed only once daily, usually on awakening and after she has emptied her bladder. The client should wear minimal clothing, such as a hospital gown, each time she is weighed. The client may attempt to place objects in her clothing to give the appearance of weight gain.

The client with bulimia is often treated on an outpatient basis. The nurse must work closely with the client to establish normal eating patterns and interrupt the binge and purge cycle. The client is encouraged to eat meals with her family or, if she lives alone, with friends. She should always sit at a table in a designated eating area such as a kitchen or dining room. It is easier for the client to follow a nutritious eating plan if it is written in advance, and groceries are purchased for the planned menus. The client must avoid buying foods frequently consumed during binges, such as cookies, candy bars, and potato chips. Food kept in desk drawers at work, in the car, or in the bedroom should be discarded or moved to the kitchen.

HELPING THE CLIENT IDENTIFY EMOTIONS AND DEVELOP COPING STRATEGIES

Because the client with anorexia has problems with self-awareness, she often has difficulty identifying her feelings. Therefore, she often expresses these feelings in terms of a somatic complaint, such as feeling fat or bloated. The nurse can help the client begin to recognize her emotions, such as anxiety or guilt, by asking her to describe how she is feeling, allowing adequate time for her to respond. The nurse should not ask, "Are you sad?" or "Are you anxious?" because the client may quickly agree rather than struggling for an answer on her own. The nurse encourages the client to describe her feelings. This approach can eventually help the client to recognize her emotions and connect them to her eating behaviors.

Self-monitoring is a cognitive-behavioral technique designed to help clients with bulimia. This technique may help clients to identify behavior patterns and then implement techniques to avoid or replace these unwanted behaviors (Wilson & Vitousek, 1999). Self-monitoring techniques raise the client's awareness about her behavior and help her regain her sense of control. The nurse should encourage the client to keep a diary of all food eaten throughout the day, including binges, and to record her moods, emotions, thoughts, circumstances, and interactions surrounding eating and bingeing or purging episodes. In this way, the client begins to see connections between emotions and situations and eating behaviors. The nurse can then help the client to develop ways to manage emotions such as anxiety by using relaxation techniques or distraction with music or another activity. This is an important step toward helping the client find ways to cope with people, emotions, or situations that do not involve food.

HELPING THE CLIENT DEAL WITH BODY IMAGE ISSUES

The nurse can help the client accept a more normal body image. This may involve the client agreeing to weigh more than she would like to be healthy and stay out of the hospital. When the client experiences relief from emotional distress, has increased self-esteem, and is meeting her emotional needs in healthy ways, she is more likely to accept her weight and body image.

The nurse can also help the client view herself in terms other than weight, size, shape, and satisfaction with body image. Helping the client to identify areas of personal strength that are not food-related helps broaden the client's perception of herself as a person. This includes identifying talents, interests, and positive aspects of her character unrelated to body shape or size.

PROVIDING CLIENT AND FAMILY EDUCATION

One primary nursing role in caring for clients with eating disorders is providing education to help the client take control of her nutritional requirements independently. This teaching can be done in the inpatient setting during discharge planning or in the outpatient setting. The nurse should provide extensive teaching about basic nutritional needs and the effects of restrictive eating, dieting, and the binge and purge cycle. Clients need encouragement to set realistic goals for eating throughout the day. Eating only salads and vegetables during the day may set up the client for a binge later on as a result of the lack of fat and carbohydrates.

For clients who purge, the most important goal is to stop this behavior. Teaching should include information about the harmful effects of purging by vomiting and laxative abuse. The nurse should explain that purging is not an effective means of weight control and only causes disruption to the neuroendocrine system. In addition, purging promotes binge eating by decreasing the anxiety that follows the binge. The nurse should explain that if the client can avoid purging, she may be less likely to engage in binge eating. The nurse also should teach the client the techniques of distraction and delay, because they are useful against both bingeing and purging. The longer the

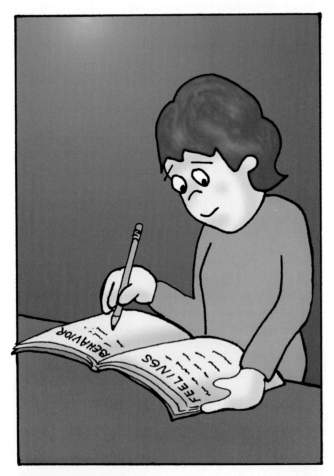

Keeping a feeling diary.

(*text continues on page 543*)

NURSING CARE PLAN: BULIMIA NERVOSA

Nursing Diagnosis

➤ **Ineffective Individual Coping** (5.1.1.1)
Impairment of adaptive behaviors and problem-solving abilities of a person in meeting life's demands and roles

ASSESSMENT DATA

- Inability to change behaviors
- Poor impulse control
- Desire for perfection
- Intolerance of self-weaknesses
- Feelings of worthlessness
- Feelings of inadequacy or guilt
- Unsatisfactory interpersonal relationships
- Low self-esteem
- Excessive need to control
- Feelings of being out of control
- Preoccupation with weight, food, or diets
- Distortions of body image
- Overuse of laxatives, diet pills, or diuretics
- Secrecy regarding eating habits or amounts eaten
- Fear of being fat
- Recurrent vomiting
- Binge eating
- Compulsive eating

EXPECTED OUTCOMES

The client will:
- Identify non–food-related methods of dealing with stress or crises
- Verbalize feelings of guilt, anxiety, anger, or an excessive need for control
- Demonstrate more satisfying interpersonal relationships
- Verbalize more realistic body image
- Demonstrate alternative methods of dealing with stress or crises
- Verbalize increased self-esteem and self-confidence

IMPLEMENTATION

Nursing Interventions	Rationale
Set limits with the client about eating habits. Food will be eaten in a dining room setting, at a table, only at conventional meal times.	These limits will discourage previous binge behavior, which involves sneaking and gulping food, hiding food, and so forth. You will help the client return to normal eating patterns. Eating three meals a day will prevent starvation and subsequent overeating in the evening.
Encourage the client to eat with other clients, when tolerated.	Eating with other people will discourage secrecy about eating, though initially the client's anxiety may be too high to join others at meal time.

continued on page 542

continued from page 541

Encourage the client to express feelings, such as anxiety and guilt about having eaten.	Verbal expression of feelings can help decrease the client's anxiety and the urge to engage in purging behaviors.
Encourage the client to keep a diary in which to write types and amounts of foods eaten and to identify feelings that occur before, during, and after eating, especially related to urges to engage in binge or purge behavior.	A diary can help the client examine his or her food intake and the feelings he or she experiences. Gradually, he or she may be able to see relationships among these feelings and behaviors. Initially, the client may be able to write about these feelings and behaviors more easily than talk about them.
Encourage the client to describe and discuss feelings verbally. Begin to separate dealing with feelings from eating or purging behaviors. Maintain a nonjudgmental approach.	You can help the client begin to express feelings in a non-threatening environment. Being nonjudgmental gives the client permission to openly discuss feelings that may be negative or unacceptable to him or her without fear of rejection or reprisal.
Discuss the types of foods that are soothing to the client and that relieve anxiety.	You may also be able to help the client see how he or she has used food to deal with feelings or to comfort himself or herself.
Help the client explore ways of relieving anxiety and expressing feelings, especially anger, frustration, and anxiety, that are not associated with eating. Help the client identify ways to experience pleasure that are not related to food or eating.	It is important to help the client separate emotional issues from food and eating behaviors.
Give positive feedback for the client's efforts.	The client may have become accustomed to judging himself or herself on accomplishments (often food related), with no regard for feelings. Your sincere praise can promote the client's attempts to deal openly and honestly with anxiety, anger, and other feelings.
Teach the client about the use of the problem-solving process.	Successful use of the problem-solving process can help increase the client's self-esteem and confidence.
Explore with the client his or her personal strengths. Making a written list is sometimes helpful.	You can help the client discover his or her strengths. It will not be useful, however, for you to list the client's strengths—he or she needs to identify them but may benefit from your supportive expectation that he or she will do so.
Discuss with the client the idea of accepting a less than "ideal" body weight.	The client's previous expectations or perception of an ideal weight may have been unrealistic, and even unhealthy.

continued on page 543

continued from page 542

Encourage the client to incorporate fattening (or "bad") foods into the diet as he or she tolerates.	This will enhance the client's sense of control of overeating.
Encourage the client to develop these skills and use them in his or her daily life. Refer the client to assertiveness training books or classes if indicated.	Many bulimic clients are passive and nonassertive in interpersonal relationships. Assertiveness training may foster a sense of increased control, confidence, and healthy relationship dynamics.
Encourage the client to express his or her feelings about family members and significant others, their roles and relationships.	Expression of feelings can help the client to identify, accept, and work through his or her feelings in a direct manner.

Adapted from Schultz, J. M., & Videbeck, S. L. (1998). Lippincott's manual of psychiatric nursing care plans (5th ed.). Philadelphia: Lippincott-Raven.

client can delay either bingeing or purging, the less likely she is to carry out the behavior.

The nurse should explain to family and friends that they can be most helpful by providing emotional support, love, and attention. They can express concern about the client's health, but it is rarely helpful to focus on food intake, calories, and weight.

Evaluation

Assessment tools such as the Eating Attitudes Test can be used to detect improvement for clients with eating disorders. Both anorexia and bulimia nervosa are chronic disorders for many clients. Residual symptoms such as dieting, compulsive exercising, and discomfort eating in a social setting are common. Treatment is considered successful if the client maintains a body weight within 5% to 10% of normal with no medical complications from starvation or purging.

COMMUNITY-BASED CARE

Treatment for clients with eating disorders usually occurs in community settings. Hospital admission is indicated only for medical necessity, such as for clients with dangerously low weight, electrolyte imbalances, or renal, cardiac, or hepatic complications. Clients who cannot control the cycle of binge eating and purging may be treated briefly in an inpatient setting. Other treatment settings include partial hospitalization or day treatment programs, individual or group outpatient therapy, and self-help groups.

Prevention and Early Detection

Nurses can educate parents, children, and young people about strategies to prevent eating disorders. Important aspects include realizing that the "ideal" figures portrayed in advertisements and magazines are unrealistic, developing realistic ideas about body size and shape, resisting peer pressure to diet, improving self-esteem, and learning coping strategies for dealing with emotions and life issues.

School nurses, student health nurses at colleges and universities, and nurses in clinics and doctors' offices may encounter clients in a variety of settings

▶ CLIENT AND FAMILY TEACHING: EATING DISORDERS

CLIENT
- Basic nutritional needs
- Harmful effects of restrictive eating, dieting, purging
- Realistic goals for eating
- Acceptance of healthy body image

FAMILY AND FRIENDS
- Provide emotional support
- Express concern about client's health
- Encourage client to seek professional help
- Avoid talking only about weight, food intake, calories
- Become informed about eating disorders
- It is not possible for family and friends to force the client to eat. The client needs professional help from a therapist or psychiatrist.

who are at risk for developing or who already have an eating disorder. In these settings, early identification and appropriate referral are primary responsibilities of the nurse. Anstine and Grinenko (2000) suggested that young women should be screened routinely for eating disorders (Box 20-1). Such early identification could result in early intervention and prevention of a full-blown eating disorder.

SELF-AWARENESS ISSUES

An emaciated, starving client with anorexia can be a shocking sight, and the nurse may want to "take care of this child" and nurse her back to health. However, when the client rejects this help and resists the nurse's caring actions, the nurse can become angry and frustrated and feel incompetent to handle the situation.

The nurse who is responsible for "making the client eat" may initially be viewed as the enemy by the client. The client may hide or throw away food or become overtly hostile as her anxiety about eating increases. The nurse must remember that the client's behavior is a symptom of the anxiety and fear she feels about gaining weight and is not personally directed toward the nurse. Taking the client's behavior personally may cause the nurse to feel angry and behave in a rejecting manner.

Because eating is such a basic part of everyday life, the nurse may wonder why the client cannot just eat "like everyone else." The nurse also may find it difficult to understand how a 75-pound client sees herself as fat when she looks in the mirror. Likewise, when working with a client who binges and purges, the nurse may wonder why the client cannot exert the will power to stop the behaviors. The nurse must remember that the client's eating behavior has gotten out of control. Eating disorders are a mental illness, just as schizophrenia or bipolar affective disorder is an illness.

Helpful Hints for Working With Clients With Eating Disorders

- Be empathetic and nonjudgmental, although this is not easy. Remember the client's perspective and fears about weight and eating.
- Avoid sounding parental when teaching the client about nutrition or why laxative use is harmful. Presenting information factually without chiding the client will obtain more positive results.
- Do not label the client as "good" when she avoids purging or eats all of her meal. Otherwise, the client will believe she is "bad" on days when she purges or fails to eat enough food.

➤ KEY POINTS

- Anorexia nervosa is a life-threatening eating disorder characterized by body weight less than 85% of normal, an intense fear of being fat, a severely distorted body image, and refusal to eat or binge eating and purging.
- Bulimia nervosa is an eating disorder that involves recurrent episodes of binge eating and compensatory behaviors such as purging, use of laxatives and diuretics, or excessive exercise.
- Ninety percent of clients with eating disorders are female. Anorexia begins at ages 14 through 18, and bulimia at age 18 or 19.
- Many neurochemical changes are present in eating disorders, but it is uncertain whether these changes cause or are a result of the eating disorder.

Box 20-1

➤ DISORDERED EATING SCREENING QUESTIONS

- How many diets have you been on in the past year?
- How often does your weight affect how you feel about yourself?
- How often do you feel you should be dieting?
- How often do you feel dissatisfied with your body size?

Reprinted with permission from Elsevier Science form *Rapid screening for disordered eating in college-aged females in the primary care setting* by Anstine, D., & Grinenko, D. Anstine, D., & Grinenko, D. Journal of Adolescent Health, 26(5), 338–342. © 2000 by the Society for Adolescent Medicine.

Critical Thinking

Questions

1. You notice a friend or family member has been losing weight, has strange eating rituals, and constantly talks about dieting. You suspect an eating disorder. How would you approach this person?
2. A client has the right to refuse treatment. How would the nurse address this right when working with a client with anorexia who doesn't want treatment?

INTERNET RESOURCES

Resource	Internet Address
▶ Anorexia Nervosa and Bulimia Association	http://www.ams.queensu.ca/anab/
▶ ANOREXIA: Information and Guidance for Patients, Families, and Friends	http://www.neca.com/~cwildes/
▶ Eating Disorders Association Resource Centre	http://www.uq.edu.au/~zzedainc/
▶ Eating Disorders Mirror Mirror	http://www.mirror-mirror.org/eatdis.htm
▶ Eating Disorders	http://www.mental-health-matters.com/eatdisord.html
▶ Eating Disorders Awareness and Prevention, Inc.	http://members.aol.com/edapinc/home.html
▶ Anorexia and Bulimia Family Support Group	http://users.iafrica.com/r/ro/ronhey/
▶ National Association of Anorexia Nervosa & Associated Eating Disorders	http://www.anad.org

- Persons with eating disorders feel unattractive and ineffective and may be poorly equipped to deal with the challenges of maturity.
- Societal attitudes regarding thinness, beauty, desirability, and physical fitness may influence the development of eating disorders.
- Severely malnourished clients with anorexia nervosa may require intensive medical treatment to restore homeostasis before psychiatric treatment can begin.
- Family therapy is effective for clients with anorexia; cognitive-behavioral therapy is most effective for clients with bulimia.
- Interventions for clients with eating disorders include establishing nutritional eating patterns, helping the client identify emotions and develop non–food-related coping strategies, helping the client deal with body image issues, and providing client and family education.

REFERENCES

Agras, W. S. (1997). Pharmacotherapy of bulimia nervosa and binge eating disorder: Long-term outcomes. *Psychopharmacology Bulletin, 33*(3), 433–436.

Agras, W. S., Walsh, B. T., Fairburn, C. G., Wilson, G. T., & Kraemer, H. C. (2000). A multicenter comparison of cognitive-behavioral therapy and interpersonal psychotherapy for bulimia nervosa. *Archives of General Psychiatry, 57*(5), 459–466.

American Psychiatric Association. (2000). *DSM-IV-TR: Diagnostic and statistical manual of mental disorders-text revision* (4th ed.). Washington, DC: American Psychiatric Association.

Anstine, D., & Grinenko, D. (2000). Rapid screening for disordered eating in college-aged females in the primary care setting. *Journal of Adolescent Health, 26*(5), 338–342.

Carrasco, J. L., Diaz-Marsa, M., Hollander, E., Cesar, J., & Saiz-Ruiz, J. (2000). Decreased platelet monoamine oxidase activity in female bulimia nervosa. *European Neuropsychopharmacology, 10,* 113–117.

Gardner, R. M., Friedman, B. N., & Jackson, N. A. (1999). Body size estimations, body dissatisfaction, and ideal size preferences in children six through thirteen. *Journal of Youth and Adolescence, 28*(5), 603–618.

Gowers, S., & North, C. (1999). Difficulties in family functioning and adolescent anorexia nervosa. *British Journal of Psychiatry, 174*(1), 63–66.

Grilo, C. M., & Masheb, R. M. (2000). Onset of dieting vs. binge eating in outpatients with binge eating disorder. *International Journal of Obesity, 24*(4), 404–409.

Halmi, K. A. (2000). Eating disorders. In B. J. Sadock & V. A. Sadock (Eds.). *Comprehensive textbook of psychiatry,* Vol. 2 (7th ed., pp. 1663–1676). Philadelphia: Lippincott, Williams & Wilkins.

Herzog, D. B., Dorer, D. J., & Keel, P. K. (1999). Recovery and relapse in anorexia and bulimia nervosa: a 7.5-year follow-up study. *Journal of the Academy of Child and Adolescent Psychiatry, 38*(7), 829–837.

Kaye, W. H., Klump, K. L., Frank, G. K. W., & Strober, M. (2000). Anorexia and bulimia nervosa. *Annual Review of Medicine, 51,* 299–313.

Matsunaga, H., Kaye, W. H., McConaha, C. Plotnicov, K., Pollice, C., Rao, R., & Stein, D. (1999). Psycho-pathological characteristics of recovered bulimics who have a history of physical or sexual abuse. *Journal of Nervous and Mental Diseases, 187*(8), 472–476.

McIntosh, V. V., Bulik, C. M., McKenzie, J. M., Luty, S. E., & Jordan, J. (2000). Interpersonal psycho-therapy for anorexia nervosa. *International Journal of Eating Disorders, 27*(2), 125–139.

North, C., Gowers, S., & Bryram V. (1997). Family functioning and life events in the outcome of adolescent anorexia nervosa. *British Journal of Psychiatry, 171*(12), 545–549.

Patel, D. R., Phillips, E. L., & Pratt, H. D. (1998). Eating disorders. *Indian Journal of Pediatrics, 65*(4), 487–494.

Peterson, C. B., & Mitchell, J. E. (1999). Psychosocial and pharmacological treatment of eating disorders: a review of research findings. *Journal of Clinical Psychology, 55*(6), 687–697.

Picard, C. L. (1999). The level of competition as a factor for the development of eating disorders in female collegiate athletes. *Journal of Youth and Adolescence, 28*(5), 583–594.

Schultz, J. M., & Videbeck, S. L. (1998). *Lippincott's manual of psychiatric nursing care plans* (5th ed.). Philadelphia: Lippincott-Raven.

Serpell, L., Treasure, J., Teasdale, J., & Sullivan, V. (1999). Anorexia nervosa: Friend or foe. 179-186.

Stice, E., Akutagawa, D., Gaggar, A., & Agras, W. S. (2000). Negative effect moderates the relation between dieting and binge eating. *International Journal of Eating Disorders, 27*(2), 218–229.

Turner, J., Batik, M., & Palmer, L. J. (2000). Detection and importance of laxative abuse in adolescents with anorexia nervosa. *Journal of the American Academy of Child and Adolescent Psychiatry, 39*(3), 378–385.

Wade, T. D., Bulik, C. M., Neale, M., & Kendler, K. S. (2000). Anorexia nervosa and major depression: shared genetic and environmental risk factors. *American Journal of Psychiatry, 157*(3), 469–471.

White, J. H. (1991). Feminism, eating, and, mental health. *Advances in Nursing Science, 13*(3), 68–80.

White, J. H. (1993). Women and eating disorders. *AWHONN, 4*(2), 227–235.

White, J. H. (1999). The development and clinical testing of an outpatient program for women with bulimia nervosa. *Archives of Psychiatric Nursing, 13*(4), 179–191.

White, J. H., & Litovitz, G. (1998). A comparison of inpatient and outpatient women with eating disorders. *Archives of Psychiatric Nursing, 12*(4), 181–194.

Wiederman, M. W. (1996). Women, sex, and food: a review of research on eating disorders and sexuality. *Journal of Sex Research, 33*(4), 301–311.

Wilson, G. T., & Vitousek, K. M. (1999). Self-monitoring in the assessment of eating disorders. *Psychological Assessment, 11*(4), 480–489.

Zipfel, S., Lowe, B., Reas, D. L., Deter, H., & Herzog, W. (2000). Long-term prognosis in anorexia nervosa: lessons from a 21-year follow-up study. *Lancet, 355,* 721–722.

ADDITIONAL READINGS

Schwitzer, A. M., Bergholz, K., & Dore, T. (1998). Eating disorders among college women: prevention, education, and treatment responses. *Journal of American College Health, 46*(5), 199–207.

Wiser, S., & Telch, C. F. (1999). Dialectic behavior therapy for binge eating disorder. *Journal of Clinical Psychology, 55*(6), 755–768.

➤ MULTIPLE-CHOICE QUESTIONS

Select the best answer for each of the following questions.

1. Treating clients with anorexia nervosa with a selective serotonin reuptake inhibitor anti-depressant such as fluoxetine (Prozac) may present which of the following problems?

   A. Clients object to the side effect of weight gain.

   B. Fluoxetine can cause appetite suppression and weight loss.

   C. Fluoxetine can cause clients to become giddy and silly.

   D. Clients with anorexia get no benefit from fluoxetine.

2. Which of the following is an example of a cognitive-behavioral technique?

   A. Distraction

   B. Relaxation

   C. Self-monitoring

   D. Verbalization of emotions

3. The nurse is working with a client with anorexia nervosa. Even though the client has been eating all her meals and snacks, her weight has remained unchanged for 1 week. Which of the following interventions is indicated?

   A. Supervise the client closely for 2 hours after meals and snacks.

   B. Increase the daily caloric intake from 1,500 to 2,000 calories.

   C. Increase the client's fluid intake.

   D. Request an order from the physician for fluoxetine.

4. Which of the following statements is true?

   A. Anorexia nervosa was not recognized as an illness until the 1960s.

   B. Cultures where beauty is linked to thinness have an increased risk for eating disorders.

   C. Eating disorders are a major health problem only in the United States and Europe.

   D. Persons with anorexia nervosa are popular with their peers as a result of their thinness.

5. All but which of the following are initial goals for treating the severely malnourished client with anorexia nervosa?

   A. Correction of body image disturbance

   B. Correction of electrolyte imbalances

   C. Nutritional rehabilitation

   D. Weight restoration

➤ TRUE-FALSE QUESTIONS

Identify each of the following statements as T (true) or F (false). Correct any false statements.

_____ 1. Satiety refers to the consumption of large amounts of calories during a binge eating episode.

_____

_____ 2. Enmeshment in families means there is a lack of clear boundaries between members.

_____

_____ 3. Comorbid psychiatric disorders are common in clients with eating disorders.

_____

_____ 4. Purging behavior refers only to self-induced vomiting after eating.

_____

_____ 5. Amenorrhea is a typical manifestation of anorexia nervosa.

_____

_____ 6. Self-monitoring is a treatment technique where clients eat whatever they choose.

_____

_____ 7. Clients with anorexia nervosa experience great distress about their bizarre eating habits.

_____

_____ 8. Clients with bulimia nervosa are in no serious medical danger as long as their weight remains near normal.

_____

➤ FILL-IN-THE-BLANK QUESTIONS

Identify each of the following characteristics as being typical of anorexia nervosa, bulimia nervosa, or both.

_____ Client puts on a pleasant and cheerful face for others.

_____ Client spends the majority of time thinking about food and food-related activities.

_____ Client believes if she starts eating, she will not be able to stop.

_____ Client believes there is no problem with her dieting behavior.

_____ Client is guilty and ashamed about her eating behavior.

1. Identify four compensatory behaviors that clients with bulimia use to avoid weight gain.

2. Describe the concept of body image disturbance.

➤ **CLINICAL EXAMPLE**

Judy is a 17-year-old high school junior who is active in gymnastics. She is 5′ 7″ tall, weighs 85 pounds, and has not had a menstrual period for 5 months. The family physician referred her to the inpatient eating disorders unit with a diagnosis of anorexia nervosa. During the admission interview, Judy is defensive about her weight loss, stating she needs to be thin to be competitive in her sport. Judy points to areas on her buttocks and thighs, saying, "See this? I still have plenty of fat. Why can't everyone just leave me alone?"

1. Identify two nursing diagnoses that would be pertinent for Judy.

2. Write an expected outcome for each identified nursing diagnosis.

3. List three nursing interventions for each nursing diagnosis.

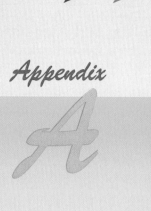

Appendix

A

DSM-IV-TR Classification

NOS = Not Otherwise Specified.

An *x* appearing in a diagnostic code indicates that a specific code number is required.

An ellipsis (. . .) is used in the names of certain disorders to indicate that the name of a specific mental disorder or general medical condition should be inserted when recording the name (eg, 293.0 Delirium Due to Hypothyroidism).

Numbers in parentheses are page numbers.

If criteria are currently met, one of the following severity specifiers may be noted after the diagnosis:

> Mild
> Moderate
> Severe

If criteria are no longer met, one of the following specifiers may be noted:

> In Partial Remission
> In Full Remission
> Prior History

Disorders Usually First Diagnosed in Infancy, Childhood, or Adolescence (39)

MENTAL RETARDATION (41)
Note: These are coded on Axis II.
317	Mild Mental Retardation (43)
318.0	Moderate Mental Retardation (43)
318.1	Severe Mental Retardation (43)
318.2	Profound Mental Retardation (44)
319	Mental Retardation, Severity Unspecified (44)

LEARNING DISORDERS (49)
315.00	Reading Disorder (51)
315.1	Mathematics Disorder (53)
315.2	Disorder of Written Expression (54)
315.9	Learning Disorder NOS (56)

MOTOR SKILLS DISORDER (56)
315.4	Developmental Coordination Disorder (56)

COMMUNICATION DISORDERS (58)
315.31	Expressive Language Disorder (58)
315.32	Mixed Receptive-Expressive Language Disorder (62)
315.39	Phonological Disorder (65)
307.0	Stuttering (67)
307.9	Communication Disorder NOS (69)

PERVASIVE DEVELOPMENTAL DISORDERS (69)
299.00	Autistic Disorder (70)
299.80	Rett's Disorder (76)
299.10	Childhood Disintegrative Disorder (77)
299.80	Asperger's Disorder (80)
299.80	Pervasive Developmental Disorder NOS (84)

ATTENTION-DEFICIT AND DISRUPTIVE BEHAVIOR DISORDERS (85)

314.xx	Attention-Deficit/Hyperactivity Disorder (85)
.01	Combined Type
.00	Predominantly Inattentive Type
.01	Predominantly Hyperactive-Impulsive Type
314.9	Attention-Deficit/Hyperactivity Disorder NOS (93)
312.xx	Conduct Disorder (93)
.81	Childhood-Onset Type
.82	Adolescent-Onset Type
.89	Unspecified Onset
313.81	Oppositional Defiant Disorder (100)
312.9	Disruptive Behavior Disorder NOS (103)

FEEDING AND EATING DISORDERS OF INFANCY OR EARLY CHILDHOOD (103)

307.52	Pica (103)
307.53	Rumination Disorder (105)
307.59	Feeding Disorder of Infancy or Early Childhood (107)

TIC DISORDERS (108)

307.23	Tourette's Disorder (111)
307.22	Chronic Motor or Vocal Tic Disorder (114)
307.21	Transient Tic Disorder (115)
	Specify if: Single Episode/Recurrent
307.20	Tic Disorder NOS (116)

ELIMINATION DISORDERS (116)

—.—	Encopresis (116)
787.6	With Constipation and Overflow Incontinence
307.7	Without Constipation and Overflow Incontinence
307.6	Enuresis (Not Due to a General Medical Condition) (118)
	Specify type: Nocturnal Only/Diurnal Only/Nocturnal and Diurnal

OTHER DISORDERS OF INFANCY, CHILDHOOD, OR ADOLESCENCE (121)

309.21	Separation Anxiety Disorder (121)
	Specify if: Early Onset
313.23	Selective Mutism (125)
313.89	Reactive Attachment Disorder of Infancy or Early Childhood (127)
	Specify type: Inhibited Type/Disinhibited Type
307.3	Stereotypic Movement Disorder (131)
	Specify if: With Self-Injurious Behavior
313.9	Disorder of Infancy, Childhood, or Adolescence NOS (134)

Delirium, Dementia, and Amnestic and Other Cognitive Disorders (135)

DELIRIUM (136)

293.0	Delirium Due to . . . *[Indicate the General Medical Condition]* (141)
—.—	Substance Intoxication Delirium *(refer to Substance-Related Disorders for substance-specific codes)* (143)
—.—	Substance Withdrawal Delirium *(refer to Substance-Related Disorders for substance-specific codes)* (143)
—.—	Delirium Due to Multiple Etiologies *(code each of the specific etiologies)* (146)
780.09	Delirium NOS (147)

DEMENTIA (147)

294.xx*	Dementia of the Alzheimer's Type, With Early Onset *(also code 331.0 Alzheimer's disease on Axis III)* (154)
.10	Without Behavioral Disturbance
.11	With Behavioral Disturbance
294.xx*	Dementia of the Alzheimer's Type, With Late Onset *(also code 331.0 Alzheimer's disease on Axis III)* (154)
.10	Without Behavioral Disturbance
.11	With Behavioral Disturbance
290.xx	Vascular Dementia (158)
.40	Uncomplicated
.41	With Delirium
.42	With Delusions
.43	With Depressed Mood
	Specify if: With Behavioral Disturbance

Code presence or absence of a behavioral disturbance in the fifth digit for Dementia Due to a General Medical Condition:

0 = Without Behavioral Disturbance
1 = With Behavioral Disturbance

294.1x*	Dementia Due to HIV Disease *(also code 042 HIV on Axis III)* (163)
294.1x*	Dementia Due to Head Trauma *(also code 854.00 head injury on Axis III)* (164)
294.1x*	Dementia Due to Parkinson's Disease *(also code 332.0 Parkinson's disease on Axis III)* (164)

*ICD-9-CM code valid after October 1, 2000.

294.1x*   Dementia Due to Huntington's Disease *(also code 333.4 Huntington's disease on Axis III)* (165)

294.1x*   Dementia Due to Pick's Disease *(also code 331.1 Pick's disease on Axis III)* (165)

294.1x*   Dementia Due to Creutzfeldt-Jakob Disease *(also code 046.1 Creutzfeldt-Jakob disease on Axis III)* (166)

294.1x*   Dementia Due to . . . *[Indicate the General Medical Condition not listed above] (also code the general medical condition on Axis III)* (167)

——.—   Substance-Induced Persisting Dementia *(refer to Substance-Related Disorders for substance-specific codes)* (168)

——.—   Dementia Due to Multiple Etiologies *(code each of the specific etiologies)* (170)

294.8   Dementia NOS (171)

AMNESTIC DISORDERS (172)

294.0   Amnestic Disorder Due to . . . *[Indicate the General Medical Condition]* (175)
    Specify if: Transient/Chronic

——.—   Substance-Induced Persisting Amnestic Disorder *(refer to Substance-Related Disorders for substance-specific codes)* (177)

294.8   Amnestic Disorder NOS (179)

OTHER COGNITIVE DISORDERS (179)

294.9   Cognitive Disorder NOS (179)

Mental Disorders Due to a General Medical Condition Not Elsewhere Classified (181)

293.89   Catatonic Disorder Due to . . . *[Indicate the General Medical Condition]* (185)

310.1   Personality Change Due to . . . *[Indicate the General Medical Condition]* (187)
    Specify type: Labile Type/Disinhibited Type/Aggressive Type/Apathetic Type/Paranoid Type/Other Type/Combined Type/Unspecified Type

293.9   Mental Disorder NOS Due to . . . *[Indicate the General Medical Condition]* (190)

*ICD-9-CM code valid after October 1, 2000.

Substance-Related Disorders (191)

The following specifiers apply to Substance Dependence as noted:

  [a]With Physiological Dependence/Without Physiological Dependence

  [b]Early Full Remission/Early Partial Remission/Sustained Full Remission/Sustained Partial Remission

  [c]In a Controlled Environment

  [d]On Agonist Therapy

The following specifiers apply to Substance-Induced Disorders as noted:

  [I]With Onset During Intoxication/[W]With Onset During Withdrawal

ALCOHOL-RELATED DISORDERS (212)

Alcohol Use Disorders (213)

303.90   Alcohol Dependence[a,b,c] (213)

305.00   Alcohol Abuse (214)

Alcohol-Induced Disorders (214)

303.00   Alcohol Intoxication (214)

291.81   Alcohol Withdrawal (215)
    Specify if: With Perceptual Disturbances

291.0   Alcohol Intoxication Delirium (143)

291.0   Alcohol Withdrawal Delirium (143)

291.2   Alcohol-Induced Persisting Dementia (168)

291.1   Alcohol-Induced Persisting Amnestic Disorder (177)

291.x   Alcohol-Induced Psychotic Disorder (338)
  .5   With Delusions[I,W]
  .3   With Hallucinations[I,W]

291.89   Alcohol-Induced Mood Disorder[I,W] (405)

291.89   Alcohol-Induced Anxiety Disorder[I,W] (479)

291.89   Alcohol-Induced Sexual Dysfunction[I] (562)

291.89   Alcohol-Induced Sleep Disorder[I,W] (655)

291.9   Alcohol-Related Disorder NOS (223)

AMPHETAMINE (OR AMPHETAMINE-LIKE)– RELATED DISORDERS (223)

Amphetamine Use Disorders (224)

304.40   Amphetamine Dependence[a,b,c] (224)

305.70   Amphetamine Abuse (225)

Amphetamine-Induced Disorders (226)

292.89   Amphetamine Intoxication (226)
    Specify if: With Perceptual Disturbances

292.0   Amphetamine Withdrawal (227)

292.81   Amphetamine Intoxication Delirium (143)

292.xx   Amphetamine-Induced Psychotic Disorder (338)

.11   With Delusions[I]
.12   With Hallucinations[I]
292.84   Amphetamine-Induced Mood Disorder[I,W] (405)
292.89   Amphetamine-Induced Anxiety Disorder[I] (479)
292.89   Amphetamine-Induced Sexual Dysfunction[I] (562)
292.89   Amphetamine-Induced Sleep Disorder[I,W] (655)
292.9   Amphetamine-Related Disorder NOS (231)

CAFFEINE-RELATED DISORDERS (231)

Caffeine-Induced Disorders (232)
305.90   Caffeine Intoxication (232)
292.89   Caffeine-Induced Anxiety Disorder[I] (479)
292.89   Caffeine-Induced Sleep Disorder[I] (655)
292.9   Caffeine-Related Disorder NOS (234)

CANNABIS-RELATED DISORDERS (234)

Cannabis Use Disorders (236)
304.30   Cannabis Dependence[a,b,c] (236)
305.20   Cannabis Abuse (236)

Cannabis-Induced Disorders (237)
292.89   Cannabis Intoxication (237)
          Specify if: With Perceptual Disturbances
292.81   Cannabis Intoxication Delirium (143)
292.xx   Cannabis-Induced Psychotic Disorder (338)
.11   With Delusions[I]
.12   With Hallucinations[I]
292.89   Cannabis-Induced Anxiety Disorder[I] (479)
292.9   Cannabis-Related Disorder NOS (241)

COCAINE-RELATED DISORDERS (241)

Cocaine Use Disorders (242)
304.20   Cocaine Dependence[a,b,c] (242)
305.60   Cocaine Abuse (243)

Cocaine-Induced Disorders (244)
292.89   Cocaine Intoxication (244)
          Specify if: With Perceptual Disturbances
292.0   Cocaine Withdrawal (245)
292.81   Cocaine Intoxication Delirium (143)
292.xx   Cocaine-Induced Psychotic Disorder (338)
.11   With Delusions[I]
.12   With Hallucinations[I]
292.84   Cocaine-Induced Mood Disorder[I,W] (405)
292.89   Cocaine-Induced Anxiety Disorder[I,W] (479)
292.89   Cocaine-Induced Sexual Dysfunction[I] (562)
292.89   Cocaine-Induced Sleep Disorder[I,W] (655)
292.9   Cocaine-Related Disorder NOS (250)

HALLUCINOGEN-RELATED DISORDERS (250)

Hallucinogen Use Disorders (251)
304.50   Hallucinogen Dependence[b,c] (251)
305.30   Hallucinogen Abuse (252)

Hallucinogen-Induced Disorders (252)
292.89   Hallucinogen Intoxication (252)
292.89   Hallucinogen Persisting Perception Disorder (Flashbacks) (253)
292.81   Hallucinogen Intoxication Delirium (143)
292.xx   Hallucinogen-Induced Psychotic Disorder (338)
.11   With Delusions[I]
.12   With Hallucinations[I]
292.84   Hallucinogen-Induced Mood Disorder[I] (405)
292.89   Hallucinogen-Induced Anxiety Disorder[I] (479)
292.9   Hallucinogen-Related Disorder NOS (256)

INHALANT-RELATED DISORDERS (257)

Inhalant Use Disorders (258)
304.60   Inhalant Dependence[b,c] (258)
305.90   Inhalant Abuse (259)

Inhalant-Induced Disorders (259)
292.89   Inhalant Intoxication (259)
292.81   Inhalant Intoxication Delirium (143)
292.82   Inhalant-Induced Persisting Dementia (168)
292.xx   Inhalant-Induced Psychotic Disorder (338)
.11   With Delusions[I]
.12   With Hallucinations[I]
292.84   Inhalant-Induced Mood Disorder[I] (405)
292.89   Inhalant-Induced Anxiety Disorder[I] (479)
292.9   Inhalant-Related Disorder NOS (263)

NICOTINE-RELATED DISORDERS (264)

Nicotine Use Disorder (264)
305.1   Nicotine Dependence[a,b] (264)

Nicotine-Induced Disorder (265)
292.0   Nicotine Withdrawal (265)
292.9   Nicotine-Related Disorder NOS (269)

OPIOID-RELATED DISORDERS (269)

Opioid Use Disorders (270)
304.00   Opioid Dependence[a,b,c,d] (270)
305.50   Opioid Abuse (271)

Opioid-Induced Disorders (271)
292.89   Opioid Intoxication (271)
          Specify if: With Perceptual Disturbances
292.0   Opioid Withdrawal (272)

292.81   Opioid Intoxication Delirium (143)

292.xx   Opioid-Induced Psychotic Disorder (338)

   .11   With Delusions[I]

   .12   With Hallucinations[I]

292.84   Opioid-Induced Mood Disorder[I] (405)

292.89   Opioid-Induced Sexual Dysfunction[I] (562)

292.89   Opioid-Induced Sleep Disorder[I,W] (655)

292.9   Opioid-Related Disorder NOS (277)

PHENCYCLIDINE (OR PHENCYCLIDINE-LIKE)– RELATED DISORDERS (278)

Phencyclidine Use Disorders (279)

304.60   Phencyclidine Dependence[b,c] (279)

305.90   Phencyclidine Abuse (279)

Phencyclidine-Induced Disorders (280)

292.89   Phencyclidine Intoxication (280)

     Specify if: With Perceptual Disturbances

292.81   Phencyclidine Intoxication Delirium (143)

292.xx   Phencyclidine-Induced Psychotic Disorder (338)

   .11   With Delusions[I]

   .12   With Hallucinations[I]

292.84   Phencyclidine-Induced Mood Disorder[I] (405)

292.89   Phencyclidine-Induced Anxiety Disorder[I] (479)

292.9   Phencyclidine-Related Disorder NOS (283)

SEDATIVE-, HYPNOTIC-, OR ANXIOLYTIC- RELATED DISORDERS (284)

Sedative, Hypnotic, or Anxiolytic Use Disorders (285)

304.10   Sedative, Hypnotic, or Anxiolytic Dependence[a,b,c] (285)

305.40   Sedative, Hypnotic, or Anxiolytic Abuse (286)

Sedative-, Hypnotic-, or Anxiolytic-Induced Disorders (286)

292.89   Sedative, Hypnotic, or Anxiolytic Intoxication (286)

292.0   Sedative, Hypnotic, or Anxiolytic Withdrawal (287)

     Specify if: With Perceptual Disturbances

292.81   Sedative, Hypnotic, or Anxiolytic Intoxication Delirium (143)

292.81   Sedative, Hypnotic, or Anxiolytic Withdrawal Delirium (143)

292.82   Sedative-, Hypnotic-, or Anxiolytic- Induced Persisting Dementia (168)

292.83   Sedative-, Hypnotic-, or Anxiolytic- Induced Persisting Amnestic Disorder (177)

292.xx   Sedative-, Hypnotic-, or Anxiolytic- Induced Psychotic Disorder (338)

   .11   With Delusions[I,W]

   .12   With Hallucinations[I,W]

292.84   Sedative-, Hypnotic-, or Anxiolytic- Induced Mood Disorder[I,W] (405)

292.89   Sedative-, Hypnotic-, or Anxiolytic- Induced Anxiety Disorder[W] (479)

292.89   Sedative-,Hypnotic-, or Anxiolytic-Induced Sexual Dysfunction[I] (562)

292.89   Sedative-, Hypnotic-, or Anxiolytic- Induced Sleep Disorder[I,W] (655)

292.9   Sedative-, Hypnotic-, or Anxiolytic- Related Disorder NOS (293)

POLYSUBSTANCE-RELATED DISORDER (293)

304.80   Polysubstance Dependence[a,b,c,d] (293)

OTHER (OR UNKNOWN) SUBSTANCE–RELATED DISORDERS (294)

Other (or Unknown) Substance Use Disorders (295)

304.90   Other (or Unknown) Substance Dependence[a,b,c,d] (192)

305.90   Other (or Unknown) Substance Abuse (198)

Other (or Unknown) Substance–Induced Disorders (295)

292.89   Other (or Unknown) Substance Intoxication (199)

     Specify if: With Perceptual Disturbances

292.0   Other (or Unknown) Substance Withdrawal (201)

     Specify if: With Perceptual Disturbances

292.81   Other (or Unknown) Substance–Induced Delirium (143)

292.82   Other (or Unknown) Substance–Induced Persisting Dementia (168)

292.83   Other (or Unknown) Substance–Induced Persisting Amnestic Disorder (177)

292.xx   Other (or Unknown) Substance–Induced Psychotic Disorder (338)

   .11   With Delusions[I,W]

   .12   With Hallucinations[I,W]

292.84   Other (or Unknown) Substance–Induced Mood Disorder[I,W] (405)

292.89   Other (or Unknown) Substance–Induced Anxiety Disorder[I,W] (479)

292.89   Other (or Unknown) Substance–Induced Sexual Dysfunction[I] (562)

292.89   Other (or Unknown) Substance–Induced Sleep Disorder[I,W] (655)

292.9   Other (or Unknown) Substance–Related Disorder NOS (295)

Schizophrenia and Other Psychotic Disorders (297)

295.xx   Schizophrenia (298)

The following Classification of Longitudinal Course applies to all subtypes of Schizophrenia:

Episodic With Interepisode Residual Symptoms (*specify if:* With Prominent Negative Symptoms)/Episodic With No Interepisode Residual Symptoms

Continuous (*specify if:* With Prominent Negative Symptoms)

Single Episode In Partial Remission (*specify if:* With Prominent Negative Symptoms)/Single Episode In Full Remission

Other or Unspecified Pattern

.30   Paranoid Type (313)
.10   Disorganized Type (314)
.20   Catatonic Type (315)
.90   Undifferentiated Type (316)
.60   Residual Type (316)
295.40   Schizophreniform Disorder (317)
   Specify if: Without Good Prognostic Features/With Good Prognostic Features
295.70   Schizoaffective Disorder (319)
   Specify type: Bipolar Type/Depressive Type
297.1   Delusional Disorder (323)
   Specify type: Erotomanic Type/Grandiose Type/ Jealous Type/Persecutory Type/Somatic Type/ Mixed Type/Unspecified Type
298.8   Brief Psychotic Disorder (329)
   Specify if: With Marked Stressor(s)/Without Marked Stressor(s)/With Postpartum Onset
297.3   Shared Psychotic Disorder (332)
293.xx   Psychotic Disorder Due to . . . *[Indicate the General Medical Condition]* (334)
   .81   With Delusions
   .82   With Hallucinations
——.—   Substance-Induced Psychotic Disorder *(refer to Substance-Related Disorders for substance-specific codes)* (338)
   Specify if: With Onset During Intoxication/With Onset During Withdrawal
298.9   Psychotic Disorder NOS (343)

Mood Disorders (345)

Code current state of Major Depressive Disorder or Bipolar I Disorder in fifth digit:

1 = Mild
2 = Moderate
3 = Severe Without Psychotic Features
4 = Severe With Psychotic Features
   Specify: Mood-Congruent Psychotic Features/Mood-Incongruent Psychotic Features
5 = In Partial Remission
6 = In Full Remission
0 = Unspecified

The following specifiers apply (for current or most recent episode) to Mood Disorders as noted:

[a]Severity/Psychotic/Remission Specifiers/[b]Chronic/[c]With Catatonic Features/[d]With Melancholic Features/[e]With Atypical Features/[f]With Postpartum Onset

The following specifiers apply to Mood Disorders as noted:

[g]With or Without Full Interepisode Recovery/[h]With Seasonal Pattern/[i]With Rapid Cycling

DEPRESSIVE DISORDERS (369)

296.xx   Major Depressive Disorder (369)
   .2x   Single Episode [a,b,c,d,e,f]
   .3x   Recurrent [a,b,c,d,e,f,g,h]
300.4   Dysthymic Disorder (376)
   Specify if: Early Onset/Late Onset
   Specify: With Atypical Features
311   Depressive Disorder NOS (381)

BIPOLAR DISORDERS (382)

296.xx   Bipolar I Disorder (382)
   .0x   Single Manic Episode [a,c,f]
   Specify if: Mixed
   .40   Most Recent Episode Hypomanic [g,h,i]
   .4x   Most Recent Episode Manic [a,c,f,g,h,i]
   .6x   Most Recent Episode Mixed [a,c,f,g,h,i]
   .5x   Most Recent Episode Depressed [a,b,c,d,e,f,g,h,i]
   .7   Most Recent Episode Unspecified [g,h,i]
296.89   Bipolar II Disorder [a,b,c,d,e,f,g,h,i] (392)
   Specify (current or most recent episode): Hypomanic/ Depressed
301.13   Cyclothymic Disorder (398)
296.80   Bipolar Disorder NOS (400)
293.83   Mood Disorder Due to . . . *[Indicate the General Medical Condition]* (401)
   Specify type: With Depressive Features/With Major Depressive–Like Episode/With Manic Features/With Mixed Features
——.—   Substance-Induced Mood Disorder *(refer to Substance-Related Disorders for substance-specific codes)* (405)
   Specify type: With Depressive Features/With Manic Features/With Mixed Features
   Specify if: With Onset During Intoxication/With Onset During Withdrawal
296.90   Mood Disorder NOS (410)

Anxiety Disorders (429)

300.01 Panic Disorder Without Agoraphobia (433)
300.21 Panic Disorder With Agoraphobia (433)
300.22 Agoraphobia Without History of Panic Disorder (441)
300.29 Specific Phobia (443)
    Specify type: Animal Type/Natural Environment Type/Blood-Injection-Injury Type/Situational Type/Other Type
300.23 Social Phobia (450)
    Specify if: Generalized
300.3 Obsessive-Compulsive Disorder (456)
    Specify if: With Poor Insight
309.81 Posttraumatic Stress Disorder (463)
    Specify if: Acute/Chronic
    Specify if: With Delayed Onset
308.3 Acute Stress Disorder (469)
300.02 Generalized Anxiety Disorder (472)
293.84 Anxiety Disorder Due to . . . *[Indicate the General Medical Condition]* (476)
    Specify if: With Generalized Anxiety/ With Panic Attacks/With Obsessive-Compulsive Symptoms
——.—— Substance-Induced Anxiety Disorder *(refer to Substance-Related Disorders for substance-specific codes)* (479)
    Specify if: With Generalized Anxiety/With Panic Attacks/With Obsessive-Compulsive Symptoms/ With Phobic Symptoms
    Specify if: With Onset During Intoxication/ With Onset During Withdrawal
300.00 Anxiety Disorder NOS (484)

Somatoform Disorders (485)

300.81 Somatization Disorder (486)
300.82 Undifferentiated Somatoform Disorder (490)
300.11 Conversion Disorder (492)
    Specify type: With Motor Symptom or Deficit/With Sensory Symptom or Deficit/With Seizures or Convulsions/With Mixed Presentation
307.xx Pain Disorder (498)
  .80 Associated With Psychological Factors
  .89 Associated With Both Psychological Factors and a General Medical Condition
    Specify if: Acute/Chronic
300.7 Hypochondriasis (504)
    Specify if: With Poor Insight
300.7 Body Dysmorphic Disorder (507)
300.82 Somatoform Disorder NOS (511)

Factitious Disorders (513)

300.xx Factitious Disorder (513)
  .16 With Predominantly Psychological Signs and Symptoms
  .19 With Predominantly Physical Signs and Symptoms
  .19 With Combined Psychological and Physical Signs and Symptoms
300.19 Factitious Disorder NOS (517)

Dissociative Disorders (519)

300.12 Dissociative Amnesia (520)
300.13 Dissociative Fugue (523)
300.14 Dissociative Identity Disorder (526)
300.6 Depersonalization Disorder (530)
300.15 Dissociative Disorder NOS (532)

Sexual and Gender Identity Disorders (535)

SEXUAL DYSFUNCTIONS (535)

The following specifiers apply to all primary Sexual Dysfunctions:

    Lifelong Type/Acquired Type
    Generalized Type/Situational Type
    Due to Psychological Factors/Due to Combined Factors

Sexual Desire Disorders (539)
302.71 Hypoactive Sexual Desire Disorder (539)
302.79 Sexual Aversion Disorder (541)

Sexual Arousal Disorders (543)
302.72 Female Sexual Arousal Disorder (543)
302.72 Male Erectile Disorder (545)

Orgasmic Disorders (547)
302.73 Female Orgasmic Disorder (547)
302.74 Male Orgasmic Disorder (550)
302.75 Premature Ejaculation (552)

Sexual Pain Disorders (554)
302.76 Dyspareunia (Not Due to a General Medical Condition) (554)
306.51 Vaginismus (Not Due to a General Medical Condition) (556)

Impulse-Control Disorders Not Elsewhere Classified (663)

312.34	Intermittent Explosive Disorder (663)
312.32	Kleptomania (667)
312.33	Pyromania (669)
312.31	Pathological Gambling (671)
312.39	Trichotillomania (674)
312.30	Impulse-Control Disorder NOS (677)

Adjustment Disorders (679)

309.xx	Adjustment Disorder (679)
.0	With Depressed Mood
.24	With Anxiety
.28	With Mixed Anxiety and Depressed Mood
.3	With Disturbance of Conduct
.4	With Mixed Disturbance of Emotions and Conduct
.9	Unspecified

Specify if: Acute/Chronic

Personality Disorders (685)

Note: *These are coded on Axis II.*

301.0	Paranoid Personality Disorder (690)
301.20	Schizoid Personality Disorder (694)
301.22	Schizotypal Personality Disorder (697)
301.7	Antisocial Personality Disorder (701)
301.83	Borderline Personality Disorder (706)
301.50	Histrionic Personality Disorder (711)
301.81	Narcissistic Personality Disorder (714)
301.82	Avoidant Personality Disorder (718)
301.6	Dependent Personality Disorder (721)
301.4	Obsessive-Compulsive Personality Disorder (725)
301.9	Personality Disorder NOS (729)

Other Conditions That May Be a Focus of Clinical Attention (731)

PSYCHOLOGICAL FACTORS AFFECTING MEDICAL CONDITION (731)

316 . . . *[Specified Psychological Factor] Affecting . . . [Indicate the General Medical Condition] (731) Choose name based on nature of factors:*

Mental Disorder Affecting Medical Condition

Psychological Symptoms Affecting Medical Condition

Personality Traits or Coping Style Affecting Medical Condition

Maladaptive Health Behaviors Affecting Medical Condition

Stress-Related Physiological Response Affecting Medical Condition

Other or Unspecified Psychological Factors Affecting Medical Condition

MEDICATION-INDUCED MOVEMENT DISORDERS (734)

332.1	Neuroleptic-Induced Parkinsonism (735)
333.92	Neuroleptic Malignant Syndrome (735)
333.7	Neuroleptic-Induced Acute Dystonia (735)
333.99	Neuroleptic-Induced Acute Akathisia (735)
333.82	Neuroleptic-Induced Tardive Dyskinesia (736)
333.1	Medication-Induced Postural Tremor (736)
333.90	Medication-Induced Movement Disorder NOS (736)

OTHER MEDICATION-INDUCED DISORDER (736)

995.2	Adverse Effects of Medication NOS (736)

RELATIONAL PROBLEMS (736)

V61.9	Relational Problem Related to a Mental Disorder or General Medical Condition (737)
V61.20	Parent-Child Relational Problem (737)
V61.10	Partner Relational Problem (737)
V61.8	Sibling Relational Problem (737)
V62.81	Relational Problem NOS (737)

PROBLEMS RELATED TO ABUSE OR NEGLECT (738)

V61.21	Physical Abuse of Child (738)
	(code 995.54 if focus of attention is on victim)
V61.21	Sexual Abuse of Child (738)
	(code 995.53 if focus of attention is on victim)
V61.21	Neglect of Child (738)
	(code 995.52 if focus of attention is on victim)
——.——	Physical Abuse of Adult (738)
V61.12	(if by partner)
V62.83	(if by person other than partner)
	(code 995.81 if focus of attention is on victim)
——.——	Sexual Abuse of Adult (738)
V61.12	(if by partner)
V62.83	(if by person other than partner)
	(code 995.83 if focus of attention is on victim)

ADDITIONAL CONDITIONS THAT MAY BE A FOCUS OF CLINICAL ATTENTION (739)

V15.81	Noncompliance With Treatment (739)
V65.2	Malingering (739)
V71.01	Adult Antisocial Behavior (740)
V71.02	Child or Adolescent Antisocial Behavior (740)
V62.89	Borderline Intellectual Functioning (740)
	Note: This is coded on Axis II.
780.9	Age-Related Cognitive Decline (740)
V62.82	Bereavement (740)
V62.3	Academic Problem (741)
V62.2	Occupational Problem (741)
313.82	Identity Problem (741)
V62.89	Religious or Spiritual Problem (741)
V62.4	Acculturation Problem (741)
V62.89	Phase of Life Problem (742)

Additional Codes (743)

300.9	Unspecified Mental Disorder (nonpsychotic) (743)
V71.09	No Diagnosis or Condition on Axis I (743)
799.9	Diagnosis or Condition Deferred on Axis I (743)
V71.09	No Diagnosis on Axis II (743)
799.9	Diagnosis Deferred on Axis II (743)

Multiaxial System

Axis I	Clinical Disorders Other Conditions That May Be a Focus of Clinical Attention
Axis II	Personality Disorders Mental Retardation
Axis III	General Medical Conditions
Axis IV	Psychosocial and Environmental Problems
Axis V	Global Assessment of Functioning

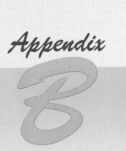

Appendix

B

NANDA-Approved Nursing Diagnoses

This list represents the NANDA-approved nursing diagnoses for clinical use and testing (1998).

PATTERN 1: EXCHANGING

1.1.2.1	Altered Nutrition: More than body requirements
1.1.2.2	Altered Nutrition: Less than body requirements
1.1.2.3	Altered Nutrition: Potential for more than body requirements
1.2.1.1	Risk for Infection
1.2.2.1	Risk for Altered Body Temperature
1.2.2.2	Hypothermia
1.2.2.3	Hyperthermia
1.2.2.4	Ineffective Thermoregulation
1.2.3.1	Dysreflexia
1.2.3.2	Risk for Autonomic Dysreflexia
1.3.1.1	Constipation
1.3.1.1.1	Perceived Constipation
1.3.1.1.2	Colonic Constipation (deleted in 1998)
1.3.1.2	Diarrhea
1.3.1.3	Bowel Incontinence
1.3.1.4	Risk for Constipation
1.3.2	Altered Urinary Elimination
1.3.2.1.1	Stress Incontinence
1.3.2.1.2	Reflex Incontinence
1.3.2.1.3	Urge Incontinence
1.3.2.1.4	Functional Incontinence
1.3.2.1.5	Total Incontinence
1.3.2.1.6	Risk for Urge Incontinence
1.3.2.2	Urinary Retention
1.4.1.1	Altered (Specify Type) Tissue Perfusion (Renal, cerebral, cardio-pulmonary, gastrointestinal, peripheral)
1.4.1.2	Risk for Fluid Volume Imbalance
1.4.1.2.1	Fluid Volume Excess
1.4.1.2.2.1	Fluid Volume Deficit
1.4.1.2.2.2	Risk for Fluid Volume Deficit
1.4.2.1	Decreased Cardiac Output
1.5.1.1	Impaired Gas Exchange
1.5.1.2	Ineffective Airway Clearance
1.5.1.3	Ineffective Breathing Pattern
1.5.1.3.1	Inability to Sustain Spontaneous Ventilation
1.5.1.3.2	Dysfunctional Ventilatory Weaning Response (DVWR)
1.6.1	Risk for Injury
1.6.1.1	Risk for Suffocation
1.6.1.2	Risk for Poisoning
1.6.1.3	Risk for Trauma
1.6.1.4	Risk for Aspiration
1.6.1.5	Risk for Disuse Syndrome
1.6.1.6	Latex Allergy Response
1.6.1.7	Risk for Latex Allergy Response
1.6.2	Altered Protection
1.6.2.1	Impaired Tissue Integrity
1.6.2.1.1	Altered Oral Mucous Membrane
1.6.2.1.2.1	Impaired Skin Integrity
1.6.2.1.2.2	Risk for Impaired Skin Integrity
1.6.2.1.2.3	Altered Dentition
1.7.1	Decreased Adaptive Capacity: Intracranial
1.8	Energy Field Disturbance

PATTERN 2: COMMUNICATING

2.1.1.1	Impaired Verbal Communication

PATTERN 3: RELATING

3.1.1	Impaired Social Interaction
3.1.2	Social Isolation
3.1.3	Risk for Loneliness
3.2.1	Altered Role Performance
3.2.1.1.1	Altered Parenting
3.2.1.1.2	Risk for Altered Parenting

561

3.2.1.1.2.1	Risk for Altered Parent/Infant/Child Attachment
3.2.1.2.1	Sexual Dysfunction
3.2.2	Altered Family Processes
3.2.2.1	Caregiver Role Strain
3.2.2.2	Risk for Caregiver Role Strain
3.2.2.3.1	Altered Family Process: Alcoholism
3.2.3.1	Parental Role Conflict
3.3	Altered Sexuality Patterns

PATTERN 4: VALUING

4.1.1	Spiritual Distress (distress of the human spirit)
4.1.2	Risk for Spiritual Distress
4.2	Potential for Enhanced Spiritual Well-Being

PATTERN 5: CHOOSING

5.1.1.1	Ineffective Individual Coping
5.1.1.1.1	Impaired Adjustment
5.1.1.1.2	Defensive Coping
5.1.1.1.3	Ineffective Denial
5.1.2.1.1	Ineffective Family Coping: Disabling
5.1.2.1.2	Ineffective Family Coping: Compromised
5.1.3.1	Potential for Enhanced Community Coping
5.1.3.2	Ineffective Community Coping
5.1.2.2	Family Coping: Potential for Growth
5.2.1	Ineffective Management of Therapeutic Regimen (Individuals)
5.2.1.1	Noncompliance (Specify)
5.2.2	Ineffective Management of Therapeutic Regimen: Families
5.2.3	Ineffective Management of Therapeutic Regimen: Community
5.2.4	Effective Management of Therapeutic Regimen: Individual
5.3.1.1	Decisional Conflict (Specify)
5.4	Health Seeking Behaviors (Specify)

PATTERN 6: MOVING

6.1.1.1	Impaired Physical Mobility
6.1.1.1.1	Risk for Peripheral Neurovascular Dysfunction
6.1.1.1.2	Risk for Perioperative Positioning Injury
6.1.1.1.3	Impaired Walking
6.1.1.1.4	Impaired Wheelchair Mobility
6.1.1.1.5	Impaired Transfer Ability
6.1.1.1.6	Impaired Bed Mobility
6.1.1.2	Activity Intolerance
6.1.1.2.1	Fatigue
6.1.1.3	Risk for Activity Intolerance

6.2.1	Sleep Pattern Disturbance
6.2.1.1.	Sleep Deprivation
6.3.1.1	Diversional Activity Deficit
6.4.1.1	Impaired Home Maintenance Management
6.4.2	Altered Health Maintenance
6.4.2.1	Delayed Surgical Recovery
6.4.2.2	Adult Failure to Thrive
6.5.1	Feeding Self Care Deficit
6.5.1.1	Impaired Swallowing
6.5.1.2	Ineffective Breast-feeding
6.5.1.2.1	Interrupted Breast-feeding
6.5.1.3	Effective Breast-feeding
6.5.1.4	Ineffective Infant Feeding Pattern
6.5.2	Bathing/Hygiene Self Care Deficit
6.5.3	Dressing/Grooming Self Care Deficit
6.5.4	Toileting Self Care Deficit
6.6	Altered Growth and Development
6.6.1	Risk for Altered Development
6.6.2	Risk for Altered Growth
6.7	Relocation Stress Syndrome
6.8.1	Risk for Disorganized Infant Behavior
6.8.2	Disorganized Infant Behavior
6.8.3	Potential for Enhanced Organized Infant Behavior

PATTERN 7: PERCEIVING

7.1.1	Body Image Disturbance
7.1.2	Self Esteem Disturbance
7.1.2.1	Chronic Low Self Esteem
7.1.2.2	Situational Low Self Esteem
7.1.3	Personal Identity Disturbance
7.2	Sensory/Perceptual Alterations (Specify) (Visual, auditory, kinesthetic, gustatory, tactile, olfactory)
7.2.1.1	Unilateral Neglect
7.3.1	Hopelessness
7.3.2	Powerlessness

PATTERN 8: KNOWING

8.1.1	Knowledge Deficit (Specify)
8.2.1	Impaired Environmental Interpretation Syndrome
8.2.2	Acute Confusion
8.2.3	Chronic Confusion
8.3	Altered Thought Processes
8.3.1	Impaired Memory

PATTERN 9: FEELING

9.1.1	Pain
9.1.1	Chronic Pain
9.1.2	Nausea

9.2.1.1	Dysfunctional Grieving		9.2.3.1.1	Rape Trauma Syndrome: Compound Reaction
9.2.1.2	Anticipatory Grieving			
9.2.1.3	Chronic Sorrow		9.2.3.1.2	Rape Trauma Syndrome: Silent Reaction
9.2.2	Risk for Violence: Self-directed or directed at others			
			9.2.4	Risk for Post-trauma Syndrome
9.2.2.1	Risk for Self-Mutilation		9.3.1	Anxiety
9.2.3	Post-trauma Syndrome		9.3.1.1	Death Anxiety
9.2.3.1	Rape Trauma Syndrome		9.3.2	Fear

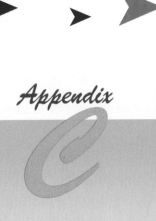

Appendix

Drug Classification Under the Controlled Substances Act

Schedule I Drugs	Schedule II Drugs	Schedule III Drugs	Schedule IV Drugs	Schedule V Drugs
OPIOIDS	**OPIOIDS**	**OPIOIDS**	**OPIOIDS**	**OPIOIDS**
Acetylmethadol	Alfentanil	Hydrocodone syrup	Pentazocine	Buprenorphine
Heroin	Codeine	Paregoric	Propoxyphene	Diphenoxylate
Normethadone	Fentanyl			plus atropine
Many others	Hydromorphone			
	Levorphanol			
	Meperidine			
	Methadone			
	Morphine			
	Opium tincture			
	Oxycodone			
	Oxymorphone			
	Sufentanil			
PSYCHEDELICS	**PSYCHOSTIMULANTS**	**STIMULANTS**	**STIMULANTS**	
Bufotenin	Amphetamine	Benzphetamine	Diethylpropion	
Diethyltryptamine	Cocaine	Phendimetrazine	Fenfluramine	
Dimethyltryptamine	Dextroamphetamine		Mazindol	
Ibogaine	Methamphetamine		Pemoline	
d-Lysergic acid	Methylphenidate		Phentermine	
diethylamide (LSD)	Phenmetrazine			
Mescaline				
3,4-Methylenedioxy-				
methamphetamine				
(MDMA)				
Psilocin				
Psilocybin				
CANNABIS DERIVATIVES	**BARBITURATES**	**BARBITURATES**	**BARBITURATES**	
Hashish	Amobarbital	Aprobarbital	Mephobarbital	
Marijuana	Pentobarbital	Butabarbital	Methohexital	
	Secobarbital	Methabarbital	Phenobarbital	
		Talbutal		
		Thiamylal		
		Thiopental		
OTHERS	**CANNABINOIDS**	**MISCELLANEOUS DEPRESSANTS**	**BENZODIAZEPINES**	
Methaqualone	Dronabinol (THC)	Glutethimide	Alprazolam	
Phencyclidine	Nabilone	Methyprylon	Chlordiazepoxide	
			Clonazepam	
			Clorazepate	
			Diazepam	

(continued)

(Continued)

Schedule I Drugs	Schedule II Drugs	Schedule III Drugs	Schedule IV Drugs	Schedule V Drugs
			Estazolam	
			Flurazepam	
		ANABOLIC STEROIDS	Halazepam	
		Fluoxymesterone	Lorazepam	
		Methyltestosterone	Midazolam	
		Nandrolone	Oxazepam	
		Oxandrolone	Prazepam	
		Stanozolol	Quazepam	
		Testosterone	Temazepam	
			Triazolam	
			MISCELLANEOUS DEPRESSANTS	
			Chloral hydrate	
			Ethchlorvynol	
			Ethinamate	
			Meprobamate	
			Paraldehyde	

Drugs in Schedule I have a high potential for abuse and have no approved medical use in the United States.
Drugs in Schedules II through V all have approved uses, and are classified based on their abuse potential.
Schedule II drugs have a higher potential for abuse.
Schedule V drugs have the lowest potential for abuse.

Answers to
Chapter Review

ANSWER KEY

CHAPTER 1

Multiple-Choice Questions

1. C
2. B
3. A
4. D
5. C

True-False Questions

1. F (Asylums in the United States were built to provide a safe refuge for mentally ill persons.)
2. T
3. T
4. F (Access to resources, intolerance of violence, and a sense of community are social/cultural factors influencing mental health.)
5. F (Persons with mental illness have not been viewed as possessed by demons since late 1800s.)
6. F (The period of enlightenment of the 1800s lasted only 100 years.)
7. T
8. T

Fill-in-the-Blank Questions

Axis I: all major psychiatric disorders except mental retardation and personality disorders

Axis II: mental retardation, personality disorders, prominent maladaptive personality features, defense mechanisms

Axis III: current medical conditions, contributing medical conditions

Axis IV: psychosocial and environmental problems

Axis V: Global Assessment of Functioning (GAF) score

Short-Answer Questions

1. The standards are used to guide nursing practice in psychiatric settings and to determine safe and acceptable practices in legal disputes.
2. Cost containment and managed care, population diversity, community-based care.
3. Fear of saying the wrong thing, not knowing what to do, being rejected by clients, handling bizarre or inappropriate behavior, physical safety, seeing a friend or acquaintance as a client.

CHAPTER 2

Multiple-Choice Questions

1. A
2. B
3. D
4. C
5. B

True-False Questions

1. F (The half-life of a drug refers to the amount of time it takes for half the drug to leave the bloodstream.)
2. T
3. F (Low-potency drugs must be given in higher dosages to be effective.)
4. T
5. F (Blocking dopamine is responsible for the extrapyramidal side effects of antipsychotic drugs.)
6. T
7. F (Clients taking MAOIs should not receive a general anesthetic for surgery.)
8. T

Fill-in-the-Blank Questions

1. Antipsychotic
2. SSRI
3. Tricyclic antidepressant
4. Anticholinergic
5. Stimulant
6. Anticonvulsant used as mood stabilizer
7. Benzodiazepine used as anxiolytic
8. Antipsychotic

Short-Answer Questions

1. Abrupt cessation results in a rebound effect (return of symptoms), recurrence of the original symptoms, or possible withdrawal symptoms. Tapering gradually alleviates or minimizes these problems.
2. A radioactive substance will be injected into the bloodstream. The client will be asked to perform "thinking" tasks while the camera takes scans of the brain working. The procedure will take 2 to 3 hours.
3. Just as kindling is used to start a larger fire, mild or small manic mood swings can eventually trigger a major, acute manic episode.

CHAPTER 3

Multiple-Choice Questions

1. D
2. D
3. C
4. B
5. A

True-False Questions

1. F (Henry Stack Sullivan described three cognitive modes: prototaxic, parataxic, and syntaxic.)
2. F (Psychiatric rehabilitation focuses on improving the client's functional abilities.)
3. T
4. F (Repressed sexual energy as the driving force in personality development was conceived by Sigmund Freud.)
5. F (Countertransference refers to the feelings a nurse might develop toward a client.)
6. F (The nursing role of surrogate involves being a substitute for another, such as a parent.)
7. T
8. F (Behaviorists believe that behavior results from reinforced past experiences.)

Fill-in-the-Blank Questions

1. Carl Rogers
2. Erik Erikson
3. Ivan Pavlov
4. Albert Ellis
5. B. F. Skinner
6. Carl Rogers
7. Frederick Perls
8. Abraham Maslow
9. Viktor Frankl
10. Albert Ellis
11. William Glasser

Short-Answer Questions

1. Clients participate in group session with members who have a shared purpose of benefiting each other and making some change. Example: family therapy to learn conflict resolution.
2. Members gather to learn about a particular topic from someone who has expertise. Example: assertiveness training group.
3. Members help themselves and each other to cope with some life stress, event, illness, or problem. Example: Survivors of Suicide (for family members of someone who has committed suicide).
4. This group is structured around a common experience that all members share and is run by the group members. Example: Alcoholics Anonymous.

CHAPTER 4

Multiple-Choice Questions

1. B
2. B
3. D
4. B
5. C

True-False Questions

1. F (ACCESS is designed for homeless clients.)
2. T
3. T
4. F (Managed care funds medically necessary services, often limited to skills training.)
5. T
6. F (The purpose is to promote full recovery.)
7. F (Success is greatly affected by the quality of the client's living environment.)
8. T

Fill-in-the-Blank Questions

Psychiatric social worker
Occupational therapist
Psychiatrist
Vocational rehabilitation specialist

Short-Answer Questions

1. Double stigma, lack of family or social support, comorbidity, adjustment problems, boundary issues
2. The evolving consumer household is a group living situation intended to transform itself into a residence where the residents fulfill their own responsibilities and function without on-site supervision from paid staff. It is intended to be a permanent residence for the client.
3. Deinstitutionalization, more rigid criteria for civil commitment, lack of adequate support, attitudes of police and society

CHAPTER 5

Multiple-Choice Questions

1. A
2. A
3. C
4. B

True-False Questions

1. F (Empathy is perceiving the meanings and feelings of another. Sympathy is showing concern and compassion for another.)
2. F (The nurse may say what town he or she lives in but should not give out his or her address.)
3. F (Unknowing is being in an open state, ready to hear another.)
4. T

Fill-in-the-Blank Questions

Empirical
Aesthetic
Personal
Ethical

Short-Answer Questions

1. Congruence: Nurse faces client, makes eye contact, and says, "My name is Mary Day, and I will be your nurse today." (verbal and nonverbal components match)

   Positive regard: Nurse sits next to client, makes eye contact, leans forward, and says, "Rosie, I am glad we have this opportunity to work on some of your problems together." (verbal and nonverbal components provide the client with a message of personal regard)

   Acceptance: Client shakes nurse's hand very hard. Nurse says, in a normal tone of voice, "Tom, I'm always pleased to shake hands when we meet, but you don't need to squeeze so hard!" (lets client know nurse likes to meet him, but places boundary)

2. Nurse: "You seem unsure of your doctor's abilities. Would you like to tell me about this concern?" Rationale: attempts to get client to expand on the comment.

   Nurse: "No, I clearly stated 6 weeks, but do you wish it were 8?" Rationale: clarifies timing with client and addresses possible underlying issue of nurse's leaving.

Clinical Example

Mr. Vittorio: "I like to choose my student nurses; otherwise, I don't get chosen."

Nurse: "I am honored that you chose me, Mr. Vittorio. My name is Sandy Moore, and I will be your student nurse for the next 6 weeks. You seem to have some experience with other groups of students." (nurse clearly states information about herself and her role and acknowledges client's previous experience)

Mr. Vittorio: "Oh, yeah, I've seen 'em come and go, but I never get picked to be their patient. I guess I'm too crazy for them!" (laughs nervously)

Nurse: "Well, I'm delighted you chose me. It makes me feel honored." (nurse makes it clear she is glad to be with client)

Mr. Vittorio: "Are you sure?"

Nurse: "Yes. I will be here on Tuesdays from 10 a.m. to 3 p.m. for the next 6 weeks. I hope we can identify and work on some issues together." (provides client with clear parameters for the relationship)

CHAPTER 6

Multiple-Choice Questions

1. D
2. C
3. A
4. D
5. B
6. A
7. B
8. C
9. A

Short-Answer Questions

1. Knowledge, values, and beliefs transmitted down through generations
2. Distance between people during interaction
3. Behavior that is inconsistent with words
4. Belief about one's place in the universe
5. Actions that agree with words
6. Process
7. Hackneyed saying
8. Descriptive comparison to help the client label similarities and differences between two items
9. The literal words spoken by an individual
10. A four-quadrant structure used to learn more about the self
11. The nurse uses the self as a tool to relate to the client in a therapeutic communication, identify with a client-centered issue, and work toward the goal of guiding the client to determine socially acceptable problem resolution.
12. The unspoken and often unconscious desires that create anxiety that prompt a person's behavior.

Cues and responses

1. Cue: I feel good.
   "What is one way you feel good?"
   "When did you start feeling good?"
   "What was going on around you just before you realized you felt good?"
2. Cues: can't take it, anymore.
   "What is it you can't take?"
   "How long have you had to take it?"
   "What is going on that you believe you have to take?"
3. Cues: two children, my wife, my girlfriend.
   Nurse: "What are the children's names and ages?"
   Client: "Taylor is 4 and Anita is 1."
   Nurse: "Tell me about the relationship between you and Taylor." After discussion concludes, try: "Tell me about your relationship with Anita."
4. Cues: we, standing, corner.
   "Who do you mean by 'we'?"
   "What corner were you standing at?"
   "What were you doing at the corner?"

5. Cues: my son, never going to understand, way his wife is ruining them.
   Nurse: "What is your son's name?"
   Client: "Paul."
   Nurse: "What is his wife's name?"
   Client: "Susan."
   Nurse: "How do you perceive Susan is ruining herself and Paul?"
   "How did you arrive at the conclusion that Paul will never understand something Susan is doing that appears perfectly clear to you?"

CHAPTER 7

Multiple-Choice Questions
1. A
2. B
3. A
4. A
5. D

True-False Questions
1. F (A belief or perception that one's personal capabilities and efforts have an effect over the events in their lives)
2. F (Affects physical as well as the emotional sustenance one receives)
3. F
4. T
5. F (Is more effective from family than health care providers)
6. F (Resiliency can be affected by relationships, education)

Fill-in-the-Blank Questions
Trust vs. Mistrust
Industry vs. Inferiority
Identity vs. Role diffusion
Intimacy vs. Isolation
Ego Integrity vs. Despair

Short-Answer Questions
1. Culturally competent nursing care means being sensitive to issues related to culture, race, gender, sexual orientation, social class, economic situation, and other factors that affect the care of the client. It means the nurse promotes the client's practice of his or her beliefs, such as spiritual practices, uses nonverbal communication that is congruent with the client, and so forth
2. Failure to successfully complete the developmental tasks at a given stage results in a negative outcome for that stage, such as mistrust rather than trust, and impedes successful completion of future tasks. Successful completion of tasks sets the stage for further success at the next developmental stage.

3. Hardiness describes the individual's ability to resist illness when under stress. Resilience refers to having healthy responses under stressful circumstances or at-risk situations.

CHAPTER 8

Multiple-Choice Questions
1. B
2. D
3. C
4. B
5. B

True-False Questions
1. F (Eventually answers the question)
2. T
3. T
4. F (Is delusional)
5. F (A depressed mood)
6. T
7. T
8. F (Can be culturally biased)

Fill-in-the-Blank Questions
Automatisms
Thought withdrawal
Psychomotor retardation
Word salad

Short-Answer Questions
1. What does the saying, "a rolling stone gathers no moss" mean to you?
2. What led you to come to the clinic?
3. How would you describe yourself as a person?
4. If you were lost downtown, what would you do?
5. In general, how are you feeling?
6. Can you tell me today's date? (time)
   Can you tell me where you are? (place)
   Can you tell me your name? (person)

Clinical Example
1. Give positive feedback for coming to the clinic to get help.
   Tell her it is all right to cry.
   Tell the client that the nurse will sit with her until she's ready to talk.
   Validate the client's feelings, ie, "I can see you're very upset."
2. What is the problem as the client sees it (to gain the client's perception of the situation)? Has the client ever felt this way before (to determine if this is a new occurrence, or recurrent)?

Does the client have thoughts of harming herself or others (to determine safety)?

Has the client been drinking alcohol, using drugs, or taking medication (to assess client's ability to think clearly or if there is impairment)?

What kind of help does the client need (to see what kind of help the client wants, eg, someone to listen, help to solve a specific problem, a referral)?

3. The client is in crisis.
The client is seeking help/treatment.
The client is not currently stable.

4. Tell the client that the nurse needs to know if the client is safe (from suicidal ideas or self-harm urges). If the client is safe, she can leave the clinic. If she is not safe, the nurse must ask her to stay, or call emergency services (911) if necessary.

CHAPTER 9

Multiple-Choice Questions
1. C
2. B
3. C
4. D
5. A

True-False Questions
1. F (Grief is a normal response to loss.)
2. F (Grieving is a unique and dynamic process; the person who is grieving may move in and out of various phases of the process while experiencing a myriad of feelings.)
3. F (Anger and depression are emotional expressions of grieving.)
4. T

Fill-in-the-Blank Questions
Emotional dimension
Behavioral dimension
Cognitive dimension
Spiritual dimension
Physiologic dimension

Short-Answer Questions
1. Styles of grieving: when a person moves from high to low distress over time in his or her grieving process.
   Adequate support: when the bereaved can identify a person or persons who are able and willing to be supportive while he or she is grieving for a loss.
   Emotional response during numbing phase of grieving: a feeling of being stunned.
2. Nurse: "This is really a shock for you, and it's difficult to believe it has happened."

Rationale: This reflection acknowledges the client's feelings and directs those feelings back to the client as a way to convey understanding as well as to encourage further verbalization of feelings.
Nurse: "Tell me more about that."
Rationale: This statement encourages exploration of the client's feelings, and a description of the client's perception can assist the nurse in understanding the client's experience. As the client speaks, feelings and perceptions shift toward a healthy integration of loss.
Nurse: "You're feeling all alone."
Rationale: This reflective statement encourages the client to express more.
Nurse: "There's absolutely no one who cares about what is happening to you?"
Rationale: Voicing doubt implies that the client's beliefs are exaggerated or false perceptions.
Nurse: "Who could we get who would be helpful to you right now?"
Rationale: This acknowledges that the client's anger is normal and most likely not a personal attack on the nurse. Using "we" suggests collaboration with the client, and focusing on the client's statement about help is a way to stay engaged and give the client the opportunity to say more.

CHAPTER 10

Multiple-Choice Questions
1. B
2. B
3. B
4. D
5. C

True-False Questions
1. F (Client must remain in the hospital until he or she is no longer dangerous to himself or herself or others.)
2. T
3. F (They often progress to the crisis phase if left alone.)
4. T
5. F (They may not be secluded unless they are imminently dangerous to themselves or others.)
6. T
7. F (Certain restrictions can be instituted by a physician's order for a documented reason.)
8. T

Fill-in-the-Blank Questions

Recovery
Postcrisis
Triggering
Escalation
Crisis

Short-Answer Questions

1. The cocktail method involves giving two medications, usually haloperidol and lorazepam, in successive doses at the time of the behavior, 30 minutes to 1 hour later, and 1 to 2 hours after the behavior until sedation is achieved. The chaser method involves giving lorazepam at the time of the behavior, 30 minutes to 1 hour later, and 1 to 2 hours after the behavior until the client is sedated. Then an antipsychotic medication, such as haloperidol, is offered.

2. The client has the right to be treated in the least restrictive environment that meets his or her needs. It means a client who can be treated in a community-based setting must be treated there and cannot be hospitalized (more restrictive) if inpatient care is not required. It also means that a client cannot be restrained or secluded unless there is no other effective way to deal with aggressive or dangerous behavior. The client's freedom cannot be restricted in any way unless there is no other way to meet his or her needs.

CHAPTER 11

Multiple-Choice Questions

1. B
2. C
3. C
4. C
5. D

True-False Questions

1. T
2. F (Self-neglect means the elder cannot manage day-to-day self-care activities.)
3. F (The most common form of child abuse is neglect.)
4. T
5. F (Reporting is mandatory in only a few states.)
6. F (Victims of trauma may have had good coping skills before the trauma.)
7. T
8. F (They desire close relationships but fear them or cannot have successful ones.)

Fill-in-the-Blank Questions

1. Child neglect
2. Elder self-neglect
3. Financial abuse
4. Psychological or emotional abuse.

Short-Answer Questions

A repeated pattern of violence in which an abusive episode is followed by a period of remorse (honeymoon period), then tension builds until the next abusive episode. *Example:* A man beats his wife, then apologizes and is loving for a few weeks, and then another battering episode occurs.

Assigning responsibility for the abuse or rape to the victim rather than to the abuser or rapist. *Example:* A woman walking alone at night is raped. Some say, "What did she expect? She should have been more careful."

When the person surviving a trauma feels ashamed or guilty about surviving. *Example:* The driver in a car crash in which two friends were killed blames himself for their deaths, saying, "Why didn't I die with the others?"

Violence in families is learned by role-modeling from one generation to the next. *Example:* A man who witnessed his father beating his mother finds himself beating his own wife when he gets angry.

CHAPTER 12

Multiple-Choice Questions

1. C
2. B
3. A
4. B
5. D

True or False

1. T
2. T
3. F
4. T

Fill-in-the-Blank

1. Severe
2. Mild
3. Panic
4. Moderate

Short Answer

1. Regression, isolation, reaction formation, undoing
2. Mild, moderate, severe, panic
3. The client is progressively exposed to the threatening object while in a safe environment until the anxiety is reduced.

Clinical Example

1. The nurse should have Mrs. Noe come up with suggestions. She is more likely to take responsibility for and act on her own solutions to problems than the suggestions of others.

2. Mrs. Noe receives secondary gain from the attention and focus Mr. Noe gives her. He is her phobic partner. The nurse could recommend that both Mr. and Mrs. Noe attend an agoraphobic self-help group in the community. Mr. Noe would benefit from attending such a group to learn about his counter-phobic partner behaviors that enable his wife to continue her agoraphobia.

3. Many medications can reduce agoraphobic behaviors, so referral to a psychiatrist or a psychiatric advanced practice nurse is appropriate.

CHAPTER 13

Multiple-Choice Questions

1. C
2. D
3. B
4. D
5. C

True-False Questions

1. F (anhedonia)
2. T
3. T
4. F (echolalia)
5. T
6. F (pseudoparkinsonism)
7. T
8. F (latency of response)

Fill-in-the-Blank Questions

1. Neologism
2. Verbigeration
3. Word salad
4. Clang association

Short-Answer Questions

1. Client believes the FBI is spying on him.
2. Client hears voices saying, "You're no good."
3. Client sees electrical cord on the floor and thinks it is a snake, but on second glance sees it is a cord.
4. *Response:* "It sounds like you're scared."
   Rationale: Focus on feeling without challenging delusion.
5. *Response:* "Tell me why you think you're in the hospital."
   Rationale: Focus on client's perceptions.
6. *Response:* "That would be very unusual."
   Rationale: Casting doubt without challenging client.
7. *Response:* "What is God telling you to do?"
   Rationale: Essential to discover content of command hallucination.

Clinical Example Questions

1. Additional assessment data (examples): discover content of any command hallucinations; ask about preferences for hygiene (for example, shower or bath); determine whether there is a thing or place that makes him feel safe and secure.

2. Altered thought processes: Client will have 5-minute interactions that are reality-based; Client will express feelings and emotions.

   Ineffective management of therapeutic regimen (medication refusal): Client will take medication as prescribed; Client will verbalize difficulties in following medication regimen.

   Self-care deficit: Client will shower or bathe, wash hair, and clean clothes every other day; Client will wear appropriate clothing for the weather or activity.

3. Altered thought processes: Engage client in present, here-and-now topics not related to delusional ideas. Focus on client's emotions and feelings.

   Ineffective management of therapeutic regimen: Offer scheduled medications in matter-of-fact manner. Allow client to open unit-dose packets. Assess for side effects and give medications or provide nursing interventions to relieve side effects. Provide factual information to the client: "This medication will decrease the voices you're hearing."

   Self-care deficit: Provide supplies and privacy for hygiene activities. Give feedback about body odor, dirty clothes, and so forth. Help client store extra clothing where he has access to it and believes it is safe.

4. John might benefit from a case manager in the community and a community support program or a clinic for possible depot injections of his medication.

CHAPTER 14

Multiple-Choice Questions

1. B
2. C
3. A
4. A

5. A
6. D
7. B
8. D
9. A
10. D
11. D

True-False Questions

1. T
2. F (People with seasonal affective disorder need more hours of light to decrease their depression.)
3. T
4. F (The nurse should always document emotional responses of mood and affect. Sadness can be from grief, but it can also be depression secondary to general medical condition.)
5. T
6. F (Suicidal ideation is a key indicator of suicide risk.)

Short-Answer Questions

1. Proper medication administration, salt and water needs, symptoms of lithium toxicity, need for periodic serum lithium monitoring
2. "You've been a good friend." "I can't do this anymore." "This is where I keep my important papers." "I'd like you to have my chess set, the one you always admired."
3. They are administered orally, usually in divided doses. The dosage is titrated by relief of symptoms.

Clinical Example

(There are other correct answers; these are just examples.)

1. The contract should state when the discussions will occur, how long they will last, and how they will be evaluated by student and faculty.
2. Altered Role Performance: client will carry out nursing duties appropriately; client will relate to fellow students and faculty appropriately
   Ineffective Individual Coping: client will sort out ability to handle school, work, and family; client will exhibit coping skills.
3. Altered Role Performance: help the student when she goes astray; communicate with her clearly, honestly, and succinctly
   Personal Coping, Ineffective: teach the student various methods of coping; help her discern when her coping is ineffective.

4. Classmates should treat her normally and remain nonjudgmental. This is a good opportunity for the other students to face their own fears of mental illness. Open discussions as part of clinical conference might prove helpful.

CHAPTER 15

Multiple-Choice Questions

1. B
2. D
3. A
4. C
5. B

True-False Questions

1. F (Confabulation is when a client makes up an answer if he or she can't remember the correct one.)
2. T
3. F (Apraxia is the inability to execute motor functions.)
4. F (A client with aphasia cannot communicate words and ideas accurately.)
5. T
6. F (Korsakoff syndrome is due to a thiamine deficiency.)
7. T
8. F (Echopraxia is the imitation of another person's behavior.)

Fill-in-the-Blank Questions

Delirium
Delirium
Dementia
Delirium
Delirium
Dementia
Dementia
Dementia

Short-Answer Questions

Distraction: shifting the client's attention and energy to a more neutral topic. *Example:* The client is yelling at someone. The nurse says, "How would you like to see the new picture in the dining room?"
Time away: leaving the client for a short time. *Example:* The client says, "Leave me alone!" The nurse leaves and then returns a short time later, not mentioning the client's request.
Going along: providing emotional reassurance without correcting the delusion or misinterpretation. *Example:* The client is expecting her dead husband to visit. The nurse says, "He'll be here later."

Reminiscence: encouraging the client to discuss pleasant memories. *Example:* Having a client talk about her childhood and her wedding day.

Clinical Example

(These are examples; there are other correct answers.)

1. What does she like to eat? What were her usual personal hygiene practices? What are her favorite activities? What personal items does she value?
2. Chronic Confusion, Impaired Socialization, Risk for Altered Nutrition: Less Than Body Requirements, Sleep Pattern Disturbance, Self-Care Deficits
3. The client will experience as little frustration as possible. *Interventions:* Point out objects, people, and the time of day to prompt the client and decrease confusion. Do not ask the client to make decisions when she is unable to; offer choices only when she can make them.

   The client will interact with the nurse. The client will participate in going for a walk with the group. *Intervention:* Involve the client in solitary activities with the nurse initially. Structure group activities that focus on intact physical abilities rather than those requiring cognition.

   The client will eat 50% of meals and snacks. *Interventions:* Provide foods the client likes; provide food in an environment where she will be likely to eat, such as her room or a table alone.

   The client will sleep 6 hours per night. *Interventions:* Provide a soothing nighttime routine every night (for example, beverage, reading aloud, dim lights). Decrease stimulation after dinner. Discourage daytime naps.

   The client will participate in hygiene routines with assistance. *Interventions:* Try to imitate the client's home hygiene routine (bath or shower, morning or evening). Develop a structured routine for hygiene.

CHAPTER 16

Multiple-Choice Questions

1. C
2. A
3. D
4. B
5. D

True-False Questions

1. F (Character is influenced by social learning, culture, and random life events unique to the individual.)
2. F (He or she would benefit from improved community functioning and contact with a single case manager.)
3. T
4. F (Clients make slow progress over a long period of time.)
5. F (A client with obsessive-compulsive disorder has a great deal of difficulty meeting deadlines at work.)
6. F (A client with narcissistic personality disorder is usually not motivated to seek treatment.)
7. T
8. T

Fill-in-the-Blank Questions

Borderline personality disorder
Antisocial personality disorder
Schizoid personality disorder
Avoidant personality disorder

Short-Answer Questions

Harm avoidance: High—fear of uncertainty, social inhibition, shyness with strangers, rapid fatigability, pessimistic worry in anticipation of problems
Harm avoidance: Low—carefree, energetic, outgoing, optimistic
Novelty seeking: High—quick-tempered, curious, easily bored, impulsive, extravagant, disorderly
Novelty seeking: Low—slow-tempered, stoical, reflective, frugal, reserved, orderly, tolerant of monotony
Reward dependence: High—tender-hearted, sensitive, sociable, socially dependent
Reward dependence: Low—practical, tough-minded, cold, socially insensitive, irresolute, indifferent if alone
Persistence: High—hard-working, persevering, ambitious, overachieving
Persistence: Low—inactive, indolent, unstable, erratic

Clinical Example

(These are examples of correct answers; others are possible.)

1. Risk for Self-Mutilation, Ineffective Individual Coping
2. Risk for Self-Mutilation: The client will be safe and free of significant injury.

Ineffective Individual Coping: The client will demonstrate increased control of impulsive behavior.

3. Risk for Self-Mutilation: Discuss presence and intensity of self-harm urges with client; negotiate a no self-harm contract with the client; help the client to identify triggers for self-harm behavior.

Ineffective Individual Coping: Help the client to identify feelings by keeping a journal; discuss ways the client can use distraction when gratification must be delayed; discuss alternative ways the client can express feelings without an exaggerated response.

4. Outpatient therapist, community support services, vocational/career counseling, self-help group

CHAPTER 17

Multiple-Choice Questions
1. B
2. A
3. B
4. B
5. A

True-False Questions
1. F (Al-Anon is for family members of alcoholics.)
2. T
3. T
4. F (Codependence refers to enabling behavior that perpetuates the substance abuse.)
5. T
6. T
7. F (Methadone is used to treat heroin dependence.)
8. F (Dual diagnosis means having two diagnoses, such as substance abuse and a major mental illness.)

Fill-in-the-Blank Questions
(These are examples; there are others.)
Stimulants: cocaine, amphetamine
Opioids: morphine, heroin
Hallucinogens: peyote, LSD
Inhalants: paint thinner, gasoline fumes

Short-Answer Questions
1. Have you ever felt you ought to Cut down on your drinking? Have people Annoyed you by criticizing your drinking? Have you ever felt bad or Guilty about your drinking? Have you ever had a drink first thing in the morning to steady your nerves or get rid of a hangover (Eye-opener)?

2. Increased reporting of "pharmacy errors," excessive amounts of narcotics are "wasted," damaged or torn packaging on controlled substances, reports of ineffective pain relief by patients, when the same medication had previously relieved pain

3. Medications are given in decreasing doses over a period of time to detoxify the user slowly and safely. The dose of medication is decreased every 2 or 3 days until the client is no longer receiving any of the medication.

Clinical Example
1. Ineffective Denial: Ineffective Individual Coping
2. Ineffective Denial: The client will abstain from alcohol or drug use; Ineffective Individual Coping: The client will identify two non-chemical ways of coping with life stressors.
3. Ineffective Denial: Teach the client about the disease of alcoholism; dispel myths about alcoholism; ask the client about recent life events (breakup, arrest) and the role of her drinking in those events; Ineffective Individual Coping: Encourage the client to express feelings directly and openly; teach the client relaxation techniques; role-play a situation (of the client's choice) that has been difficult for her to handle.

CHAPTER 18

Multiple-Choice Questions
1. D
2. A
3. C
4. A
5. A

True-False Questions
1. F (Conduct disorder is the most common.)
2. T
3. F (Enuresis is usually not related to underlying psychological problems.)
4. T
5. F (A tic is a sudden, rapid, recurrent, non-rhythmic, stereotyped motor movement or vocalization.)
6. T
7. T
8. F (Children with the disinhibited type would be expected to accept contact from anyone.)

Fill-in-the-Blank Questions
Pica
Rumination disorder

Reactive attachment disorder
Selective mutism

Short-Answer Questions

1. Limit setting involves informing the client of the rule or limit, explaining the consequences if the limit is exceeded, and consistently enforcing the limit, with no exceptions.
2. Time-out is a retreat to a neutral place so the client can regain control. It is not a punishment. It can be initiated by staff until the client can institute it for himself or herself.

Clinical Example

(These are sample answers.)

1. Ritalin is a stimulant medication that is effective for 70% to 80% of children with ADHD by decreasing hyperactivity and impulsivity and improving the child's attention. Ritalin can cause appetite suppression and should be given after meals to encourage proper nutrition. Substantial, nutritious snacks between meals are helpful. Giving the medication in the daytime helps avoid the side effect of insomnia. The parents should notice improvements in the next day or two. Notify the physician or return to the clinic if no improvements in behavior are noted.
2. The exact cause of ADHD is not known, but it is not due to faulty parenting or anything the parents have done. Taking medications will be helpful with behavioral symptoms, but other strategies are needed as well. The medication will help control symptoms so Dixie can participate in school, make friends, and so forth.
3. Provide supervision when Dixie is with her brother, and help her learn to play gently with him. Do not forbid her to touch him, but teach her the proper ways to do so. Give Dixie directions in a clear, step-by-step manner, and assist her to follow through and complete tasks. Provide a quiet place with minimal distraction for activities requiring concentration, such as homework. Try to establish a routine for getting up and dressing, eating meals, going to school, doing homework, and playing; don't change the routine unnecessarily. Structured expectations will be easier for Dixie to follow. Remember to recognize Dixie's strengths and provide positive feedback frequently to boost her self-esteem and foster continued progress.
4. The parents should contact Dixie's teacher, principal, and guidance counselor to inform them of this diagnosis so that special education classes or tutoring can be made available. It would also be helpful to meet with the school nurse who will be giving Dixie her medication at noon on school days. The nurse can refer the parents to a local support group for parents of children with ADHD and provide pamphlets, books, or other written materials, and Internet addresses if the parents have access to a computer.

CHAPTER 19

Multiple-Choice Questions

1. B
2. C
3. D
4. B
5. A

True-False Questions

1. F (Clients with hypochondriasis are not reassured by negative findings.)
2. F (Conversion disorders occur between the ages of 10 and 35 years.)
3. T
4. T
5. T
6. F (Narcotics are not effective in treating pain disorder.)
7. T
8. F (Somatization, pain, and conversion disorders are more common in women.)

Fill-in-the-Blank Questions

Body dysmorphic disorder
Somatization disorder
Conversion disorder
Pain disorder
Hypochondriasis

Short-Answer Questions

Primary gain is the direct benefit clients experience, such as relief from anxiety, conflict, or distress. *Example:* If the client is physically sick, she doesn't have to deal with problems with the children.

Secondary gain is the personal benefit derived from illness, such as special attention or comfort received from others. *Example:* When the client has physical symptoms, she gets breakfast in bed.

La belle indifference is the indifference about physical symptoms seen in clients with a conversion disorder. *Example:* A man who is paralyzed and cannot walk is cheerful and seems unconcerned about the paralysis.

Clinical Example

(These are sample answers; others are possible.)

1. Ineffective Individual Coping, Pain, Anxiety
2. The client will identify the relationship between stress and increased pain; the client will be able to perform activities of daily living.
3. Have the client keep a journal about emotional feelings and the quality or intensity of pain; teach the client relaxation exercises; help the client make a daily schedule of activities, beginning with simple tasks; encourage the client to listen to music or engage in other distracting activities she may enjoy; talk with the client about her feelings of frustration and anxiety in a sensitive and supportive manner.
4. Physical therapy, vocational rehabilitation, nutrition services
5. Support group for persons with chronic pain/pain disorder, exercise group, social or volunteer opportunities

CHAPTER 20

Multiple-Choice Questions

1. B
2. C
3. A
4. B
5. A

True-False Questions

1. F (Satiety means the satisfaction of appetite.)
2. T
3. T
4. F (Purging involves not only self-induced vomiting but also use of laxatives, diuretics, and enemas.)
5. T
6. F (Self-monitoring is a technique that allows clients to identify behavior patterns so they can avoid or change those patterns.)

7. F (Clients with bulimia experience great distress, not clients with anorexia. Clients with anorexia do not see their behavior as a problem.)
8. F (Clients with bulimia can be in medical danger as a result of repeated vomiting.)

Fill-in-the-Blank Questions

Bulimia
Both
Both
Anorexia
Bulimia

Short-Answer Questions

1. Self-induced vomiting; fasting; use of laxatives, diuretics, enemas; excessive exercise
2. Body image is how one sees oneself, a mental picture of the physical body. Body image disturbance involves an extreme discrepancy between one's own perception of body image and the perceptions of others. There is also extreme dissatisfaction with one's body image.

Clinical Example

(These are examples; there are other correct answers.)

1. Altered Nutrition: Less Than Body Requirements and Ineffective Individual Coping
2. (Nutrition) The client will eat all of her meals and snacks with no purging behaviors. (Coping) The client will identify two non–food-related mechanisms.
3. (Nutrition) Sit with the client while eating; monitor client 1 to 2 hours after meals and snacks; supervise client's use of the bathroom. (Coping) Ask the client how she is feeling, and continue to focus on feelings if the client gives a somatic response; have the client keep a journal including emotions, feelings, and food eaten; teach the client the use of relaxation and distraction, such as music and activities.

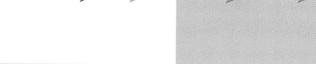

Index

Page numbers followed by "b" indicate boxed material; page numbers followed by "f" indicate figures; page numbers followed by "t" indicate tabular material.